Women's Health
and Wellness Across the Lifespan

10/15

Women's Health
and *Wellness Across*
the Lifespan

Ellen F. Olshansky,
PHD, RN, WHNP-BC, NC-BC, FAAN

Professor and Founding Director
Program in Nursing Science
University of California
Irvine, California

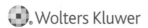

. Wolters Kluwer

Philadelphia · Baltimore · New York · London
Buenos Aires · Hong Kong · Sydney · Tokyo

Acquisitions Editor: Shannon W. Magee
Product Development Editor: Maria M. McAvey
Developmental Editor: Franny Murphy
Senior Marketing Manager: Mark Wiragh
Editorial Assistant: Zachary Shapiro
Production Project Manager: David Saltzberg
Design Coordinator: Teresa Mallon
Manufacturing Coordinator: Kathleen Brown
Prepress Vendor: S4Carlisle

Library of Congress Cataloging-in-Publication Data
Women's health and wellness across the lifespan / [edited by] Ellen F. Olshansky. — First edition.
    p. ; cm.
  Includes bibliographical references and index.
  ISBN 978-1-4511-9200-1
  I. Olshansky, Ellen Frances, 1949- , editor.
  [DNLM: 1. Women's Health. 2. Age Factors. 3. Health Behavior. 4. Sex Factors. WA 309.1]
  RA778
  613'.04244—dc23

                                                                          2014026947

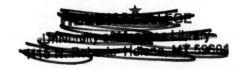
RRS1409

Contributors

Judith A. Berg, PhD, RN, WHNP-BC, FAAN, FAANP
Clinical Professor
University of Arizona
College of Nursing
Tucson, Arizona

Barbara B. Cochrane, PD, RN, FAAN
Professor and Director
Rheba de Tornyay Endowed Professor
  for Healthy Aging
School of Nursing
University of Washington
Seattle, Washington

Susan M. Cohen, PhD, CRNP, FAAN
Associate Professor
Department of Health Promotion and
  Development
University of Pittsburgh
Pittsburgh, Pennsylvania

Stephanie Deible, BSN, RN, RYT 200
Registered Nurse, Teaching Fellow, Doctoral
  Student
University of Pittsburgh Medical Center
Shadyside Hospital Emergency Department
School of Nursing
University of Pittsburgh
Pittsburgh, Pennsylvania

Diana Diefenderfer, PMA, CPT
Lecturer
Claire Trevor School of the Arts
Ballet, Pilates Director
Department of Dance Wellness
University of California
Irvine, California

Anastasia Fisher, PhD, RN
Psychiatric Liaison Nurse
John Muir Medical Center
Walnut Creek, California

Cindy Smith Greenberg, DNSc, RN,
  PNP-BC, FAAN
Professor and Director
School of Nursing
California State University
Fullerton, California

Diane C. Hatton, PhD, RN
Consultant
Women and Health Justice
Reno, Nevada

Mahtab Jafari, PharmD
Associate Professor, Director
Pharmaceutical Sciences
  Undergraduate Program
University of California
Irvine, California

Versie Johnson-Mallard, PhD, WHNP-BC
Associate Professor
College of Nursing
University of South Florida
Tampa, Florida

Julia Lange Kessler, CM, DNP, FACNM
Program Director, Nurse-Midwifery
WHNP Program
Georgetown University
School of Nursing and Health Studies
Washington, DC

Elizabeth A. Kostas-Polston, PhD, APRN,
WHNP-BC, FAANP
Assistant Professor
Robert Wood Johnson Foundation Nurse
Faculty Scholar
Woman's Health Nurse Practitioner
College of Nursing
University of South Florida
Tampa, Florida

Diane N. Krause, PhD
Adjunct Professor
Department of Pharmacology
School of Medicine
University of California
Irvine, California

Madeleine M. Lloyd, PhD, RN, FNP-BC,
PMHNP-BC
Clinical Director, Nurse Practitioner
College of Nursing
New York University
New York, New York

Ruth Mielke, PhD, CNM, WHNP
Assistant Professor
School of Nursing
California State University
Fullerton, California

Nancy Lieberman Neudorf,
MSN, RN, FNP
Clinical Instructor
Program of Nursing Science
University of California
Planning Commissioner
Irvine, California

Ellen F. Olshansky, PhD, RN, WHNP-BC,
NC-BC, FAAN
Professor and Founding Director
Program in Nursing Science
University of California
Irvine, California
before Gabriel Orenstein.

Gabriel Orenstein, BS
Martial Arts Instructor
United Studios of Self Defense
Research Assistant
Pharmaceutical Sciences
University of California
Los Angeles, California

Karla Parsons, RN, DNP, FNP-BC
Assistant Professor
School of Nursing
California State University
Fullerton, California

JoAnne Reifsnyder, PhD, RN
Senior Vice President
Clinical Operation, Chief Nursing Officer
Genesis HealthCare
Kennett Square, Pennsylvania

Joan L. F. Shaver, PhD, RN, FAAN
Dean and Professor
College of Nursing
University of Arizona
Tucson, Arizona

Diana Taylor, PhD, RNP, FAAN
Professor Emerita
School of Nursing
Research Faculty
Bixby Center for Global Reproductive Health
Department of Family Health Care Nursing
Advancing New Standards for Reproductive
Health Program
University of California
San Francisco, California

Susan Thrane, RN, MSN, OCN
Pre-doctoral Fellow
School of Nursing
Department of Health Promotion and
Development
University of Pittsburgh
Pittsburgh, Pennsylvania

Nancy Fugate Woods, PhD, RN, FAAN
Professor
Biobehavioral Nursing and Health Systems
Dean Emerita, School of Nursing
University of Washington
Seattle, Washington

Heather M. Young, PhD, RN, FAAN
Associate Vice Chancellor for Nursing
Dean and Professor
Betty Irene Moore School of Nursing
University of California
Sacramento, California

Robynn Zender, MS
Research Assistant
Program in Nursing Science
University of California
Irvine, California

Preface

I t is not an understatement to say that health care is changing in the United States. Hospital stays are shorter, more health care occurs in the community, and there is a greater emphasis on promoting health and preventing illness. Many previously uninsured people are becoming insured. With a critical lack of primary health-care providers, we not only need to increase the number of providers, but need providers who reflect the ethnicities and backgrounds of their patients. We need providers in urban and rural areas, in private practices and community clinics. We need a variety of providers who work as an interprofessional team, where the skills of each profession complement the others and ultimately the patient receives the highest quality care.

The patient, in fact, ought to be the center of the health care provided and the center of a health-care system that engages with patients, responding to their concerns and working on behalf of their health and welfare. Women as patients bring unique issues that must be addressed based on current evidence. Women's health as a specialty actually includes men and families, as women's health is influenced by their social contexts and everyday life experiences.

The role of nursing is a major focus of *Women's Health and Wellness across the Lifespan*, with a particular emphasis on nursing's history and contributions to women's health. This book aims to provide comprehensive information for a variety of health-care providers, especially those in primary care and community settings, who care for women and their families. Furthermore, women who seek information that will facilitate their good health will also find this book useful.

Women's Health and Wellness across the Lifespan addresses women's health from a holistic and life span perspective, incorporating various modalities of care. The overall goal is to highlight approaches to care, grounded in scientific evidence, which promote optimal wellness in women at all stages of their lives, recognizing individual differences and health conditions that women experience. I invite you to join the contributors to this book, and me, in our journey toward optimizing women's health and health care.

Acknowledgments

An effort such as this one is never accomplished alone. I have many people who deserve sincere thanks. First, I want to thank Shannon Magee, Acquisitions Editor at Wolters Kluwer, with whom I shared my initial idea for the book. I remember our breakfast at the American Academy of Nursing in 2012, when I brought a rough draft of my proposal and she was very enthusiastic and encouraging. As I proceeded with the book, I have been fortunate to work closely with Franny Murphy, Development Editor, Maria McAvey, Product Development Editor at Wolters Kluwer, and Shailaja Subramanian, Project Manager at S4Carlisle Publishing Services. Franny was my direct contact person, and she always answered my questions and my emails promptly. She encouraged and supported me, often indicating that she was so interested in the topic of women's health. She was able to communicate with all the contributors to the book, and together, along with all the amazing contributors, we were able to complete this book in a timely manner. I also thank all the others at Wolters Kluwer who do so much "behind the scenes."

I want to give a heartfelt thanks and gratitude to the contributors to the book. The people whom I invited to write chapters are all busy and accomplished professionals who agreed to make time to write. I felt much support from the contributors who all share a passion for women's health. Franny Murphy even commented on how responsive the contributors were when we were under a deadline or needed more information. This book could not have been written without the expertise and commitment of these wonderful colleagues who so graciously agreed to contribute to this effort.

I also want to thank the University of California, Irvine, for granting me a 3-month sabbatical so that I could focus on the book. Granted, I ended up on jury duty for 2 1/2 months, with 1 month being part of my 3-month sabbatical, but doing my civic duty was also important! And so, in fact, I would like to thank my fellow jurors who always asked me about how I was progressing on the book.

I thank my family and friends who supported and encouraged me throughout this entire process. They were always interested in the progress and gave me the time and space to work. My husband, Richard Pattis, was constantly and unwaveringly supportive. My sons, Alex and Mark Pattis, seemed to be truly proud that their mom was writing a book!

Ellen F. Olshansky, PHD, RN, WHNP-BC, NC-BC, FAAN

Contents

Preface   ix

Acknowledgments   xi

Section i   Introduction to Women's Wellness Care   1

Chapter **1**   Introduction: Holistic, Life-span Approach to Women's Wellness as Guiding Framework   2
Ellen F. Olshansky

Chapter **2**   Women's Health in the 21st Century   7
Ellen F. Olshansky

Chapter **3**   Women's Health: Evolution of the Science and Clinical Specialty   12
Nancy Fugate Woods, Versie Johnson-Mallard, Elizabeth A. Kostas-Polston, Diana Taylor, Judith A. Berg, Joan L. F. Shaver, and Ellen F. Olshansky

Section ii   Specific Wellness Issues for Women across the Life Span   29

Chapter **4**   Puberty through Early Adulthood   30
Ruth Mielke, Karla Parsons, and Cindy Smith Greenberg

Chapter **5**   Women at Midlife   68
Judith A. Berg, Diana Taylor, and Nancy Fugate Woods

Chapter **6**   Healthy Aging for Women   96
Heather M. Young and Barbara Cochrane

Section iii Promoting Women's Wellness across the Life Span   123

Chapter **7**   Wellness for Special Populations of Women   124
Ellen F. Olshansky and Robynn Zender

Chapter **8**   Body Composition: Enhancing Health through Exercise and Nutrition   133
Robynn Zender

Chapter **9**   Oral Health   157
Madeleine M. Lloyd and Julia Lange Kessler

Chapter **10**   Resilience in Women   181
Anastasia Fisher, Diane C. Hatton, and Ellen F. Olshansky

Chapter **11**   Self-care: Healing Energy and Other Complementary Therapies   188
Susan Thrane, Stephanie Deible, and Susan M. Cohen

Chapter **12**   Women and Herbal Medicine   203
Mahtab Jafari and Gabriel Orenstein

Chapter **13**   Pharmacologic Approaches to Wellness and Disease Prevention in Women over the Life Span   223
Diana N. Krause

Chapter **14**   Healing Arts: Movement in the Form of Pilates   246
Diane Diefenderfer

Chapter **15**   Healing Environments   262
Nancy Lieberman Neudorf

Chapter **16**   Healing Relationships   285
Robynn Zender and Ellen F. Olshansky

Chapter **17**   Promoting Healthy Sleep   309
Joan L. F. Shaver

Chapter **18**   Peaceful Dying   334
JoAnne Reifsnyder

Index   355

Introduction to Women's Wellness Care

Chapter **1** Introduction: Holistic, Life-span Approach to Women's Wellness as Guiding Framework

Chapter **2** Women's Health in the 21st Century

Chapter **3** Women's Health: Evolution of the Science and Clinical Specialty

Introduction: Holistic, Life-span Approach to Women's Wellness as Guiding Framework

Ellen F. Olshansky

Health and wellness have always been of keen interest to both the lay public and professionals of all backgrounds. Most people care about being healthy, staying healthy, and managing a healthy lifestyle. It is not always easy, however, especially in the face of many external and internal challenges, to achieve optimal health. Women, in particular, face a myriad of complex health challenges, often complicated by broad social factors as well as individual health risks. Nurses and other health-care providers are well positioned to assist women, by partnering with them in their care through listening, empathizing, advising/coaching, and providing specific health-care interventions in order for them to achieve their own level of optimal health.

Current trends in health care embrace not only prevention of illness, but also promotion of optimal health and wellness. Preventing illnesses means understanding root causes and how to either eliminate or ameliorate them. Promoting wellness means understanding how to encourage individuals and groups to develop and maintain healthy lifestyle habits, but it goes beyond lifestyle habits. Dossey and Keegan (2012, p. 3) define optimal health as "an individually defined state or process wherein the individual experiences a sense of well-being, harmony, unity, in which subjective experiences about health beliefs and values are honored; process of becoming an expanding consciousness – integrated, congruent functioning toward reaching one's highest potential." The Samueli Institute (2012) focuses on the interrelationship among social, psychological, spiritual, physical, and behavioral aspects of organizations with the goal of creating optimal healing environments that can influence and enhance the capacity to heal.

Holistic/Integrated Approach to Health and Wellness

Holistic, or integrated, health is reflected in a combination of various approaches to well-being, including allopathic and alternative methods, resulting in a true complementary and comprehensive health-care system. Such an approach includes a continuum of preventive and curative services and is individualized over time and across different levels of the health system. The term "integrated" is often used interchangeably with "holistic." A holistic approach to women's health is very important to enhance the likelihood that women will achieve their optimum level of wellness. Traditionally, our health-care system has focused on treating people based on their symptoms, which form a diagnosis that leads to a prognosis and specific interventions/treatment. A holistic approach emphasizes the whole person, who is much more than his or her symptoms and is much more than the sum of his or her body parts. A holistic approach embraces the importance of mind/body interaction as well as spiritual and emotional aspects of a person (Olshansky, 2000). Such an approach also includes the environment, nutrition, and epigenetics, as these factors influence a woman's health. In taking a holistic approach, it is also important to recognize that sometimes women often pursue treatments, such as supplements, vitamins, herbs, and minerals, some of which have support for their use, but others need more scientific evidence (Lloyd & Hornsby, 2009). This book includes treatments and approaches that are supported by the latest scientific evidence.

Life-span Approach to Health and Wellness

A life-span approach is very important in the quest to achieve optimal wellness. Earlier experiences influence later experiences in regard to health. This is so for all people, but, once again, women encounter unique experiences across the spans of their lives that influence their ongoing health and wellness. Understanding the various life stages and how a woman experienced her health in the past at those life stages provides a foundation for a comprehensive understanding of her current health. At certain life stages, women may be able to engage in specific lifestyle behaviors that contribute to the prevention of health conditions later in life. Current research supports the wisdom of understanding women's health across her life span (Fine, Kotelchuck, Adess, & Pies, 2009; Halfon, 2009). A life-span approach is actually part of a holistic approach in that it takes into account the woman's life circumstances, past and present, social and environmental determinants of health, as well as bio-psycho-social-spiritual aspects in early life that may affect later life.

Unique Aspects of Women's Health and Wellness

Although the health of all persons is a concern for our health-care system, delineating women's health as a specialty remains an important area for health-care providers and consumers. Clearly, women's health issues overlap with men's health and children's and families' health, but women also experience unique aspects of health that deserve focused attention. The past two decades have witnessed a shift in focus on women's health from that of breast and cervical cancer and reproductive health, which remain central to the health of women, to a broader definition of health that encompasses additional aspects such as cardiovascular health, metabolic health, and oral health, to name just a few. These health conditions affect women and men, although there may be unique ways in which women experience these conditions (Pinn & Kravitz, 2011). The health of women, who are often central to families and communities, can influence entire communities. Fontenot and Hawkins (2011) aptly stated that women's health-care nurse practitioners provide education for women about their own health so that, ultimately, they can influence the development of healthier communities. In some areas of women's health, we may have developed some complacency, for example in the area of preventing unintended pregnancies (Berg, Olshansky, Taylor, Shaver, & Woods, 2012). We must continue to be vigilant in supporting health policies that provide access to care for women in this area. We have learned from past experiences that we cannot simply apply a general understanding of health to the health of women. For example, research has revealed that women often experience symptoms of cardiac disease differently from the way men experience such symptoms. Women sometimes respond to specific medications differently than do men. Women also experience certain social determinants of health in a way that men do not.

The Office of Research on Women's Health (ORWH) was established in 1990 to respond to the mission of women as well as minorities, who were not systematically included in clinical research (Pinn & Kravitz, 2011; Shaver, Olshansky, & Woods, 2013). Building on the recommendations of the ORWH, as well as the Institute of Medicine, Shaver et al. (2013) recommended a research agenda for women's health. Accompanying that article, Berg, Taylor, and Woods (2013) recommended a clinical services and policy agenda for women based on the Affordable Care Act, the National Prevention Council and Strategy, the Institute of Medicine, and the World Health Organization. Both of these articles, sanctioned by the Expert Panel on Women's Health of the American Academy of Nursing, support the need for a focus on women's health as a significant category of health issues. More detail, including a historical overview and perspective, to support the need for identifying women's health as a specialty area of practice and scholarship is presented in Chapter 3 by Woods and colleagues.

Health-Care Providers' Roles in Health and Wellness

For both prevention of illness and promotion of optimal wellness it is critical that health-care professionals provide encouragement to clients to make constructive changes on their journey to wellness. Often this encouragement is in the form of facilitating decision making and goal setting by clients and, in collaboration with them, assessing periodically how well they are meeting their goals, sometimes modifying goals and strategies to meet those revised goals. The health-care provider is often the "coach," who is likely a nurse, nurse practitioner, or other health-care professional who creates a professional partnership with a client as she moves forward on her trajectory toward optimal wellness (Hess et al., 2013). Clients must have a sense of "agency" and be active participants in their health rather than passive recipients. In the realm of optimal wellness, the role of the health-care provider is that of a knowledgeable, sensitive, empathic professional who builds on the strengths of each individual client to facilitate, in partnership with the client, the attainment of what is optimal for each individual.

Organization and Purpose of This Book

The purpose of this book is to provide a guide to women's health and optimal wellness from a holistic perspective that encompasses life-span considerations.

With the focus being on wellness, the emphasis of the book is on promotion of health rather than on pathology, emphasizing individualized/personalized wellness.

The book is organized according to three sections. The first section addresses women's health within our newly reformed health-care system, providing the foundation for the book. The second section presents common concerns of women at various life stages related to the promotion of wellness. The third section presents strategies for promoting various aspects of wellness for women.

In Section One, the framework that guides this book is presented. That framework is a combination of a holistic, integrated approach to health and health care and a life-span approach to understanding common health concerns of women in their quest to attain optimal wellness. A discussion of trends in approaches to health care and wellness in the 21st century is presented, along with an in-depth discussion of why it is significant and important to distinguish women's health as a specialty area in practice and scholarship. The history of women's health in the United States, with a particular focus on nursing's contributions to women's health, is presented.

In Section Two, common health concerns for women across the life span are described. This section is organized according to three chapters. The first chapter addresses health concerns of young girls through adolescence and young womanhood; the second chapter addresses middle-aged women, and the third chapter addresses older women. All of these chapters are focused on maintaining wellness, while recognizing risk factors for various health conditions and how best to screen for and manage risk factors.

In Section Three, specific issues related to attaining and maintaining optimal wellness, are discussed, with some interventions described. Such topics include specific wellness issues for special populations of women, resilience, healthy body composition, oral health, environmental health, relationships, resilience, self-care and energy healing, pharmacological approaches, herbal supplements, healing arts (with Pilates as the exemplar), environment, sleep, and peaceful dying.

This book is intended for primary care providers and wellness coaches who work with women. It can be used for educators who are teaching students to work clinically in the area of women's health. It can also be used by women themselves to learn more about their own bodies and how to maintain their health at optimum levels. The aim of the book is to provide comprehensive, integrated evidence-based information that is helpful to enhance women's health.

References

Berg, J. A., Olshansky, E., Taylor, D., Shaver, J., & Woods, N. F. (2012). Women's health in jeopardy: Failure to curb unintended pregnancies: A statement from the AAN Women's Health Expert Panel. *Nursing Outlook, 60*(3), 163–164.

Berg, J. A., Taylor, D., & Woods, N. F. (2013). Where we are today: Prioritizing women's health services and health policy. A report by the Women's Health Expert Panel of the American Academy of Nursing. *Nursing Outlook, 61*, 5–15.

Dossey, B. M., & Keegan, L. (2012). *Holistic nursing: A handbook for practice.* Topeka, KS: American Holistic Nurses Association.

Fine, A., Kotelchuck, M., Adess, N., & Pies, C. (2009). *Policy brief: A new agenda for MCH policy and programs: Integrating a life course perspective.* Martinez, CA: Contra Costa Health Services.

Fontenot, H., & Hawkins, J. W. (2011). The evolution of specialists in women's health across the lifespan: Women's health nurse practitioners. *Journal of the American Academy of Nurse Practitioners, 23*, 314–319.

Halfon, N. (2009). *Life course health development: A new approach for addressing upstream determinants of health and spending.* Washington, DC: Expert Voices, NIHCM Foundation.

Hess, D. R., Dossey, B. M., Southard, M. E., Luck, S., Schaub, B. G., & Bark, L. (2013). *The art and science of nurse coaching: The providers' guide to coaching scope and competencies.* Silver Spring, MD: Nurses books.org (Publishing program of the American Nurses Association).

Lloyd, K. B., & Hornsby, L. B. (2009). Complementary and alternative medications for women's health issues. *Nutrition in Clinical Practice, 24*(5), 589–608.

Olshansky, E. F. (2000). *Integrative women's health: A comprehensive approach*. Sudbury, MA: Jones & Bartlett.

Pinn, V. W., & Kravitz, J. Y. (2011). Expanding the evidence base for women's health across the lifespan. *Journal of Dental Education, 75*(Suppl. 3), S11–S19.

Samueli Institute. (2012). Optimal healing environments. Retrieved from http://www.samueliinstitute. org/our-research/optimal-healing-environments/ohe-framework

Shaver, J., Olshansky, E., & Woods, N. F. (2013). Women's health research agenda for the next decade: A report by the Women's Health Expert Panel of the American Academy of Nursing. *Nursing Outlook, 61*(1), 16–24.

Chapter 2

Women's Health in the 21st Century

Ellen F. Olshansky

The 21st century has brought with it significant changes in health and health care, but more importantly, it has brought with it a critical need to continue to make significant changes and advances in order that health care is accessible and of high quality for all people. Health-care reform is a major topic of conversation among politicians, health policy experts, health-care professionals, and the public. Scientific advances have improved diagnostic and treatment abilities, but equal access to health care continues to be a challenge. In addition to providing optimum health care for all persons, specific challenges to providing optimal health care for women remain and must be addressed.

In envisioning a transformed health-care system of the 21st century that emphasizes the attainment of optimal health and wellness, several key aspects are essential. Most important of these are as follows:

- Equal access to high-quality health care
- New roles in health care
- Interprofessional health-care workforce
- Focus on prevention of illness and promotion of health
- Holistic, comprehensive approach to care

The purpose of this chapter is to emphasize many of the key aspects of a transformed health-care system, a health-care system to which we aspire as soon as possible. With that description as context, discussion is included on specific aspects of women's health that are envisioned to be part of a transformed health-care system.

Equal Access to High-Quality Health Care

We continue to suffer significant disparities in the access to and quality of health care. The Institute of Medicine (IOM, 2001), in their now classic publication, *Crossing the Quality Chasm: A New Health System for the 21st Century*, delineated the important aspects of health care now and in the future as being safe, effective, efficient, timely, patient-centered, and equitable. In 2010, the IOM convened a workshop to assess the advances we have made subsequent to the 2001 report, and in 2012, it reported on that workshop (IOM, 2012). Among the findings were that significant disparities in health and health care continue, poverty is a major concern, institutional racism still exists, and there is a continuing need to increase awareness of the magnitude of health disparities.

In our country with great advances in health care, there are still those who do not have access to this care. In fact, it is often poor families, often headed by women, and children who suffer the most in this regard. Former Surgeon General C. Everett Koop (2006) admonished us, as a society, to address the issue of lack of access to health care with great urgency.

New Roles in Health Care

There is an increasing appreciation of the need for a diverse health-care workforce. Many health-care professionals and patients have embraced a holistic approach to health and health care, incorporating traditional methods, such as healing touch, mindfulness meditation, visualization, herbs, acupuncture, acupressure, and other approaches. Our health-care professionals would do well to learn about the appropriate use of some of these holistic approaches. We need to emphasize health promotion and illness prevention. New roles in health care will become more important as we better embrace health promotion approaches. For example, the integrative nurse coach is a new role, developed by a group of nurses, that focuses on holistic care (Hess et al., 2013), as mentioned in chapter 1. Approximately 100 nurses have become board certified as nurse coaches. Many large corporations and other employers have hired nurse coaches in an effort to keep their employees well.

Interprofessional Health-Care Workforce

The necessity for more primary care providers has led to the recognition that advanced practice nurses, physician assistants, nurse wellness coaches and other coaches, social workers, and others can meet important needs in primary care in addition to primary care and family practice physicians. Health care is taking a more deliberate interprofessional approach, recognizing the importance of strong teams of health-care providers, each with unique contributions, who can work together to enhance optimal wellness in patients. Our educational programs in health care must embrace such an interprofessional approach in order that health-care providers of the future have a deep understanding of and respect for their colleagues within the larger health-care system.

Embracing a true interprofessional health-care workforce starts with education of the health-care workforce. Nursing, medical, dental, pharmacy, public health, social work students, and others can be educated together in some courses. One of the great values in doing this is that each of the various health-care providers will better understand the roles of each of their colleagues and better respect one another. The Macy Foundation (2013) strongly advocates the need to support interprofessional health-care education as a way of transforming how health care is delivered, making it based on an interprofessional team approach. Cortese (2013) urges us to embrace teams of health-care providers that provide care that is integrated and coordinated in order to deliver the best care possible to patients.

Focus on Prevention of Illness and Promotion of Health

As a result of the amazing technological advances in health care that we have witnessed over the past several decades, we are fortunate to be able to cure diseases that were not curable earlier, to prevent diseases that were not preventable earlier, and to lengthen the average life span of a person. We are able to prolong life through intricate technology. Along with these advances has come an increase in chronic illness, often experienced by individuals as comorbid chronic illnesses. Our health-care system of the future is challenged to focus on how to help people enhance their quality of life while managing chronic conditions. Better yet, we are challenged to prevent the development of chronic illnesses, most of which are caused by lifestyle behaviors.

With the Patient Protection and Affordable Care Act (PPACA), there is an increasing focus on health promotion and illness prevention. Much of prevention is aimed at chronic illnesses. There is much that can be modified in a person's lifestyle to help prevent chronic illnesses. As well, there are ways to manage chronic illnesses such that a person can achieve a level of wellness in spite of the presence of a chronic illness. Despite our knowledge on how to better prevent and manage chronic illness, the Centers for Disease Control and Prevention (CDC, 2009) describe chronic illness as the major challenge of the 21st century, noting that 75% of our health-care dollars are directed at chronic illness, and yet the life expectancy in the United States is lower than that in several other countries who actually spend less money on health care.

Holistic Approach to Care

We are also challenged to maintain and even increase our caring, human approach to health care within a context of technology. We can't forget the patient, who is at the center of the care. A holistic approach to health care includes the use of various modalities for healing and also a personalized approach to care. Holistic care, also noted in chapter 1, encompasses a bio–psycho–social–emotional–cultural–environmental–spiritual approach, meaning that multifaceted aspects of a person must be considered (Dossey & Keegan, 2013). The new Patient-Centered Outcomes Research Institute (PCORI), which was authorized by Congress as part of the PPACA, emphasizes the importance of clinicians truly engaging with their patients to understand their patients' perspectives of their health conditions (PCORI, 2014, http://www.pcori.org/). By better understanding patients' individual perspectives, we can, in partnership with patients, develop and tailor approaches to their care that may include various modalities or approaches.

Nursing's Future in Health Care

When we look at the future of health care, one of the documents that are helpful is specific to nursing. In 2010, the IOM commissioned the Robert Wood Johnson Foundation (RWJF) to develop recommendations for the future of the nursing profession. Cochaired by Dr. Linda Burnes Bolton and President of the University of Miami, Donna Shalala, this task force produced a document titled "The Future of Nursing," in which the following four key messages were formulated (IOM, 2010):

1. Nurses should practice to the full extent of their education and training.
2. Nurses should achieve higher levels of education and training through an improved education system that promotes seamless academic progression.
3. Nurses should be full partners with physicians and other health-care professionals in redesigning health care in the United States.
4. Effective workforce planning and policy making require better data collection and improved information infrastructure.

Although these recommendations are specific to nursing, they also clearly embrace an interprofessional approach to health care. We can use this document to think about other professions as well. The Josiah Macy Foundation has published several key documents on the critical need for interprofessional education and practice.

We, as health-care professionals, must become more facile with technology, must understand the roles and responsibilities of our colleagues in different fields of health care, and must better communicate with patients, putting them at the center of care. In summary, health care in the 21st century must be accessible to all, provide quality care to the population, and be cost-effective.

Relevance to Health and Wellness for Women

In order to promote optimal wellness for women, there are several strategies that reflect health care in the 21st century. One is a focus on embracing women as partners in their own health care. Women must be encouraged to have a voice in their own care and to see their health-care providers as partners. Such an approach requires that health-care providers educate not only their individual patients but the larger population about wellness. Women must also be encouraged to employ various strategies to promote their health, both allopathic and alternative approaches. For health-care providers to encourage this, they themselves must learn about and be open to various approaches.

We must understand women's health from a larger, societal perspective, recognizing the importance of the social context and social factors/determinants of health that affect the health of individual women and their families. Thus, a holistic approach to understanding the health of women and to providing health care for women is needed.

While it is important to understand and conceptualize women's health from a comprehensive perspective, recognizing that women's health is more than reproductive health, we must also not neglect the importance of women's reproductive health. In fact, it is imperative that sexual and reproductive health be a routine part of comprehensive primary care.

Issues related to the health of women continue to be an important area of concern for the 21st century. The entire book addresses specific issues related to how best to promote optimum health and wellness in women across the life span.

This chapter has presented a very brief overview of health-care concerns for the 21st century. The purpose is to provide a context for the remaining chapters in the book. Chapter 3 provides an in-depth historical look at women's health and emphasizes why we continue to need a specialty in women's health and why it is so important to continue to focus on the unique needs of women in order to foster optimum health and wellness across the life span.

In sum, we have made amazing strides in health care over the years. However, we must remain vigilant in working strategically and thoughtfully to meet the continuing challenges in health care. Women's health must be understood within the context of our larger health-care system. By ensuring equal access to high-quality health care for all, we will improve not only the health of women but the health of our nation.

References

Centers for Disease Control and Prevention. (2009). *The power of prevention: Chronic disease—The public health challenge of the 21st century*. Washington, DC: Department of Health and Human Services, National Center for Chronic Disease Prevention and Health Promotion. Retrieved from http://www.cdc.gov/chronicdisease/pdf/2009-power-of-prevention.pdf

Cortese, D. A. (2013). A health care encounter of the 21st century. *Journal of the American Medical Association, 310*(18), 1937–1938.

Dossey, B. M., & Keegan, L. (2013). *Holistic nursing: A handbook for practice* (6th ed.). Burlington, MA: Jones and Bartlett Learning.

Hess, D. R., Dossey, B. M., Southard, M. E., Luck, S., Schaub, B. G., & Bark, L. (2013). *The art and science of nurse coaching: A provider's guide to coaching scope and competencies.* Silver Spring, MD: Nursesbooks.org.

Institute of Medicine. (2001, March). *Crossing the quality chasm: A new health system for the 21st century.* Washington, DC: National Academy Press. Retrieved from http://www.iom.edu/~/media/Files/Report%20Files/2001/Crossing-the-Quality-Chasm/Quality%20Chasm%202001%20%20report%20brief.pdf

Institute of Medicine. (2010). *The future of nursing: Leading change, advancing health.* Washington, DC: National Academies of Sciences.

Institute of Medicine. (2012). *How far have we come in reducing health disparities? Progress since 2000: Workshop summary.* Washington, DC: National Academies Press.

Koop, C. E. (2006). Health and health care for the 21st century: For all the people. *American Journal of Public Health, 96*(12), 2090–2092.

Macy Foundation. (2013). *Transforming patient care: Aligning inter-professional education with clinical practice redesign* [Conference recommendations]. Atlanta, GA: Author. Retrieved from http://macyfoundation.org/docs/macy_pubs/TransformingPatientCare_ConferenceRec.pdf.

Patient-Centered Outcomes Research Institute (2014). http://www.pcori/org/

Women's Health: Evolution of the Science and Clinical Specialty

Nancy Fugate Woods, Versie Johnson-Mallard, Elizabeth A. Kostas-Polston, Diana Taylor, Judith A. Berg, Joan L. F. Shaver, and Ellen F. Olshansky

Evolution of the field of women's health as a specialty in the United States can be traced to the first wave of the women's movement in the early part of the 20th century. Development of a distinct specialty in women's health in nursing in Europe and the United States can be tracked to the work of Florence Nightingale, whose text, Notes on Nursing, provided guidance for women in their health ministrations to their families (Nightingale, 1859). During the early part of the 20th century, there was a focus on the need for social reforms to improve the health of women and children. Early in that century, public health efforts focused on the major cause of mortality among women: maternal death associated with childbirth. In fact, during the first decade of the 20th century, the average life span for women was approximately 50 years, much shorter than that for men, owing to high rates of childbirth-related death (National Center for Health Statistics, 2005). Not surprisingly, in public health the conjoined field of "maternal child health" focused on health-care needs of women in their roles as mothers and caregivers for their children. Lillian Wald's work among poor women in New York, Margaret Sanger's efforts to help women control their fertility, and Mary Breckenridge's efforts to provide maternity care to poor women exemplify early 20th century nursing's efforts in women's health. For several ensuing decades the notion of women's health conjured visions of maternal health and pregnancy care, emphasizing prevention of maternal sepsis and other complications of labor and delivery. Early efforts of midwifery, an early specialty in nursing, were targeted at reducing maternal death rates through provision of education for pregnant women to promote safe delivery and optimum health during pregnancy (Weissman, 1998; Wertz & Wertz, 1989).

Many of the historical moments in the history of women's health were appropriately associated with the improvement of reproductive and public health outcomes. Consequently, the nature of women's health became defined as synonymous with reproductive health. Public health improvements parallel those improvements in health services for poor and pregnant women. The late 1880s and early 1900s witnessed a growing concern for the high rate of maternal and infant mortality, combined with the need to address the emerging public health problems due to burgeoning urban immigrant populations. Solutions and health-care delivery models were borrowed from European systems, particularly the United Kingdom, the Netherlands, and Scandinavian countries. Nurses were influential in developing new models of care and borrowing new practices from the Europeans.

Women's health has its roots in the work of Florence Nightingale who, during the mid-1850s in Europe, not only elevated nursing and midwifery status, but founded the first public health system focused on the plight of poor women and children. Lillian Wald is considered the founder of public health nursing in the United States, working with women and children as well as others. In 1916, Margaret Sanger, a public health nurse, turned to Europe, where the battle for the right to talk openly about birth control had already been won, as women began to discuss the diaphragm and fertility rhythm method, and sexual education and rights were integrated into the public health system. What she learned in the Dutch system—run by physicians and nurses—later became the Planned Parenthood Federation of America (Planned Parenthood Federation, 2009). Development, testing, and introduction of oral contraceptives to US women awaited the national changes in policy and politics that enabled women to limit family size and to time their pregnancies (Weissman, 1998). In 1970, the Title X Family Planning Program was enacted by President Nixon to fund a range of preventive health-care services free of charge to patients at or below the poverty level. As part of the US Public Health system, services included breast and pelvic exams, Pap smears and other cancer screenings, HIV testing (after the onset of the HIV/AIDS epidemic), pregnancy testing and counseling, and affordable birth control. However, owing to Congressional action (the Hyde Amendment), pregnancy termination services were not included in these federally funded programs.

In 1973, the US Supreme Court decision, Roe v Wade (US Reports, 1973), provided a watershed moment in women's health as the highest court in the land protected a woman's right to choose whether or not to continue a pregnancy. Despite political efforts to reverse the right to choose, women continue to have this right, although access to pregnancy termination and even contraceptive services continues to be severely limited in some parts of the United States.

Concurrent with these advances in public health services, a vision of women's health as more than obstetrics and gynecology was advanced by the popular women's health movement of the 1960s and 1970s, which was linked to both the second wave of the feminist movement and the popular health movement (Weissman, 1998). Self-help for women originated with public health nurses and sex education advocates Margaret Sanger and Lillian Wald. During this era, women-centered clinics, such as the Los Angeles Feminist Women's Health Center, were created by women activists, with the "Jane Movement" providing impetus for their efforts (Ruzek, 1978; Weissman, 1998). The Chicago-based Abortion Counseling Service of Women's Liberation, a pre-Roe v Wade abortion referral service, included an underground "Jane Movement" (Kaplan, 1997) that sent activists into women's living rooms to educate them about reproductive health and help them "bring on their periods" through the use of menstrual extraction (a technique still used today in many parts of the world to terminate early pregnancies). With the help of volunteer nurses and experienced activists, women could learn to safely perform the procedure themselves, using a cannula, or tube, to suction out blood during a heavy menstrual period—or a fertilized egg (Chicago Women's Liberation Union, n.d.; Kaplan, 1997). It is important to note that these activities were done before the historic Roe v Wade decision, which allowed women to seek care from their health-care providers for safe pregnancy termination.

In addition, women activists made remarkable efforts to publish information for women about their bodies and health in an effort to help women demystify their bodies.

The classic *Our Bodies, Ourselves*, first published in the early 1970s as a pamphlet, and even before that as a course (Women and Their Bodies: A course, 1970), remains as a feminist text now circulated globally (Boston Women's Health Book Collective, 1971/2011). In addition to creating new health-care institutions such as feminist clinics and birthing centers, women also engaged with formal health-care systems in an effort to transform them. Although some efforts resulted only in superficial change, others were truly transformative, such as the development of birthing centers and integration of midwifery care within traditional health-care systems and health-care plan coverage for women's primary health-care needs (Federal Register, 2013). Midwifery and federally funded contraceptive/fertility management services were also created through Title X clinics, and professional organizations concerned with reproductive health, including Nurse Practitioners in Women's Health, Association of Reproductive Health Professionals, Office of Women's Health, United States Public Health Service.

In the early efforts to transform women's health, nurses were often invisible despite the fact that many were engaged as political and community activists in collaboration with feminist groups, self-help groups, and community organizations. Public health nurses and nurse scholars focused on women's health from an ecological perspective, in which women and children's health and illness derived from interaction with a healthy family, community, and society. Aside from our nurse midwifery and obstetrical nursing colleagues who advocated for improving and humanizing obstetrical care, much of the work to enlarge the view of women's health did not have voice in women's health science until the 1980s. This decade marked a transition—one when nursing voices began to surface in the published literature. The social and political activists of the 1970s became the women's health scholars of the 1980s and ensuing decades. A feminist nurse–scholar, Wilma Scott Heide, served as president of the National Organization for Women. Her writings about social and political activism were directed to all health professionals (Heide, 1985). Nursing textbooks focusing on women's health care (as distinct from only obstetrical nursing) began to be published during the 1970s and 1980s, and research on women's health exploded (Taylor & Woods, 2001). At the same point in history, the growth of women's health as a specialty practice in nursing occurred concurrently with the growth of women's health as an emphasis in medicine (Harrison, 1994). During ensuing years, development of women's health in several disciplines occurred with growth of science, educational programs, and new models of health care for women.

With this brief historical background as context, this chapter aims to:

1. Describe women's health as a specialty, including a redefinition of women's health for the 21st century.
2. Review evidence for women's health as a distinct field of scholarship in health disciplines.
3. Review evidence for women's health as a distinct practice specialty in health care and nursing.
4. Outline contemporary challenges to women's health care.

Women's Health Redefined

Definitions of women's health in nursing and medicine had emphasized, appropriately, reproductive health care during the early portion of the 20th century. With the resurgence of a women's health movement in the 1970s, women's health advocates emphasized the importance of demystifying women's health and enhancing women's ability to receive appropriate health care. This resurgence contributed to a broader vision of women's health, replacing one that fragmented women's health and focused only on disease. In the 1980s, dialogue initiated by nurses promoted several efforts to broaden the focus on women's health from reproductive health to a much more comprehensive view. McBride and McBride (1991), in addressing theoretical underpinnings for women's health, admonished us to consider health as well-being rather than focused only on diseases, essentially expanding the definition of women's health. They also urged us to consider health as more than reproductive health, although they identified reproductive health as an important component of women's health. In her later work, McBride (1993) suggested that those who were working to transform women's health care should consider transformation from gynecology to "Gyn Ecology." By doing so, women's health would now be framed within the context of a woman's life. This shift resulted in broadening women's health from only a biopsychosocial and cultural perspective (Woods, 1985) to now redefining it to include an integrative perspective that emphasized the unique health experiences of women, providing an important foundation for research during the 1980s. Work by pioneer sociologists, Virginia Olesen and Ellen Lewin, birthed the Women's Health and Healing Program at the University of California San Francisco School of Nursing in 1982, along with a seminar series. During this same period, Alice Dan led development of a women's health program at the University of Illinois, Chicago. Both efforts provided an opportunity for critical examination of women's health literature, services, and academic programs, leading to the emergence of the Society for Menstrual Cycle Research as well as pointing to future reforms (Dan, 1994; Ruzek, Olesen, & Clarke, 1997).

In 1985, the United States Public Health Service (USPHS) Task Force on Women's Health Issues published a two-volume report that recommended the expansion of biomedical and behavioral research to specifically include conditions uniquely relevant to women across the life span. This recommendation identified conditions for which current medical interventions were different or the health risks greater for women than for men (USPHS, 1985). In 1986, the National Institutes of Health Advisory Committee on Women's Health recommended that researchers: (1) include women in research, particularly in clinical trials; (2) explain the exclusion of women from research when appropriate; and (3) evaluate gender differences in their findings. It quickly appeared that the USPHS's recommendations had fallen on deaf ears, as a few years later, a Government Accounting Office study found that recommendations and resulting policies had not been implemented. In 1990, the Congressional Caucus on Women's Issues drafted the Women's Health Equity Act. The Act set in motion a series of events leading to House and Senate hearings on women's health research funded by the NIH, and in 1990 the establishment of an Office of Research on Women's Health (ORWH) at the NIH (Baird, Davis, & Christensen, 2009). The initial objectives of the ORWH were to ensure that issues pertaining to women were adequately addressed, especially conditions that are specific to women, including situations in which risk factors are different for women as well as approaches to care. In addition, the ORWH was to ensure the appropriate participation of women in research, including clinical trials, and to foster increased involvement of women in conducting biomedical research, especially in decision-making roles in clinical medicine and research environments (USPHS, 1992).

In 1991, NIH's ORWH convened a Task Force on Opportunities for Research on Women's Health to develop recommendations on research for all US women (USPHS, 1992). The initial focus of this work included a life-span view of women's health and dimensions of science that intersected with the life span, such as reproductive biology, early developmental biology, aging processes, cardiovascular function and disease, malignancy, and immune function and infectious disease. The framework for this agenda was significant in its efforts to transcend the boundaries of the institutes that constituted the NIH by naming areas of nonreproductive and reproductive health that were significant for women. In essence, the NIH adopted definitions of women's health that would shape biomedical research for decades to come. In 1997, the NIH created an agenda for research on women's health for the 21st century (USPHS, 1999).

The attempts of women's health scholars, advocates, and government to redefine women's health provided a significant foundation on which to build and transform the practice of women's health care and the education of professionals who would provide this care as well as study women's health. The ORWH research agenda marked an important transition in federal policy: recommendations for studying women's health would be translated into research funding decisions. Moreover, the redefined field would inform the provision of health care for women.

Women's Health Scholarship: An Evolving Field of Study in Health Disciplines

Consistent with a redefinition of women's health, new knowledge began to challenge dominant beliefs about women's health and health care. Milestones that reflect significant events in women's health are included in the Timeline of Significant Events in Women's Health in Table 3.1. Fragmentation of women's health care across medical specialties challenged women's abilities to obtain holistic care that spanned dimensions of their reproductive, somatic and mental health. The nursing profession responded to the fragmentation of women's health care with holistic scholarship and promoted the diffusion of the new science of women's health by contributing to research, transforming conceptual frameworks for studying women, and employing new methodologies and methods to study women's health. New conceptual frameworks for women's health research put women at the center of the inquiry, integrated feminist theory in the frameworks, employed theoretical models of health and illness specific to women, and emphasized health, holism, person–environment relationships, and social determinants of health. Integration of biological with psychosocial and cultural dimensions of health, and emphasis on life-span development characterized women's health scholarship, which emphasized life transitions rather than disease, as the focus of nursing scholarship (Andrist & MacPherson, 2001; Taylor & Woods, 2001). Attention to the social context of women's lives led to consideration of racism, sexism, classism, and heterosexism in this body of work (Taylor, Olesen, Ruzek, & Clarke, 1997; Taylor &Woods, 1996).

Following the publication of the first NIH women's health research agenda, investigators were cautioned that merely reproducing mainstream science would not transform research about women. Simply adding a cohort of women to studies designed with men as the norm would not contribute to a deep understanding of women's health. Investigators were asked to reexamine the nature of science that would serve emancipatory ends by searching for a more complete understanding of diversity of women's health and health experiences. Changes in methodology from solely empiricist to integration of interpretive, naturalistic methodologies marked the body of nursing scholarship that became more prevalent in women's health during the 1980s. Critical methodology also became more evident, emphasizing the development of knowledge **for** women instead of **about** women, using new knowledge to empower and liberate women (Andrist & MacPherson,

TABLE 3.1	Timeline of Significant Events in Women's Health: Public and Professional Efforts		
Timeline	Historical/ Contemporary Events	Public	Professional
ERA	Public effort to advance Women's Health	Women's Health Approaches/Strategies	Practice of Women's Health Specialty Care
1960	Great Society Programs	Cover primary care needs not met by MDs	Expanded scope of practice for RNs
1960s	Second Wave of Feminist Movement in US popular health movement	Jane Abortion Movement Feminist Women's Health Clinics develop	
1965	First Certificate Nurse Practitioner (CNP) program at University of Colorado	Provide family planning & reproductive health care to women	Expand specialty skills of experienced RNs
1969	Nurses Association of American College of Obstetrics & Gynecologists (NAACOG) established	CNP collaboration with MD to manage normal patients & abnormal states only after a MD had treated abnormal findings	Educational opportunities & enhancement of Women's Health, OB, & Neonatal practice standards
1970	Title X of the Public Health Service Act	Meet family planning & reproductive needs of women	Educate experienced RNs in family planning & reproductive care
1970	**January 22, 1973**: Roe vs. Wade Supreme Court Decision **1971**: Publication of *Our Bodies, Ourselves*	More information available to women within the public domain and more women's health publications available professionally	**1971**: Publication of *Journal of Obstetric, Gynecologic, & Neonatal Nursing* (JOHNN) **1979**: *Health Care for Women International* published
1975	Family Planning Nurse Practitioner programs created	Underserved & low income communities have family planning & reproductive health-care services provided by NPs	Traineeship money: $20 million invested in education & training
1979	Master's NP programs	Public health needs becoming more complex; need for integration of NP programs into graduate education	Division of Nursing began funding schools of nursing in support of master's prepared NP education

(continued)

TABLE 3.1

Timeline of Significant Events in Women's Health: Public and Professional Efforts *(continued)*

Timeline	Historical/ Contemporary Events	Public	Professional
1980	National Certification Corporation (NCC) Exam for WHNPs	Certification needed to ensure quality of care and to expand components of care provided by WHNPs	National Certification Corporation (NCC) first available. Components of certification shifted from women's reproductive care only to also include male exam, obstetrics, and primary care
1980	Public & Professional Organizations	**1985:** *USPHS Task Force Report on Women's Health* published. **1989:** NINR funds first *Center for Women's Health Research* at University of Washington	**1980:** First meeting of NONPF. **1980:** NPWH formed. **2000:** AWHONN & NPWH defined WHNP role. **1984**: First International Congress on Women's Health Issues (ICOWHI) meeting
1990	Congressional Women's Caucus requests GAO study of Women's Health Research	**1990**: *NIH Office on Women's Health Research*. **1991**: *NIH Research Agenda on Women's Health*. **1991**: Initiation of *Women's Health Initiative* (WHI) Study. **1991**: Dr. Bernadine Healey first woman to direct NIH	Publication of: **1990**: *Women's Health Issues* **1991**: *Journal of Women's Health* **1990**: *Center for Research on Women & Gender*, University of Illinois
1993	NAACOG separates from ACOG	Holistic care by WHNPs to span reproductive, somatic, and mental health	AWHONN established as independent association
1996	Centers of Excellence in Women's Heath established by USPHS		
1999	Globalization prompts USA to increase focus on global women's health	*ORWH Research Agenda for the 21st Century (1999)*	
2005	Expansion to master's degree as entry into NP practice for WHNPs.	Obtain professional education of sufficient complexity and scope to reflect required license and certification	Endorsed by National Certification Corporation (NCC)

TABLE 3.1	Timeline of Significant Events in Women's Health: Public and Professional Efforts *(continued)*		
Timeline	Historical/ Contemporary Events	Public	Professional
2007	Master's degree mandated	Advanced level of education required to ensure safe, high quality care and to publicly demonstrate expertise to employers, patients, and colleagues	Mandated by NCC
2010	US foreign policy focuses on the status of women	**2010**: *IOM Report on Women's Health Research* **2010**: *ORWH Research Agenda 3* **2010**: *IOM Report on Clinical Preventive Services*	**2011**: *Center on Global Women's Health established* at University of Pennsylvania
2010	*Affordable Care Act* signed by President Obama	Women's preventive health services covered without cost sharing	DHHS & IOM define preventive services specific to women's health
2009–2014	NP education programs specific to Women's Health difficult to locate	Access to providers qualified to manage complex reproductive, sexual health issues, and contraceptive services are extremely limited	Decline in NP programs specific to women's health; movement to integrate Women's Health into primary care

2001). Investigators were encouraged to engage in reflexivity by considering the impact of their relationships with the women who participated in studies and recognizing that knowledge is cocreated between the women and the investigators. Awareness of being a "situated knower" and its impact on the knowledge produced became part of the methods used to gather data. Andrist (1998) asserted that the evolution of women's health as a specialty was marked by grassroots activism, public policy, and government institutions making women's health a priority in education, policy, research, and health care that prompted change. In addition, increased attention to women in federally sponsored research (marking a change in funding priorities), and the growth of women's health centers in the United States (marking a change in delivery models) reflected changes in institutional priorities and practices.

By 2000, nurse researchers had made significant contributions to women's health research in a variety of areas, including but not limited to parenting, employment, caregiving, disparities of health such as experienced by lesbians, menstrual cycle, menopause, stress, fatigue and sleep, violence against women, and women's decision making related to their health (Taylor & Woods, 2001). Developing women's health scholarship within the discipline of nursing and including interdisciplinary approaches contributed to new perspectives and enhanced understanding in caring for women, leading to the creation of new models of health care that placed women at the center of the service. One federal effort was USPHS support for Centers of Excellence in Women's Health, established in 1996 in several academic health centers and communities. The vision for these Centers was to create models for integrated approaches to clinical practice, education, and research related to women's health. Components of these Centers of Excellence were envisioned to advance clinical services, enhance teaching, improve public outreach, and promote women in academic health careers, as well as multidisciplinary women's health research (Mazure, Espeland, Douglas, Champion, & Killien, 2000). Advancing research with underrepresented populations of women, including a focus on ethical approaches to women as research participants, was a specific focus of this work.

Women's Health Practice: An Evolving Area of Specialization

Specialty practice in maternal child health nursing and midwifery established an important foundation for future specialty practice in women's health care that considered women's needs for family planning, perinatal care, and reproductive health. What is known today as a specialty in women's health care can be traced to the *Great Society* programs of the 1960s that emphasized the need for increased resources in primary care. (Youngkin, Davis, Schadewald, & Juve, 2013). During the 1970s, funding of Family Planning Certificate Nurse Practitioner programs by the Department of Health, Education, and Welfare (DHEW) supported the education of Family Planning Nurse Practitioners. These nurse practitioners were public health nurses prepared to provide family planning services in public health settings. Planned Parenthood Federation of America provided support for the first Family Planning NP program in the United States in 1972, in collaboration with the Department of Obstetrics and Gynecology of the New Jersey College of Medicine and Dentistry (Auerbach et al., 2012). In 1979, Title X supported the role of the women's health nurse practitioner (WHNP), which, at that time consisted of a 4-month in-residence training program followed by a 6-month clinical residency. In 2005, national nursing education standards changed. Education and training for entry into the profession now consisted of academic preparation at the master's level. This change triggered state boards of nursing to begin to require national certification for entry into NP practice (Kass-Wolff & Lowe, 2009). Three years later, as the NP role continued to evolve, the American Association of Colleges of Nursing (AACN) and the National Organization of Nurse Practitioner Faculties (NONPF) together endorsed entry-level academic preparation for the NP at the Doctor of Nursing Practice (DNP) level. Simultaneously, a major shift in the focus of NP core competencies occurred moving toward a population-based focus (Kass-Wolff & Lowe, 2009; NCC, 2013; NONPF, 2012).

Early WHNP certification focused on family planning and reproductive health care, but later, obstetrics, general physical assessment, primary care topics, and assessment of the male genitourinary system were added. This expansion signified the expanding role of the WHNP (Wysocki, 2013).

The Nurses Association of American College of Obstetricians and Gynecologist (NAACOG) was formed within the physician group American College of Obstetrician and Gynecologist (ACOG) (Kass-Wolfe & Lowe, 2009). Registered nurses were trained by physicians to manage (not diagnose) low-risk patients. In addition, physicians defined the role and set the standards for practice. The education of women's health nurses experienced a paradigm shift from medicine to nursing in the 1980s. Movement from apprenticeship to certificate programs to degree programs ensued gradually. WHNP certificate programs partnered or merged with degree granting programs in Schools of Nursing. An impetus for the decrease in WHNP certificate programs and the increase in WHNP graduate degree programs was the decline in Title X funding, which had been available since 1970, for health professional training combined with a shift to primary care NP funding by the Division of Nursing (HRSA, USPHS).

By 1980, the National Association of Nurse Practitioners in Reproductive Health (NANPRH), now called the National Association of Nurse Practitioners in Women's Health (NPWH), was formed by Susan Wysocki. In 1993, the Association of Women's Health, Obstetric, and Neonatal Nursing (AWHONN) was formed to replace NAACOG, and was created as an organization independent of ACOG. In 1997, the Expert Panel on Women's Health of the American Academy of Nursing (AAN) recommended expanding nursing education, evolving practice models and advancing reimbursement for care delivered to women across the life span, including primary and specialty care. In 2000, AWHONN and Nurse Practitioners in Women's Health (NPWH) formulated shared goals of quality care provided by nurse practitioners through graduate education and clear practice guidelines (AWHONN & NPWH, 2002). In 2013, Berg, Taylor and Woods addressed the need to prioritize women health services and policy. Shaver, Olshansky, and Woods (2013) emphasized the need for a women's health research agenda to include the various clinical services necessary for comprehensive women's health care, which was reiterated in a Call to Action by the Women's Health Expert Panel of the American Academy of Nursing (Berg, Shaver, Olshansky, Woods, & Taylor, 2013). While emphasizing comprehensive primary care, a concern remains as to whether or not education for NPs in the United States includes sufficient content to prepare primary care providers to assume the full array of sexual and reproductive health care (Berg, Woods, Kostas-Polston, & Johnson-Mallard, 2014).

In recent years, in order to be eligible for the certification examination, graduates are required to have a master's degree, DNP, or postmaster's certificate from a program that incorporates the National Task Force on Quality Nurse Practitioner Education criteria for evaluation of NP programs (National Task Force on Quality Nurse Practitioner Education, 2012; NCC, 2013). In 2010, national certification maintenance programs were revamped to support an increasingly complex health-care environment. These highly educated practitioners are needed to meet the challenge of creating a competent workforce to implement preventive services and meet national health goals (Berg et al., 2013). Fontenot and Hawkins (2011) have made a strong case for the need for current NPs in women's health to mentor the next generation.

The recent Licensure, Accreditation, Certification, and Education (LACE) Consensus Project coordinated by the National Council of State Boards of Nursing (NCSBN) has provided a framework by which specialization will be recognized across the nation (Consensus Model for APRN Regulations, 2008). The LACE Report defines an Advanced Practice Registered Nurse (APRN) in the United States as a nurse who has

- completed an accredited graduate-level education program preparing him/her for one of the four recognized APRN roles (certified registered nurse anesthetist [CRNA], certified nurse-midwife [CNM], clinical nurse specialist [CNS], or certified nurse practitioner [CNP]
- passed a national certification examination that measures APRN role and population-focused competencies and maintains continued competence as evidenced by recertification in the role and population through the national certification program.

Further, the *LACE Report* indicates that APRNs have acquired **advanced clinical knowledge and skills** preparing them to provide direct care to patients and populations, as well as a component of indirect care. APRN practice **builds on the competencies of registered nurses (RNs)** by demonstrating greater depth and breadth of knowledge, synthesis of data, increased complexity of skills and interventions, and greater role autonomy than RN preparation provides. APRNs are educationally prepared to assume responsibility and accountability for:

- health promotion and/or maintenance and
- assessment, diagnosis, and management of patient problems, including use and prescription of pharmacologic and nonpharmacologic interventions

The Consensus Model for APRN Regulations (2008) also includes a new framework in which individual states are able to award licensure. LACE recommendations include licensure for practice in a specific role (nurse practitioner, nurse midwife, nurse anesthetist, clinical specialist) while focusing on a specific population (family/individual across the life span, neonatal, pediatrics, women's health/gender-related, psychiatric/mental health, and adult/geriatric). In addition to the population-specific certification requirements, APRNs may pursue study in specialty areas that might include further certification in an area of the specialty.

The pathway for preparation as a nurse practitioner is outlined in Table 3.2. Organizational resources for WHNPs are outlined in Table 3.3.

Consistent with the Affordable Care Act is a growing emphasis on health promotion and wellness. In that effort, a new role for nursing has been created—that of the Integrative Nurse Coach. The International Nurse Coach Association (INCA, n.d.) has developed an educational curriculum for nurses to become board-certified nurse coaches, focusing on the promotion of optimal health and wellness (Hess et al., 2013). This work has relevance for a holistic approach to health (Dossey & Keegan, 2012), and has global implications (Dossey & Hess, 2013). The website for INCA is http://inursecoach.com. Some nurse coaches focus on women's health specifically, using integrative approaches to working in partnership with women to attain an optimal level of wellness.

Contemporary Challenges to Women's Health Scholarship and Women's Health Care

In the United States, sexual and reproductive health services for men and women are fragmented and not integrated into a health-care system of public health and primary care services. Furthermore, unlike other countries, most of our national health goals have not been achieved, specifically reduction of unintended pregnancies and sexually transmitted infections (Healthy People 2020, n.d.).

Two models are likely to drive a coordinated system of women's health services within a public and private primary care system in the United States. These models are the World Health Organization (WHO) definition of sexual and reproductive health (SRH) care (WHO, nd), including the necessary standards and provider competencies (WHO, 2011), and the United Kingdom (UK) application of the WHO model of SRH specialty care delivered by primary care and public health nurses, nurse practitioners, midwives, and generalist physicians within the UK National Health Service (Faculty of Sexual & Reproductive Health, 2012).

Just as Lillian Wald, Margaret Sanger, and Mary Breckinridge learned from the advances in health care in Europe, lessons learned from countries with national health services can inform the advancement of a coherent, high-quality model of population health delivery. The challenge and opportunity will be to continue the development of women's

TABLE 3.2	Accreditation, Education, Certification, and Licensure: Resources		
Accreditation	**Education: Completion of Degree Requirements/ Competencies**	**Certification: Specialty Knowledge and Competencies**	**Licensure as APRN**
Commission on Collegiate Nursing Commission (CCNE)	National Organization of Nurse Practitioner Faculties (NONPF): Population-Focused NP Competencies (2013) • Family/Across the Life span • Neonatal Acute Care Pediatric • Primary Care Pediatric • Psychiatric-Mental Health • Women's Health/ Gender Related	American Nurses Credentialing Center (ANCC) • Family Acute Care Adult-Gero Acute Care • Adult-Gero Primary Care • Adult Psychiatric- Mental Health • Gero • Pediatric • School NP National Certification Corporation (NCC) • Women's Health • Neonatal American Academy of Nurse Practitioners Certification Program (AANPCP) • Adult Gero Family Pediatric Nursing Certification (PNCB) • Pediatric Primary Care • Acute Care Pediatric	Each state has its own requirements for licensing nurse practitioners • All states require some form of advance training beyond undergraduate RN training • 27 states require a master's degree in nursing • 35 states require national certification
Accreditation Commission for Education in Nursing (ACEN) Accreditation	American Association of Colleges of Nursing (AACN) • The Essentials of Master's Education in Nursing (2011) • The Essentials of Master's Education for Advance Practice Nursing (1996) • The Essentials of the Doctoral Education for Advanced Nursing Practice (2006)		

TABLE 3.3	Organizational Resources for Women's Health Nurse Practitioners	
Professional Organizations	**Resources/Mission**	**Journal**
Association of Women's Health, Obstetric and Neonatal Nurses (AWHONN)	www.awhonn.org Our mission is to improve and promote the health of women and newborns and to strengthen the nursing profession through the delivery of superior advocacy, research, education, and other professional and clinical resources to nurses and other health-care professionals.	*Journal of Women's Health, Obstetric, and Neonatal Nursing*
National Association of Nurse Practitioners in Women's Health (NPWH)	www.npwh.org NPWH's mission is to ensure the provision of quality primary and specialty health care to women of all ages by women's health and women's health–focused nurse practitioners. Our mission includes protecting and promoting a woman's right to make her own choices regarding her health within the context of her personal, religious, cultural, and family beliefs.	*Women's Healthcare: A Clinical Journal for NPs.*
Association of Reproductive Health Professional (ARHP)	www.arhp.org The Association of Reproductive Health Professionals (ARHP), founded in 1963, is a multidisciplinary association of professionals who provide reproductive health services or education, conduct reproductive health research, or influence reproductive health policy.	*The Official Journal of ARHP, Contraception: An International Reproductive Health Journal*
The American Congress of Obstetricians and Gynecologists (ACOG)	www.acog.org The ACOG Continuing Medical Education program supports the mission of the College to advance women's health through lifelong education of its members.	*Obstetrics & Gynecology* is the Official Publication of the American College of Obstetricians and Gynecologists (ACOG).
North American Menopause Society (NAMS)	www.menopause.org	Menopause is the official publication of NAMS

health scholarship focused on women's health needs as well as the study of integrating gender-based SRH care within primary care and public health services.

Contemporary curricula invite further thinking about pathways to providing women's health care and point to the need for further elaboration. Prompted by the continuing challenges of fragmentation of sexual and reproductive care (SRH) in the primary care setting, there has been increased examination of current trends in graduate education for nurse practitioners preparing to practice in the area of women's health care. SRH care has been redefined to include preconception care, contraception, pregnancy and unintended pregnancy care, women's health/common gynecology care, genitourinary conditions of men, assessment of specialty gynecology/male GU problems, including infertility, sexual health promotion, and coordination with public health and primary care services (Auerbach et al., 2012). With an increasing emphasis on primary care as the focus in graduate programs preparing NPs, concern exists about educating NPs to provide SRH care as outlined by the WHO's SRH Core Competencies in Primary Care (2011) and the Royal College of Nursing's (2009, 2010) Sexual Health Competencies: An Integrated Career and Competence Framework for Sexual and Reproductive Health Nursing across the United Kingdom.

A recent Rand Corporation study of SRH care provided by nurse practitioners identified workforce changes threatening the supply of nurse practitioners who were educated appropriately to provide SRH services (Auerbach et al., 2012). This concern has grown from a notable and significant reduction in the number of US graduate programs that prepare WHNPs. With an emphasis on preparing primary care NPs for the purpose of meeting the demand for health-care providers necessary to successfully implement the 2010 Patient Protection and Affordable Care Act, many nursing schools have decided to discontinue women's health specialty programs, instead subsuming reproductive and sexual health curricula within primary care concentration curricula. As a result of the increasing emphasis on preparing NPs for comprehensive primary care practice, we are challenged to meet the needs for SRH care workforce development. A recent editorial by members of the American Academy of Nursing Expert Panel on Women's Health and Robert Wood Johnson Nurse Faculty Scholar colleagues recommends the following avenues for assuring the adequacy of preparation of nurse practitioners to deliver SRH care:

1. Assess the adequacy of SRH content in current educational programs preparing primary care NPs to develop the necessary competencies for SRH care as determined by the WHO and Royal College of Nursing;
2. Obtain feedback from graduates about the adequacy of their preparation to meet the SRH needs of men and women in their practices;
3. Ascertain whether or not SRH care in the context of primary care is meeting the needs of women and men;
4. Work with certification and accreditation programs to establish educational standards to measure SRH competencies in primary care specialties; and
5. Consider offering residency programs to augment SRH knowledge among primary care NPs (Berg et al., 2014, pp. 3–4).

Summary

This chapter has reviewed the evolution of women's health as a distinct specialty, serving as a foundation for the focus of this book. The scope of this book is on the promotion of wellness in women across the life span, recognizing that wellness must include a comprehensive approach to women's health. Nurses have a strong history in the development of women's health as a specialty. A myriad of health professionals, in addition to nurses, can make an important and positive difference in the lives of women. In fact, a new nursing role, that of a board-certified holistic/integrated nurse wellness coach, can make an important contribution in working with women to help them attain and maintain their own level of optimal wellness.

Historically, women's health has been marginalized, both in practice and research. Although advances have been made, we must continue to be vigilant in assuring that women's health care as a specialty is valued and support for women's health research continues to advance science to support care. At the same time that we are examining the adequacy of resources to prepare future specialists to provide women's health care, including SRH, we face multiple challenges to the scholarship of women's health. With the recent Institute of Medicine (IOM) study of Women's Health Research (IOM, 2010) and the recently released ORWH research agenda (USPHS, 2010), we face challenges of bridging significant knowledge gaps in the face of fiscal challenges threatening all health research. Women warrant investment of research dollars in advancing their health given their own value and their value to society as a whole. Moreover, given the challenges inherent in delivering services to women and men, the opportunities to provide optimal health care to both depend on the quality of emerging science undergirding practice.

References

Andrist, L. C. (1998). Women's health: Where are nurse practitioner programs headed? *Clinical Excellence for Nurse Practitioners, 2,* 286–292.

Andrist, L. C., & Mac Pherson, K. I. (2001). Conceptual models for women's health research: Reclaiming menopause as an exemplar of nursing's contributions to feminist scholarship. *Annual Review of Nursing Research, 19,* 29–60.

Association of Women's Health, Obstetric and Neonatal Nurses, & Nurse Practitioners in Women's Health. (2002). *The women's health nurse practitioner: Guidelines for practice and education* (5th ed.). Washington, DC: Authors.

Auerbach, D. I., Pearson, M. L., Taylor, D., Battistelli, M., Sussell, J., Hunter, L. E., … Schneider, C. (2012). *Nurse practitioners and sexual and reproductive health services. Technical report.* Santa Monica, CA: RAND Health Corporation. Retrieved from http://www.rand.org/pubs/technical_reports/TR1224.html

Baird, K. L., Davis, D. A., & Christensen, K. (2009). *Beyond reproduction: Women's health, activism, and public policy.* Madison, NJ: Fairleigh Dickinson University Press.

Berg, J., Shaver, J., Olshansky, E., Woods, N. F., & Taylor, D. (2013). A call to action: Expanded research agenda for women's health. *Nursing Outlook, 61*(4), 252.

Berg, J., Taylor, D., & Woods, N. F. (2013). Where we are today: Prioritizing women's health services and health policy. A report by the Women's Health Expert Panel of the American Academy of Nursing. *Nursing Outlook, 61*(1), 5–15.

Berg, J. A., Woods, N. F., Kostas-Polston, E., & Johnson-Mallard, V. (2014). Breaking down silos: The future of sexual and reproductive health care—An opinion from the women's health expert panel of the American Academy of Nursing. *Journal of the American Association of Nurse Practitioners, 26*(1), 3–4.

Boston Women's Health Collective. (1970). *Women and their bodies: A course.*

Boston Women's Health Book Collective. (2005). *Our bodies, ourselves.* Boston, MA: Author. (Original work published 1971).

Chicago Women's Liberation Union. (n.d.). *Herstory project: A history of the Chicago Women's Liberation Union.* http://www.cwluherstory.org

Consensus Model for APRN Regulations: Licensure, Accreditation, Certification & Education. (2008). *APRN Joint Dialogue Group Report.* Retrieved from http://www.aacn.nche.edu/education-resources/evalcriteria2012.pdf

Dan, A. J. (1994). *Reframing women's health: Multidisciplinary research and practice*. Thousand Oaks, CA: SAGE.

Dossey, B. M., & Hess, D. R. (2013). Professional nurse coaching: Advances in national and global healthcare transformation. *Global Advances in Health and Medicine*, 2(4), 10–16.

Dossey, B. M., & Keegan, L. (2012). *Holistic nursing: A handbook for practice*. Topeka, KS: American Holistic Nurses Association.

Faculty of Sexual & Reproductive Health. (2012). *Community sexual & reproductive health curriculum* (2nd ed.). London, UK: FSRH. Retrieved from http://www.fsrh.org/pages/CSRH_Curriculum.asp

Federal Register. (2013). Department of Health and Human Services 45 CFR Parts 147 and 156 Coverage of Certain Preventive Services Under the Affordable Care Act Final Rules.

Fontenot, H., & Hawkins, J. W. (2011). The evolution of specialists in women's health across the lifespan: Women's health nurse practitioners. *Journal of the American Academy of Nurse Practitioners*, 23, 314–319.

Harrison, M. (1994). Women's health: New models of care and a new academic discipline. In A. Dan (Ed.), *Reframing women's health: Multidisciplinary research and practice*. Thousand Oaks, CA: SAGE.

Healthy People 2020. (n.d.). *Healthy People 2020 final review*. Centers for Disease Control and Prevention. Retrieved from http://www.cdc.gov/nchs/data/hpdata2010/hp2010_final_review.pdf

Heide, W. S. (1985). *Feminism for the health of it*. Buffalo, NY: Margaretdaughters.

Hess, D. R., Dossey, B. M., Southard, M. E., Luck, S., Schaub, B. G., & Bark, L. (2013). *The art and science of nurse coaching: The provider's guide to coaching scope and competencies*. Silver Spring, MD: Nurses Books.org, American Nurses Association.

Institute of Medicine. (2010). *Women's Health Research: Progress, pitfalls, and promise*. Washington, DC: The National Academies Press.

International Nurse Coach Association. (n.d.). Retrieved from http://inursecoach.com

Kaplan, L. (1997). *The story of Jane: The legendary underground feminist abortion service*. Chicago, IL: University of Chicago Press.

Kass-Wolff, J. H., & Lowe, N. K. (2009). A historical perspective on the women's health nurse practitioner. *Nursing Clinics of North America*, 44, 271–280. Retrieved from http://www.nursingconsult.com/nursing/journals/0029-6465/full-text/PDF/s0029646509000395.pdf?issn=0029-6465&full_text=pdf&pdfName=s0029646509000395.pdf&spid=22416509&article_id=708719

Mazure, C. M., Espeland, M., Douglas, P., Champion, V., & Killien, M. (2000). Multidisciplinary women's health research: The national centers of excellence in women's health. *Journal of Women's Health & Gender-Based Medicine*, 9(7), 717–724.

McBride, A. B. (1993). *Women's health scholarship: From critique to assertion. Journal of Women's Health*, 2, 43–47.

McBride, A. B., & McBride, W. L. (1991). Theoretical underpinning for women's health. *Women and Health*, 6, 37–55.

National Center for Health Statistics. (2005). Figure 26. Life expectancy in years by year for women and men. Health, United States.

National Certification Corporation. (2013). *NP-BC Nurse Practitioner Board Certified Women's Health Care Nurse Practitioner and Neonatal Nurse Practitioner*. Retrieved from www.nccwebsite.org

National Institutes of Health. (1986). Inclusion of women in study populations. *NIH Guide for Grants and Contracts*, 15(22), 1.

National Organization of Nurse Practitioner Faculties. (2012). *Nurse practitioner core competencies amended 2012*. Washington, DC: NONPF. Retrieved from http://c.ymcdn.com/sites/www.nonpf.org/resource/resmgr/competencies/npcorecompetenciesfinal2012.pdf

National Task Force on Quality Nurse Practitioner Education. (2012). *Criteria for evaluation of nurse practitioner programs*. Washington, DC: National Organization of Nurse Practitioner Faculties.

Nightingale, F. (1859). *Notes on nursing: What it is and what it is not*. London, UK: Dover.

Planned Parenthood Federation of America. (2009). *Margaret Sanger—20th Century hero*. PPFA Report. New York, NY: PPFA Katherine Dexter McCormick Library. Retrieved from http://www.plannedparenthood.org/files/PPFA/Margaret_Sanger_Hero_1009.pdf

Royal College of Nursing. (2009). *Sexual health competencies: An integrated career and competence framework for sexual and reproductive health nursing across the U.K*. London, UK: Author.

Royal College of Nursing. (2010). *Sexual health specialty*. London, UK: Author. Retrieved from http://www.rcn.org.uk/development/practice/public_health/topics/sexual_health

Ruzek, S. B. (1978). *The women's health movement: Feminist alternatives to medical control*. New York, NY: Praeger.

Ruzek, S. B., Olesen, V. L., & Clarke, A. (1997). *Women's health: Complexities and difference.* Columbus: Ohio State University Press.

Shaver, J., Olshansky, E., & Woods, N. F. (2013). Women's health research agenda for the next decade. A report by the Women's Health Expert Panel of the American Academy of Nursing. *Nursing Outlook, 61*(1), 16–24.

Taylor, D., Olesen, V., Ruzek, C., & Clarke, A. (1997). Strengths and strongholds in women's health research. In C. Ruzek, V. Olesen & A. Clarke (Eds.), *Women's health: complexities and differences* (pp. 580–606). Columbus: Ohio State University Press.

Taylor, D., & Woods, N. (2001). What we know and how we know it: Contributions from nursing to women's health research and scholarship. *Annual Review of Nursing Research, 19,* 3–28.

Taylor, D. L., & Woods, N. F. (1996). Changing women's health, changing nursing practice. *Journal of Obstetric, Gynecologic, and Neonatal Nursing, 25,* 791–802.

US Public Health Services. (1992). *Opportunities for research on women's health.* Bethesda, MD: National Institutes of Health.

US Public Health Services. (1999). *Agenda for Research on Women's Health for the 21st Century. A Report of the Task Forces on the NIH Women's Health Research Agenda for the 21st Century, Volume 5. Sex and Gender Perspectives for Women's Health Research.* Bethesda, MD: National Institutes of Health. Retrieved from http://britecenter.org/wp-content/uploads/2013/02/Psychological-Differences-Between-Men-and-Women-Implications-for-a-Research-Agenda-on-Women's-Physical-and-Mental-Health.pdf

US Public Health Services. (2010). *Moving into the future with new dimensions and strategies: A vision for 2020 for women's health research.* Bethesda, MD: National Institutes of Health.

US Public Health Service Task Force on Women's Health Issues. (1985). *Women's health: Report of the Public Health Services.* Washington, DC: US Department of Health and Human Services, US Public Health Service.

US Reports. (1973). Roe v. Wade, 410 US 113.

Weissman, C. S. (1998). *Women's health care: Activist traditions and institutional change.* Baltimore, MD: Johns Hopkins Press.

Wertz, R. W., & Wertz, D. C. (1989). *Lying-in: A history of childbirth in America.* New Haven, CT: Yale University Press. (Original work published 1977).

Woods, N. F. (1985). New models of women's health care. *Health Care for Women International, 6,* 193–208.

World Health Organization. (2011). *Sexual and reproductive health core competencies in primary care.* Geneva: Author.

World Health Organization. (n.d.). *Sexual and reproductive health strategic plan 2010–2015 and proposed programme budget for 2010–2011.* Geneva: Author.

Writing Group for the 1996 AAN Expert Panel on Women's Health Issues. (1997). Women's health and women's health care: Recommendations of the 1996 AAN expert Panel on Women's Health. *Nursing Outlook, 45,* 7–15.

Wysocki, S. (2013). Nurse practitioners in women's health? Where is the future headings. In E. Q. Youngkin, M. S. Davis, D. M. Schadewald & C. Juve (Eds.), *Women's health: A primary care clinical guide* (4th ed.). Boston, MA: Pearson.

Youngkin, E. Q., Davis, M. S., Schadewald, D. M., & Juve, C. (Eds.). (2013). *Women's health: A primary care clinical guide* (4th ed.). Boston, MA: Pearson.

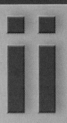

Specific Wellness Issues for Women across the Life Span

Chapter **4** Puberty through Early Adulthood

Chapter **5** Women at Midlife

Chapter **6** Healthy Aging for Women

Puberty through Early Adulthood

Ruth Mielke, Karla Parsons, and Cindy Smith Greenberg

A Life Course Perspective (LCP) is necessary for clinicians to identify multiple determinants of health that interact across the life span to produce health outcomes (Kuh, Ben-Shlomo, Lynch, Hallqvist, & Power, 2003; Lynch & Smith, 2005). The pubescent or young woman, in particular, possesses intergenerational health determinants. Her baseline health in early adulthood not only portends future health as an older woman, but through childbearing, she also influences the health of the next generation (Santelli, Sivaramakrishnan, Edelstein, & Fried, 2013). Therefore, optimizing preconception and interconception health is a critical theme in the care of adolescent and young women. As defined by the Centers for Disease Control and Prevention (CDC), preconception and interconception care is a set of interventions that aim to identify and modify biomedical, behavioral, and social risks to a woman's health or pregnancy outcome through prevention and management.

Preconception care is more than a single visit to a health-care provider and less than all well-woman care, as defined by including the full scope of preventive and primary care services for women before a first pregnancy or between pregnancies (i.e., commonly known as interconception care) (Johnson et al., 2006, p. 3).

The definition suggests a clinical approach that is proactive, consistent, and pervasive throughout all encounters with the young woman. This is evident in that 5 of the 10 core CDC recommendations to improve preconception and interconception health for women are clinician-driven: (a) encourage women to develop a reproductive life plan (RLP), (b) offer risk assessment and counseling to all women of childbearing age as a routine part of preventive care visits, (c) provide interventions to counter or minimize preconception risk factors, (d) provide additional intensive interventions in the interconception period for women with prior adverse pregnancy outcomes, and (e) offer prepregnancy planning visits to couples planning pregnancy (Johnson et al., 2006).

Well-Woman Care: Common Conditions and Treatment Approaches

Clinicians who provide well-woman care may do so as early as the onset of puberty and continue throughout adolescence and into young womanhood. Biologically, adolescence is marked with a usual sequence of pubertal changes and spans 8 to 10 years. At ages 11 to 12, a growth spurt in height and weight is usually seen followed by development of secondary sex characteristics; thelarche (breast development), adrenarche (growth of pubic and axillary hair), and menarche (onset of menstruation). Chronologically, stages of adolescence are categorized as early adolescence (ages 11 to 14), mid-adolescence (ages 15 to 17), and late adolescence (ages 18 to 21).

Beyond their biological influence, the hormonal changes of adolescence concurrently influence the social–cognitive and social–affective areas of the brain, resulting in evolving ability to forge healthy relationships, make prudent decisions, problem solve, set goals for the future, and become more independent. Adolescence is a phase of development during which neural systems may result in windows of time when the brain is biologically prepared for learning (Crone & Dahl, 2012). Further, the recent recognition of the plasticity of the adolescent brain highlights the need for exposure to healthy environmental influences in order to facilitate healthy transition to young adulthood (Konrad, Firk, & Uhlhaas, 2013). The clinician who provides care to adolescent girls is afforded a unique opportunity to identify risky behaviors such as unhealthy eating, physical inactivity, substance use, those that contribute to unintentional injuries, violence, unintended pregnancies, and sexually transmitted infections (CDC, 2012); and to promote healthy behaviors during the transition from childhood to young adulthood. See Table 4.1 for a summary of risky behavior in the youth population.

The annual examination or well-woman visit provides the young woman with an opportunity to learn about her body, to better care for herself, and to develop a collaborative relationship with a health-care provider. Although physical assessment is often the young woman's focus in the annual examination, the visit should also include risk-sensitive screening, education, counseling, and immunizations in order to promote gynecologic as well as general health. If the young woman is new to the practice and/or the clinician, this first well-woman visit will include a comprehensive history and examination, but as important, it is an opportunity to establish a new relationship with the clinician, and, in so doing, to be empowered to identify her strengths, vulnerabilities, and opportunities for improved health. If the clinician has already established a relationship with the young woman, the well-woman visit can be used to follow the progress on issues previously identified as well as attending to developing issues. Ongoing points of contact with the adolescent/young woman will range from episodic focused examinations (contraceptive follow-up, test results, single chief complaint such as vaginal discharge/urinary symptoms) to performance of a comprehensive physical examination for purposes of routine surveillance and others such as sports clearance, college entry, pre-employment screening, or preoperative history and physical. Most visits concurrently are opportunities to counsel the young woman on immunizations appropriate for her and to provide those that will optimize her health. Based on the most current Advisory Committee on Immunization Practices schedule, for adults these may include Tdap, annual influenza, a meningococcal booster, and the human papilloma virus (HPV) vaccine series.

The interval for the well-woman visit and the scope of services included may vary depending on the ambulatory setting. Although the physical examination is a key element of the visit, components of the examination should be tailored to the woman's age,

TABLE 4.1	Summary of Results from the Youth Risk Behavior Surveillance*—United States 2011
Health-risk behaviors associated with leading causes of death in persons aged 10–24 years in the last 30 days	
Texted or e-mailed while driving	32.8%
Had drunk alcohol	38.7%
Had used marijuana	23.1%
Health-risk behaviors associated with leading causes of death in 12 months prior to survey	
Had been in a physical fight	32.8%
Had ever been bullied on school property	20.1%
Had attempted suicide	7.8%
Sexual risk behaviors in the 3 months prior to the survey	
Had ever had sexual intercourse	47.4%
Had sexual intercourse during the 3 months before the survey (i.e., currently sexually active)	33.7%
Had sexual intercourse with four or more people during their life	15.3%
Among those currently sexually active, had used a condom during their last sexual intercourse	60.2%
Health-risk behaviors associated with the leading causes of death among adults aged ≥25 years	
In the last 30 days	
Had smoked cigarettes	18.1%
Had used smokeless tobacco	7.7%
In the last 7 days	
Had not eaten fruit or drunk 100% fruit juices	4.8%
Had not eaten vegetables	5.7%.
Had played video or computer games for 3 or more hours on an average school day	31.1%

*Youth Risk Behavior Surveillance System (YRBSS) monitors six categories of priority health-risk behaviors among youth and young adults: (1) behaviors that contribute to unintentional injuries and violence; (2) tobacco use; (3) alcohol and other drug use; (4) sexual behaviors that contribute to unintended pregnancy and sexually transmitted diseases (STDs), including human immunodeficiency virus (HIV) infection; (5) unhealthy dietary behaviors; and (6) physical inactivity. In addition, YRBSS monitors the prevalence of obesity and asthma. YRBSS includes a national school-based Youth Risk Behavior Survey (YRBS) conducted by CDC and state and large urban school district school-based YRBSs conducted by state and local education and health agencies. This table summarizes results from the 2011 national survey, 43 state surveys, and 21 large urban school district surveys conducted among students in grades 9–12.

Adapted from Centers for Disease Control and Prevention, (2012). Youth risk behavior surveillance—United States, 2011, Morbidity and Mortality Weekly Report, 61(4), 1–168.

risk factors, and elements of care already received. For instance, in some systems, the young woman will present having had an annual general examination by a primary care provider that did not include pelvic and breast examination. In this instance, the clinician will perform pelvic and breast examination as indicated. For many women, the focus of the well-woman examination is on pelvic and breast assessment. However, for young women in particular, the clinician needs to understand when it is appropriate to include breast and pelvic examinations as opposed to times when they are not warranted because they will likely not add useful information to the examination.

The pelvic examination includes three elements: (a) visual inspection of the external genitalia (mons pubis, labia majora and minora) and external structures (urethra [including urethral milking to assess for discharge], clitoris, glandular structures), vaginal introitus, and perianal region including (b) visual examination of vagina and cervix with a speculum, and (c) a bimanual examination in which uterus, cervix, ovaries, and adnexa are assessed with palpation. In certain circumstances, a rectovaginal examination may also be performed (American College of Obstetrics and Gynecology [ACOG], 2012b), and in some cases assessment of vaginal secretion odors will also be important (Fogel, 2013). The ACOG (2012b) recommends annual pelvic examination for women 21 years of age or older. For women younger than 21, pelvic examination is not necessary unless there are symptoms or complaints suggestive of urogenital, pelvic, or rectal disorders.

Breast Health

The occurrence of breast cancer is rare in women younger than 20 years of age and uncommon in women before 30 years of age (ACOG, 2011). Therefore, in the care of the young woman, the role of the clinician will rarely be to identify malignancy, but will be to promote breast health by (a) helping her to become aware of the characteristics of her breasts, (b) assisting her to identify factors that may impact later risk for developing breast cancer, and (c) identifying the small subset of younger women who have hereditary risk factors for breast cancer and therefore require special testing.

Efforts to increase breast cancer awareness in the United States have been successful. In the past several decades, clinical breast examination (CBE) and self-breast examination (SBE) have been highly publicized for their potential to identify potential malignancies. More recently, the appropriateness of both CBE and SBE have been reexamined in terms of breast cancer detection in women of all ages. With respect to the asymptomatic, low-risk young woman, there are no specific recommendations as to when CBE should be initiated or even if it should even be utilized routinely. The United States Preventive Services Task Force (USPSTF, 2009b) does not address CBE in younger women, while ACOG, American Cancer Society (ACS), and National Comprehensive Cancer Network (NCCN) recommend a CBE every 1–3 years in women aged 20–39 years (ACOG, 2011; ACS, 2011) or in women from 25 to 39 years of age (NCCN, 2013).

The USPSTF (2009b) recommends against clinicians teaching women how to perform breast self-examination (Grade D) as there is "moderate certainty that the harms outweigh the benefits." Such harms resulting from using SBE include psychological harms, unnecessary imaging tests and biopsies in women without cancer, and inconvenience due to false-positive screening results. While the USPSTF recommends against clinicians teaching women how to perform SBE, the ACS and ACOG endorse *breast self-awareness,* which is defined as "the woman's awareness of the normal appearance and feel of her breasts" (ACOG, 2011). This is further qualified by NCCN (2013), which emphasizes the clinician's role in breast self-awareness by assisting the young woman to become familiar with her breasts via "periodic, consistent BSE," which in premenopausal women, should be done at the end of menses.

When the younger woman has a breast concern, for example, pain or "something doesn't feel right" or "my partner wonders if this is normal," the clinician can use the CBE during the physical examination to assist with breast self-awareness. Mastalgia, or breast pain, is a common breast concern in the younger woman. Most of the time, this is cyclic and occurs premenstrually as it is related to the hormonal changes of the menstrual cycle. The pain is usually bilateral, not localized, and is described as "achy" rather than sharp (Aliotta & Schaeffer, 2013). Fibrocystic breast changes—tender, nodular, "cobblestone" feeling areas—can accompany mastalgia. If fibrocystic areas are palpated on CBE, the clinician can guide the young woman to palpate them as well while explaining that they are normal variations of her breasts.

Another concern for the young woman as well as the clinician is palpation of a breast mass. Fibroadenomas are nontender, round, movable, and firm, and are the most common mass found in adolescents and young women (Argy, Hughes, & Roche, 2002). Although identification of a breast mass in any age woman warrants follow-up with mammogram or ultrasound, in women younger than 30 years, observation of the mass over one or two menstrual cycles is an option as there is such a low index of suspicion for malignancy. If the mass resolves, the young woman returns to normal screening, but if it persists, ultrasound should be performed (NCCN, 2013). When CBE is performed or if the young woman expresses concern over the possibility of developing breast cancer, factors associated with later breast cancer risk can also be discussed so that she can consider potential lifestyle changes such as reduction in alcohol intake or increasing exercise. Table 4.2 summarizes factors that may increase or decrease risk for breast cancer development.

TABLE 4.2	**Factors that Increase or Reduce Risk for Development of Breast Cancer**	
	Factors that Increase Risk	
	Comments	**Magnitude of Effect**
Combination hormone therapy	Combination hormone therapy (HT; estrogen–progestin) is associated with an increased risk of developing breast cancer.	Approximately a 26% increase in incidence of invasive breast cancer; number needed to harm for every 237 patients participating in the Women's Health Initiative (WHI) trial and randomly assigned to the combination HT arm: one invasive breast cancer occurred beyond those that happened in the placebo arm of the trial.
Ionizing radiation	Exposure of the breast to ionizing radiation is associated with an increased risk of developing breast cancer, starting 10 years after exposure and persisting lifelong. Risk depends on dose and age at exposure, with the highest risk occurring during puberty.	Variable, but approximately a six-fold increase in incidence overall.

TABLE 4.2	**Factors that Increase or Reduce Risk for Development of Breast Cancer** *(continued)*

Factors that Increase Risk

	Comments	Magnitude of Effect
Obesity	Obesity is associated with an increased breast cancer risk in postmenopausal women who have not used HT. It is uncertain whether reducing weight would decrease the risk of breast cancer	The WHI observational study of 85,917 postmenopausal women found body weight to be associated with breast cancer. Comparing women weighing more than 82.2 kg with those weighing less than 58.7 kg, the relative risk (RR) was 2.85 (95% confidence interval [CI], 1.81–4.49).
Alcohol	Exposure to alcohol is associated with an increased breast cancer risk in a dose-dependent fashion. It is uncertain whether decreasing alcohol exposure would decrease the risk of breast cancer.	The RR for women consuming approximately four alcoholic drinks per day compared with nondrinkers is 1.32 (95% CI, 1.19–1.45). The RR increases by 7% (95% CI, 5.5%–8.7%) for each drink per day.
Major inheritance susceptibility	Women who inherit gene mutations associated with breast cancer have an increased risk.	Variable, depending on gene mutation, family history, and other risk factors affecting gene expression.

Factors that Reduce Risk

	Comments	Magnitude of Effect
Estrogen-only use among women with a hysterectomy	Based on fair evidence, estrogen-only use after menopause among women with a hysterectomy is associated with a decreased risk of breast cancer incidence and mortality.	Based on one RCT of estrogen-only therapy with conjugated equine estrogen, there was a 23% decrease in incidence of invasive breast cancer (0.27% per year with a median of 5.9 years of use, compared with 0.35% per year among those taking a placebo).
Exercise	Based on solid evidence, exercising strenuously for more than 4 hours per week is associated with reduced breast cancer risk.	Average RR reduction is 30%–40%. The effect may be greatest for premenopausal women of normal or low body weight.
Early pregnancy	Women who have a full-term pregnancy before age 20 years have decreased breast cancer risk.	50% decrease in breast cancer compared with nulliparous women or those who give birth after age 35 years.

Adapted from National Cancer Institute. Breast Cancer Prevention. Retrieved from http://www.cancer.gov/ cancertopics/pdq/prevention/breast/HealthProfessional#Section_188.

In the general population, 12.3% of women will develop breast cancer during their lifetime, and 2.74% will die of the disease (Howlader et al., 2013). Most breast cancers are *sporadic* and are due to a variety of factors such as environmental exposures or random cellular events. Another 15% to 20% are *familial* in that there is a family history of the same or related type of cancer that can be associated with environmental or other exposures that relatives have in common. The smallest subset, approximately 5% to 10%, is due to an *inherited germline genetic mutation*, BRCA1 and BRCA2, which increases cancer susceptibility significantly (Lashley, 2005). Clinicians can use risk assessment tools such as http://www.cancer.gov/bcrisktool/ or the construction of three generation pedigrees to help identify familial or inherited patterns of breast cancer risk. Recently, the USPSTF recommended (Grade B) that primary care providers screen women who have family members with breast, ovarian, tubal, or peritoneal cancer with one of several screening tools designed to identify a family history that may be associated with an increased risk for potentially harmful mutations in breast cancer susceptibility genes (BRCA1 or BRCA2). Women with positive screening results should receive genetic counseling and, if indicated after counseling, BRCA testing (Moyer, 2014).

Menstrual Health

The menstrual cycle expresses the status of both the reproductive and general health of the young woman. However, as many adolescent or young women cannot assess what constitutes normal menstrual cycles, some will seek medical attention for cycle variations that fall within the normal range, while others are unaware that their bleeding patterns are abnormal and may be due to medical issues with the potential for long-term health consequences. The American Academy of Pediatrics (AAP) and ACOG (AAP & ACOG, 2006; ACOG, 2006) have suggested that evaluation of the menstrual cycle should be considered an additional vital sign so that clinicians will reinforce its importance in assessing overall health status for young women.

Identification of abnormal patterns of menstrual bleeding or amenorrhea is critical in the care of the young woman. Adolescent or young women may be hesitant to discuss their cycles or if amenorrheic, may be relieved not to have menses and not feel the need to discuss. It is well known that adolescents have greater menstrual irregularity due to fewer ovulatory cycles than do adults as ovulatory regularity develops (AAP & ACOG, 2006; ACOG, 2006; Rosenfield, 2013). However, there is a widespread misconception that any degree of menstrual irregularity is acceptable. This misconception must be dispelled because disorders with long-term health consequences may underlie adolescent anovulation and are often overlooked at a critical developmental stage.

Clinicians should be aware of normal ranges related to variations in the menstrual cycle from adolescence through young adulthood so that they convey accurate information more frequently and with less prompting. Characteristics of normal menstrual cycles in young females are: menarche (median age) is 12.43 years; mean cycle interval is 32.2 days in the first year after menarche; menstrual cycle interval (range) is 21 to 45 days; menstrual flow length is ≤ 7 days, and 3 to 6 pads/tampons are used during each day of the menses (AAP & ACOG, 2006).

In reality, anovulation causes only minor menstrual cycle irregularity in young women. In the first year after menarche, 75% of adolescents have cycles ranging from 21 to 45 days, with 95% having cycles of 21 to 40 days by five gynecologic years. During the first two gynecologic years, half of the cycles are ovulatory, increasing to 75% by

5 years, and ultimately to 80% in the next several years when the mature menstrual pattern is achieved (Metcalf, Skidmore, Lowry, & Mackenzie, 1983). Approximately half of menstrual irregularity in adolescents is due to immaturity of the hypothalamic–pituitary axis, and usually resolves spontaneously. However, the other half, seen more often in the young woman who is obese, is associated with increased androgen levels and may mimic or be related to polycystic ovary syndrome (PCOS) (Rosenfield, 2013; Tsai & Goldstein, 2012). Although anovulation is the most common cause of irregular bleeding, adolescents with heavy menstrual bleeding may have an underlying hematologic disorder. Von Willebrand disease and platelet dysfunction account for most such disorders.

Amenorrhea is the other category of menstrual cycle problems that must be identified in the care of the young woman. In the adolescent, primary amenorrhea is assessed when there is lack of menarche by age 15 or by 3 years after the onset of breast development, and secondary amenorrhea is assessed in the adolescent or young woman when no menstrual period has occurred in over 90 days after initially menstruating (AAP & ACOG, 2006; ACOG, 2006). However, in an adolescent or young woman with secondary amenorrhea, pregnancy must be considered first, even when she has "only missed one period."

When amenorrhea is identified in the young woman, consider lifestyle causes. Amenorrhea, low energy availability (with or without eating disorders), and low bone mineral density—termed the *female athlete triad*—can, alone or in combination, pose significant immediate and long-term health risks to physically active girls and women (American College of Sports Medicine, 2007; Thein-Nissenbaum, 2013). Athletes involved in "lean sports" (those that emphasize weight categories or aesthetics, such as ballet, gymnastics, or endurance running) are at highest risk, but components can also occur in recreational exercisers (Javed, Tebben, Fischer, & Lteif, 2013). Substantial bone mass is acquired during adolescence (Misra, 2008), and by age 22, nearly all (92%) bone mineral density has been attained (Teegarden et al., 1995). In the long term, low estrogen levels (from menstrual dysfunction), and inadequate calcium and vitamin D (from negative energy balance) negatively affect bone density and preclude the young woman from acquiring bone mass during critical years of growth.

Considering evaluation of the menstrual cycle as a "vital sign," clinicians should inquire at every visit for the first day of the young women's last menstrual period and for characteristics of her cycles. When amenorrhea or variations in menstrual cycles persist, assessment of lifestyle factors must be considered as well as hypothalamic–pituitary–gonadal function or hematological disease.

Reproductive Life Plan

The CDC recommends that young women take individual responsibility across their life span via a RLP. A RLP is "a set of personal goals regarding the conscious decision about whether or not to bear children" (Files et al., 2011, p. 468) from which the clinician and young woman develop a plan to achieve these goals. It is well known that approximately 50% of all pregnancies are unintended, but these proportions are even higher in adolescent and young women; women with lower levels of education and income; and women of racial/ethnic minorities. Further, unintended pregnancies in women in these groups increase the risk of poor maternal and infant outcomes more so than in women in general (Finer & Zolna, 2011).

Ongoing assessment of pregnancy intention is critical in supporting adolescent and young women in development of a RLP. Pregnancy intention ranges from the desire for pregnancy either soon or in the future, to ambivalence, as well as lack of intention to become pregnant. Intended pregnancies are those reported to have occurred at the "right" time or later than hoped for because of difficulties in conceiving. In contrast, unintended pregnancies are those reported to be either unwanted or mistimed. Women with an unintended pregnancy may choose to terminate the pregnancy; continue the pregnancy and offer the infant for adoption; or if ambivalent, may continue the pregnancy (Santelli et al., 2003).

In the young woman, simple lead questions for developing the RLP are "Do you plan to have (more) children?" and/or "Do you have plans for conceiving a child in the next 1 to 5 years?" (Moos, 2003; Moos et al., 2008; Stern, Larsson, Kristiansson, & Tydén, 2013). It is useful to start the discussion as to whether having children is an eventual desire and if desired, the hoped for time frame. In the pubescent girl, the concept of a RLP can be introduced in the context of age-appropriate life planning (Holland Wade, Herrman, & McBeth-Snyder, 2012). If childbearing is desired, the elements of the RLP should include: (a) age of the woman and her partner, (b) maternal health (c) number and spacing of children, (d) pregnancy risk tolerance, (e) family history, and (f) life context (Files et al., 2011). Table 4.3 presents elements of the RLP with corresponding patient education.

TABLE 4.3	Considerations for the Reproductive Life Plan with Clinician Discussion Points
Reproductive Life Plan Elements	**Discussion Points**
Age	
Woman	Advancing maternal age positively associated with more fetal and maternal risk: • spontaneous abortion • genetic anomalies • multiple gestation • comorbidities during pregnancy (e.g., hypertension, diabetes) Advancing maternal age associated with reduced fertility: • By age 35, a woman has 30% probability of pregnancy (on most fertile cycle day) compared with 50% in women 19–26 years of age
Male Partner	Increasing paternal age associated with more fetal and maternal risk: • male partners aged 45 years and older at 4–5 times increased risk of having offspring with a new autosomal dominant condition than men aged 20–25 years • male partners aged 40 years and older, increased pregnancy-associated complications in their partners (spontaneous abortion, preeclampsia, preterm births, and surgical deliveries) and an increase in adverse outcome in the offspring* Increasing paternal age associated with lower fertility*
Number and Spacing of Children	Interpregnancy interval (time between 2 consecutive births minus gestational age of the second infant) of 18–23 months has lowest risk of adverse perinatal outcomes.

TABLE 4.3	Considerations for the Reproductive Life Plan with Clinician Discussion Points *(continued)*
Reproductive Life Plan Elements	**Discussion Points**
Risk Tolerance	Each woman possesses a set of unique risks based on lifestyle choices, baseline health, prior pregnancy outcomes, and age at time of conception.
	Maternal prematurity and low birth weight are associated with decreased fertility and increased risk of having preterm or small for gestational age infant[†]
	Fragile X premutation carriers have median age of menopause 6–8 years earlier than most women, and about 20% have ovarian failure before 40 years of age.
Family History	Genetic factors: - primary ovarian insufficiency (no menses for at least 4 to 12 months and FSH levels in menopausal range) will compromise fertility[‡] - heritable conditions such as cystic fibrosis, Huntington's Disease should be addressed by genetic counseling for the woman and her partner
Life Context	Planning for pregnancy allows the woman to consider her life/career trajectory within the context of her expected fertility and personal risk factors.
	Sensitivity to women who are more vulnerable to the negative effects of unintended pregnancy (adolescents, uninsured, or single) is essential, but simultaneously, clinicians should not prejudge women who are not prepared to discuss a RLP.

* Sartorius, G. A., & Nieschlag, E. (2010). Paternal age and reproduction. *Human Reproduction Update, 16(1),* 65–79. doi:10.1093/humupd/dmp027

†Sydsjö, G. (2011). Long-term consequences of non-optimal birth characteristics. *American Journal of Reproductive Immunology, 66,* 81–87. doi:10.1111/j.1600-0897.2011.01035.x

‡Baker, V. (2011). Life plans and family-building options for women with primary ovarian insufficiency. *Seminars in Reproductive Medicine, 29(04),* 362–372. doi:10.1055/s-0031-1280921

Adapted from Files, J. A., Frey, K. A., David, P. S., Hunt, K. S., Noble, B. N., & Mayer, A. P. (2011). Developing a reproductive life plan. *Journal of Midwifery & Women's Health, 56(5),* 468–474. doi:10.1111/j.1542-2011.2011.00048.x

Risk Assessment and Counseling

Clinicians must acknowledge risk factors that are unique to young women as well as the likelihood of engaging in harmful and beneficial health behaviors. The Pregnancy Risk Assessment Monitoring System (PRAMS) provides such data on maternal behaviors, health conditions, and experiences for women in the United States who have delivered a live birth in selected states and cities in the United States. As an ongoing state- and population-based surveillance system, PRAMS includes data on 28 indicators that were selected on the basis of their potential health impact and relevance to preconception and interconception health (D'Angelo et al., 2007). Table 4.4 summarizes 2004 PRAMS data.

Behaviors such as the use of tobacco (23.2%) and alcohol (50.1%) in women overall prior to pregnancy necessitates an active role by the clinician to provide behavioral and/or pharmacological smoking cessation options and to screen for alcohol abuse. The

Indicator		% Women with Private Insurance	% Women with Medicaid
Preconception Factors (Risk and Protective)	Tobacco use	17.3	36.0
	Alcohol use	37.7	37.1
	Multivitamin use	21.4	45.9
	Nonuse of contraception	52.2	54.9
	Dental visit	84.9	73.1
	Health counseling (preconception visit)	39.5	20.9
	Physical abuse	1.8	8.0
	Stress	11.1	33.8
Preconception Health Condition	Underweight*	12.1	14.5
	Overweight*	12.9	14.4
	Obesity*	23.3	32.7
	Anemia	7.6	19.5
	Asthma	6.5	10.7
	Diabetes	2.9	1.4
	Hypertension	2.2	2.4
	Heart problem	0.9	2.4
History of Adverse Outcome	LBW	8.8	15.6
	Preterm	11.7	13.7
Postpartum/Inter-conception Factors (Risk and Protective)	Tobacco use	10.9	26.8
	Contraceptive use	85.5	85.1
	Postpartum depression	10.2	22.5
	Postpartum social support	91.1	79.7
	Recent LBW	6.5	8.8
	Recent preterm	9.9	11.1
	Postpartum examination	93.6	84.7
	Contraceptive use counseling	89.8	88.6
	Dental visit	41.5	18.1
	WIC participation	20.3	88.5

*Body mass index (BMI) categories: underweight <19.8; overweight 26.0–29.0; and obese> 29.0.

Adapted from D'Angelo, D., Williams, L., Morrow, B., Cox, S., Harris, N., Harrison, L., . . . Zapata, L. (2007). Preconception and interconception health status of women who recently gave birth to a live-born infant—Pregnancy Risk Assessment Monitoring System (PRAMS), United States, 26 reporting areas, 2004. Morbidity and Mortality Weekly Report, 56(SS10), 1–35.

PRAMs data also demonstrates that women who are poor (i.e., using Medicaid) experience a greater degree of physical conditions; anemia, asthma, and psychosocial stressors; stress, abuse, and depression in preconception and postpartum periods, which are likely to be associated with more adverse birth outcomes than women of greater means (i.e., with private insurance). The fact that over half of this group of childbearing women was not using contraception, even though not trying to get pregnant, suggests that clinicians should consider offering contraceptive methods with rates of high adherence such as long-acting reversible contraceptives (LARC).

Delaying/Preventing Pregnancy

Approximately half of women with unintended pregnancies report not using contraception at the time they became pregnant, and the other half report that they became pregnant despite use of contraception (Finer & Henshaw, 2006). In 2006 to 2010, 43% of never-married adolescent women (15 to 19 years of age) had experienced sexual intercourse at least once, and of those, 78% had used some form of contraception, the majority (68%) using a condom (Martinez, Copen, & Abma, 2011). Figure 4.1 depicts various family planning methods, including their effectiveness rates.

For young women who wish to delay pregnancy and have no contraindications, the use of LARC (contraceptive implants and intrauterine devices [IUDs]) should be encouraged and made readily available. As LARCs require only a single act of clinician placement for long-term use (3 years for etonorgestrel implant, 5 years for levonorgestrel IUD, and 10 years for inert copper IUD) and are independent of user motivation and adherence, their typical use failure rates (< 1%) are significantly lower than those of more commonly used methods such as oral contraceptives (8%) and condoms (15%) (Hatcher

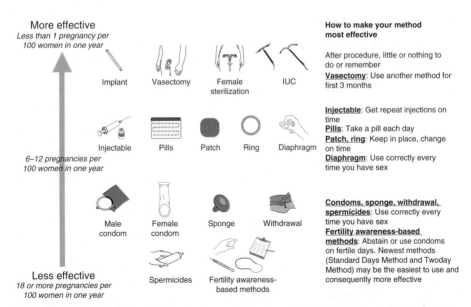

FIGURE 4.1 Effectiveness of family planning methods. From Hatcher, R. A., Trussell, J., Nelson, A., Cates, W., Kowal, D., & Policar, M. S. (2011). *Contraceptive technology* (20th ed.). New York, NY: Ardent Media. Retrieved from https://us-mg6.mail.yahoo.com/neo/launch?retry_ssl=1 - _msocom_1#_ msocom_1;; https://us-mg6.mail.yahoo.com/neo/launch?retry_ssl=1 - _msocom_2#_msocom_2.

et al., 2011; Trussell, 2011) (Fig. 4.1). In a prospective cohort study (*n* = 7486) of contraceptive effectiveness, the contraceptive failure rate in women using pills, patch, or ring was 4.55 per 100 participant-years, as compared with 0.27 among those using long-acting reversible contraception (after adjustment for age, educational level, and history with respect to unintended pregnancy). Further, younger women (less than 21 years of age) who used pills, patch, or ring had a risk of unintended pregnancy that was almost twice as high as the risk when these methods were used in older women (Winner et al., 2012). This study demonstrates the efficacy of LARC in women of all ages, but, in particular, highlights the benefit of LARCs in adolescents and younger women, who are at greater risk for unintended pregnancy.

As the effectiveness of long-acting reversible contraception is superior to that of contraceptive pills, patch, or ring and is not altered in adolescents and young women, clinicians should be proactive in offering LARC methods to young women (Russo, Miller, & Gold, 2013). A recent study reported that although clinic staff did not generally equate being a teen with ineligibility for IUDs, one quarter of the young women did perceive that their age rendered them ineligible. Common challenges to providing LARC-specific services to younger patients included extra time required to counsel young patients about LARC methods, outdated clinic policies requiring multiple visits to obtain IUDs, and a perceived higher removal rate among young women (Kavanaugh, Frohwirth, Jerman, Popkin, & Ethier, 2013).

Therefore, prevention of unintended pregnancy in women at risk must include several strategies. These strategies include: (a) identification of safe and most efficacious methods based on the woman's risk profile and that suit their lifestyle and RLP, (b) accurate education and follow-up visits to ensure best use of barrier and short-term contraceptive methods such as pills, patches, and rings, (c) increased accessibility of LARCs via clinician training and patient-friendly approaches such as same-day insertion.

Planning Pregnancy

Less than a third of women receive prepregnancy health counseling (D'Angelo et al., 2007). The preconception health visit may not necessarily be termed as such nor be the reason that the young woman seeks care. However, any visit in which the young woman indicates that she has not been using contraception or is considering having a baby is an opportunity to promote health access, and initiate behaviors that will best prepare her for an optimal pregnancy outcome. On average, 85% of healthy couples who are having regular, unprotected intercourse will conceive within 1 year (Trussell, 2011). Therefore, engaging the young woman in discussion of areas of risk or vulnerability prior to actively attempting pregnancy is critical.

An ongoing theme in the care of the young woman should be promotion of healthy weight. One third of US adolescent girls aged 13 to 19 are overweight or obese (Ogden, Carroll, Kit, & Flegal, 2012), and 56% of young women aged 20 to 39 are overweight or obese (Flegal, Carroll, Kit, & Ogden, 2012). A key modifiable risk factor in pregnancy planning is achieving normal prepregnancy body mass index (BMI). Extremes of BMI reflect baseline health of the young woman and can significantly influence maternal complications; gestational diabetes, pregnancy-related hypertension, and neonatal complications; prematurity, low birthweight, or macrosomia (Baeten, Bukusi, & Lambe, 2001; Catalano & Ehrenberg, 2006; Kosa et al., 2011; Rosenberg, Garbers, Chavkin, & Chiasson, 2003). A comprehensive resource for clinicians that addresses general aspects of care as well as specific health conditions, "Guidelines for Preconception and Interconception Care," is available at http://www.everywomancalifornia.org/content_display.cfm?categoriesID=97&contentID=360.

Folic Acid Supplementation

It is well known that periconceptional folic acid supplements reduce the risk of neural tube defects (NTD) in children (Czeizel & Dudás, 1992; MRC Vitamin Study Research Group, 1991; Safi, Joyeux, & Chalouhi, 2012; Smithells, Sheppard, Wild, & Schorah, 1989). Besides NTD, folic acid supplementation may reduce other anomalies: cardiovascular defects and urogenital anomalies (Canfield et al., 2005; Czeizel, 2009), orofacial clefts (Canfield et al., 2005; Tolarova, 1982), and limb reductions (Canfield et al., 2005).

Neural tube closure is normally complete 6 weeks after the woman's last period, a time when many women are unaware of early pregnancy (ACOG, 2003). Only 35.1% of women in the United States used a multivitamin four or more times a week in the month before their most recent pregnancy (D'Angelo et al., 2007). The USPSTF recommends (Grade A) that all "women planning or capable of pregnancy take a daily supplement containing 0.4 to 0.8 mg (400 to 800 µg) of folic acid" at least one month before conception and through the first 2 to 3 months of pregnancy (USPSTF, 2009a). Higher doses of folic acid (4 mg) are recommended in women with a history of infant with NTD, or for those taking antiseizure medications with an antifolate effect (ACOG, 2003).

Young women should be taking a multivitamin containing folic acid as a routine part of their daily life. Foods rich in folate, or vitamin B9, are dark leafy vegetables, legumes, nuts, asparagus, and strawberries. However, food folate is not as bioavailable as folic acid, the synthetic form of folate. It is important to convey that the prepregnancy/early pregnancy supplementation of folic acid either alone or in the prenatal vitamin ensures the dietary recommendation even though some young women may insist that their dietary intake has sufficient folate (Simpson, Bailey, Pietrzik, Shand, & Holzgreve, 2010).

Promoting Healthy Behaviors

Healthy decisions and behaviors promote achievement of optimal health. As such, the goal is to foster health-promoting decisions and reduce participation in risky behaviors. Adolescents, in particular, are governed by their perception of invincibility and thus invulnerable to the consequences of risky behavior. In adolescents, personal goals for the future (Wickman, Anderson, & Greenberg, 2008) and future expectations (how much one presumes something will occur) (Sipsma, Ickovics, Lin, & Kershaw, 2013) can protect against risky behaviors. To effect optimal health, it is important to provide knowledge and skills for the client to make healthy decisions.

Immunizations

Each year, the Advisory Committee on Immunization Practices (ACIP) develops recommendations for routine use of vaccines in children, adolescents, and adults in the United States. Updated guidelines are readily available for clinicians and in consumer-oriented formats. It is important to reinforce with women that vaccinations not only confer protection on the young woman, but also on her family and the community in which she and her children live.

Two concepts that can help young women in understanding the importance of immunization are that of *herd immunity* and *cocooning*. "Herd immunity" is based on the premise that when enough individuals in the population (herd) have been vaccinated, protection is provided to all others, whether or not vaccinated themselves. The term "cocooning" means vaccinating anyone who cares for or comes in close contact with babies who are too young to receive a particular vaccine. A cocooning strategy should include not only the young woman, but also her family members, and other caregivers (daycare facility workers, nannies, teenage babysitters, etc.).

Reducing Substance Use

Alcohol-related harms are a public health issue worldwide (Humeniuk, Henry-Edwards, Ali, Poznyak, & Monteiro, 2010a). In women and girls in the United States during 2001 to 2005, an estimated 23,000 deaths were attributed to excessive alcohol use (CDC, 2013a). Among adult women, binge drinking (consuming 4 or more drinks per occasion) is most prevalent in those aged 18 to 24 at 24.2% (CDC, 2013a). Binge drinking puts women at risk for sexual victimization (Testa & Hoffman, 2012), unintentional injuries, violence, sexually transmitted infections (STIs), unintended and alcohol-exposed pregnancy, and breast cancer (CDC, 2013a). Alcohol use is also associated with increased tobacco use (Piasecki et al., 2012).

The issue of substance use in adolescents is a concern on many dimensions. Altering cognition leads to other risky behaviors that target multiple risk pathways. Subclinical alcohol use is associated with deviations in neurodevelopment (Luciana, Collins, Muetzel, & Lim, 2013). Early initiation and use of alcohol is associated with an increased risk of subsequent alcohol use disorders, and increased risk of involvement in violent behaviors, suicide attempts, and a variety of other problematic activities. Youth who perceive greater harm in using substances report lower usage (SAMHSA, 2013). An inverse relationship exists between religiosity and substance use in adolescents (Kub & Solari-Twadell, 2013), suggesting that religious affiliation may confer some protective benefit from substance use.

Clinicians can impact alcohol use in young women (Gebarra, Bhona, Ronzani, Lourenço, & Noto, 2013). First, it is essential to assess for substance use. Numerous tools are available for clinicians who work with specific populations of women to screen for substance abuse. The CRAFFT screener is a tool with adequate psychometrics to detect alcohol and substance use in adolescents (Dhalla, Zumbo, & Poole, 2011), and is presented in Table 4.5. The CRAFFT may be useful in identifying prenatal alcohol and drug use in pregnant women up to age 25 (Chang et al., 2011). Another tool, the ASSIST (Alcohol, Smoking and Substance Involvement Screening Test) is a culturally neutral tool to screen for use of multiple substances including tobacco, alcohol, and other drugs (Humeniuk et al., 2010a).

It is equally essential to provide an avenue to discuss without shame as the goal is to reroute the young woman to abstain, then to refer to mental health counseling or to an

TABLE 4.5	CRAFFT Screener
1. Have you ever ridden in a car driven by someone (including yourself) who was high or had been using alcohol or drugs?
2. Do you ever use alcohol or drugs to relax, feel better about yourself, or fit in?
3. Do you ever use alcohol or drugs when you are by yourself, alone?
4. Do you ever forget things you did while using alcohol or drugs?
5. Do your family or friends ever tell you that you should cut down on your drinking or drug use?
6. Have you ever gotten into trouble while you were using alcohol or drugs?

intervention resource such as a detoxification center or inpatient rehabilitation center. Using simple questions can lead to more specific questions, if indicated.

Integrated screening and Brief Intervention (BI), consisting of providing risky drinkers with feedback on their alcohol use, information on harmful consequences of use, and benefits of intake reduction, and techniques to reduce consumption using an empathetic attitude, stressing individual responsibility for consumption, decreases alcohol consumption in women (Gebarra et al., 2013). The World Health Organization provides guidance for providing BI (Humeniuk et al., 2010b). Offer handouts (accessible on line from state or community health services clinics at no charge) that provide knowledge and skills to resist pressures to drink or use other substances. It is important to discuss with the client, and family as appropriate, the importance of factors that may protect against substance use.

For adolescents, interventions include clear house rules that are enforced, discussion about the dangers of drug and alcohol use, involvement in religious and community programs, and eating family meals together. Community- and school-based programs exist for both parents and youth, along with parenting classes that include signs and symptoms of use in the young person. An example of an effective program is Project Northland (http://www.epi.umn.edu/projectnorthland/schoolba.html), a research-based curriculum designed for the school setting that offers social behavior activities, peer leadership, parenting involvement, and community links to support the concept of "one message, many messengers."

Preventing Sexually Transmitted Infections

Nearly 50% of the STIs in the United States occur in young people (ages 15 to 24), although this group represents only 25% of the sexually experienced population (Satterwhite et al., 2013). Historically, men were thought to be more affected by STIs, but women and children can have more symptoms and sequelae than men (Fogel, 2013). Although the annual number of new infections among young women and young men is roughly equal (51% vs. 49%) (Satterwhite et al., 2013), the consequences of untreated STIs in young women, such as infertility and the potential for perinatal transmission are significant not only for their own health but that of their offspring.

Chlamydia and gonorrhea are the most reported STIs in the United States, but many cases of chlamydia, gonorrhea, and syphilis continue to go undiagnosed and therefore unreported. Screening for STIs includes exploring aspects of a sexual risk history at each encounter with the young woman; the initial encounter, a more extensive sexual risk history and subsequent visits to identify if there have been changes in sexual practices. The easiest question to ask may be "Have there been any changes in your sexual life?" Follow the recommendations of the USPSTF, to screen for chlamydia in all sexually active nonpregnant young women aged 24 and younger and for older nonpregnant women who are at increased risk (Grade A), and screen for gonorrhea infection in all sexually active women, including those who are pregnant, if they are at increased risk for infection (Grade B). However, the USPSTF is in the process of updating and consolidating these guidelines with one recommendation for both of these as chlamydial and gonorrheal infections often coexist (CDC, 2010a). If pelvic examination is indicated, endocervical cultures for chlamydia and gonorrhea can be obtained, but current evidence demonstrates that screening can be performed by nucleic acid amplification testing from urine specimens (Cook, Hutchison, østergaard, Braithwaite, & Ness, 2005), affording a more acceptable means of screening to the young woman.

Other STIs, such as HPV, herpes simplex virus, and trichomoniasis, are not routinely reported to CDC but are associated with morbidity (CDC, 2011b; Gantt & Muller, 2013). In the United States, the most prevalent STIs in women are genital herpes (herpes simplex virus-2 [HSV-2]) and HPV (Satterwhite et al., 2013).

Genital Herpes. Herpes simplex virus types 1 and 2 (HSV-1 and HSV-2) are lifelong infections. HSV-1 has typically been thought to be transmitted nonsexually during childhood, while HSV-2 is almost always transmitted sexually. Therefore, in young women, the prevalence of HSV-2 increases with sexual exposure: ages 14 to 19 (2.1%), 20 to 29 (14.4%), and 30 to 39 (25.2%) (CDC, 2010c). It is important to note that, in recent years, HSV-1 has been recognized as an increasingly important cause of genital herpes in the United States (Bradley, Markowitz, Gibson, & McQuillan, 2014).

Besides the discomfort and shame of symptomatic infection, HSV-2 infection is a concern because of the strong association between HSV-2 and HIV infections. Even in subclinical HSV-2 infections, microulcerations are believed to provide access to the HIV virus (Freeman et al., 2006). Further, in women of childbearing age, genital HSV infection during pregnancy can lead to serious infection in neonates through vertical transmission (Gantt & Muller, 2013).

Young women should be aware that most viral shedding and transmission occur with active herpes lesions, but shedding can also occur when asymptomatic. Therefore, ways to protect an uninfected partner are abstinence from sexual contact from the onset of the prodrome until the lesions are completely healed and during asymptomatic periods, use of latex condoms and suppressive therapy. She should also be advised that during outbreaks, her partner should not share any intimate articles that may have come into contact with the lesions (CDC, 2013a, 2013b).

Human Papilloma Virus. While HPV is the most prevalent STI in US women overall (32.9%), its prevalence peaks in younger women; in 15 to 19-year-olds, 38.9%, and in 20 to 24-year-olds, 53.8% (Satterwhite et al., 2013). Prevention of HPV is critical as it is the cause of most anogenital cancers and warts (Chelimo, Wouldes, Cameron, & Elwood, 2013). Young women will express concern over the finding that they have a "bump down there," often a genital wart, but the young woman must also be educated to have as much concern over the potential for developing cervical cancer.

Risk factors for HPV infection, genital warts, and ultimately for cervical cancer are related to sexual practices and health behaviors. Sexual behaviors are those that increase viral exposure to HPV: increasing number of lifetime partners, increase in the age difference between a woman and her first partner, having male partners who have been sex workers, and coinfection with other STIs such as HSV-2, chlamydia, or HIV. Health behaviors associated with HPV infection include long-term oral contraceptive use (5 or more years), high parity (five or more term pregnancies), and cigarette smoking (Chelimo et al., 2013).

Since 2006, a quadrivalent HPV vaccine has been available in the United States for females aged 9 to 26 years and in 2009, was available for males. The quadrivalent vaccine protects against HPV subtypes 6, 11, 16, and 18. Types 6 and 11 are responsible for about 90% of anogenital warts, while types 16 and 18 are high-risk oncogenic types associated with anogenital (cervical) cancers. In 2009, a bivalent HPV vaccine that provides protection against types 16 and 18 was licensed for use in females aged 10–25 years (CDC, 2011b). As only 32% of girls aged 13 to 17 years received the recommended regimen of HPV 3 vaccine series over 6 months in comparison with 91.6% who received the hepatitis B, also a 3 vaccine series (CDC, 2011a), this presents an opportunity for clinicians to educate adolescents and their parents on the benefits of the vaccine, which is widely available in the United States.

In developed countries, cervical cancer is largely preventable. For cervical cancer to develop, there is first the initial infection with HPV via sexual contact, and then if the HPV infection is not resolved, it progresses to precancerous and cancerous lesions. However, in terms of cervical cancer prevention, key points for the clinician to understand are that (a) for the most part, healthy young women less than 21 years old have an immune response that clears most HPV in an average of 8 months after infection, (b) fewer than 10% of new HPV infections will persist and become precancerous, usually over 5–10 years, (c) invasive cancer arises over many years or even decades, and (d) in the minority of women with precancer, the peak or plateau in risk is at about 35–55 years of age (Ho, Bierman, Beardsley, Chang, & Burk, 1998; Schiffman, Castle, Jeronimo, Rodriguez, & Wacholder, 2007; Woodman et al., 2001).

With these points in mind, ACOG, ACS, and the USPSTF recommend that cervical cancer screening be done every 3 years between ages 21 and 29, and in women aged 30 to 65 every 3 years or if HPV co-testing is done, every 5 years (ACOG, 2012a; Moyer, 2012; Saslow et al., 2012). Therefore, the role of the clinician in prevention of anogenital warts and cervical cancer is threefold: identify risky practices and promote practices that diminish HPV exposure; educate young women, and if very young, their parents, on the benefits of the HPV vaccine; incorporate age-appropriate cervical cancer screening within a system that affords follow-up for women with abnormal screening results.

Finally, the role of the clinician in prevention of STIs in the young woman includes ongoing verbal screening, risk-driven clinical screening, and consistent discussion of practices (abstinence, condoms, HPV vaccine) that will reduce her exposure to STIs.

Promoting Healthy Body Image

Healthy Weight

A key aspect of the role of the clinician who cares for the young woman is to encourage positive behaviors and to identify potential threats to a healthy self-image. Promotion of healthy weight is one critical aspect of a healthy self-image. Weight appropriate for one's height, based on BMI, and age, helps maintain optimal health. Being overweight or obese is risky as is being underweight. Health risks associated with underweight include amenorrhea, fertility problems, miscarriage, and osteoporosis. Individuals who are obese have an increased risk of developing type 2 diabetes, cardiovascular disease, and asthma. Other issues involve burden on the growing frame with strain on joints and ligaments.

Unhealthy weight-loss behaviors (diet pills, laxatives, and diuretics, employing self-induced vomiting, and skipping meals) are more likely to occur among overweight or obese female adolescents and among female adolescents who perceive themselves to be overweight or obese (Paxton, Valois, & Drane, 2004). A recent study reported that 23% of normal weight US female adolescents perceived themselves to be overweight or obese, while of those who were overweight or obese, 21% did not perceive themselves to have a high BMI (Yost, Krainovich-Miller, Budin, & Norman, 2010). Further, weight perception in young women differs across ethnicities; African American adolescents had less than half the likelihood of White adolescents of perceiving themselves as overweight, while Asian Americans were significantly more likely than Whites to perceive themselves as overweight (Boyd, Reynolds, Tillman, & Martin, 2011). Assessing the young woman's perception of her body weight is a necessary first step in promoting healthy weight. This can be done with BMI charts or smart phone applications such as "My BMI Calculator," available from the National Heart, Lung and Blood Institute, to show that she is in a "healthy" weight category (green) or in a less healthy BMI category, for example, obese (red).

Discussing weight can be a sensitive subject. As a health-care provider, bringing up the subject provides an opportunity to discuss excess weight or underweight and the associated health risks. The SCOFF questionnaire (Sick, Control, One stone [weight], Fat, Food) (Morgan, Reid, & Lacey, 1999) presented in Table 4.6, and the Eating disorder Screen for Primary care (ESP) (Cotton, Ball, & Robinson, 2003), validated in those 18 and older, provide questions to screen for eating disorders. The clinician needs to explore the client's concerns and ask questions that come from the client's perspective. Providing a safe and matter-of-fact approach to weight issues can start a dialogue on eating habits and exercise, and provides an opportunity for exploring body image and weight concerns. After rapport is established, it is helpful to review strategies using a team approach for long-term weight management, which will guide follow-up appointments and referrals to nutritionists as appropriate. Recommendations to help prevent eating disorders and obesity in adolescents have been delineated by Neumark-Sztainer (2009) and include the following: (a) encourage and support the use of eating and physical activity behaviors that can be maintained on an ongoing basis to discourage unhealthy dieting; (b) promote a positive body image, (c) encourage enjoyable family meals, (d) encourage families to focus less on weight and more on providing an environment at home to facilitate healthy eating and physical activity; and (e) assume that overweight teens have experienced mistreatment because of their weight (e.g., teasing, being excluded from activities) and discuss this issue with the teen and their family. These recommendations help with a more sustained behavioral change (Neumark-Sztainer, 2009). The USPSTF found that moderate- to high-intensity weight-management programs that include dietary, physical activity, and behavioral counseling were effective in those aged 6 to 18 years (USPSTF, 2010). For obese adults, the most effective interventions were high intensity (12 to 26 sessions in a year) and comprehensive, including setting weight-loss goals, self-monitoring, dealing with barriers to change, and strategizing on how to maintain long-term lifestyle changes (USPSTF, 2012). It was not determined which of the components were associated with sustained weight loss.

TABLE 4.6	The SCOFF Questions
Do you make yourself **S**ick because you feel uncomfortably full?
Do you worry you have lost **C**ontrol over how much you eat?
Have you recently lost more than **O**ne stone in a 3-month period?
Do you believe yourself to be **F**at when others say you are too thin?
Would you say that **F**ood dominates your life?

From Morgan, J. F., Reid, F., & Lacey, J. H. (1999). The SCOFF questionnaire: Assessment of a new screening tool for eating disorders. BMJ, 319(7223), 1467–1468. One stone is from the British = 14 lbs or 6.5 kg.

Healthy Skin

Acne vulgaris is a common skin condition that may negatively impact the young woman's body image. Body image issues associated with acne include depression, anxiety, social isolation, and low self-esteem (Smithard, Glazebrook, & Williams, 2001). Some degree of acne affects most adolescents (Ghodsi, Orawa, & Zouboulis, 2009; Law, Chuh, Lee, & Molinari, 2010) and 64% and 43% of individuals in their 20s and 30s, respectively (Bhate & Williams, 2013). Young women are affected more than young men (Collier et al., 2008), probably due to premenstrual cycling, and are more likely to have acne that continues into middle age (Goulden, Stables, & Cunliffe, 1999). Of young adults, 11% to 14% experience moderate to severe acne (Ghodsi et al., 2009; Smithard et al., 2001).

It is important to counsel the young woman that acne is a condition that is both associated with normal hormonal changes and also inheritable (Bhate & Williams, 2013). Acne severity risk increases with family history, specifically maternal history of acne, and with increasing pubertal maturity (Ghodsi et al., 2009). Suicidal ideation and completion is more common in those with moderate to severe acne compared with mild acne (Picardi, Lega, & Tarolla, 2013). It is important to take the young woman's concerns about her skin appearance seriously, and in the case of moderate to severe acne, comanage or refer to a specialist.

Acne vulgaris is a disease of hair follicles in the skin that have oil glands. Clinical features of acne are seborrhea (excess grease), noninflammatory lesions (open comedones [blackheads] and closed comedones [whiteheads]), inflammatory lesions (papules and pustules), and various degrees of scarring (Degitz, Placzek, Borelli, & Plewig, 2007). Therefore, pharmacological treatment includes topical and systemic measures to decrease bacterial load to break down comedones and to minimize scarring (Well, 2013). In a young woman with severely cystic acne that has not responded to other treatments, Isotretinoin (Accutane) can be used, but because it is teratogenic, she must use two forms of contraception and cannot fill new prescriptions without documented monthly pregnancy tests (Strauss et al., 2007). Young women with premenstrual flares of acne or with the diagnosis of polycystic ovarian syndrome, associated with excess androgen, may benefit from combined oral contraceptives with low androgenic activity (Schindler, 2013). However, it is always important to ask adolescent and adult women presenting with acne about irregular menses, hirsutism, or unexplained weight gain. Consider evaluation for polycystic ovary syndrome or other endocrine disorders in young women with acne resistant to conventional treatment or with sudden onset of severe acne (Well, 2013).

Health education for the young woman with acne should include: (a) use of mild cleansers and noncomedogenic moisturizers in combination with topical acne medications to avoid skin irritation, (b) avoidance of abrasive exfoliants and picking that rupture comedones, and (c) minimal use of cosmetics or if used, only anticomedogenic preparations (Well, 2013). It is not clear whether dietary intake is associated with acne although there is some evidence that high glycemic index and high dairy diets may increase hyperinsulinemia with subsequent increase in androgen availability (Burris, Rietkerk, & Woolf, 2013; Mahmood & Bowe, 2014).

Body Art and Body Modification

In women, body art refers to tattoos and piercing other than the earlobes. Body modification is a term more often used for less mainstream practices, such as genital piercing, branding, cutting, digit amputation, beading, stretching, and braiding (Griffith, 2009; Myers, 1992). In the United States, most states have laws prohibiting minors (defined by the state; varies from 14 to 21 years of age) from getting tattoos or body piercings, and of these, many prohibit body art even with parental consent (National Conference of State Legislatures, 2012). However, body art in adolescents and young people is increasingly considered a mainstream activity (Mayers & Chiffriller, 2008). In addition to self-expression, body art commemorates special occasions and fosters a sense of community such as membership in gangs, fraternities, sororities, religious organizations, or military service (McGuinness, 2006).

Tattoos are created when pigment is lodged in the dermis deliberately or as a result of trauma. Of the five categories, professional, amateur, cosmetic, traumatic, and medical, young women will likely have professional tattoos, which are placed by the vibrating needle of a tattoo machine, or amateur tattoos made from substances such as charcoal, pen ink, soot, or whatever pigment the home tattooist has on hand. Cosmetic tattoos or "permanent makeup" have also become increasingly popular with young women in recent years (Kent & Graber, 2012).

Unlike piercings, which are reversible, young women should understand that tattoos are largely permanent. Nearly all college freshmen (87.3%) believed that it was possible to remove a tattoo (Quaranta et al., 2011); however, although the tattoo removal industry is well known, it is less known that removal is painful, expensive, requires multiple (6 to 10) treatments and that success in removal is variable. In some cases, the laser may even darken the pigment. Certain colors, such as yellow and orange, are resistant to laser, and red and green may respond variably (Kent & Graber, 2012).

The clinician should consider that the degree of body art on the young woman may be associated with risk-taking behaviors. Body art has become mainstream, and those with tattoos or piercings have been reported to be no different from others regarding high school and college graduation rates (Tate & Shelton, 2008). However, recent studies have reported that those with four or more tattoos, seven or more body piercings, or piercings located in their nipples or genitals, were more likely to binge drink, use illegal drugs, have first sexual encounter at age 15 or younger, have multiple sex partners, and have a history of being arrested for a crime (Koch, Roberts, Armstrong, & Owen, 2010; Owen, Armstrong, Koch, & Roberts, 2013). Intimate (genital or nipple) piercings have been associated with a history of forced sexual activity and physical abuse (Owen et al., 2013; Young, Armstrong, Roberts, Mello, & Angel, 2010). However, the young woman's decision to have intimate piercing has been described as "a marker, a celebration, and/or a symbol of moving from victim to survivor" (Young et al., 2010, p. 79) and therefore may signify her own strength to overcome the past trauma.

For many young women, body art is an expression of individualism and a means of improving physical attractiveness. A recent study of young people showed that most of the reasons for body art were associated with enhancement of physical attractiveness, specifically improvement in aesthetic aspect (28.4%), fashion (12.3%), and individualism (18.4%) with only a minority "unable to explain it" (23.8%) (Quaranta et al., 2011). Engaging the young woman in discussion about her body art can be a powerful point of connection between the young woman and the clinician. During the physical examination, stating simply, "Tell me about this," indicating the tattoo on her lower right abdomen "RIP Elijah Duane 07/01/2012 to 06/20/2013," may give you information not only about her own child or a sibling that died but perhaps even more about her family context. You may also learn about the circumstances in which the body art was done; "I was high on . . . or "I was depressed after . . ."

In some instances, the clinician may have an opportunity to provide accurate information on body art. Although a study reported that many college freshmen were aware that

HIV was a possible infection (60.3%), fewer knew that body art was associated with other infections such as hepatitis C (38.2%), hepatitis B (33.7%) and tetanus (34.3%). Further, 28.1% of the freshmen were not aware that there are also noninfectious complications (Quaranta et al., 2011). Young women may be aware that early complications of oral piercings include infection and difficulty with speaking and eating, but less aware of common chronic problems such as tooth fracture; gingival recession, periodontitis infection/abscess, nerve damage, and metal hypersensitivity reactions (Chismark, 2013). Besides regular teeth brushing and flossing, young women with oral piercings should be advised to use a mouthwash rinse after every meal and remove piercings before playing sports (American Dental Association, 2013).

Healthy Sexual Identity

Developmentally, adolescence and young adulthood is a period of experimentation with new roles and relationships and establishment of intimate attachments. It is also a time when sexual identity is differentiated, although Lesbian, Gay, Bisexual, Transgender, Queer (LGBTQ) youth often report knowing they were attracted to those of the same gender at 10 years or younger (Ryan, 2009). Sexual identity development consists of identity formation (awareness of one's developing sexual orientation, questioning if one might be of a sexual minority [lesbian, gay, bisexual], participating in a sexual relationship with someone of the same gender) and identity integration (accepting and incorporating one's sexual identity) (Rosario, Schrimshaw, & Hunter, 2008).

The negative consequences of being in a sexual minority group include higher risk than in the case of those who are heterosexual for psychosocial stress (including harassment, discrimination, victimization), school difficulties, risky sexual behavior, substance abuse, mental disorder, sadness/depression, deliberate self-harm, suicidal ideation, suicide, and even reduced safety belt use (Birkett, Espelage, & Koenig, 2009; Dube, 2000; King et al., 2008; Lewis, Kholodkov, & Derlega, 2012; Reisner, Van Wagenen, Gordon, & Calzo, 2014; Shields, Whitaker, Glassman, Franks, & Howard, 2012; Talley, Hughes, Aranda, Birkett, & Marshal, 2014). Gay and lesbian students in grades 9 to 12 report greater prevalence of health-risk behaviors (behaviors that contribute to violence, behaviors related to attempted suicide, tobacco use, alcohol use, other drug use, sexual behaviors, and weight management); in addition to these, among bisexual youth there was a higher prevalence of behaviors that contribute to unintentional injuries (Kann et al., 2011).

Negative outcomes can be reduced by parental (Needham & Austin, 2010) and family support (Ryan, Russell, Huebner, Diaz, & Sanchez, 2010). Factors in schools that can produce more positive outcomes are a more protective school climate (safe spaces for sexual minority youth and Gay-Straight Alliances), a positive climate with no tolerance for homophobic teasing/victimization (Birkett et al., 2009; Hatzenbuchler, Birkett, Van Wagenen, & Meyer, 2014), comprehensive antibullying policies, and supportive school personnel. Health-care providers should include discussion of sexuality when obtaining a health history. Physicians were found to discuss sexuality with adolescents during health maintenance visits an average of 36 seconds; one third did not mention sexuality issues at all (Alexander et al., 2014). Discussion can assist in normalizing the process and promoting healthy development, sexual health, and informed decisions. Convey an open, accepting, respectful approach using nonjudgmental language (e.g., use partner vs. referring to the opposite gender). It is important to be specific and follow-up on statements; young women may interpret the question "are you sexually active?" as moving vigorously during intercourse. The question "are your sex partners men, women, or both?" indicates openness to any answer. The CDC has a guide for discussing sexual health at http://www.cdc.gov/std/treatment/SexualHistory.pdf. By assessing for strengths in addition to risks, the health-care provider can both help the young woman recognize her worth and provide a base for intervention.

Promoting Healthy Relationships

The clinician has a unique role in the young woman's development of healthy relationships. While adolescent young women are redefining their relationships with parents, forging alliances with peer groups, and experiencing early romantic relationships, the young woman is more likely to be in a committed romantic relationship and less dependent on her parents. Care of the young woman must include assessment of where she is on the continuum of dependence–interdependence–independence with her parents and on the health of her peer and romantic relationships. In addition, the clinician must be astute to identify areas of potential risk or relationships that are toxic.

During the transition to greater independence, parents still matter to their adolescent children (Rew, Arheart, Thompson, & Johnson, 2013), so it is important to include parents in efforts to promote adolescents' healthy behaviors. While monitoring is important, parents must be reminded that they are powerful role models of health behaviors for their children.

During adolescence, young people learn how to form safe and healthy relationships with friends, parents, teachers, and romantic partners. Both young boys and girls often experiment with different identities and roles during this time, and relationships contribute to their development. Peers, in particular, play a big role in identity formation, but relationships with caring adults—parents, teachers, clinicians, and coaches—are also important to healthy development.

The parent–adolescent relationship often informs how a young person handles other relationships. The National Longitudinal Study of Adolescent Health (Resnick et al., 1997) surveyed over 90,000 adolescents to measure behaviors that promote good health. The major finding was that adolescents who feel a "connectedness" to their parents were the least likely to engage in risk-taking behaviors. This includes feeling close to, cared for, and protected. Adolescents whose parents had high expectations for their children's school performance also reported fewer indicators for emotional distress, such as depression or suicide attempts. In addition, a sense of connection to the school when their classmates are not prejudiced and when they feel their teachers care about them also protects young people from a variety of other risk behaviors (Resnick et al., 1997).

The development of health-promoting behaviors in puberty helps to lay an essential framework for a healthy lifestyle later in adulthood. Understanding the powerful prevention safety nets that parents, clinicians, and the community can provide has an effect on reducing risk-taking activities.

Parents

Parent/adolescent relationships vary greatly as the adolescent moves from a dependent to an independent status as maturity takes place. During the adolescent years, there is both harmony and conflict on many levels. However, the need for support, stability, and encouragement from the family remains constant. A study of early-to-middle adolescence (ages 12 to 16) and middle-to-late adolescence (ages 16 to 20) examined the links over time between an adolescent's perception of relationship quality with parents and with friends (De Goede, Branje, Delsing, & Meeus, 2009). Overall, the perceptions of parents were as positive at the age of 12 as they were at the age of 16. When adolescents perceived their parents as more supportive, they also perceived their friends as more supportive (De Goede et al., 2009). This is generalizable to suggest that perceptions of relationships with parents generalize to friendships, which is an important concept to share with parents. Thus, reminding parents of their powerful role in teaching interpersonal skills through their own role-modeling, by setting good examples, and helping adolescents nurture positive friendships can be built into the conversation during wellness and episodic examinations.

Clinicians

The clinician has a role in helping the young woman identify teachable moments so that health promotion can be transferred to the next generation. *Teachable moments* are those times when it is comfortable for both the parent and the teen. It can be because an everyday topic or a current event is discussed with a natural segue into asking the teen about what they feel about the situation, or if they know someone with the same circumstance. From there dialogue can occur with insight and guidance (Table 4.7). This will also give the teen something of a reference point for issues that may occur in her life. Choosing the appropriate teachable moment is an important factor.

Another practical guide that parents can access online is Connected Kids, a program of the AAP to address the important issue of violence prevention. The format is user-friendly and geared to the provider as well as the parents who want to know more about how to approach topics and communicate with young people of all ages. This website can be found at: http://www2.aap.org/connectedkids/ClinicalGuide.pdf.

Friendships

Friendships play a major role in the lives of adolescents. A circle of caring and supportive friends can have a positive influence on healthy development, while, conversely, the absence of caring and respectful friends can have negative effects. Therefore, parents, teachers, and other adult role models can help young people learn how to make and keep good friends. Peer pressure, both good and bad, often affects decisions young people make.

Adolescence is a period of rapid physical, emotional, and social development and can be separated into three different groups: Preadolescence, Mid-adolescence, and Late adolescence. The relationship patterns change as the young person matures. In Preadolescence, relationships are typically with groups of same sex peers with whom they most constantly associate. In Mid-adolescence, peer groups help to define an identity that is unique and independent. The social support of camaraderie is significant. Although parents still have an important role with support and advice, peer influence, in large part, fosters ideas and thoughts during this time. In Late adolescence, friendships are more stable, more tolerant, and typically include both genders. Attitudes, values, and behaviors are derived from these close associations. The impact is significant, and the influence may

TABLE 4.7	Conversation Starters and Conversation Tips for Parents of Adolescents

Setting the Stage

Think of a scene from a movie or TV show. Perhaps it's a song lyric or a news story. Or it could be something that has happened in the neighborhood. These, or anything else that seems timely, can be effective conversation starters.

Starting the Conversation	Continuing the Conversation
"What do you think about that?" And "that" might be regarding: • A peer or family member learns she is pregnant • A television show discusses teen relationships • A news report on something involving teens • A popular song on the radio that talks about relationships	If your son or daughter answers, "I dunno" or something like that, say, "Well, let me share what I think." Don't lecture. Just use it as a jumping-off point to talk about your views and feelings. You might also ask, "Do you know anybody that has happened to? It is important not to lecture or scold. This may shut off active dialogue, and cause uneasiness when the subject is discussed again. Also, it is wise for a parent to give an opinion over time, instead of unloading one large lecture session.

Conversation Tips	Responses to Adolescent
Keep your composure. Remain calm. Becoming angry or overreacting to a question or mistake can upset your teen, or, worse, silence any hope of future dialogue. Instead, listen and ask open-ended questions. Teens say that they are uncomfortable talking about sex with their parents because they worry it will make their parents angry, or that their parents will assume they are doing some things they might not actually be doing. In other words, teens say they are afraid their parents will "freak out." You may be freaking out on the inside, but on the outside, try to keep calm.	It means a lot to me that you told me about the problem you're having with your friends. Being a teen is tough sometimes. But you are doing great. Remember, I'm here to talk more about it if you want to.
Be present. Parents have a lot going on these days. When you have a chance to talk with your teen, though, try to put some of those worries and activities aside. Pay attention to the conversation, and don't do too many other things at the same time. You don't have to drop everything; you can cook or do laundry while you talk. Just be sure to listen and make certain your teen knows you are hearing every word.	It was great meeting your boyfriend last night! It felt great that you wanted me to get to know him. I'm always here to talk about the relationships in your life. Thanks for making dinner with me last night. It was great to get to hear about what's going on with your friends and to spend time with you one-on-one. Love you!

TABLE 4.7	Conversation Starters and Conversation Tips for Parents of Adolescents *(continued)*
Conversation Tips	**Responses to Adolescent**
Be sympathetic. Let your teen know you understand how challenging life as an adolescent can be. Your teen may not believe you can really relate. Help teens know that you understand that the social pressures and obligations of a teen can feel like a lot. Encourage them to stay focused on school and other priorities.	Good luck on your Math exam today. Proud of you for all the time you spent studying! Your performance yesterday at the concert/in the game was amazing. Let's go out tonight and celebrate! Keep being true to yourself! Thanks for being honest with me about trying cigarettes. I think it's important to have open communication but for you to remember that smoking is really harmful.
Stress safety. Regardless of your views on the timing of sex, safety is an important part of the message to give your teen. Stress the absolute necessity of using a condom every single time. And stress the importance of using birth control. Don't lecture or nag, but don't be too shy to emphasize this point.	Hope you'll think more about what we talked about yesterday, and that you'll wait until you're a bit older to have sex. There is no rush, and I want to make sure you are ready for it. Have fun at the dance! Remember, I'm always happy to give you a ride— call or text me if your ride home has been drinking.

Adapted from DHHS Office of Adolescent Health. Retrieved from http://www.hhs.gov/ash/oah/resources-and-publications/info/parents/conversation-tools/

be positive or negative. Engaging the young woman in a dialogue about her friends and associations is an important avenue to assess elements of peer pressure and to determine risks associated with these relationships.

Romantic Relationships

Clinicians who provide care for the young woman have a unique opportunity to promote positive romantic relationships. Much of the emphasis in US public health programs for adolescent and young adults is related to what sexual behaviors should be avoided, for example, abstinence-only programs (Santelli et al., 2006) or the negative outcomes (STIs, HIV, and pregnancy) associated with risky sexual behaviors (Michaud, 2006). The approach has been proscriptive rather than being prescriptive and in some sense stigmatizes discussions related to her emerging sexuality. An alternative approach, termed the ABC-and-D model, can be adopted by the clinician to promote positive adolescent sexual experiences and outcomes (Schalet, 2011).

The "A" refers to *autonomy* of the sexual self. The transition to young adulthood is marked with increasing autonomy, but this is rarely applied to sexuality. The encounter with the young woman should be a safe place for her to gain information on sexual desire and pleasure, and to recognize her power in determining sexual wishes and boundaries. If a pelvic examination is included in the visit, the young woman can be given information on the aspects of her own genitalia. Offering her a hand mirror is a good way to show her normal variations, for example, irritated hair follicle from shaving, nevi, etc. as well as conditions that need treatment such as genital warts, or irritations/erosions from yeast infections.

The "B" is *building* good romantic relationships. Healthy romantic relationships will more likely result when there are not extreme age differences (Senn & Carey, 2011) and if the couple discusses use of contraception (Widman, Welsh, McNulty, & Little, 2006). The clinician can ask what types of intimate behaviors she is engaged in, and whether she is comfortable with these. If acceptable to the young woman, her partner can be part of the contraceptive option discussion.

The "C" is *connectedness* with parents and caregivers. The young woman may come for the visit with her mother or a grandmother. If she is comfortable having a parent/grandmother with her when discussing the reason for the visit, for example, vaginal discharge, receiving HPV vaccine, this normalizes topics that otherwise may be considered too sensitive to discuss with parents. Adolescents engaging in more frequent communication with their parents on sexual topics feel closer to their parents, and are more able to communicate with their parents in general and about sex specifically (Martino, Elliott, Corona, Kanouse, & Schuster, 2008).

Finally, "D" is recognizing *diversities* and removing *disparities* in terms of access to resources. It is difficult not to judge a young woman who says that she is trying to become pregnant during her senior year of high school so that she has something to do when she graduates. This is a rich opportunity to discuss what pregnancy and mothering means in her cultural or familial context. It also paves the way for developing a RLP that recognizes her career goals within the context of optimal fertility and health. Removing *disparities* includes clustering services at an encounter rather than insisting that the young woman return on subsequent visits for contraception refills, vaccines, and laboratory results. Increasing access to resources also includes increasing clinician availability to the young woman. For instance, after an annual well-woman examination, suggesting that she return to the clinic for review of her laboratory results instead of getting these over the phone or by mail creates another point of contact with the clinician and increases her comfort in accessing health care.

Preventing Bullying

Bullying is a serious problem, but it can be prevented or stopped when those involved know how to address it. The definition of bullying is an imbalance of power, intent to hurt, and repetition of threatening or hurtful behavior (Olweus, 1993). This also includes cyberbullying, which is effected through the use of electronic means such as computers, iPhones, and other electronic devices. Many adolescents and younger adults have experienced bullying (Vessey, DiFazio, & Strout, 2013), whether they were bullied by someone else or saw someone being bullied. A high percentage of college students report bullying at school (43%) and work (33%) (Rospenda, Richman, Wolff, & Burke, 2013).

Bullying is associated with short- and long-term health issues (Vessey et al., 2013). Bullying may be a particular health risk as social connections and relationships are very important to the young person. With limited cognitive understanding of why bullying occurs, the young person is at high risk for serious distress, which can lead to decreased academic performance and social isolation. In adolescents, bullying is associated with increased alcohol and substance use, and in college students with increased alcohol consumption and binge drinking (Rospenda et al., 2013). Being involved in childhood bullying has been linked with suicide (Cooper, Clements, & Holt, 2012), which is ranked the second leading cause of death in 15 to 24 year-olds (CDC, 2010b).

It is important to understand that bullying behaviors differ by gender. Adolescent girls are more often involved in verbal and relational bulling, such as social exclusion or rumor spreading, while boys more often bullied by physical as well as verbal means. (Carbone-Lopez, Esbensen, & Brick, 2010). This may make it more elusive to identify that the young woman is being bullied in contrast to the young man with a black eye or obvious contusion. In the young woman, dating violence is a form of partner bullying and is associated with increased risk of smoking, depressive symptoms, eating disorders, and having multiple (5+) sexual partners (Bonomi, Anderson, Nemeth, Rivara, & Buettner, 2013). If these behaviors are assessed in the young woman, the clinician should probe more deeply into the characteristics of her relationships. She may not want to disclose negative aspects the first time she is asked whether she "feels safe" in her relationship, but eventually she will know that she can trust her clinician to listen to what she becomes comfortable with disclosing. It is important to screen for bullying and victimization, including dating and intimate partner violence, at every health-care visit. Questions that can be used in the clinical setting to assess for bullying include:

Have you been bullied in the past 12 months?
When did the bullying last happen?
What kind of bullying was it? Physical, verbal, indirect (group exclusion), cyber?
Have you talked to anyone about the bullying?
How did the bullying make you feel?

Positive responses to any of these questions should prompt further questioning. In adolescents, parental support can be protective against all forms of bullying (Wang, Iannotti, & Nansel, 2009), so it is essential that the clinician partner with the parents as appropriate so that they can support their teen and work with school officials to address the problems. Although antibullying initiatives are becoming commonplace, the issue remains pervasive. Relationships in which the young woman can share feelings and be supported must be supported. Referral to mental health services for those affected can help reduce emotional distress.

Summary

Caring for women in pubescence through young womanhood affords a rich opportunity for clinicians to partner with and provide guidance for the young woman and sometimes for her parents. During this span of transition from childhood through young womanhood, the clinician is privy to both observe and intervene when necessary in her process of achieving biological, psychological, and cognitive maturity. Caring for the young woman of childbearing age needs to be nonjudgmental and respectful. This relationship can be fun and rewarding, using guidance and empowerment to help young women take responsibility for their own health. Clinicians must be able to identify variations of normal physical and emotional health, assess for destructive behaviors or pathologic conditions, and possess skills in accessing resources to prevent harm and facilitate health. As a summary, Table 4.8 presents an overview of the USPSTF screening recommendations for adolescents and young women. There is some information included for middle-age and older women as well. Chapters 5 and 6 discuss in detail health and wellness for middle-age and older women.

TABLE 4.8	USPSTF Grade A B Recommendations for Adolescents and Women	
Topic	**Description**	**Grade**
Alcohol misuse counseling	The USPSTF recommends screening and behavioral counseling interventions to reduce alcohol misuse by adults, including pregnant women, in primary care settings.	B
Anemia screening: pregnant women	The USPSTF recommends routine screening for iron deficiency anemia in asymptomatic pregnant women.	B
Aspirin to prevent CVD: women	The USPSTF recommends the use of aspirin for women age 55–79 years when the potential benefit of a reduction in ischemic strokes outweighs the potential harm of an increase in gastrointestinal hemorrhage.	A
Bacteriuria screening: pregnant women	The USPSTF recommends screening for asymptomatic bacteriuria with urine culture for pregnant women at 12–16 weeks' gestation or at the first prenatal visit, if later.	A
Blood pressure screening	The USPSTF recommends screening for high blood pressure in adults aged 18 and older.	A
BRCA screening, counseling about	The USPSTF recommends that women whose family history is associated with an increased risk of deleterious mutations in BRCA1 or BRCA2 genes be referred for genetic counseling and evaluation for BRCA testing.	B
Risk assessment, genetic counseling, and genetic testing for BRCA-related cancer in women	NEW! The USPSTF recommends that primary care providers screen women who have family members with breast, ovarian, tubal, or peritoneal cancer with one of several screening tools designed to identify a family history that may be associated with an increased risk of potentially harmful mutations in breast cancer susceptibility genes (BRCA1 or BRCA2). Women with positive screening results should receive genetic counseling and, if indicated after counseling, BRCA testing.	B
Breast cancer preventive medication	The USPSTF recommends that clinicians discuss chemoprevention with women at high risk for breast cancer and at low risk for adverse effects of chemoprevention. Clinicians should inform patients of the potential benefits and harms of chemoprevention.	B
Breast cancer screening	The USPSTF recommends screening mammography for women, with or without clinical breast examination, every 1–2 years for women aged 40 and older.	B
Breastfeeding counseling	The USPSTF recommends interventions during pregnancy and after birth to promote and support breastfeeding.	B
Cervical cancer screening	The USPSTF recommends screening for cervical cancer in women ages 21–65 years with cytology (Pap smear) every 3 years or, for women ages 30–65 years who want to lengthen the screening interval, screening with a combination of cytology and human papillomavirus (HPV) testing every 5 years. See the Clinical Considerations for discussion of cytology method, HPV testing, and screening interval.	A

TABLE 4.8	USPSTF Grade A B Recommendations for Adolescents and Women *(continued)*	
Topic	**Description**	**Grade**
Chlamydial infection screening: nonpregnant women	The USPSTF recommends screening for chlamydial infection for all sexually active nonpregnant young women aged 24 and younger and for older nonpregnant women who are at increased risk.	A
Chlamydial infection screening: pregnant women	The USPSTF recommends screening for chlamydial infection for all pregnant women aged 24 and younger, and for older pregnant women who are at increased risk.	B
Cholesterol abnormalities screening: women 45 and older	The USPSTF strongly recommends screening women aged 45 and older for lipid disorders if they are at increased risk for coronary heart disease.	A
Cholesterol abnormalities screening: women younger than 45	The USPSTF recommends screening women aged 20–45 for lipid disorders if they are at increased risk for coronary heart disease.	B
Colorectal cancer screening	The USPSTF recommends screening for colorectal cancer using fecal occult blood testing, sigmoidoscopy, or colonoscopy, in adults, beginning at age 50 years and continuing until age 75 years. The risks and benefits of these screening methods vary.	A
Depression screening: adolescents	The USPSTF recommends screening of adolescents (12–18 years of age) for major depressive disorder when systems are in place to ensure accurate diagnosis, psychotherapy (cognitive–behavioral or interpersonal), and follow-up.	B
Depression screening: adults	The USPSTF recommends screening adults for depression when staff-assisted depression care supports are in place to assure accurate diagnosis, effective treatment, and follow-up.	B
Diabetes screening	The USPSTF recommends screening for type 2 diabetes in asymptomatic adults with sustained blood pressure (either treated or untreated) greater than 135/80 mm Hg.	B
Folic acid supplementation	The USPSTF recommends that all women planning or capable of pregnancy take a daily supplement containing 0.4–0.8 mg (400–800 µg) of folic acid.	A
Gonorrhea screening: women	The USPSTF recommends that clinicians screen all sexually active women, including those who are pregnant, for gonorrhea infection if they are at increased risk for infection (that is, if they are young or have other individual or population risk factors).	B
Healthy diet counseling	The USPSTF recommends intensive behavioral dietary counseling for adult patients with hyperlipidemia and other known risk factors for cardiovascular and diet-related chronic disease. Intensive counseling can be delivered by primary care clinicians or by referral to other specialists, such as nutritionists or dietitians.	B

(continued)

TABLE 4.8	USPSTF Grade A B Recommendations for Adolescents and Women *(continued)*	

Topic	Description	Grade
Hepatitis B screening: pregnant women	The USPSTF strongly recommends screening for hepatitis B virus infection in pregnant women at their first prenatal visit.	A
HIV screening	The USPSTF strongly recommends that clinicians screen for HIV all adolescents and adults at increased risk for HIV infection.	A
Obesity screening and counseling: adults	The USPSTF recommends that clinicians screen all adult patients for obesity and offer intensive counseling and behavioral interventions to promote sustained weight loss for obese adults.	B
Obesity screening and counseling: children	The USPSTF recommends that clinicians screen children aged 6 years and older for obesity and offer them or refer them to comprehensive, intensive behavioral interventions to promote improvement in weight status.	B
Osteoporosis screening: women	The USPSTF recommends that women aged 65 and older be screened routinely for osteoporosis. The USPSTF recommends that routine screening begin at age 60 for women at increased risk for osteoporotic fractures.	B
Rh incompatibility screening: first pregnancy visit	The USPSTF strongly recommends Rh (D) blood typing and antibody testing for all pregnant women during their first visit for pregnancy-related care.	A
Rh incompatibility screening: 24–28 weeks' gestation	The USPSTF recommends repeated Rh (D) antibody testing for all unsensitized Rh (D)-negative women at 24–28 weeks' gestation, unless the biological father is known to be Rh (D)-negative.	B
STIs counseling	The USPSTF recommends high-intensity behavioral counseling to prevent sexually transmitted infections (STIs) for all sexually active adolescents and for adults at increased risk for STIs.	B
Tobacco use counseling: nonpregnant adults	The USPSTF recommends that clinicians ask all adults about tobacco use and provide tobacco cessation interventions for those who use tobacco products.	A
Tobacco use counseling: pregnant women	The USPSTF recommends that clinicians ask all pregnant women about tobacco use and provide augmented, pregnancy-tailored counseling to those who smoke.	A
Syphilis screening: nonpregnant persons	The USPSTF strongly recommends that clinicians screen persons at increased risk for syphilis infection.	A
Syphilis screening: pregnant women	The USPSTF recommends that clinicians screen all pregnant women for syphilis infection.	A

Adapted from United States Preventive Services Task Force. (2012). The guide to clinical preventive services, 2012; Recommendations of the US Preventive Services Task Force (AHRQ Pub. No. 12-05154).

References

Alexander, S. C., Fortenberry, J. D., Pollack, K. I., Bravender, T., Davis, J. K., Østbye, T., . . . Shields, C. G. (2014). Sexuality talk during adolescent health maintenance visits. *JAMA Pediatrics*, *168*(2):163–169. doi:10.1001/jamapediatrics.2013.4338

Aliotta, H. M., & Schaeffer, N. J. (2013). Breast conditions. In K. Schuiling & F. Kikis (Eds.), *Women's gyncecologic health* (pp. 485–533). Burlington, MA: Jones & Bartlett Learning.

American Academy of Pediatrics, & American College of Obstetrics and Gynecology. (2006). Menstruation in girls and adolescents: Using the menstrual cycle as a vital sign. *Pediatrics*, *118*(5), 2245–2250. doi:10.1542/peds.2006-2481

American Cancer Society. (2011). *Breast cancer: Early detection*. Retrieved from http://www.cancer.org/acs/groups/cid/documents/webcontent/003165.pdf

American College of Obstetrics and Gynecology. (2003). ACOG practice bulletin no. 44: Neural tube defects. *International Journal of Gynecology & Obstetrics*, *83*(1), 123–133. doi:10.1016/S0020-7292(03)00390-4

American College of Obstetrics and Gynecology. (2006). Committee opinion no. 349: Menstruation in girls and adolescents: Using the menstrual cycle as a vital sign. *Obstetrics & Gynecology*, *108*(5), 1323–1328.

American College of Obstetrics and Gynecology. (2011). Practice bulletin no. 122: Breast cancer screening. *Obstetrics & Gynecology*, *118*(2, Pt. 1), 372–382.

American College of Obstetrics and Gynecology. (2012a). Practice bulletin no. 131: Screening for cervical cancer. *Obstetrics & Gynecology*, *120*(5), 1222–1238.

American College of Obstetrics and Gynecology. (2012b). Committee opinion no. 534: Well-woman visit. *Obstetrics & Gynecology*, *120*, 421–424.

American College of Sports Medicine. (2007). The female athlete triad. *Medicine & Science in Sports & Exercise*, *39*(10), 1867–1882.

American Dental Association. (2013). *Mouth healthy: Oral piercings*. Retrieved from http://www.mouthhealthy.org/en/az-topics/o/oral-piercings

Argy, O., Hughes, K., & Roche, C. (2002). Managing the patient with a breast mass. In I. Atoi (Ed.), *Manual of breast diseases*. Philadelphia, PA: Lippincott Williams & Wilkins.

Baeten, J. M., Bukusi, E. A., & Lambe, M. (2001). Pregnancy complications and outcomes among overweight and obese nulliparous women. *American Journal of Public Health*, *91*(3), 436–440.

Bhate, K., & Williams, H. C. (2013). Epidemiology of acne vulgaris. *British Journal of Dermatology*, *168*(3), 474–485. doi:10.1111/bjd.12149

Birkett, M., Espelage, D. L., & Koenig, B. (2009). LGB and questioning students in schools: The moderating effects of homophobic bullying and school climate on negative outcomes. *Journal of Youth and Adolescence*, *38*(7), 989–1000. doi:10.1007/s10964-008-9389-1

Bonomi, A. E., Anderson, M. L., Nemeth, J., Rivara, F. P., & Buettner, C. (2013). History of dating violence and the association with late adolescent health. *BMC Public Health*, *13*, 821. doi:10.1186/1471-2458-13-821

Boyd, E. M., Reynolds, J. R., Tillman, K. H., & Martin, P. Y. (2011). Adolescent girls' race/ethnic status, identities, and drive for thinness. *Social Science Research*, *40*(2), 667–684. doi:10.1016/j.ssresearch.2010.11.003

Bradley, H., Markowitz, L. E., Gibson, T., & McQuillan, G. M. (2014). Seroprevalence of herpes simplex virus Types 1 and 2—United States, 1999–2010. *Journal of Infectious Diseases*, *209*(3), 325–333. doi:10.1093/infdis/jit458

Burris, J., Rietkerk, W., & Woolf, K. (2013). Acne: The role of medical nutrition therapy. *Journal of the Academy of Nutrition and Dietetics*, *113*(3), 416–430. doi:10.1016/j.jand.2012.11.016

Canfield, M. A., Collins, J. S., Botto, L. D., Williams, L. J., Mai, C. T., Kirby, R. S., . . . Mulinare, J. (2005). Changes in the birth prevalence of selected birth defects after grain fortification with folic acid in the United States: Findings from a multi-state population-based study. *Birth Defects Research Part A: Clinical and Molecular Teratology*, *73*(10), 679–689. doi:10.1002/bdra.20210

Carbone-Lopez, K., Esbensen, F.-A., & Brick, B. T. (2010). Correlates and consequences of peer victimization: Gender differences in direct and indirect forms of bullying. *Youth Violence Juvenile Justice*, *8*(4), 332–350. doi:10.1177/1541204010362954

Catalano, P. M., & Ehrenberg, H. M. (2006). The short- and long-term implications of maternal obesity on the mother and her offspring. *BJOG*, *113*, 1126–1133.

Centers for Disease Control and Prevention. (2010a). Sexually transmitted diseases treatment guidelines—2010. *Morbidity and Mortality Weekly Report. Recommendations and Reports, 59*(RR-12), 1–110.

Centers for Disease Control and Prevention. (2010b). *Leading causes of death in females.* Retrieved from http://www.cdc.gov/women/lcod

Centers for Disease Control and Prevention. (2010c). Seroprevalence of herpes simplex virus Type 2 among persons aged 14–49 years—United States, 2005–2008. *Morbidity and Mortality Weekly Report, 59*(15), 456–459.

Centers for Disease Control and Prevention. (2011a). National and state vaccination coverage among adolescents aged 13 through 17 years—United States, 2010. *Morbidity and Mortality Weekly Report, 60*(33), 1117–1123.

Centers for Disease Control and Prevention. (2011b). *Sexually transmitted disease surveillance 2010.* Atlanta, GA: US Department of Health and Human Services.

Centers for Disease Control and Prevention. (2012). Youth risk behavior surveillance—United States, 2011. *Morbidity and Mortality Weekly Report, 61*(4), 1–168.

Centers for Disease Control and Prevention. (2013a). Vital signs: Binge drinking among women and high school girls—United States, 2011. *Morbidity and Mortality Weekly Report, 62*(1), 9–13.

Centers for Disease Control and Prevention. (2013b). *Genital herpes—CDC fact sheet.* Retrieved from http://www.cdc.gov/std/herpes/stdfact-herpes.htm

Chang, G., Orav, E. J., Jones, J. A., Buynitsky, T., Gonzalez, S., & Wilkins-Haug, L. (2011). Self-reported alcohol and drug use in pregnant young women: A pilot study of prevalence and associated factors. *Journal of Addiction Medicine, 5*(3), 221–226. doi:10.1097/ADM.0b013e318214360b

Chelimo, C., Wouldes, T. A., Cameron, L. D., & Elwood, J. M. (2013). Risk factors for and prevention of human papillomaviruses (HPV), genital warts and cervical cancer. *Journal of Infection, 66*(3), 207–217. doi:10.1016/j.jinf.2012.10.024

Chismark, A. (2013). Oral piercing and body art—Century realities and safety issues. *Journal of the California Dental Hygienists' Association, 28*(1), 16–34.

Collier, C. N., Harper, J. C., Cantrell, W. C., Wang, W., Foster, K. W., & Elewski, B. E. (2008). The prevalence of acne in adults 20 years and older. *Journal of the American Academy of Dermatology, 58*(1), 56–59. doi:10.1016/j.jaad.2007.06.045

Cook, R. L., Hutchison, S. L., østergaard, L., Braithwaite, R. S., & Ness, R. B. (2005). Systematic review: Noninvasive testing for chlamydia trachomatis and neisseria gonorrhoeae. *Annals of Internal Medicine, 142*(11), 914–925.

Cooper, G. D., Clements, P. T., & Holt, K. E. (2012). Examining childhood bullying and adolescent suicide: Implications for school nurses. *Journal of School Nursing, 28*(4), 275–283. doi:10.1177/1059840512438617

Cotton, M. A., Ball, C., & Robinson, P. (2003). Four simple questions can help screen for eating disorders. *Journal of General Internal Medicine, 18*(1), 53–56.

Crone, E. A., & Dahl, R. E. (2012). Understanding adolescence as a period of social-affective engagement and goal flexibility. *Nature Reviews Neuroscience, 13*(9), 636–650. doi:10.1038/nrn3313

Czeizel, A. E. (2009). Periconceptional folic acid and multivitamin supplementation for the prevention of neural tube defects and other congenital abnormalities. *Birth Defects Research Part A: Clinical and Molecular Teratology, 85*(4), 260–268. doi:10.1002/bdra.20563

Czeizel, A. E., & Dudás, I. (1992). Prevention of the first occurrence of neural-tube defects by periconceptional vitamin supplementation. *New England Journal of Medicine, 327*(26), 1832–1835. doi:10.1056/NEJM199212243272602

D'Angelo, D., Williams, L., Morrow, B., Cox, S., Harris, N., Harrison, L., . . . Zapata, L. (2007). Preconception and interconception health status of women who recently gave birth to a live-born infant—Pregnancy Risk Assessment Monitoring System (PRAMS), United States, 26 reporting areas, 2004. *Morbidity and Mortality Weekly Report, 56*(SS10), 1–35.

Degitz, K., Placzek, M., Borelli, C., & Plewig, G. (2007). Pathophysiology of acne. *JDDG: Journal der Deutschen Dermatologischen Gesellschaft, 5*(4), 316–323. doi:10.1111/j.1610-0387.2007.06274.x

De Goede, I. H., Branje, S. J., Delsing, M. J., & Meeus, W. H. (2009). Linages over time between adolescents' relationships with parents and friends. *Journal of Youth and Adolescence, 38*(10), 1304–1315. doi:10.1007/s10964-009-9403-2

Dhalla, S., Zumbo, B. D., & Poole, G. (2011). A review of the psychometric properties of the CRAFFT instrucment: 1999–2010. *Current Drug Abuse Reviews, 4*(1), 57–64.

Dube, E. M. (2000). The role of sexual behavior in the identification process of gay and bisexual males—Statistical data included. *Journal of Sex Research. 37*(2), 123–132.

Files, J. A., Frey, K. A., David, P. S., Hunt, K. S., Noble, B. S., & Mayer, A. P. (2011). Developing a reproductive life plan. *Journal of Midwifery & Women's Health, 56*(5), 468–474. doi:10.1111/j.1542-2011.2011.00048.x

Finer, L. B., & Henshaw, S. K. (2006). Disparities in rates of unintended pregnancy in the United States, 1994 and 2001. *Perspectives on Sexual & Reproductive Health, 38*(2), 90–96.

Finer, L. B., & Zolna, M. R. (2011). Unintended pregnancy in the United States: Incidence and disparities, 2006. *Contraception, 84*(5), 478–485. doi:10.1016/j.contraception.2011.07.013

Flegal, K. M., Carroll, M. D., Kit, B. K., & Ogden, C. L. (2012). Prevalence of obesity and trends in the distribution of body mass index among us adults, 1999–2010. *Journal of the American Medical Association, 307*(5), 491–497. doi:10.1001/jama.2012.39

Fogel, C. I. (2013). Sexually transmitted infections. In K. Schuiling & F. Kikis (Eds.), *Women's gynecologic health* (pp. 485–533). Burlington, MA: Jones & Bartlett Learning.

Freeman, E. E., Weiss, H. A., Glynn, J. R., Cross, P. L., Whitworth, J. A., & Hayes, R. J. (2006). Herpes simplex virus 2 infection increases HIV acquisition in men and women: Systematic review and meta-analysis of longitudinal studies. *AIDS, 20*(1), 73–83.

Gantt, S., & Muller, W. J. (2013). The immunologic basis for severe neonatal herpes disease and potential strategies for therapeutic intervention. *Clinical and Developmental Immunology, 2013,* 16. doi:10.1155/2013/369172.

Gebarra, C. F., Bhona, F. M., Ronzani, T. M., Lourenço, L. M., & Noto, A. R. (2013). Brief intervention and decrease of alcohol consumption among women: A systematic review. *Substance Abuse Treatment, Prevention, and Policy, 8*(31). doi:10.1186/1747-597X-8-31

Ghodsi, S. Z., Orawa, H., & Zouboulis, C. C. (2009). Prevalence, severity, and severity risk factors of acne in high school pupils: A community-based study. *Journal of Investigative Dermatology, 129*(9), 2136–2141. doi:10.1038/jid.2009.47

Goulden, V., Stables, G. I., & Cunliffe, W. J. (1999). Prevalence of facial acne in adults. *Journal of the American Academy of Dermatology, 41*(4), 577–580. doi:10.1016/S0190-9622(99)80056-5

Griffith, R. (2009). Legal regulation of body art in children and young people. *British Journal of School Nursing, 4*(6), 293–297.

Hatcher, R. A., Trussell, J., Nelson, A., Cates, W., Kowal, D., & Policar, M. S. (2011). *Contraceptive technology* (20th ed.). New York, NY: Ardent Media.

Hatzenbuchler, M. L., Birkett, M., Van Wagenen, A., & Meyer, I. H. (2014). Protective school climates and reduced risk for suicide ideation in sexual minority youths. *American Journal of Public Health, 104*(2):279–286.

Ho, G. Y. F., Bierman, R., Beardsley, L., Chang, C. J., & Burk, R. D. (1998). Natural history of cervicovaginal papillomavirus infection in young women. *New England Journal of Medicine, 338*(7), 423–428. doi:10.1056/NEJM199802123380703

Holland Wade, G., Herrman, J., & McBeth-Snyder, L. (2012). A preconception care program for women in a college setting. *MCN: The American Journal of Maternal Child Nursing, 37*(3), 164–172. doi:10.1097/NMC.0b013e31824b59c7

Howlader, N., Noone, A., Krapcho, M., Garshell, J., Neyman, N., Altekruse, S., . . . Cronin, K. A. (2013). *SEER cancer statistics review, 1975–2010.* Bethesda, MD: National Cancer Institute. Retrieved from http://seer.cancer.gov/csr/1975_2010

Humeniuk, R. E., Henry-Edwards, S., Ali, R. L., Poznyak, V., & Monteiro, M. (2010a). The alcohol, smoking and substance involvement screening test (ASSIST): Manual for use in primary care. Geneva: World Health Organization.

Humeniuk, R.E., Henry-Edwards, S., Ali, R.L., Poznyak, V., & Monteiro, M. (2010b). The ASSIST-linked brief intervention for hazardous and harmful substance use: Manual for use in primary care. Geneva: World Health Organization.

Javed, A., Tebben, P. J., Fischer, P. R., & Lteif, A. N. (2013). Female athlete triad and its components: Toward improved screening and management. *Mayo Clinic Proceedings, 88*(9), 996–1009. doi:10.1016/j.mayocp.2013.07.001

Johnson, K., Posner, S. F., Biermann, J., Cordero, J. F., Atrash, H. K., Parker, C. S., . . . Curtis, M. G. (2006). Recommendations to improve preconception health and health care—United States: A report of the CDC/ATSDR Preconception Care Work Group and the Select Panel on Preconception Care. *Morbidity and Mortality Weekly Report. Recommendations and Reports, 55*(RR-6), 1–23.

Kann, L., Olsen, E. O., McManus, T., Kinchen, S., Chyen, D., Harris, W. A., & Wechsler, H.; Centers for Disease Control and Prevention. (2011). Sexual identity, sex of sexual contacts, and health-risk behaviors among students in grades 9–12—youth risk behavior surveillance, selected sites, United States, 2001–2009. *Morbidity and Mortality Weekly Report. Surveillance Summaries, 60*(7), 1–133.

Kavanaugh, M. L., Frohwirth, L., Jerman, J., Popkin, R., & Ethier, K. (2013). Long-acting reversible contraception for adolescents and young adults: Patient and provider perspectives. *Journal of Pediatric and Adolescent Gynecology, 26*(2), 86–95.

Kent, K. M., & Graber, E. M. (2012). Laser tattoo removal: A review. *Dermatologic Surgery, 38*(1), 1–13. doi:10.1111/j.1524-4725.2011.02187.x

King, M., Semlyen, J., Tai, S. S., Killaspy, H., Osborn, D., Popelyuk, D., & Nazareth, I. (2008). A systematic review of mental disorder, suicide, and deliberate self harm in lesbian, gay and bisexual people. *BMC Psychiatry, 8*, 70. doi:10.1186/1471-244X-8-70

Koch, J. R., Roberts, A. E., Armstrong, M. L., & Owen, D. C. (2010). Body art, deviance, and American college students. *Social Science Journal, 47*(1), 151–161. doi:http://dx.doi.org/10.1016/j.soscij.2009.10.001

Konrad, K., Firk, C., & Uhlhaas, P. J. (2013). Brain development during adolescence. *Deutsches Aerzteblatt International, 110*(25), 425–431. doi:10.3238/arztebl.2013.0425

Kosa, J., Guendelman, S., Pearl, M., Graham, S., Abrams, B., & Kharrazi, M. (2011). The association between pre-pregnancy BMI and preterm delivery in a diverse southern California population of working women. *Maternal and Child Health Journal, 15*(6), 772–781. doi:10.1007/s10995-010-0633-4

Kub, J., & Solari-Twadell, P. A. (2013). Religiosity/spirituality and substance use in adolescence as related to positive development: A literature review. *Journal of Addictions Nursing, 24*(4), 247–262. doi:10.1097/JAN.0000000000000006

Kuh, D., Ben-Shlomo, Y., Lynch, J., Hallqvist, J., & Power, C. (2003). Life course epidemiology. *Journal of Epidemiology and Community Health, 57*(10), 778–783. doi:10.1136/jech.57.10.778

Lashley, F. R. (2005). *Clinical genetics in nursing practice* (3rd ed.). New York, NY: Springer.

Law, M. P. M., Chuh, A. A. T., Lee, A., & Molinari, N. (2010). Acne prevalence and beyond: Acne disability and its predictive factors among Chinese late adolescents in Hong Kong. *Clinical and Experimental Dermatology, 35*(1), 16–21. doi:10.1111/j.1365-2230.2009.03340.x

Lewis, R. J., Kholodkov, T., & Derlega, V. J. (2012). Still stressful after all these years: A review of lesbians' and bisexual women's minority stress. *Journal of Lesbian studies, 16*(1), 30–44. doi:10.1080/1089 4160.2011.557641.

Luciana, M., Collins, P. F., Muetzel, R. L., & Lim, K.O. (2013). Effects of alcohol use initiation on brain structure in typically developing adolescents. *American Journal of Drug and Alcohol Abuse, 39*(6), 345–355. doi:10.3109/00952990.2013.837057

Lynch, J., & Smith, G. D. (2005). A life course approach to chronic disease epidemiology. *Annual Review of Public Health, 26*(1), 1–35. doi:10.1146/annurev.publhealth.26.021304.144505

Mahmood, S.N. & Bowe, W.P. (2014). Diet and acne update: Carbohydrates emerge as the main culprit. *Journal of Drugs in Dermatology, 13*(4), 428–435.

Martinez, G., Copen, C. E., & Abma, J. C. (2011). Teenagers in the United States: Sexual activity, contraceptive use, and childbearing, 2006–2010 National Survey of Family Growth. *Vital Health Statistics, 23*(31), 1–44.

Martino, S. C., Elliott, M. N., Corona, R., Kanouse, D. E., & Schuster, M. A. (2008). Beyond the "Big Talk": The roles of breadth and repetition in parent-adolescent communication about sexual topics. *Pediatrics, 121*(3), e612–e618. doi:10.1542/peds.2007-2156

Mayers, L. B., & Chiffriller, S. H. (2008). Body art (Body piercing and tattooing) among undergraduate university students: "Then and now." *Journal of Adolescent Health, 42*(2), 201–203. doi:10.1016/j.jadohealth.2007.09.014

McGuinness, T. M. (2006). Youth in mind. Teens & body art. *Journal of Psychosocial Nursing & Mental Health Services, 44*(4), 13–16.

Metcalf, M. G., Skidmore, D. S., Lowry, G. F., & Mackenzie, J. A. (1983). Incidence of ovulation in the years after the menarche. *Journal of Endocrinology, 97*(2), 213–219. doi:10.1677/joe.0.0970213

Michaud, P.-A. (2006). Adolescents and risks: Why not change our paradigm? *Journal of Adolescent Health, 38*(5), 481–483. doi:10.1016/j.jadohealth.2006.03.003

Misra, M. (2008). Long-term skeletal effects of eating disorders with onset in adolescence. *Annals of the New York Academy of Sciences, 1135*(1), 212–218. doi:10.1196/annals.1429.002

Moos, M.-K. (2003). Unintended pregnancies: A call for nursing action. *MCN, American Journal of Maternal Child Nursing, 28*(1), 24–30.

Moos, M.-K., Dunlop, A. L., Jack, B. W., Nelson, L., Coonrod, D. V., Long, R., . . . Gardiner, P. M. (2008). Healthier women, healthier reproductive outcomes: Recommendations for the routine care of all women of reproductive age. *American Journal of Obstetrics and Gynecology, 199*(6, Suppl. B), S280–S289. doi:10.1016/j.ajog.2008.08.060

Morgan, J. F., Reid, F., & Lacey, J. H. (1999). The SCOFF questionnaire: Assessment of a new screening tool for eating disorders. *BMJ, 319*(7223), 1467–1468.

Moyer, V. A. (2012). Screening for cervical cancer: US Preventive Services Task Force Recommendation Statement. *Annals of Internal Medicine, 156*(12), 880–891.

Moyer, V. A. (2014). Risk assessment, genetic counseling, and genetic testing for BRCA-related cancer in women: US Preventive Services Task Force Recommendation Statement. *Annals of Internal Medicine, 160*(4). doi:10.7326/m13-2747

MRC Vitamin Study Research Group. (1991). Prevention of neural tube defects: Results of the Medical Research Council Vitamin Study. *Lancet, 338*(8760), 131–137.

Myers, J. (1992). Nonmainstream body modification: Genital piercing, branding, burning, and cutting. *Journal of Contemporary Ethnography, 21*(3), 267–306. doi:10.1177/089124192021003001

National Comprehensive Cancer Network (2013). Breast cancer screening and diagnosis. In NCCN Clinical Practice Guidelines in Oncology. Available from: http://www.nccn.org/professionals/physician_gls/f_guidelines.asp

National Conference of State Legislatures. (2012). *Tattoos and body piercings for minors.* Retrieved from http://www.ncsl.org/research/health/tattooing-and-body-piercing.aspx

Needham, B. L., & Austin, E. L. (2010). Sexual orientation, parental support, and health during the transition to young adulthood. *Journal of Youth and Adolescence, 39*(10), 1189–1198. doi:10.1007/s10964-010-9533-6

Neumark-Sztainer, D. (2009). Preventing obesity and eating disorders in adolescent: What can health care providers do? *Journal of Adolescent Health, 44*(3), 206–213. doi:10.1016/j.jadohealth.2008.11.005

Ogden, C. L., Carroll, M. D., Kit, B. K., & Flegal, K. M. (2012). Prevalence of obesity and trends in body mass index among US children and adolescents, 1999–2010. *Journal of the American Medical Association, 307*(5), 483–490. doi:10.1001/jama.2012.40

Olweus, D. (1993). Victimization by peers: Antecedents and long-term outcomes. In K. Rubin & J. Asendorpf (Eds.), *Social withdrawal, inhibition, and shyness in childhood* (pp. 315–341). Hillsdale, NJ: Lawrence Erlbaum Associates.

Owen, D. C., Armstrong, M. L., Koch, J. R., & Roberts, A. E. (2013). College students with body art. *Journal of Psychosocial Nursing & Mental Health Services, 51*(10), 20–28. doi:10.3928/02793695-20130731-03

Paxton, R. J., Valois, R. F., & Drane, J. W. (2004). Correlates of body mass index, weight goals, and weight-management practices among adolescents. *Journal of School Health, 74*(4), 136–143.

Piasecki, T. M., Jahng, S., Wood, P. K., Robertson, B. M., Epier, A. J., Rohrbaugh, J. W., . . . Sher, K. J. (2012). The subjective effects of alcohol-tobacco co-use: An ecological momentary assessment investigation. *Journal of Abnormal Psychology, 120*(3), 557–571. doi:10.1037/a0023033

Picardi, A., Lega, I., & Tarolla, E. (2013). Suicide risk in skin disorders. *Clinics in Dermatology, 31*(1), 47–56. doi:10.1016/j.clindermatol.2011.11.006

Quaranta, A., Napoli, C., Fasano, F., Montagna, C., Caggiano, G., & Montagna, M. T. (2011). Body piercing and tattoos: A survey on young adults' knowledge of the risks and practices in body art. *BMC Public Health, 11*(1), 774–781. doi:10.1186/1471-2458-11-774

Reisner, S. L., Van Wagenen, A., Gordon, A., & Calzo, J. P. (2014). Disparities in safety belt use by sexual orientation identity among US high school students. *American Journal of Public Health, 104*(2), 311–318.

Resnick, M. D., Bearman, P. S., Blum, R. W., Bauman, K. E., Harris, K. M., Jones, J., . . . Udry, J. R. (1997). Protecting adolescents from harm. Findings from the National Longitudinal study on Adolescent Health. *Journal of the American Medical Association, 278*(10), 823–832.

Rew, L., Arheart, K. L., Thompson, S., & Johnson, K. (2013). Predictors of adolescents' health-promoting behaviors guided by primary socialization theory. *Journal for Specialists in Pediatric Nursing, 18*(4), 277–288. doi:10.1111/jspn.12036

Rosario, M., Schrimshaw, E. W., & Hunter, J. (2008). Predicting different patterns of sexual identity development over time among lesbian, gay, and bisexual youths: A cluster analytic approach. *American Journal of Community Psychology, 42*(3), 266–282. doi:10.1007/s10464-008-9207-7

Rosenberg, T. J., Garbers, S., Chavkin, W., & Chiasson, M. A. (2003). Prepregnancy weight and adverse perinatal outcomes in an ethnically diverse population. *Obstetrics & Gynecology, 102*(5), 1022-1027.

Rosenfield, R. L. (2013). Adolescent anovulation: Maturational mechanisms and implications. *Journal of Clinical Endocrinology & Metabolism, 98*(9), 3572–3583. doi:10.1210/jc.2013-1770

Rospenda, K. M., Wolff, J. M., Richman, J. A., & Burke, L. A. (2013). Bullying victimization among college students: Negative consequences for alcohol use. *Journal of Addictive Diseases, 32*(4), 325–342. doi:10.1080/10550887.2013.859023

Russo, J. A., Miller, E., & Gold, M. A. (2013). Myths and misconceptions about long-acting reversible contraception (LARC). *Journal of Adolescent Health, 52*(4), S14–S21.

Ryan, C. (2009). *Helping families support their lesbian, gay, bisexual, and transgender (LGBT) children.* Washington, DC: National Center for Cultural Competence, Georgetown University Center for Child and Human Development.

Ryan, C., Russell, S. T., Huebner, D., Diaz, R. M., & Sanchez, J. (2010). Family acceptance in adolescence and the health of LGBT young adults. *Journal of Child and Adolescent Psychiatric Nursing, 23*(4), 205–213. doi:10.1111/j.1744-6171.2010.00246.x

Safi, J., Joyeux, L., & Chalouhi, G. E. (2012). Periconceptional folate deficiency and implications in neural tube defects. *Journal of Pregnancy, 2012,* 9. doi:10.1155/2012/295083

SAMHSA (Substance Abuse and Mental Health Services Administration). (2013). *Results from the 2012 National Survey on Drug Use and Health: Summary of National Findings* (NSDUH Series H-46, HHS Publication No. [SMA] 13-4795). Rockville, MD: Substance Abuse and Mental Health Services Administration.

Santelli, J., Ott, M. A., Lyon, M., Rogers, J., Summers, D., & Schleifer, R. (2006). Abstinence and abstinence-only education: A review of US policies and programs. *Journal of Adolescent Health, 38*(1), 72–81. doi:10.1016/j.jadohealth.2005.10.006

Santelli, J., Rochat, R., Hatfield-Timajchy, K., Gilbert, B. C., Curtis, K., Cabral, R., . . . Schieve, L. (2003). The measurement and meaning of unintended pregnancy. *Perspectives on Sexual and Reproductive Health, 35*(2), 94–101. doi:10.1363/3509403

Santelli, J. S., Sivaramakrishnan, K., Edelstein, Z. R., & Fried, L. P. (2013). Adolescent risk-taking, cancer risk, and life course approaches to prevention. *Journal of Adolescent Health, 52*(5, Suppl.), S41–S44. doi:10.1016/j.jadohealth.2013.02.017

Saslow, D., Solomon, D., Lawson, H. W., Killackey, M., Kulasingam, S. L., Cain, J., . . . Myers, E. R.; ACS-ASCCP-ASCP Cervical Cancer Guideline Committee. (2012). American Cancer Society, American Society for Colposcopy and Cervical Pathology, and American Society for Clinical Pathology screening guidelines for the prevention and early detection of cervical cancer. *CA Cancer Journal for Clinicians, 62*(3), 147–172. doi:10.3322/caac.21139

Satterwhite, C. L., Torrone, E., Meites, E., Dunne, E., Mahajan, R., Ocfemia, M. C. B., . . . Weinstock, H. (2013). Sexually transmitted infections among US women and men: Prevalence and incidence estimates, 2008. *Sexually Transmitted Diseases, 40*(3), 187–193. doi: 10.1097/OLQ.0b013e318286bb53

Schalet, A. T. (2011). Beyond abstinence and risk: A new paradigm for adolescent sexual health. *Women's Health Issues, 21*(3, Suppl.), S5–S7. doi:10.1016/j.whi.2011.01.007

Schiffman, M., Castle, P. E., Jeronimo, J., Rodriguez, A. C., & Wacholder, S. (2007). Human papillomavirus and cervical cancer. *Lancet, 370*(9590), 890–907. doi:10.1016/S0140-6736(07)61416-0.

Schindler, A. E. (2013). Non-contraceptive benefits of oral hormonal contraceptives. *International Journal of Endocrinology and Metabolism, 11*(1), 41–47. doi:10.5812/ijem.4158

Senn, T. E., & Carey, M. P. (2011). Age of partner at first adolescent intercourse and adult sexual risk behavior among women. *Journal of Women's Health (Larchmt), 20*(1), 61–66. doi:10.1089/jwh.2010.2089

Shields, J. P., Whitaker, K., Glassman, J., Franks, H. M., & Howard, K. (2012). Impact of victimization on risk of suicide among lesbian, gay, and bisexual high school students in San Francisco. *Journal of Adolescent Health, 50*(4), 418–420. doi:10.1016/j.jadohealth.2011.07.009

Simpson, J. L., Bailey, L. B., Pietrzik, K., Shane, B., & Holzgreve, W. (2010). Micronutrients and women of reproductive potential: Required dietary intake and consequences of dietary deficiency or excess. Part I—Folate, Vitamin B12, Vitamin B6. *Journal of Maternal-Fetal & Neonatal Medicine, 23*(12), 1323–1343. doi:10.3109/14767051003678234

Sipsma, H. L., Ickovics, J. R., Lin, H., & Kershaw, T. S. (2013). The impact of future expectations on adolescent sexual risk behavior. *Journal of Youth and Adolescence,* doi:10.1007/s10964-013-0082-7

Smithard, A., Glazebrook, C., & Williams, H. C. (2001). Acne prevalence, knowledge about acne and psychological morbidity in mid-adolescence: A community-based study. *British Journal of Dermatology, 145*(2), 274–279. doi:10.1046/j.1365-2133.2001.04346.x

Smithells, R. W., Sheppard, S., Wild, J., & Schorah, C. J. (1989). Prevention of neural tube defect recurrences in Yorkshire: Final report. *Lancet, 334*(8661), 498–499. doi:10.1016/S0140-6736(89)92103-X

Stern, J., Larsson, M., Kristiansson, P., & Tydén, T. (2013). Introducing reproductive life plan-based information in contraceptive counselling: An RCT. *Human Reproduction, 28*(9), 2450–2461. doi:10.1093/humrep/det279

Strauss, J. S., Krowchuk, D. P., Leyden, J. J., Lucky, A. W., Shalita, A. R., Siegfried, E. C., . . . Bhushan, R. (2007). Guidelines of care for acne vulgaris management. *Journal of the American Academy of Dermatology, 56*(4), 651–663. doi:10.1016/j.jaad.2006.08.048

Talley, A. E., Hughes, T. L., Aranda, F., Birkett, M., & Marshal, M. P. (2014). Exploring alcohol-use behaviors among heterosexual and sexual minority adolescents: Intersections with sex, age, and race/ethnicity. *American Journal of Public Health, 104*(2), 295–303.

Tate, J. C., & Shelton, B. L. (2008). Personality correlates of tattooing and body piercing in a college sample: The kids are alright. *Personality and Individual Differences, 45*(4), 281–285. doi:10.1016/j.paid.2008.04.011

Teegarden, D., Proulx, W. R., Martin, B. R., Zhao, J., McCabe, G. P., Lyle, R. M., . . . Weaver, C. M. (1995). Peak bone mass in young women. *Journal of Bone and Mineral Research, 10*(5), 711–715. doi:10.1002/jbmr.5650100507

Testa, M., & Hoffman, J. H. (2013). Naturally occurring changes in women's drinking from high school to college and implicatinos for sexual victimization. *Journal of Studies on Alcohol and Drugs, 73*(1), 26–33.

Thein-Nissenbaum, J. (2013). Long term consequences of the female athlete triad. *Maturitas, 75*(2), 107–112. doi:10.1016/j.maturitas.2013.02.010

Tolarova, M. (1982). Periconceptional supplementation with vitamins and folic acid to prevent recurrence of cleft lip. *Lancet, 320*(8291), 217. doi:10.1016/S0140-6736(82)91063-7

Trussell, J. (2011). Contraceptive failure in the United States. *Contraception, 83*(5), 397–404. doi:10.1016/j.contraception.2011.01.021

Tsai, M. C., & Goldstein, S. R. (2012). Office diagnosis and management of abnormal uterine bleeding. *Clinical Obstetrics and Gynecology, 55*(3), 635–650. doi:10.1097/GRF.0b013e31825d3cec

US Preventive Services Task Force. (2009a). Folic acid for the prevention of neural tube defects: US Preventive Services Task Force recommendation statement. *Annals of Internal Medicine, 150*(9), 626–631. doi:10.7326/0003-4819-150-9-200905050-00009

US Preventive Services Task Force. (2009b). Screening for breast cancer: US Preventive Services Task Force recommendation statement. *Annals of Internal Medicine, 151*(10), 716–726, W-236.

US Preventive Services Task Force. (2010). *Screening for obesity in children and adolescents: Recommendation statement* (AHRQ Publication No. 10-05144-EF-2). Retrieved from http://www.uspreventiveservicestaskforce.org/uspstf10/childobes/chobesrs.htm

US Preventive Services Task Force. (2012). *Screening for and management of obesity in adults: US Preventive Services Task Force Recommendation Statement* (AHRQ Publication No. 11-05159-EF-2). Retrieved from http://www.uspreventiveservicestaskforce.org/uspstf11/obeseadult/obesers.htm

Vessey, J. A., DiFazio, R. L., & Strout, T. D. (2013). Youth bullying: A review of the science and call to action. *Nursing Outlook, 61*(5), 337–345. doi:10.1016/j.outlook.2013.04.011

Well, D. (2013). Acne vulgaris: A review of causes and treatment options. *Nurse Practitioner, 38*(10), 22–31.

Wickman, M. E., Anderson, N. L., & Greenberg, C. S. (2008). The adolescent perception in invincibility and its influence on teen acceptance of health promotion strategies. *Journal of Pediatric Nursing, 23*(6), 460–468. doi:10.1016/j.pedn.2008.02.003

Widman, L., Welsh, D. P., McNulty, J. K., & Little, K. C. (2006). Sexual communication and contraceptive use in adolescent dating couples. *Journal of Adolescent Health, 39*(6), 893–899. doi:10.1016/j.jadohealth.2006.06.003

Winner, B., Peipert, J. F., Zhao, Q., Buckel, C., Madden, T., Allsworth, J. E., & Secura, G. M. (2012). Effectiveness of long-acting reversible contraception. *New England Journal of Medicine, 366*(21), 1998–2007. doi:10.1056/NEJMoa1110855

Woodman, C. B. J., Collins, S., Winter, H., Bailey, A., Ellis, J., Prior, P., . . . Young, L. S. (2001). Natural history of cervical human papillomavirus infection in young women: A longitudinal cohort study. *Lancet, 357*(9271), 1831–1836. doi:10.1016/S0140-6736(00)04956-4

Yost, J., Krainovich-Miller, B., Budin, W., & Norman, R. (2010). Assessing weight perception accuracy to promote weight loss among US female adolescents: A secondary analysis. *BMC Public Health, 10*, 465–475.

Young, C., Armstrong, M. L., Roberts, A. E., Mello, I., & Angel, E. (2010). A triad of evidence for care of women with genital piercings. *Journal of the American Academy of Nurse Practitioners, 22*(2), 70–80. doi:10.1111/j.1745-7599.2009.00479.x

Chapter 5

Women at Midlife

Judith A. Berg, Diana Taylor, and Nancy Fugate Woods

Major Issues and Challenges Midlife Women Face in Maintaining Health

Midlife women have many of the health needs of their younger counterparts as well as those of aging women. For example, fertility management remains an issue until menopause, defined as twelve consecutive months of amenorrhea, as do issues related to sexual activity. Midlife women are at possible increased risk for sexually transmitted infections and unintended pregnancy perhaps because of recent separation, divorce, or widowhood, making them single again (Idso, 2009). Taylor and James (2012) also suggest midlife women are at increased risk for pregnancy owing to a limited knowledge of safer sexual practices, less regular menstrual cycles, a health-care provider who may not evaluate sexual health risks, and a growing use of medications for erectile dysfunction in men that has created increased numbers of available sexual partners. At the same time, midlife women transition to higher risk categories related to cancer, cardiovascular disease, depression, abnormal bereavement, and physical abuse or neglect in common with older women, which require implementation of more aggressive screening guidelines and prevention strategies (Cobb, 1998).

Although midlife women are far from a homogeneous group, the context of their lives is an important determinant of health. For example, midlife women are more likely than men to take on the role of primary caregiver, care for a spouse or a parent, and spend more hours caring for sick relatives while simultaneously caring for children living in the household (Berg, 2011). They are also more likely to provide assistance to relatives with housework and meal preparation (Navaie-Waliser, Spriggs, & Feldman, 2002). Add to that the possibility that a midlife woman might be a single mother, single head of household, and employed full time. These women might be simultaneously dealing with symptoms related to the menopausal transition and managing chronic health issues, such as obesity, diabetes, cardiovascular disease, asthma, and other chronic conditions. Together, these multiple roles and health-related issues provide context for women's attitudes toward their own health and health promotion activities.

In this chapter, common health conditions encountered by women aged 40 to 65 years will be discussed along with various treatment approaches. Recommended health promotion behaviors will be detailed, as will ways to promote a positive self-image and self-esteem. All of these aspects of midlife women's health will be viewed through a lens that recognizes the complexity and multiplicity of roles women occupy simultaneously.

Well-Woman Care: Common Health Conditions and Treatment Approaches

Data on selected conditions that influence women's morbidity and mortality as they move into midlife (defined as ages 40 to 65 years) were examined as background to this discussion. The conditions discussed in this chapter were selected on the basis of their prevalence among women, but also because prevention and early detection play a significant role in the status of women's health (National Institute for Health Care Management [NIHCM] Foundation, 2005). The conditions discussed are cardiovascular disease, breast and cervical cancer, mental illness and depression, osteoporosis, and obesity and overweight. These common health conditions are followed by a discussion of the menopausal transition and menstrual issues, sexual and reproductive health needs of midlife women, and role issues that may impact health, such as employment and informal caregiving.

Cardiovascular Disease

The number one cause of death and disability among women in the United States is cardiovascular disease (Go et al., 2013; Kones, 2013). Heart disease and stroke are the most prevalent forms of cardiovascular disease that share similar risk factors including hypertension, hypercholesterolemia, smoking, and being overweight (NIHCM Foundation, 2005). Additional risk factors include physical inactivity and diabetes. All of the risk factors for cardiovascular disease in women are considered modifiable by adopting healthy behaviors. Yet nationally representative data have shown an increase in the prevalence of stroke and myocardial infarction among middle-aged women (Towfighi, Zheng, & Ovbiagele, 2009, 2010), which parallels an increase in obesity and abdominal obesity rates in women compared with men (Ford, Zhao, Li, Pearson, & Mokdad, 2008). In 2005, it was estimated the annual health-care expenditures for treatment of heart disease and stroke in the United States were $209 billion and $28 billion, respectively (Centers for Disease Control and Prevention [CDC], 2010). Symptoms of heart attack and stroke may be atypical in women, and this has spearheaded a national campaign by the American Heart Association (AHA) to raise public awareness of these hard to recognize symptoms that include fatigue, shortness of breath, back pain, jaw pain, and nausea (AHA, 2013).

Risk Factors

Hypertension. Considered one of the most important risk factors for heart disease and stroke, hypertension affects women and men about equally during midlife. The percentage of women experiencing hypertension ranges from 35% of women age 45–54 to 53.3% of women age 55–65 years. Normal blood pressure is defined as a systolic pressure less than 120 mm Hg and diastolic less than 80 mm Hg (Roger et al., 2012). In 2009, Americans visited their health-care providers more than 55 million times to treat their blood pressure (Roger et al., 2012), and about 7 in 10 US adults (69.9%) with high blood pressure use medications to treat it (CDC, 2011) (see Box 5.1).

Box 5.1 Recommendations/Guidelines to Control Hypertension

- Follow your health-care provider's instructions and stay on your medications.
- Eat a healthy diet that is low in salt; low in total fat, saturated fat, and cholesterol; and rich in fresh fruits and vegetables.
- Take a brisk 10-minute walk, 3 times a day, 5 days a week.

Don't smoke. If you smoke, quit as soon as possible. Visit http://www.cdc.gov/blood pressure/ for tips on quitting (CDC, 2013).

Treatment. Hypertension is treated by a combination of lifestyle modification and pharmacologic treatment. An optimal blood pressure is < 120/80, and pharmacotherapy is indicated when blood pressure is ≥ 140/90 mm Hg. Thiazide diuretics are generally part of the drug regimen for most patients unless contraindicated or if there are compelling indications for other agents such as β-blockers and/or angiotensin converting enzyme (ACE) inhibitors/angiotension II receptor blockers (ARBs) with addition of other drugs such as thiazides as needed to achieve goal blood pressure (Mosca et al., 2011).

High Cholesterol (hypercholesterolemia). Excess cholesterol in the blood can lead to cardiovascular disease, which, as noted, is the number one cause of death in the United States. Approximately 2,200 Americans die of cardiovascular disease each day, an average of one death every 39 seconds. Lowering cholesterol can reduce women's risk of heart disease and stroke. Encouraging women to take responsibility for managing their cholesterol levels can have a positive impact on their future morbidity and mortality. Cholesterol is a waxy, fat-like substance that is needed in the body, but when there is too much in the blood, it can build up on the walls of arteries. This can lead to heart disease and stroke (US Department of Health and Human Services [USDHHS], Office of Women's Health, 2013). Particles called lipoproteins carry cholesterol in the blood. There are two kinds of lipoproteins:

- Low-density lipoproteins (LDL) cholesterol make up the majority of the body's cholesterol. LDL is known as "bad" cholesterol because having high levels can lead to a buildup in the arteries and result in heart disease.
- High-density lipoproteins (HDL) cholesterol absorb cholesterol, and carry it back to the liver, which flushes it from the body. High levels of HDL, or "good" cholesterol, reduce the risk of heart disease and stroke.

There are generally no symptoms of high cholesterol. Many women have never had their cholesterol checked, so they don't know they're at risk. A simple blood test can determine the level of LDL and HDL in the blood. The key is to prevent high cholesterol—or to reduce levels if they are high.

Risk Reduction. The USDHHS, Office of Women's Health (2013) has developed several recommendations to reduce the risk of hypercholesterolemia (see Box 5.2).

Smoking. Smoking is a major cause of coronary heart disease (CHD), and the risk increases with number of cigarettes smoked and the duration of smoking. Although fewer women smoke than men, the percentage difference between the two has continued to decrease. Today, with a much smaller gap between men's and women's smoking rates, women share a much larger burden of smoking-related diseases (American Lung Association,

---

Box 5.2 Recommendations/Guidelines to Control Hyperlipidemia

- Maintain a healthy weight—simply losing weight can help lower total cholesterol and LDL.
- Eat better—eat foods low in saturated fats, trans fats, and cholesterol.
- Eat more—fish, poultry.
- Broil, bake, roast, or poach foods. Remove the fat and skin before eating.
- Drink/eat skim (fat-free) or low-fat (1%) milk and cheese and low-fat or nonfat yogurt.
- Try to eat five servings a day of fruits and vegetables.
- Eat cereals, breads, rice, and pasta made from whole grains.
- Eat less—organ meats (liver, kidney, brains), egg yolks, fats (butter, lard) and oils, packaged and processed foods.
- Two diets that may help lower cholesterol are:
  - Heart Healthy Diet (http://www.mayoclinic.org/diseases-conditions/heart-disease/in-depth/heart-healthy-diet/art-20047702) and
  - Therapeutic Lifestyles Changes (TLC) Diet (https://www.nhlbi.nih.gov/health/public/heart/chol/chol_tlc.pdf)
- Exercise can help lower LDL and raise HDL. Exercise at a moderate intensity for at least 2 hours and 30 minutes each week, or get 1 hour and 15 minutes of vigorous intensity physical activity each week.
- Take medication if prescribed to lower cholesterol. Take exactly as prescribed.

2013). It is known that women smokers are nearly 13 times more likely to die from chronic obstructive pulmonary disease (COPD) compared with women who've never smoked (US Department of Health and Human Services [DHHS], 2004). Smoking is directly responsible for 80% of lung cancer deaths in women each year, and lung cancer surpassed breast cancer as the leading cause of cancer deaths among women in the United States. Further, women have been targeted in tobacco marketing with themes such as social desirability, independence, weight control, and positive smoking messages in advertisements (DHHS, 2004).

Risk Reduction. The primary way to reduce risks associated with smoking is to stop smoking. The many avenues available to assist with smoking cessation include counseling, nicotine replacement, and other pharmacologic therapies. Many of these therapies accompanied by a formalized smoking cessation program with group counseling can help women quit smoking (Turk, Tuite, & Burke, 2009).

Physical Inactivity. Physical inactivity is an important risk factor in CHD. Significant research has supported the use of exercise in decreasing the risk of CHD (Lawrence, 2008; Thompson et al., 2003). In addition, the Women's Health Initiative Observation Study enrolled 73,743 postmenopausal women to examine total physical activity scores, walking, vigorous exercise, and hours spent sitting or sleeping as predictors of cardiovascular events (Manson et al., 2002). Conclusions were that at least 1 hour of walking per week predicted a lower risk for CHD, so even light to moderate activity is associated with lower CHD rates in women. Yet despite the evidence, fewer than 30% of women engage in the recommended levels of physical activity (Health Resources and Services Administration [HRSA], 2004). Brown, Heesch, and Miller (2009) found that the effects of recent life events, such as decreased income or the illness of a child or family member may be different on middle-aged women's physical activity engagement compared with the effects on younger or older women's physical activity engagement.

Risk Reduction. Increasing women's physical activity is an important step toward reducing risk for CHD. However, a number of studies suggest perceived barriers such as lack of time, fatigue, lack of motivation, and perception of work as sufficient physical activity (Berg, Cromwell, & Arnett, 2002; Cromwell & Berg, 2006; Im, Lee, Chee, & Stuifbergen, 2011). Interventions that bolster women's physical activity must address perceived barriers and benefits, cultural beliefs, and busy lives in ways that maximize their ability to engage in and maintain levels of physical activity that reduce CHD risk.

Overweight and Obesity. Women are advised to maintain an appropriate body weight (BMI $< 25kg/m^2$) (Mosca et al., 2011) as excess body weight is linked to cardiac arrhythmias, congestive heart failure, ischemic heart disease, and sudden death (Klein et al., 2004). Therefore, overweight and obesity pose significant risk for developing CHD. Efforts to avoid weight gain may need to be intensified over women's lifetimes to adjust for physiologic and age-related changes (Kumanyika et al., 2008). See Chapter 8 for more extensive discussion on body composition in women.

For weight loss, Berkel, Poston, Reeves, & Foreyt (2005) recommended a weight loss program that includes a 500 calorie per day reduction in food intake and a 1,000 calorie per week expenditure in physical activity to obtain a weight loss of 0.5 to 1.0 kg per week. Women frequently serve as a keystone in the family's diet, and understanding factors that shape women's dietary behaviors can give insight into dietary patterns of the entire family (Brown, Smith, & Kromm, 2012).

Risk Reduction. Women should consume a diet rich in fruits and vegetables, wholegrains and, high-fiber. It is recommended that they consume fish, especially oily fish, at least twice a week, limit intake of saturated fat, cholesterol, alcohol, sodium, and sugar, and avoid trans-fatty acids (Mosca et al., 2011).

Treatment. There are several approaches to weight management and obesity treatment, including behavioral strategies, pharmacotherapy, and surgical treatment. Behavioral approaches include goal setting for dietary intake and physical activity, self-monitoring, problem solving, stimulus control, cognitive restructuring, and relapse prevention (Berkel et al., 2005; Wadden, Butryn, & Wilson, 2007). Pharmacotherapy is appropriate for some women and is currently approved for persons with a BMI of 30 kg/m^2 or more or BMI of 27 kg/m^2 with comorbidities such as sleep apnea, diabetes, or hypertension (Turk et al., 2009). Medications approved for the purpose of weight loss maintenance are types that block the reuptake of serotonin and noradrenaline in the central nervous system (e.g., Sibutramine) and those that decrease fat absorption by approximately 30% through gastrointestinal tract inhibition of gastric and pancreatic lipases essential for digestion of fats (e.g., Orlistat) (Turk et al., 2009). Both drug types should be prescribed with caution owing to potential side effects. Surgical treatment of obesity may be indicated in women with BMI >40 kg/m^2 or a BMI of 35 kg/m^2 or more with comorbidities such as sleep apnea, diabetes, or hypertension (National Institute of Health [NIH] Consensus Development Panel, 1991). Several bariatric surgical techniques are used for weight loss using restrictive or malabsorptive methods, for example gastric bypass, vertical banded gastroplasty, adjustable gastric banding, and biliopancreatic diversion (Mango & Frishman, 2006).

Diabetes. Type 1 diabetes is currently not preventable, but type 2 diabetes can be (Food and Drug Administration [FDA], 2013). If not preventable, diabetes is treatable (AHA, 2013).

For the remainder of this discussion, the term diabetes refers to type 2 only. Heart disease and stroke are the leading causes of death and disability among people with type 2 diabetes; in fact, at least 65% of people with diabetes die from some form of heart disease or stroke. Adults with diabetes are two to four times more likely to have heart disease or a stroke than adults without diabetes, and the AHA considers diabetes to be one of the seven major controllable risk factors for cardiovascular disease (AHA, 2012). It is known that 12.5 million, or 10.8% of all women aged 20 years or older, have diabetes (American Diabetes Association, 2011). The AHA (2012) explains that people with diabetes, particularly type 2 diabetes, are at increased risk for developing cardiovascular disease because they often have comorbid conditions of hypertension, abnormal cholesterol and high triglycerides, obesity, lack of physical activity, poorly controlled blood glucose, and may be smokers. Individuals with insulin resistance or diabetes in combination with one or more of these risk factors are more likely to have heart disease or stroke. However, by controlling these risk factors, women with diabetes may avoid or delay the development of cardiovascular disease (AHA, 2012).

Midlife is the period in which chronic diseases emerge as a major burden on the adult US population, and the prevalence of diabetes increases with age (Sabolsi, Solomon, & Manson, 2001). According to data from the National Health Interview Survey (NHIS), an estimated 135,000 newly diagnosed cases of diabetes were reported by women aged 45 to 64 years in 1996 (CDC, 2000), and diabetes is a leading cause of death among middle-aged American women (Peters, Kochanek, & Murphy, 1998).

Risk Reduction. Type 2 diabetes results from a combination of genetic predisposition (nonmodifiable), behavioral, and environmental risk factors (Yoon, Kwok, & Magkidis, 2013). In a systematic review of randomized controlled trials using lifestyle interventions to avert type 2 diabetes in individuals with impaired glucose tolerance, lifestyle interventions had a beneficial effect on the incidence of diabetes. However, several of the studies found the effect of lifestyle intervention decreased after the intervention was terminated, and no long-term benefit in mortality and morbidity was found (Yoon et al., 2013). Dietary and physical activity intervention strategies were utilized across the clinical trials studied. Observation studies associate a healthy lifestyle (regular physical activity, moderate alcohol consumption, abstinence from smoking, healthy diet, and avoidance of overweight) with a greatly reduced risk for developing type 2 diabetes (Glauber & Karnieli, 2013). In the US Diabetes Prevention Program, the strongest predictor of type 2 diabetes prevention was weight loss, and risk of diabetes was 16% lower for every kilogram of weight lost (Knowler et al., 2009). Gillies et al. (2007) analyzed 21 randomized controlled trials that evaluated interventions to delay or prevent type 2 diabetes in individuals with impaired glucose tolerance and found that lifestyle and pharmacological interventions (oral diabetes drugs and antiobesity drugs) reduce the rate of progression to type 2 diabetes in people with impaired glucose tolerance. Lifestyle interventions seemed to be at least as effective as drug treatment (Gillies et al., 2007).

Treatment. Comprehensive diabetes risk factor management must include blood pressure control, lipid management, weight reduction in overweight or obese individuals, and smoking cessation (Giorgino, Leonardini, & Laviola, 2013). The general goal of lowering hemoglobin A_{1c} (HbA$_{1c}$) to <7.0% is the norm, but for selected individuals, lower HbA$_{1c}$ can be considered if it can be achieved without significant hypoglycemia or other adverse effects of treatment. The individuals who might benefit from this target are those with short duration of diabetes, long life expectancy and no significant CHD (Giorgino et al., 2013). A new class of glucose-lowering drugs, such as the incretin-based therapies, may hold promise among therapeutic options, not only as add-on treatments, but also as a strategy to reduce the burden of diabetes and its vascular complications (Giorgino et al., 2013).

In all cases, pharmacologic treatment options must be accompanied by important lifestyle changes that are aimed at lowering blood pressure, managing lipids, reducing weight in overweight individuals, and smoking cessation.

Osteoporosis

Osteoporosis is the most common bone disease, with about 10 million persons in the United States over age 50 years diagnosed with osteoporosis and another 34 million determined to be at risk (NIHCM Foundation, 2005). Osteoporosis is characterized by low bone mass and deterioration of structural bone tissue in aging adults, with women four times more likely than men to develop it (NIHCM Foundation). Often named a silent disease, osteoporosis may not present until fractures occur following minimal trauma (National Osteoporosis Foundation [NOF], 2013). The World Health Organization diagnostic classification defines osteoporosis as bone mineral density at the hip or lumbar spine that is less than or equal to 2.5 standard deviations below the mean bone mineral density of a young-adult reference population (Kanis, 2008). For women at midlife, osteoporosis becomes a serious consideration as there is known to be dramatic loss of bone following the menopausal transition.

The National Osteoporosis Foundation (NOF) recommends risk assessment, diagnosis, and treatment of osteoporosis in postmenopausal women and men age 50 and older (NOF, 2013). A number of risk factors cause or contribute to osteoporosis and fractures. These include lifestyle factors such as alcohol abuse, low calcium intake, vitamin D insufficiency, excess vitamin A, high salt intake, inadequate physical activity, immobilization, smoking, falling, and excessive thinness. In addition, genetic factors such as cystic fibrosis, parental history of hip fracture, homocystinuria, and many others contribute. For a complete listing of conditions, diseases, and medications that cause or contribute to osteoporosis and fractures, see the NOF (2013) clinician's guide.

Risk Reduction. NOF has developed a list of universal recommendations to prevent or reduce osteoporosis, which are a combination of lifestyle changes, including weight-bearing exercises and cessation of smoking if the woman does smoke, as well as dietary changes. Calcium (1,200 mg daily for women 51 and older) and Vitamin D supplements (800–1,000 mg daily for women 50 and older) are also recommended. In additional early detection through bone mineral density testing as well as more extensive testing (vertebral imaging) for women at higher risk.

Treatment. Treatment recommendations from the NOF (2013) form clinical guidelines related to osteoporosis, which consist predominantly of pharmacotherapy. More detailed discussion of pharmacologic treatment of osteoporosis is included in Chapter 13.

Breast and Cervical Cancer

Although women suffer from any number of forms of cancer, this discussion is limited to breast and cervical cancer owing to the important role of screening in promoting health and preventing morbidity from these cancers.

Breast Cancer

Breast cancer is the most frequently diagnosed cancer in women in the United States, not including skin cancer, and is second to lung cancer as a cause of cancer deaths

(US Preventive Services Task Force [USPSTF], 2009). Increasing age is the most important risk factor for breast cancer for most women, but women without the genetic mutations BRCA1 or BRCA2 may have other demographic, physical, or historical risk factors, although none conveys a clinically important absolute increased risk (USPSTF, 2009). The 10-year risk for breast cancer is 1 in 69 for women age 40 years, 1 in 42 at age 50 years, and 1 in 29 at age 60 years (Horner et al., 2009). According to the USPSTF (2009), the incidence rate has increased since the 1970s; however, recent data show this rate seems to be decreasing. In 2003, the incidence rate was 124.2 per 100,000, a 6.7% decrease from the previous year, which some speculate may be due to discontinuation of hormone replacement therapy (Ravdin et al., 2007). Nelson et al. (2009) confirmed that screening mammography reduces mortality with improvements in the relative risk of death due to breast cancer similar in women age 39 to 49 years and 50 to 59 years. Digital mammography has been shown to perform similarly to film mammography. But magnetic resonance imaging (MRI) has not been evaluated for its potential benefit in screening average risk women, while clinical breast examination has not been compared with no screening, nor has the risk of clinical breast examination plus mammography been compared with mammography alone. Importantly, two large trials of teaching breast self-examination outside the United States demonstrated no mortality benefit (Ravdin et al., 2007). Examination of screening data led to the USPSTF recommendations for breast cancer screening published in 2009 (see Table 5-3). And, although they are controversial and make many changes to previously held views, these recommendations are evidence-based and currently utilized in clinical practice. Further, false-positive results are common with mammography, and cause anxiety, and lead to additional imaging studies and procedures such as biopsy or fine-needle aspiration. False-positive and false-negative results were both considered when the USPSTF examined evidence upon which the recommendations were made.

Table 5.1 describes what the recommendation grades mean and suggestions for practice, while Table 5.2 details the USPSTF-defined levels of certainty regarding net benefit. Table 5.3 provides a summary of breast cancer screening recommendations and evidence (USPSTF, 2012).

Risk Reduction. Risk reduction strategies for breast cancer include following cancer screening guidelines as recommended by the USPSTF (2009), limiting the amount of alcohol, being physically active and maintaining a healthy body weight, stopping smoking, and following guidelines related to hormone therapy during the menopausal transition (Canadian Cancer Society, 2013). For women at high risk for developing breast cancer (known to have the BRCA gene), their specialist physician might recommend chemoprevention in the form of selective estrogen-receptor modulators (SERMs), which are antiestrogen drugs that block the effects of estrogen in some tissues (e.g., breast) and act like estrogen in other tissues (Canadian Cancer Society, 2013; Chlebowski, Collyar, Somerfield, & Pfister, 1999). Chlebowski and colleagues suggested tamoxifen could be used for reducing breast cancer risk, but it was premature to recommend raloxifene for that purpose. In 2002, Chlebowski suggested breast cancer risk reduction is an achievable medical objective using SERMs, prophylactic surgery, and lifestyle change (weight loss, dietary change, and increased physical activity) (Chlebowski, 2002). According to the Canadian Cancer Society (2013), prophylactic mastectomy results in a 90% decrease in the risk of breast cancer in high-risk women. In addition, prophylactic oophorectomy can decrease the risk of breast cancer in women with BRCA mutations and can also decrease women's risk of ovarian cancer. However, there should be very good indications for doing these types of preventive surgeries.

TABLE 5.1	What the Grades Mean and Suggestions for Practice

The USPSTF updated its definition of and suggestions for practice for the grade C recommendation. This new definition applies to USPSTF recommendations voted on after July 2012. Describing the strength of a recommendation is an important part of communicating its importance to clinicians and other users. Although most of the grade definitions have evolved since the USPSTF first began, none has changed more noticeably than the definition of a C recommendation, which has undergone three major revisions since 1998. Despite these revisions, the essence of the C recommendation has remained consistent: at the population level, the balance of benefits and harms is very close, and the magnitude of net benefit is small. Given this small net benefit, the USPSTF has either not made a recommendation "for or against routinely" providing the service (1998), recommended "against routinely" providing the service (2007), or recommended "selectively" providing the service (2012). Grade C recommendations are particularly sensitive to patient values and circumstances. Determining whether or not the service should be offered or provided to an individual patient will typically require an informed conversation between the clinician and the patient.

Grade	Definition	Suggestions for Practice
A	The USPSTF recommends the service. There is high certainty that the net benefit is substantial.	Offer or provide this service.
B	The USPSTF recommends the service. There is high certainty that the net benefit is moderate or there is moderate certainty that the net benefit is moderate to substantial.	Offer or provide this service.

Grade	Definition	Suggestions for Practice
C	The USPSTF recommends selectively offering or providing this service to individual patients based on professional judgment and patient preferences. There is at least moderate certainty that the net benefit is small.	Offer or provide this service for selected patients depending on individual circumstances.
D	The USPSTF recommends against the service. There is moderate or high certainty that the service has no net benefit or that the harms outweigh the benefits.	Discourage the use of this service.
I Statement	The USPSTF concludes that the current evidence is insufficient to assess the balance of benefits and harms of the service. Evidence is lacking, of poor quality, or conflicting, and the balance of benefits and harms cannot be determined.	Read the clinical considerations section of USPSTF Recommendation Statement. If the service is offered, patients should understand the uncertainty about the balance of benefits and harms.

TABLE 5.2	Levels of Certainty Regarding Net Benefit
Level of Certainty*	**Description**
High	The available evidence usually includes consistent results from well-designed, well-conducted studies in representative primary care populations. These studies assess the effects of the preventive service on health outcomes. This conclusion is therefore unlikely to be strongly affected by the results of future studies.
Moderate	The available evidence is sufficient to determine the effects of the preventive service on health outcomes, but confidence in the estimate is constrained by such factors as: • The number, size, or quality of individual studies. • Inconsistency of findings across individual studies. • Limited generalizability of findings to routine primary care practice. • Lack of coherence in the chain of evidence. As more information becomes available, the magnitude or direction of the observed effect could change, and this change may be large enough to alter the conclusion.
Low	The available evidence is insufficient to assess effects on health outcomes. Evidence is insufficient because of: • The limited number or size of studies. • Important flaws in study design or methods. • Inconsistency of findings across individual studies.
	• Gaps in the chain of evidence. • Findings not generalizable to routine primary care practice. • Lack of information on important health outcomes. More information may allow estimation of effects on health outcomes.

*The USPSTF defines certainty as "likelihood that the USPSTF assessment of the net benefit of a preventive service is correct." The net benefit is defined as benefit minus harm of the preventive service as implemented in a general, primary care population. The USPSTF assigns a certainty level based on the nature of the overall evidence available to assess the net benefit of a preventive service.

Treatment. Effective treatments are available for invasive breast cancer that include radiation, chemotherapy (including hormonal treatment), and surgery. There is debate about the standard treatments women receive for ductal carcinoma in situ (DCIS), but those approaches currently include surgery, radiation, and hormonal therapy (USPSTF, 2009).

Cervical Cancer

Cervical cancer is the third most common cancer among women worldwide (15%) and the second most common in developing countries (Appleby et al., 2007). Scientists have made great strides toward identifying the cause of cervical cancer. Human papilloma virus (HPV) causes the production of two proteins known as E6 and E7 that turn off some tumor suppressor genes. This may allow the cervical lining cells to grow too much and to

TABLE 5.3	Screening for Breast Cancer: Summary of Recommendation and Evidence

- The USPSTF recommends biennial screening mammography for women aged 50 to 74 years. Grade: B recommendation
- The decision to start regular, biennial screening mammography before the age of 50 years should be an individual one and take patient context into account, including the patient's values regarding specific benefits and harms. Grade: C recommendation
- The USPSTF concludes that the current evidence is insufficient to assess the additional benefits and harms of screening mammography in women 75 years or older. Grade: I Statement
- The USPSTF recommends against teaching breast self-examination (BSE). Grade: D recommendation
- The USPSTF concludes that the current evidence is insufficient to assess the additional benefits and harms of clinical breast examination (CBE) beyond screening mammography in women 40 years or older. Grade: I Statement
- The USPSTF concludes that the current evidence is insufficient to assess the additional benefits and harms of either digital mammography or magnetic resonance imaging (MRI) instead of film mammography as a screening modality for breast cancer. Grade: I Statement

develop changes in additional genes, which in some cases will lead to cancer. However, HPV does not completely explain what causes cervical cancer because most women with HPV don't get cervical cancer. Certain other risk factors, such as smoking and HIV infection, which may be correlated with HPV in women, may contribute to the development of cervical cancer. Cervical cancer tends to occur in midlife; most cases are found in women younger than 50, and more than 20% of cases of cervical cancer are found in women over age 65 years (American Cancer Society, 2013a). Risk factors that increase chances of developing cervical cancer are age, family history, smoking, HPV infection, immunosuppression, current or past chlamydia infection, diet low in fruits and vegetables, long-term use of oral contraceptives, multiple full-term pregnancies (three or more), young age at the first full-term pregnancy, poverty, and being a daughter of a mother who took diethylstilbestrol (DES). Signs and symptoms of cervical cancer and precancer are rare, but can include abnormal vaginal bleeding, such as bleeding after intercourse, bleeding after menopause, bleeding and spotting between periods, and having menstrual periods that are longer or heavier than usual. In addition, there may be an unusual discharge from the vagina or pain during intercourse (American Cancer Society, 2013c).

The ultimate goal of cervical cancer screening is to decrease the incidence of and subsequent mortality from invasive cervical cancer (Peirson, Fitzpatrick-Lewis, Ciliska, & Warren, 2013). Pooled evidence from a dozen case-control studies indicated a significant protective effect of cytology screening, although the review found no conclusive evidence for establishing optimal ages to start and stop cervical cancer screening, nor for determining how often to screen. However, data suggest substantial protective effects against mortality from screening women 30 years and older at intervals of up to 5 years (Peirson et al., 2013).

Cervical cancer can be prevented by finding and treating precancers before they become true cancers and by preventing the precancers. The Pap test and the HPV test are used to find cervical precancers. If a precancer is found, it can be treated, thus stopping cervical cancer before it really starts (American Cancer Society, 2013b). Prevention of precancers is possible with a combination of lifestyle changes and vaccination. Lifestyle changes must include avoidance of exposure to HPV. This is an increasingly important issue for midlife women who might be newly single and dating. Use of condoms is extremely important in this population, as they provide some protection against HPV. Smoking cessation is another important lifestyle change that can prevent precancers of the cervix. Perhaps the most important breakthrough in cervical cancer prevention was vaccine development that can protect women from HPV infections. To date, a vaccine that protects against HPV types 6, 11, 16, and 18 (Gardasil) and one that protects against types 16 and 18 (Cervarix) is available in the United States. Both vaccines require a series of three injections over a 6-month period. In clinical trials, both vaccines prevented cervical cancers and precancers caused by HPV types 16 and 18 (American Cancer Society, 2013b). At the present time, the American Cancer Society's guidelines do not address the use of the vaccine in older women and men. However, midlife women may be in a position to recommend HPV vaccination to their daughters and/or granddaughters.

Risk Reduction. Risk reduction focuses on the already mentioned early detection, lifestyle changes, and vaccination. For midlife women, finding cervical precancers is an important risk reduction activity. Details of the procedures utilized to diagnose cervical precancers and cancer can be found at http://www.cancer.org/cancer/cervicalcancer/detailedguide/cervical-cancer-diagnosis.

Treatment. Options for treating patients with cervical cancer depend on the stage of the disease, which indicates how far the cancer has spread. Information from diagnostic tests is used to determine the size of the tumor, how deeply the tumor has invaded tissues within and around the cervix, and the spread to lymph nodes or distant organs (metastasis). In 2012, a group of 47 experts representing 23 professional societies, national and international health organizations and federal agencies met in Bethesda, Maryland, to revise the 2006 American Society for Colposcopy and Cervical Pathology Consensus Guidelines (Massad et al., 2013). The resultant consensus document from the American Society for Colposcopy and Cervical Pathology provides updated guidelines for the management of abnormal cervical cancer screening tests and cancer precursors (Massad et al., 2013). This document was collaboratively created and endorsed by coauthor delegates, nonauthor delegates, and participating organizations and is utilized in clinical practice.

Depression and Anxiety

Mental illnesses affect women and men differently as some disorders are more common in women, and some express themselves with different symptoms (National Institute of Mental Health [NIMH], 2013a). The focus of this discussion will be on depression (major depressive disorder, dysthymic disorder, minor depression) and anxiety disorders (general anxiety disorder, obsessive–compulsive disorder, panic disorder, posttraumatic stress disorder, and social anxiety disorder).

The cause of mood and anxiety disorders is not precisely known, but may be triggered by stressful life events and enduring stressful social conditions, and is affected by biologic, genetic, and psychosocial factors (brain chemistry, hormonal balance, socioeconomic status, support network, diet, premorbid medical conditions, cognition, personality, and gender) (USDHHS, 1999). Depression and anxiety often occur together, as about one half of those with a primary diagnosis of major depression also have an anxiety disorder (USDHHS, 1999). Major depressive disorder is one of the most common mental disorders in the United States. Each year about 6.7% of US adults experience major depressive disorder, with women 70% more likely than men to experience depression during their lifetime. Non-Hispanic blacks are 40% less likely than non-Hispanic whites to experience depression during their lifetime. Average age of onset is 32 years (Kessler, Chiu, Demler, & Walters, 2005). At the same time, women are 60% more likely than men to experience an anxiety disorder over their lifetime. Non-Hispanic blacks are 20% less likely, and Hispanics are 30% less likely than non-Hispanic whites to experience an anxiety disorder during their lifetime (Kessler et al., 2005).

Depression

Depression is most likely caused by a combination of genetic, biological, environmental, and psychological factors. All depressive illnesses are disorders of the brain; brain-imaging technologies, such as magnetic resonance imaging, have shown that the brains of people who have depression look different than those of people without depression (NIMH, 2013b). Some types of depression tend to run in families; however, it can occur in people without family histories of depression. Research into depression includes the study of certain genes that may make some individuals more prone to depression, but some genetics research indicates that depression risk is the result of the influence of several genes acting together with contextual factors such as environment, trauma, loss of a loved one, a difficult relationship, or any stressful situation that might trigger a depressive episode (NIMH, 2013b). The NIMH lists signs and symptoms of depression (see Box 5.3).

Not all women with depressive disorders experience the same symptoms, but all have some symptoms, as indicated above (NIMH, 2013b).

Risk factors. Risk factors for depression in midlife women include family history, personal history of depression, history of postpartum depression, history or presence of anxiety disorders, alcohol and other substance abuse or dependence, and depression may occur with other serious medical illnesses such as heart disease, stroke, cancer, HIV/AIDS, diabetes, and Parkinson's disease (NIMH, 2013b). Research has indicated depression is consistently associated with increased use of health services (Simon, Ormel, VonKorff, & Barlow, 1995), obesity (Simon et al., 2008), smoking (Holahan et al., 2011), and intimate partner violence (Devries et al., 2013). Risk factors are not generally modifiable unless associated with lifestyle, such as physical inactivity and obesity, smoking, and intimate partner violence. Of importance is early detection and treatment.

Box 5.3 Signs and Symptoms of Depression

- Persistent sad, anxious, or "empty" feelings
- Feelings of hopelessness or pessimism
- Feelings of guilt, worthlessness, or helplessness
- Irritability, restlessness
- Loss of interest in activities or hobbies once pleasurable, including sex
- Fatigue and decreased energy
- Difficulty concentrating, remembering details, and making decisions
- Insomnia, early-morning wakefulness, or excessive sleeping
- Overeating, or appetite loss
- Thoughts of suicide, suicide attempts
- Aches or pains, headaches, cramps, or digestive problems that do not ease even with treatment

Treatment. The most common treatments for depression are medication and psychotherapy. Medications include antidepressants, which primarily work on brain chemicals known as neurotransmitters—particularly serotonin and norepinephrine. Other antidepressants work on the neurotransmitter dopamine. Antidepressant medication categories include serotonin reuptake inhibitors (SSRIs), norepinephrine reuptake inhibitors (SNRIs), tricyclics, and monoamine oxidase inhibitors (MAOIs). SSRIs and SNRIs tend to have fewer side effects than older antidepressants, but they can cause headaches, nausea, jitters, or insomnia when first taken. These symptoms tend to fade with time. Sexual problems experienced with SSRIs or SNRIs may be ameliorated by dosage adjustments or switching to another medication. Tricyclics are older antidepressants less utilized today in view of their potential side effects. MAOIs are the oldest class of antidepressant medications and are more commonly utilized in atypical depression and may be of assistance with associated anxiety (NIMH, 2013b). The latest information on medications used for treating depression is available on the US Food and Drug Administration (FDA) website, http://www.fda.gov. Also, further discussion is included in Chapter 13 on Pharmacotherapies.

Two main types of psychotherapies—cognitive–behavioral therapy (CBT) and interpersonal therapy (IPT) are effective in treating depression. Psychotherapy helps people restructure negative thought patterns and assists with troubled relationships. The NIMH recommends psychotherapy as the best option for women with mild to moderate depression. However, for severe depression, psychotherapy may need to be accompanied by pharmacologic treatment (NIMH, 2013a). Additional information on psychotherapy is available on the NIMH website: http://www.nimh.nih.gov/health/topics/psychotherapies/index.shtml.

Anxiety

Although anxiety is a normal reaction to stress and can be beneficial, it can become excessive. While the anxious individual may realize their anxiety is too much, they have difficulty controlling it to the degree that it negatively affects their daily living (NIHM, 2013c). Current scientific knowledge about anxiety disorders, indeed all mental illnesses, is they are complex and probably result from a combination of genetic, environmental, psychological, and developmental factors (NIMH, 2013c). Brain-imaging technology and neurochemical techniques have led to the discovery that the amygdala and hippocampus play significant roles in most anxiety disorders. As already described, women are 60% more likely than men to experience an anxiety disorder over their lifetime. Mild, brief anxiety caused by a stressful event may last at least 6 months and can get worse if not treated. Generalized anxiety is not necessarily related to on specific stressful event. Anxiety disorders commonly occur with other mental or physical illnesses, including alcohol or substance abuse, and these may mask symptoms or heighten them.

Risk Reduction. Like all mental illnesses, specific risk reduction is not applicable. However, early diagnosis and intervention is the most effective way to treat.

Treatment. Anxiety disorders are most often treated with medication, specific types of psychotherapy, or both. Medication must be prescribed by physicians, usually psychiatrists, or psychiatric–mental health nurse practitioners. The principal medications used for anxiety disorders are antidepressants, antianxiety drugs, and beta-blockers to control some of the physical symptoms. Antidepressants, originally developed to treat depression, are also effective for anxiety disorders. Although these medications begin to alter brain chemistry after the first dose, their full effect requires about 4 to 6 weeks before symptoms begin to fade. SSRIs and tricyclics are commonly utilized for anxiety disorders, although tricyclics are not effective with obsessive–compulsive disorder. MAOIs are the oldest class of antidepressant medications, and a few (phenelzine and tranylcypromine, and isocarboxazid) are useful in treating panic disorder and social phobia. Individuals who take MAOIs cannot eat a variety of foods and beverages (including cheese and red wine) or take some medications, including some types of birth control pills, pain relievers (Advil, Motrin, or Tylenol), cold and allergy medications, and herbal supplements as these substances can interact with MAOIs to cause dangerous increases in blood pressure. High-potency benzodiazepines combat anxiety and have few side effects other than drowsiness. Because there may be a habituating effect, benzodiazepines are generally prescribed for short periods of time, especially for people who have abused drugs or alcohol and who become easily dependent on medication. However, people who have panic disorder can take benzodiazepines for up to a year without harm (NIMH, 2013c).

CBT is useful in treating anxiety disorders. The cognitive aspect helps people change the thinking patterns that support their fears, and the behavioral part helps people change the way they react to anxiety-provoking situations. Exposure-based behavioral therapy has been used for many years to treat specific phobias. The person gradually encounters the object or situation that is feared in increments often accompanied by the therapist. Both forms of therapy often last about 12 weeks and are conducted both individually and in groups. To be effective, the therapy must be directed at the person's specific anxieties and must be tailored to her needs. The only side effects are the discomfort of temporarily increased anxiety. Most often, therapy is combined with medication use and seems to be the most effective approach for the majority of people (NIMH, 2013c).

Coping with anxiety disorders might be enhanced by the inclusion of a self-help or support group of individuals sharing their problems and achievements. Internet chat rooms are also thought to be useful for this, but caution should be used in accepting advice or treatment recommendations from this modality. Trusted friends, family, or clergy can also be of support, although not considered a substitute for help from a mental health professional (NIMH, 2013c).

Menopausal Transition and Menstrual Issues

Menopausal Transition

The menopausal transition is frequently the focal point of research of midlife women. It usually begins with menstrual irregularity, and the diagnosis of menopause is a specific time point, which is 12 consecutive months of amenorrhea (Utian, 2005). The menopausal transition is a natural life occurrence for all women who live long enough. Over the past two decades, there has been a significant amount of research that focused on symptoms, symptom management, symptom clusters, and the debate about use of hormone therapy in women and cardiovascular disease (Valdiviezo, Lawson, & Ouyang, 2013). It is known that women at midlife experience symptoms associated with both menopause and aging (Dennerstein et al., 2007). Often, the focus is on vasomotor symptoms, such as hot flashes and night sweats, but women also report symptoms such as pain, shortness of breath, headaches, fatigue, palpitations, dizziness, musculoskeletal aches, and joint stiffness (Sievert & Obermeyer, 2012). Women have used a variety of management strategies for these symptoms, including Chinese herbal medicine, yoga, exercise, and acupuncture, but the most widely researched is hormone therapy.

Hot flashes and night sweats are considered primary menopausal symptoms that may also be associated with sleep and mood disturbances and cognitive symptoms (forgetfulness and difficulty concentrating) (Utian, 2005). The timing and frequency of hot flashes have been reviewed by many scholars (Nachtigall & Nachtigall, 2004). Data from the Study of Women Across the Nation (SWAN) indicated that vasomotor symptoms were more frequently reported by women in late perimenopause, and frequency varies across women, but tends to remain consistent for an individual (North American Menopause Society [NAMS], 2004, 2012).

There is evidence that midlife women will utilize complementary and alternative practices such as physiotherapists, chiropractors, osteopaths, acupuncturists, and massage therapists for back pain (Broom, Kirby, Sibbritt, Adams, & Refshauge, 2012). Critical analysis of the efficacy and side effects of Chinese herbal medicine (CHM) for menopausal symptom management found that such approaches may be effective for at least some menopausal symptoms with side effects less likely than those from hormone therapy (Xu et al., 2012). However, much of the research on use of CHM for menopausal symptoms found herbs not effective on somatic, vasomotor, or urogenital symptoms. This may be due to a mismatch between the therapeutic methods utilized (Chinese Herbal Medicine) which target specific symptoms related to heat and cold, etc., and the measurement of outcomes (allopathic) (Xu et al., 2012). To best discover the effectiveness of CHM, researchers must develop ways to measure the outcomes it is intended to positively affect. This mismatch may explain why the herbs were not effective on somatic, vasomotor, or urogenital symptoms. There is moderate evidence for short-term effectiveness of yoga for psychological symptoms of menopausal women, but no evidence was found for effectiveness with total menopausal symptoms, somatic symptoms, vasomotor symptoms, or urogenital symptoms (Cramer, Lauche, Langhorst, & Dobos, 2012). Using the Menopausal Quality of Life Questionnaire (MENQOL), investigators found yoga treatment did improve vasomotor symptoms and sexual domain scores on the MENQOL (Reed et al., 2014). A twelve week yoga class plus home practice, compared with usual activity, did not improve vasomotor symptoms or frequency or both, but did reduce insomnia symptoms (Newton et al., 2013). Acupuncture has been studied and is thought to affect serotonin and beta-endorphin activity in the central nervous system, and may thus influence the thermoregulatory center and make it more stable (Andersson & Lundeberg, 1995; Borud, et al., 2009). It has been shown to reduce hot flashes due to natural or artificial menopause greater than natural remission alone, and the evidence suggests this might be due to a general effect of needling, not restricted to acupuncture points (Borud & White, 2010).

Over the past two decades, opinions on menopausal hormone therapy have ranged from considering it a public health measure and "fountain of youth" to beliefs that it increases cancer and cardiovascular risk (Valdiviezo et al., 2013). The Women's Health Initiative (WHI), the largest randomized clinical trial ever conducted, was stopped early as risks outweighed benefits (Rossouw et al., 2002). Debate remains on whether the effect of hormone therapy on the cardiovascular system differs if administered closer to menopause in healthier younger women (the Timing Theory), using lower doses (the Dosage Theory), and whether the hormone formulation alters the risk–benefit profile (Rossouw et al., 2002). The USPSTF recently reviewed hormone therapy for primary prevention of chronic conditions, and systematically reviewed studies published up to November 2011 (Nelson, Walker, Zakher, & Mitchell, 2012) and the Cochrane review of long-term hormone therapy studies published up to February 2012 (Marjoribanks, Farquhar, Roberts, & Lethaby, 2012). Findings from these two comprehensive reviews support that menopausal hormone therapy is not indicated for primary or secondary prevention of CHD. The consensus is that hormone therapy may be used to relieve moderate to severe menopausal symptoms among women who have recently entered menopause.

This is supported by the opinion of the American College of Obstetricians and Gynecologists (ACOG), USPSTF, and the NAMS (Valdiviezo et al., 2013). The consensus is that estrogen and progesterone should be used for a short duration, not longer than 3 to 5 years, because of increased risk of breast cancer and breast cancer mortality associated with prolonged use (ACOG, 2008; NAMS, 2012). Since oral preparations are associated with increased risk of thrombosis owing to effects on proteins in the coagulation pathway, transdermal routes may be recommended since these risks are avoided by first pass hepatic metabolism (Valdiviezo et al., 2013). Currently under study is the use of different estrogens and progestins to reduce potential side effects. Valdiviezo et al. (2013) suggest that, in light of accumulating data, health-care practitioners should feel comfortable prescribing hormone therapy for menopausal symptoms using the lowest dose necessary for the shortest period possible. They also point to the need to implement evidence-based guidelines on reduction of cardiovascular disease through well-proven interventions such as lifestyle changes of exercise, weight management, and blood pressure and lipid control to prevent and reduce cardiovascular disease risk.

Menstrual Changes. Recognizing the importance of clearly defining the stages of reproductive aging and identifying valid, reliable, and clinically useful criteria for the onset of each stage of the menopausal transition, the Stages of Reproductive Aging Workshop (STRAW) was convened in 2001. Based on a consensus of the scientific evidence, STRAW recommended that reproductive life be characterized by seven stages (Soules et al., 2001). Prior to menopause, reproductive life was divided into the reproductive years (three stages) and the transition years (two stages). Postmenopausal years (two stages) follow the final menstrual period. The STRAW group reconvened in 2010 to revisit the reproductive staging criteria. STRAW+10 revised and extended the STRAW recommendations to include additional criteria for defining specific stages of reproductive life (Harlow et al., 2012). The applicatioin of these criteria are intended to improve guidance for classifying ovarian status of midlife women in research, but also in the clinical setting for both clinicians and their patients (Harlow et al., 2012).

Early menopause transition is defined as a persistent difference in consecutive menstrual cycle length of 7 or more days, beginning on average 6 to 8 years before the final menstrual period. Late transition is defined by an episode of 60 or more days of amenorrhea beginning on average 2 years before the final menstrual period (Harlow & Paramsothy, 2011). Although the classic description of the menopausal transition as first marked by increased variability in menstrual cycle lengths followed by increasing frequency of very long cycles until permanent amenorrhea occurs describes the majority of women's experiences, about 15% to 25% of women experience minimal or no change in menstrual regularity prior to their final menstrual period (Harlow & Paramsothy, 2011). The duration and amount of blood loss during the menopausal transition is more variable, and women are most likely to experience excessive blood loss during this reproductive life stage, particularly in the late menopausal transition. Excessive bleeding is often associated with ovulatory cycles, although spotting and bleeding more than 8 days is associated with anovulatory cycles. Heavy bleeding is more commonly found in obese women and women with leiomyomas or uterine fibroids (Harlow & Paramsothy, 2011). Evidence suggests the STRAW stages are applicable to women who smoke and to women of all body sizes; however, it may be difficult to identify onset of the menopause transition and final menstrual period in women with chronic diseases associated with nutritional compromise or in women taking medications that alter hormone profiles. Polycystic ovary syndrome appears to be associated with a later age at menopause, but more research is needed to fully understand how women with this condition experience the menopause transition. Medical conditions and medical treatments that may increase menstrual blood loss or alter menstrual cycles must be considered when treating midlife women (Harlow & Paramsothy, 2011).

Promoting Health

Healthy Behaviors

Poor lifestyle behaviors, including suboptimal diet, physical inactivity, and tobacco use, are leading causes of preventable diseases globally (Mozaffarian et al., 2012). A healthy lifestyle is one of the most basic of health promotion strategies suggested for midlife women (Enjezab, Farajzadegan, Taleghani, & Aflatoonian, 2012). However, research indicates that history and early life events and trajectories influence women's dietary behaviors. Women in midlife often face many challenges related to shifts in family and work-related roles, economic stability, and health status (Moen, 1996; Moen, Dempster-McClain, & Williams, 1992). These shifts, challenges, and multiple roles may affect middle-aged women's physical activity engagement and dietary behaviors, which in turn, can have profound effects upon a woman's overall healthy lifestyle. In a study of perceptions of the relationship of recent life transitions and events to dietary decisions made for themselves and their families, 43 women aged 40 to 64 years suggested that transitions and events related to household structure, health status, phases of motherhood, and shifts in financial and employment status all had the potential to have profound and immediate effects on dietary decisions and resulting dietary behaviors (Enjezab et al., 2012). Women's ability to engage in discussions or joint decision making with other household members regarding food preferences may improve dietary outcomes for women and their family members (Schafer, Schafer, Martin, & Keith, 1999). Building capacity related to dietary selections that benefit health may be an important factor (Brown et al., 2012).

A healthy lifestyle is defined in various ways, but commonalities exist for preventing heart disease, cancer, diabetes, and a number of chronic diseases. As defined by the US National Library of Medicine, National Institutes of Health (2013), a healthy lifestyle includes several behaviors, as indicated in Box 5.4.

Specifics of good nutrition are included in Box 5.5. Chapter 8 also presents information on nutrition.

Box 5.4 Elements of a Healthy Lifestyle

- Do not smoke or use tobacco.
- Get plenty of exercise. Women who need to lose or keep off weight should get at least 60 to 90 minutes of moderate-intensity exercise on most days. To maintain your health, get at least 30 minutes of exercise a day, preferably at least 5 days a week.
- Maintain a healthy weight. Women should strive for a body mass index (BMI) between 18.5 and 24.9 and a waist smaller than 35 inches.
- Get checked and treated for depression, if necessary.
- Women with high cholesterol or triglyceride levels may benefit from omega-3 fatty acid supplements.
- If you drink alcohol, limit yourself to no more than one drink per day.

Good nutrition is important to your heart health, and it will help control some of your heart disease risk factors.

Box 5.5 Guidelines for Healthy Nutrition

- Eat a diet that is rich in fruits, vegetables, and whole grains.
- Choose lean proteins, such as chicken, fish, beans, and legumes.
- Eat low-fat dairy products, such as skim milk and low-fat yogurt.
- Avoid sodium (salt) and fats found in fried foods, processed foods, and baked goods.
- Eat fewer animal products that contain cheese, cream, or eggs.

Read labels, and stay away from "saturated fat" and anything that contains "partially hydrogenated" or "hydrogenated" fats. These products are usually loaded with unhealthy fats.

Several factors are involved in promoting healthy behaviors in midlife women, including attitudes and barriers and benefits. In some cultures, motivating self to engage in physical activity goes beyond knowledge that it would improve health (Im et al., 2011). Issues like making it a routine, finding a companion with whom to exercise, and getting more involved in social interactions were ways to bolster physical activity. At the same time, Mexican American women were found to place their own health below that of family, so engaging in health behaviors took second place or even last place (Berg et al., 2002).

Studies do demonstrate improvement in health indicators when a healthy lifestyle intervention is employed. In a study that evaluated the effectiveness of an integrated personalized health-care system that provided instant biofeedback on measured body weight, BMI, body fat and blood pressure, participants utilizing the system for 8 weeks experienced significantly decreased body weight, BMI, and blood pressure, but participants' perceived health status and health promoting behavior did not significantly improve (Lee et al., 2012). However, two evidence-based programs demonstrated strategies that highlighted the importance of weight reduction and physical activity in the prevention of cardiovascular disease in women and men. The Diabetes Prevention Program randomized participants to receive metformin or an intensive lifestyle intervention that promoted calorie control and 150 min/week of physical activity. Fifty percent of the intensive lifestyle intervention group lost 7% of their body weight and reduced their risk of developing diabetes over 3 years by nearly 60%, which surpassed the findings in the metformin group (Knowler et al., 2002). Another study compared the effects on cardiovascular disease risk factors of an intensive lifestyle-intervention program in diabetic patients with the effects of routine diabetes support and education in a control group. The lifestyle intervention group had greater weight loss and significantly greater improvement in blood glucose, blood pressure, and lipids (Pi-Sunyer et al., 2007).

Employment

Empirical evidence suggests paid employment improves the health of unmarried women and married women who have positive attitudes toward employment (Repetti, Matthews, & Waldron, 1989). There is evidence to support that increased social support from coworkers and supervisors may be an important mediator of the beneficial health effects of employment. At the same time, negative health consequences from employment may be related to overload or multiple role strain (Repetti et al., 1989) or to stress, although midlife women who are employed report better health, lower anxiety, less depression, and greater subjective well-being than women who stay at home (National Association of Social Workers [NASW], 2013). Employment could lead to behavior changes that influence health, such as smoking and drinking alcohol; however, several older studies suggest there is no difference in the prevalence of cigarette smoking between employed and nonemployed women (Waldron, 1980). There are studies that suggest employed young women are more likely to be problem drinkers or heavy drinkers (Hazuda, Haffner, Stern, & Eifler, 1988), but this could be linked to historical trends in women's employment that appear to have contributed to the liberalization of norms concerning women's behavior (Repetti et al., 1989).

Women's work histories are often erratic because of parenting and caretaking duties (Berg, 2011; Berg & Woods, 2009; NASW, 2013). Many women leave work for periods of time, work part-time or take low-paying jobs (Repetti et al., 1989), and this contributes to lost opportunity for income and retirement and health insurance benefits (Berg & Woods, 2009). Therefore, it would seem obvious that income is an important mediating variable and could account for some of the health benefits of employment (Repetti et al., 1989). For example, working mothers might have sufficient income to hire household help, or the added income might relieve some of the stress related to financing family and household needs.

Health promotion related to employment must consider the benefits of employment versus role burden and stress. Since there is evidence to support the health benefits of paid employment for midlife women, it seems prudent for health professionals to be prepared to discuss this with their patients. Social networks and social support have been found to be beneficial to the health of individuals in a variety of ways—reducing mortality rates, improving recovery from serious illness, and increasing use of preventive health practices. Social relationships appear to be particularly important to women (Hurdle, 2001), and many enjoy social relationships with coworkers. At the same time, already working women should be queried about their job satisfaction and the overall multiplicity of roles they occupy simultaneously. Women whose employment is a source of stress might benefit from employment counseling or conflict resolution-type training as a way to reduce the situational stress.

Sexuality

The sexual health of midlife women is frequently overlooked by health-care providers (Taylor & James, 2012). As well, sexual function and sexual well-being in midlife women is multifaceted and not completely understood (Prairie, Scheier, Matthews, Chang, & Hess, 2011). Participation in partnered sexually intimate activities has been associated with more social support and better emotional well-being (Prairie et al., 2011). However, it is also known that midlife women who are sexually active are at risk for both unintended pregnancy and STIs. An important aspect of sexual health promotion is to ascertain women's satisfaction with their sexuality and sexual partner and to initiate conversations with women about contraception, testing for STIs, sexual relationships, and concerns about sexuality. It is also important to initiate conversations about risky behaviors that can lead to unintended pregnancy, STI acquisition, and STI transmission.

Women in troubled relationships need encouragement to seek counseling or resources related to improving their relationships, self-esteem, and choices. Since many primary care providers neglect this aspect of midlife women's health, it is prudent for nurses and advanced practice nurses to make sexual assessments part of their routine examinations.

Caregiving

Social expectations place midlife women in the caregiving role for children, spouses, parents, other relatives, or a mix of these individuals (Berg, 2011). For example, the typical caregiver for older adults is female, married, and middle-aged, and caregiving has been identified as a chronic stressor that may have negative health consequences, restricting personal life, social life, and paid employment (Given & Sherwood, 2006; Navaie-Waliser et al., 2002; Pinquart & Sorensen, 2003). Morbidity, mortality, and financial problems have been associated with informal caregiving, defined as "unpaid provision of assistance to someone who is incapacitated or needs help" (McGuire, Anderson, Talley, & Crews, 2007). Perhaps the most serious long-term effect for female informal caregivers is financial, as this role often results in loss of paid employment, accrual of Social Security benefits, retirement benefits, and health insurance (Berg & Woods, 2009; McGuire et al., 2007).

Health promotion related to caregiving must be multifaceted. Health policy makers must collectively provide accessible, affordable, and innovative support services and programs that remove some of the strain associated with informal caregiving (Berg, 2011). At the same time, caregivers themselves need to be involved in local, regional, and national policy-making endeavors, as their perspective is critical. Clinicians need to be familiar with the Family and Medical Leave Act, which provides some employees as much as 12 weeks of unpaid leave per year and includes job protection (US Department of Labor, 2011). Caregivers need to acquaint themselves with respite resources and utilize them to avoid burnout, psychological and physical stress, and reduce economic consequences of assuming an informal caregiving role. Being aware of the emotional and physical issues related to caregiving is the first step toward reducing the negative impact. The second step is to apply resources, including other family members, to ameliorate some of the negative consequences of caregiving.

Positive Body Image and Healthy Self-Esteem

When women enter middle age, they may need help in acknowledging changes in physical appearance and dealing with associated emotions (American Counseling Association, 2004). The emphasis on youth and beauty in advertising, television, movies, and print media bombard midlife women and constantly remind them they vary from these ideals that prevail in society. The relevance of this issue depends on how much a woman bases her identity on physical/sexual attractiveness (American Counseling Association, 2004). Health promotion related to body image and self-esteem includes women working on obtaining a self-identity that is not dependent on the views of others (Pearlman, 1993). Assertiveness training has been suggested as an important component of bolstering a positive self-image (McBride, 1990). In addition, values clarification can help women realize that incongruence of values with behavior and circumstances can cause conflicting emotions about who they really are. Women with values congruent with their behaviors and circumstances reported feeling happy, satisfied, and comfortable (Howell, 2001). Counselors and clinicians can guide women to think of midlife as a time for reevaluations rather than crisis. One way is to encourage them to be more realistic and to reappraise their goals and their ability to meet them (Mackin, 1995). Often called the journey to self-awareness, this process of reevaluation and separation from externally driven self-image can be extremely rewarding. Nurses and other clinicians are integral to facilitating this process, and can help women learn to value themselves for their inner selves rather than their outer shells (American Counseling Association, 2004).

Mental Health Promotion

Midlife women are stereotyped as irritable, depressed, or moody (National Women's Health Resource Center, 2014). Since midlife is a time of change, both mentally and physically, it's no wonder that moods swing from high to low. Fluctuating hormones are often blamed for mood swings and changes, but no differences have been found in blood levels of reproductive hormones in women with perimenopausal depression and those without (National Women's Health Resource Center, 2014). Therefore, it is prudent to assess depression and anxiety in women who report new onset of symptoms during the menopausal transition. The first step to promoting mental health in midlife women is to determine that the woman does not have clinical anxiety or depression. The next step is to reassure her if these conditions are ruled out. Promoting mental health involves all aspects of health promotion already discussed, and if each of these areas is addressed, it is likely that midlife women will enjoy this time in their lives.

Healthy Relationships

As discussed in the chapters on young women and older women (Chapters 4 and 5 respectively), as well in chapter 16, relationships are key contributors to health. Women at midlife are at varying stages of relationships with children (if they have children), especially since some women who give birth do so at an early age and others give birth in their late 30s and early 40s. As a result, not only do women have varying relationships with their children, they also have varying relationships with their peers. It is not uncommon for a new mother to be peers with a new grandmother.

The mother–daughter relationship has been studied, and blamed, for many problems. Classic psychoanalysis has suggested that this relationship is the foundation for conflict later in life, described by Miller (1986) in her now classic book "Toward a New Psychology of Women." Conflict, however, does not always have to be negative. Miller (1986, p. 132) coined the phrase "waging good conflict," wherein persons in authentic, reciprocal relationships are able to disagree with one another within a safe environment without fear of retribution. Women at midlife have many relationships, and being able to cultivate healthy, growth-fostering relationships are key to both psychological and physiological health (Miller, 1986; Zender & Olshansky, 2012).

Summary

Overall, women at midlife can benefit from living healthy lifestyles. By eating a cardioprotective diet, adding physical activity to their everyday lives, stopping smoking, and drinking alcohol in moderation, midlife women can positively affect their health. Virtually all who recommend nutrition, physical activity, and reducing risk from smoking and alcohol consumption, agree upon healthy lifestyle characteristics for modifiable risk reduction related to cardiovascular disease, diabetes, hypertension and hyperlipidemia, osteoporosis and cancer. Healthy relationships, too, contribute to overall health at midlife.

References

American Cancer Society. (2013a). *What are the key statistics about cervical cancer?* Retrieved from http://www.cancer.org/cancer/cervicalcancer/detailedguide/cervical-cancer-key-statistics

American Cancer Society. (2013b). *Can cervical cancer be prevented?* Retrieved from http://www.cancer.org/cancer/cervicalcancer/detailedguide/cervical-cancer-prevention

American Cancer Society. (2013c). *How are cervical cancers and pre-cancers diagnosed?* Retrieved from http://www.cancer.org/cancer/cervicalcancer/detailedguide/cervical-cancer-diagnosis

American College of Obstetricians & Gynecologists. (2008). ACOG Committee Opinion No. 420, November 2008: Hormone therapy and heart disease. *Obstetrics and Gynecology, 112,* 1189–1192.

American Counseling Association. (2004). *Midlife and beyond: Issues for aging women.* Retrieved from http://www.redorbit.com/news/health/109713/midlife_and_beyond_issues_for_aging_women

American Diabetes Association. (2011). *Data from the 2011 National Diabetes Fact Sheet.* http://www.diabetes.org/diabetes-basics/diabetes-statistics/

American Heart Association. (2012). *Cardiovascular disease & diabetes.* Retrieved from http://www.heart.org/HEARTORG/Conditions/Diabetes/WhyDiabetesMatters/CardiovascularDisease

American Heart Association. (2013). *Hard to recognize heart attack symptoms in women.* Retrieved from https://www.goredforwomen.org/about-heart-disease/symptoms_of_heart_disease_in_women/hard-to-recognize-heart-attack-symptoms/

American Lung Association. (2013). *Women and tobacco use.* Retrieved from http://www.lung.org/stop-smoking/facts-figures/women-and-tobacco-use/

Andersson, S., & Lundeberg, T. (1995). Acupuncture—From empiricism to science: Functional background to acupuncture effects in pain and disease. *Medical Hypotheses, 45*(3), 271–281.

Appleby, P., Beral, V., deGonzalez, A., Colin, D., Franceschi, S., Goodhill, A., . . . Sweetland, S. (2007). Cervical cancer and hormonal contraceptives: Collaborative reanalysis of individual data for 16,573 women with cervical cancer and 35,509 women without cervical cancer from 24 epidemiological studies. *Lancet, 370*(9599), 1609–1621.

Berg, J. (2011). The stress of caregiving in midlife women. *The Female Patient, 36,* 33–36.

Berg, J., Cromwell, S., & Arnett, M. (2002). Physical activity: Perspectives of Mexican American and Anglo American midlife women. *Healthcare for Women International, 23*(8), 894–904.

Berg, J., & Woods, N. (2009). Global women's health: A spotlight on caregiving. *Nursing Clinics of North America, 44,* 375–384. doi:10.1016/j.cnur.2009.06.003

Berkel, L., Poston, W., Reeves, R., & Foreyt, J. P. (2005). Behavioral interventions for obesity. *Journal of the American Dietary Association, 105*(5 Suppl. 1), S35–S43.

Borud, E., Alraek, T., White, A., Fonnebo, V., Eggen, A. E., Hammar, M., . . . Grimsgaard, S. (2009). The acupuncture on hot flushes among menopausal women (ACUFLASH) study, a randomized controlled trial. *Menopause, 16*(3), 484–493.

Borud, E., & White, A. (2010). A review of acupuncture for menopausal problems. *Maturitas, 66,* 131–134. doi:10.1016/j.maturitas.2009.12.010

Broom, A., Kirby, E., Sibbritt, D., Adams, J., & Refshauge, K. (2012). Use of complementary and alternative medicine by mid-age women with back pain: A national cross-sectional survey. *BMC Complementary and Alternative Medicine, 12,* 98. doi:10.1186/1472-7882-12-98

Brown, N., Smith, K., & Kromm, E. (2012). Women's perceptions of the relationship between recent life events, transitions, and diet in midlife: Findings from a focus group study. *Women's Health, 52*(3), 234–251.

Brown, W., Heesch, K., & Miller, Y. (2009). Life events and changing physical activity patterns in women at different life stages. *Annals of Behavioral Medicine, 37,* 294–305.

Canadian Cancer Society. (2013). *Risk reduction strategies for breast cancer.* Retrieved from http://www.cancer.ca/en/cancer-information/cancer-type/breast/risks/risk-reductionstrategies

Centers for Disease Control and Prevention. (2000). Retrieved from http://www.cdec.gov/diabetes/statistic/surv199/chap2/table23.htm

Centers for Disease Control and Prevention. (2010). *Healthy People 2010*. US Department of Health and Human Services. Office of Disease Prevention and Health Promotion. Healthy People 2020. Washington, DC. http://www.cdc.gov/nchs/healthy_people/hp/2010.htm.

Centers for Disease Control and Prevention. (2011). Vital signs: Prevalence, treatment and control of hypertension—United States, 1999–2002 and 2005–2008. *Morbidity and Mortality Weekly Report*, *60*(4), 103–108.

Centers for Disease Control and Prevention. (2013). *High blood pressure facts*. Retrieved from http://www.cdc.gov/bloodpressure/facts.htm

Chlebowski, R. (2002). Breast cancer risk reduction: Strategies for women at increased risk. *Annual Review of Medicine*, *53*, 519–540.

Chlebowski, R., Collyar, D., Somerfield, M., & Pfister, D. (1999). American Society of Clinical Oncology technology assessment on breast cancer risk reduction strategies: Tamoxifen and raloxifene. *Journal of Clinical Oncology*, *17*(6), 1939. doi:10-46/annurev.med.53.082901.103925

Cobb, M. (1998). CNS role in women's health promotion and maintenance in a collaborative practice. *Clinical Nurse Specialist*, *12*(3), 112–116.

Cramer, H., Lauche, R., Langhorst, J., & Dobos, G. (2012). Effectiveness of yoga for menopausal symptoms: A systematic review and meta-analysis of randomized controlled trials. *Evidence-Based Complementary and Alternative Medicine*. doi:10.1155/2012/863905

Cromwell, S., & Berg, J. (2006). Lifelong physical activity patterns of sedentary Mexican American women. *Geriatric Nursing*, *27*(4), 209–213.

Dennerstein, L., Lehert, P., Koochaki, P., Graziottin, A., Leiblum, S., & Alexander, J. (2007). A symptomatic approach to understanding women's health experiences: A cross-cultural comparison of women aged 20 to 70 years. *Menopause*, *14*(4), 688–696.

Department of Health and Human Services. (2004). *Health consequences of smoking: A report of the surgeon general*.

Devries, K., Mak, J., Bacchus, L., Child, J., Falder, G., Petzold, M., . . . Watts, C. (2013). Intimate partner violence and incident depressive symptoms and suicide attempts: A systematic review of longitudinal studies. *PLoS Medicine*, *10*(5), e1001439. doi:10.1371/journal.pmed.1001439

Enjezab, B., Farajzadegan, Z., Taleghani, F., & Aflatoonian, A. (2012). Internal motivations and barriers effective on the healthy lifestyle of middle-aged women: A qualitative approach. *Iranian Journal of Nurse Midwifery Research*, *17*(5), 390–398.

Food and Drug Administration. (2013). *Diabetes prevention*. Retrieved from http://www.fda.gov/ForConsumers/ByAudience/for PatientAdvocates/diabetesInfo/ucm30

Ford, E., Zhao, G., Li, C., Pearson, W., & Mokdad, A. (2008). Trends in obesity and abdominal obesity among hypertensive and nonhypertensive adults in the United States from 1999–2008. *International Journal of Obesity*, *35*, 736–743.

Gillies, C., Abrams, K., Lambert, P., Cooper, N., Sutton, A., Hsu, R. T., & Khunti, K. (2007). Pharmacological and lifestyle interventions to prevent or delay type 2 diabetes in people with impaired glucose tolerance: Systematic review and meta-analysis. *British Medical Journal*, *334*(7588), 299–308. doi:10.1136/bmj.39063.689375.55

Giorgino, F., Leonardini, A., & Laviola, L. (2013). Cardiovascular disease and glycemic control in type 2 diabetes: Now that the dust is settling from large clinical trials. *Annals of the New York Academy of Sciences*, *1281*, 36–50. doi:10.1111/nyas.12044

Given, B., & Sherwood, P. (2006). Family care for the older person with cancer. *Seminars in Oncology Nursing*, *22*(1), 43–50.

Glauber, H., & Karnieli, E. (2013). Preventing type 2 diabetes mellitus: A call for personalized intervention. *Permanente Journal*, *17*(3), 74–79.

Go, A., Mozaffarian, D., Roger, V., Benjamin, E., Berry, J., Borden, W. B., . . . Turner, M. B. (2013). Heart disease and stroke statistics—2013 update: A report from the American Heart Association. *Circulation*, *127*, e6–e245.

Harlow, S. D., Gass, M., Hall, J. E., Lobo, R., Maki, P., Rebar, R. W., . . . de Villiers, T. J.; for the STRAW +10 Collaborative Group (2012). Executive summary of the Stages of Reproductive Aging Workshop+10: Addressing the unfinished agenda of staging reproductive aging. *Menopause: The Journal of the North American Menopause Society*, *19*(4), 1–9. doi: 10.1097/gme.0b013e31824d8f40

Harlow, S., & Paramsothy, P. (2011). Menstruation and the menopause transition. *Obstetrics & Gynecology Clinics of North America*, *38*(30), 595–607. doi:10.1016/j.ogc.2011.05.010

Hazuda, H., Haffner, S., Stern, M., & Eifler, C. (1988). Effect of acculturation and socioeconomic status on obesity and diabetes in Mexican Americans. The San Antonio Heart Study. *American Journal of Epidemiology*, *128*(6), 1289–1301.

Health Resources and Services Administration. (2004). *Women's Health USA 2004.*

Holahan, C., Holahan, C., Powers, D., Hayes, R., Marti, N., & Ockene, J. (2011). Depressive symptoms and smoking in middle-aged and older women. *Nicotine and Tobacco Research, 13*(8), 722–731. doi:10.1093/ntr/ntr066

Horner, M., Ries, L., Krapcho, M., Neyman, N., Aminou, R., Howlader, N., . . . Edwards, B. K. (2009). *SEER cancer statistics review, 1975–2006.* Bethesda, DD: National Cancer Institute.

Howell, L. (2001). Implications of personal values in women's midlife development. *Counseling and Values, 46,* 54–65.

Hurdle, D. (2001). Social support: A critical factor in women's health and health promotion. *Health & Social Work, 26*(2), 72–79.

Idso, C. (2009). Sexually transmitted infection prevention in newly single older women: A forgotten health promotion need. *Journal of Nurse Practitioners, 5*(6), 440–446.

Im, E., Lee, B., Chee, W., & Stuifbergen, A. (2011). Attitudes toward physical activity of white midlife women. *Journal of Obstetric, Gynecologic & Neonatal Nursing, 40*(3), 312–321.

Kanis, J. (on behalf of the World Health Organization Scientific Group). (2008). *Assessment of osteoporosis at the primary health care level: 2008 Technical report.* University of Sheffield, UK: WHO Collaborating Center.

Kessler, R., Chiu, W., Demler, O., & Walters, E. (2005). Prevalence, severity, and comorbidity of twelve-month DSM-IV disorders in the National Comorbidity Survey Replication (NCS-R). *Archives of General Psychiatry, 62*(6), 617–627.

Klein, S., Burke, L., Bray, G., Blair, S., Allison, D. B., Pi-Sunyer, X., . . . Eckel, R. H. (2004). Clinical implications of obesity with specific focus on cardiovascular disease. A statement for professionals from the American Heart Association Council on nutrition, physical activity, and metabolism. *Circulation, 110,* 2952–2967.

Knowler, W., Barrett-Connor, E., Fowler, S., Hamman, R. F., Lachin, J. M., Walker, E. A., & Nathan, D. M. (2002). Reduction in the incidence of type 2 diabetes with lifestyle intervention or metformin. *New England Journal of Medicine, 346*(6), 393–403.

Knowler, W., Fowler, S., Hamman, R., Christophi, C. A., Hoffman, H. J., Brenneman, A. T., . . . Nathan, D. M.; Diabetes Prevention Program Research Group. (2009). 10-year follow-up of diabetes incidence and weight loss in the Diabetes Prevention Program Outcomes Study. *Lancet, 374*(9702), 1677–1686. doi:http://dx.doi.org.ezproxy2.library.arizona.edu/10.1016/S0140-6736(09)61457-4

Kones, R. (2013). *Primary prevention of coronary heart disease: Integration of new data, evolving views, revised goals, and role of rosuvastatin in management. A comprehensive survey.* Retrieved from http://www-ncbi-nlm-nih-gov.ezproxy1.library.arizona.edu/pmc/articles/PMC3140289

Kumanyika, S., Obarzanek, E., Stettler, N., Bell, R., Field, A. E., Fortmann, S. P., . . . Hong, Y. (2008). Population-based prevention of obesity: The need for comprehensive promotion of healthful eating, physical activity, and energy balance: A scientific statement from American Heart Association council on epidemiology and prevention, interdisciplinary committee for prevention. *Circulation, 118*(4), 428–464.

Lawrence, C. (2008). Healthy practices: Exercise intervention. In C. Fogel & N. F. Woods (Eds.), *Women's health care in advanced practice nursing.* New York, NY: Springer.

Lee, H., Kang, K., Park, S., Ju, S., Jin, M., & Park, B. (2012). Effect of integrated personalized health care system on middle-aged and elderly women's health. *Healthcare Informatics Research, 18*(3), 199–207. doi:10.4258/hir.2012.18.3.199

Mackin, J. (1995). Women, stress and midlife. *Human Ecology Forum, 23*(4), 20–22.

Mango, V., & Frishman, W. (2006). Physiologic, psychologic, and metabolic consequences of bariatric surgery. *Cardiology Reviews, 14*(5), 232–237.

Manson, J., Greenland, P., LaCroix, A., Stefanick, M. L., Mouton, C. P., Oberman, A., . . . Siscovick, D. S. (2002). Walking compared with vigorous exercise for the prevention of cardiovascular events in women. *New England Journal of Medicine, 347*(10), 716–725.

Marjoribanks, J., Farquhar, C., Roberts, H., & Lethaby, A. (2012). Long term hormone therapy for perimenopausal and postmenopausal women. *Cochrane Database Systematic Review, 7,* CD004143.

Massad, L., Einstein, M., Huh, W., Katki, H. A., Kinney, W. K., Schiffman, M., . . . Lawson, H. W. (2013). 2012 Updated consensus guidelines for the management of abnormal cervical cancer screening tests and cancer precursors. *Journal of Lower genital Tract Disease, 17*(5), S1–S27.

McBride, M. (1990). Autonomy and the struggle for female identity: Implications for counseling women. *Journal of Counseling & Development, 69,* 22–26.

McGuire, L., Anderson, L., Talley, R., & Crews, J. (2007). Supportive care needs of Americans: A major issue for women as both recipients and providers. *Journal of Women's Health, 16*(6), 784–789.

Miller, J. B. (1986). *Toward a new psychology of women.* Boston, MA: Beacon Press.

Moen, P. (1996). A life course perspective on retirement, gender, and well-being. *Journal of Occupational Health Psychology, 1*(2), 131–144.

Moen, P., Dempster-McClain, D., & Williams, R. (1992). Successful aging: A life-course perspective on women's multiple roles and health. *American Journal of Sociology, 97*(6), 1612–1638.

Mosca, L., Benjamin, E., Berra, K., Bezanson, J., Dolor, R., Lloyd-Jones, D. M., . . . Wenger, N. K. (2011). Effectiveness-based guidelines for the prevention of cardiovascular disease in women—2011 update: A guideline from the American Heart Association. *Circulation, 123,* 1243–1262.

Mozaffarian, D., Afshin, A., Benowitz, N., Bittner, V., Daniels, S. R., Franch, H. A., . . . Zakai, N. A. (2012). Population approaches to improve diet, physical activity, and smoking habits: A scientific statement from the American Heart Association. *Circulation, 126,* 1514–1563.

Nachtigall, L., & Nachtigall, M. (2004). Menopausal changes, quality of life, and hormone therapy. *Clinical Obstetrics & Gynecology, 47,* 485–488. doi:10.1097/00003081-200406000-00023

National Association of Social Workers. (2013). *Women at midlife.* Retrieved from http://www.naswdc .org/diversity/women/032503.asp

National Institute for Health Care Management Foundation. (2005). *Women's health prevention and promotion.* Washington, DC: Author.

National Institutes of Health Consensus Development Panel. (1991). Gastrointestinal surgery for severe obesity. *Annals of Internal Medicine, 115*(12), 956–961.

National Institute of Mental Health. (2013a). *Women and mental health.* Retrieved from http://www.nimh .nih.gov/health/topics/women-and-mental-health/index.shtml

National Institute of Mental Health. (2013b). *Depression.* Retrieved from http://www.nimh.nih.gov/ health/topics/depression/index.shtml

National Institute of Mental Health. (2013c). *Anxiety disorders.* Retrieved from http://www.nimh.nih.gov/ health/topics/anxiety-disorders/index.shtml

National Osteoporosis Foundation. (2013). *2013 Clinician's guide to prevention and treatment of osteoporosis.* Washington, DC: National Osteoporosis Foundation.

National Women's Health Resource Center. (2014). *Your mental health at midlife.* Retrieved from http:// www.healthywomen.org/content/article/your-mental-health-midlife?context

Navaie-Waliser, M., Spriggs, A., & Feldman, P. (2002). Informal caregiving: Differential experiences by gender. *Medical Care, 40*(12), 1249–1259.

Nelson, H. D., Tyne, K., Naik, A., Bougatsos, C., Chan, B.K., & Humphrey, L. (2009). Screening for breast cancer: An update for the US Preventive Services Task Force. *Annals of Internal Medicine, 151* (10), 716–826. doi: 10.7326/0003-4819-151-10-200911170-00008

Nelson, H., Walker, M., Zakher, B., & Mitchell, J. (2012). Menopausal hormone therapy for the primary prevention of chronic conditions: A systematic review to update the US Preventive Services Task Force recommendations. *Annals of Internal Medicine, 157,* 104–113.

Newton, K. M., Reed, S. D., Guthrie, K. A., Sherman, K. J., Booth-LaForce, C., Caan, B., . . . LaCroix, A. Z. (2013). Efficacy of yoga for vasomotor symptoms: A randomized controlled trial. *Menopause: The Journal of the North American Menopause Society, 21*(4), 1–8.

North American Menopause Society. (2004). Treatment of menopause-associated vasomotor symptoms: Position statement of The North American Menopause Society. *Menopause, 11,* 11–33. doi:10.1097/01.GME.0000108177.85442.71

North American Menopause Society. (2012). The 2012 hormone therapy position statement of The North American Menopause Society. *Menopause, 19,* 257–271. doi: 10.1097/gme.ob013e31824b970a

Pearlman, S. (1993). Late mid-life astonishment: Disruptions to identity and self-esteem. In N. D. Davis, E. Cole & E. D. Rothblum (Eds.), *Faces of women and aging* (pp. 1–23). Binghamton, NY: The Haworth Press.

Peirson, L., Fitzpatrick-Lewis, D., Ciliska, D., & Warren, R. (2013). Screening for cervical cancer: A systematic review and meta-analysis. *Systematic Reviews, 2,* 35–49. doi:10.1186/2046-4053-2-35

Peters, K., Kochanek, K., & Murphy, S. (1998). Deaths: Final data for 1996. *National Vital Statistics Report, 47*(9), 1–100.

Pinquart, M., & Sorensen, S. (2003). Differences between caregivers and noncaregivers in psychological health and physical health: A meta-analysis. *Psychology and Aging, 18*(2), 250–267.

Pi-Sunyer, X., Blackburn, G., Brancati, F., Bray, G. A., Bright, R., Clark, J. M., . . . Yanovski, S. Z. (2007). Reduction in weight and cardiovascular disease risk factors in individuals with type 2 diabetes: One-year results of the look AHEAD trial. *Diabetes Care, 30*(6), 1374–1383.

Prairie, B., Scheier, M., Matthews, K., Chang, C., & Hess, R. (2011). A higher sense of purpose in life is associated with sexual enjoyment in midlife women. *Menopause, 18*(8), 839–844.

Ravdin, P., Cronin, K., Howlader, N., Berg, C. D., Chlebowski, R. T., Feuer, E. J., . . . Berry, D. A. (2007). The decrease in breast cancer incidence in 2003 in the United States. *New England Journal of Medicine, 356,* 1670–1674.

Reed, S. D., Guthrie, K. A., Newton, K. M., Anderson, G. L., Booth-LaForce, C., Caan, B., . . . LaCroix, A. Z. (2014). Menopause and quality of life: Randomized clinical trial of yogal, exercise, and omega-3 supplements. *American Journal of Obstetrics and Gynecology, 210,* 1–11.

Repetti, R., Matthews, K., & Waldron, I. (1989). Employment and women's health. Effects of paid employment on women's mental and physical health. *American Psychologist, 44*(11), 1394–1401.

Roger, V., Go, A., Lloyd-Jones, D., Benjamin, E., Berry, J., Borden, W. B., . . . Turner, M. B. (2012). Heart disease and stroke statistics—2012 update: A report from the American Heart Association. *Circulation, 125*(1), e2–e220.

Rossouw, J., Anderson, G., Prentice, R., LaCroix, A. Z., Kooperberg, C., Stefanick, M. L., . . . Ockene, J. (2002). Risks and benefits of estrogen plus progestin in healthy postmenopausal women: Principal results from the Women's Health Initiative randomized controlled trial. *Journal of the American Medical Association, 288,* 321–333.

Sabolsi, M., Solomon, C., & Manson, J. (2001). The middle years. In G. Beckles & P. Thompson-Reid (Eds.), *Diabetes and women's health across the life stages: A public health perspective* (pp. 105–145). Atlanta, GA: US Department of Health and Human Services, Centers for Disease Control and Prevention, National Center for Chronic Disease Prevention and Health Promotion, Division of Diabetes Translation.

Schafer, R., Schafer, E., Martin, D., & Keith, P. (1999). Marital food interaction and dietary behavior. *Social Science & Medicine, 48*(6), 787–796.

Sievert, L., & Obermeyer, C. (2012). Symptom clusters at midlife: A four-country comparison of checklist and qualitative responses. *Menopause, 19*(2), 133–144. doi:10.1097/gme.0b013e3182292af3

Simon, G., Ludman, E., Linde, J., Operskalski, B. H., Ichikawa, L., Rohde, P., . . . Jeffery, R. W. (2008). Association between obesity and depression in middle-aged women. *General Hospital Psychiatry, 30*(1), 32–39. doi:10.1016/j.genhosppsych.2007.09.001

Simon, G., Ormel, J., VonKorff, M., & Barlow, W. (1995). Health care costs associated with depressive and anxiety disorders in primary care. *American Journal of Psychiatry, 152,* 352–357.

Soules, M., Sherman, S., Parrott, E., Rebar, R., Santoro, N., Utian, W., & Woods, N. (2001). Executive summary: Stages of Reproductive Aging Workshop (STRAW). *Fertility & Sterility, 76*(5), 874–878.

Taylor, D., & James, E. (2012). Risks of being sexual in midlife: What we don't know can hurt us. *The Female Patient, 37,* 17–20.

Thompson, P., Buchner, D., Pina, I., Balady, G. J., Williams, M. A., Marcus, B. H., . . . Wenger, N. K. (2003). Exercise and physical activity in the prevention and treatment of atherosclerotic cardiovascular disease: A statement from the council on Clinical Cardiology (Subcommittee on Exercise, Rehabilitation, and Prevention) and the Council on Nutrition, Physical Activity, and Metabolism (Subcommittee on Physical Activity). *Circulation, 107*(24), 3109–3116.

Towfighi, A., Zheng, L., & Ovbiagele, B. (2009). Sex-specific trends in midlife coronary heart disease risk and prevalence. *Archives of Internal Medicine, 169,* 1762–1766.

Towfighi, A., Zheng, L., & Ovbiagele, B. (2010). Weight of the obesity epidemic: Rising stroke rates among middle-aged women in the United States. *Stroke, 41,* 1371–1375.

Turk, M., Tuite, P., & Burke, L. (2009). Cardiac health: Primary prevention of heart disease in women. *Nursing Clinics of North America, 44,* 315–325.

US Department of Health and Human Services, Office on Women's Health. (2013). *Frequently asked questions.* Retrieved from http://www.womenshealth.gov

US Department of Health and Human Services, Substance Abuse and Mental Health Services Administration. (1999). *Mental health: A report of the surgeon general—executive Summary.* Rockville, MD: US Department of Health and Human Services, Substance Abuse and Mental Health Services administration, Center for Mental Health Services, National Institutes of Health, National Institute of Mental Health.

US Department of Labor. (2011). *Family and medical leave act.* Retrieved from http://www.dol.gov/dol/topic/benefits-leave/fmla.htm

US National Library of Medicine, National Institutes of Health. (2013). Retrieved from http://nim.nih.gov/medlineplus/ency/article/007188.htm

US Preventive Services Task Force. (2009). Screening for breast cancer. Recommendation statement. *Annals of Internal Medicine, 151,* 716–726.

US Preventive Services Task Force. (2012, July). Retrieved from http://www.uspreventiveservicestask-force.org/uspstf/gradespost.htm

Utian, W. (2005). Psychosocial and socioeconomic burden of vasomotor symptoms in menopause: A comprehensive review. *Health and Quality of Life Outcomes, 3*, 47–58.

Valdiviezo, C., Lawson, S., & Ouyang, P. (2013). An update on menopausal hormone replacement therapy in women and cardiovascular risk. *Current Opinion in Endocrinology, Diabetes, & Obesity, 20*(2), 148–155. doi:10.1097/MED.0b013e32835ed58b

Wadden, T., Butryn, M., & Wilson, C. (2007). Lifestyle modification for the management of obesity. *Gastroenterology, 132*(6), 2226–2238.

Waldron, I. (1980). Employment and women's health: An analysis of causal relationships. *International Journal of Health Services, 10*, 435–454.

Xu, L., Jia, M., Salchow, R., Kentsch, M., Cui, X., Deng, H., . . . Kluwe, L. (2012). Efficacy and side effects of Chinese Herbal Medicine for menopausal symptoms: A critical review. *Evidence-Based Complementary and Alternative Medicine.* doi:10.1155/2012/568106

Yoon, U., Kwok, L., & Magkidis, A. (2013). Efficacy of lifestyle interventions in reducing diabetes incidence in patients with impaired glucose tolerance: A systematic review of randomized controlled trials. *Metabolism, 62*, 303–314.

Zender, R., & Olshansky, E. (2012). The biology of caring: Researching the health effects of stress response regulation through relational engagement. *Biological Research in Nursing, 14* (4), 419–430.

Chapter 6

Healthy Aging for Women

Heather M. Young and Barbara Cochrane

Major Issues and Challenges for Older Women

Adults over 65 are the fastest expanding segment of the population, growing by 15.1% in the past decade, compared with the total population growth of 9.7%, with women comprising 56.9% of the over 65 population (US Census, 2011). With greater longevity, there are three generations of women included in the 65-and-older age group, contributing to increasing heterogeneity of social circumstance, functional ability, and life priorities. The population of older women is becoming more diverse, and despite awareness of the issue, health disparities persist and are exacerbated by issues of gender, race, and class.

The lives of women over 65 reflect many paths and priorities—many are still working, some are still caring for children and grandchildren, others are caring for their parents and older relatives or their partners, some are pursuing a new vocation or avocation. Health trajectories are also highly variable, as genetics as well as behaviors and risks from across the life span influence expression of health and illness. Older women face common transitions of late life, including retirement, changes in living situation and social roles, and changes in health and function.

Each woman makes her own meaning of her transitions and goes through an adjustment process as these transitions intensify and increase with older age. There are seven elements to healthy transition processes (Meleis, Sawyer, Im, Messias, & Schumacher, 2010): redefining meanings; modifying expectations; restructuring life routines; developing new knowledge and skills; maintaining whatever continuity is possible in identity, relationships, and environment; being open to exploring new choices; and finding opportunities for personal growth. Older women and health-care professionals can anticipate many of the psychological and physiological changes that come with age, and can partner to optimize health and function, and increase meaningful engagement and well-being.

Some of the conditions presented in this chapter are also mentioned in Chapter 5 on Women at Midlife. There is some overlap in risk factors for certain conditions, but it is important to emphasize these conditions at both stages of a woman's life.

Common Health Conditions and Treatment Approaches

Mental Health

Older women have accumulated a lifetime of experience, and many have developed effective coping strategies as they face new challenges, building resilience that can mitigate the impact of late-life transitions and losses. In comparison with younger women, older women report higher self-ratings of successful aging and greater resilience, even with worse physical health and lower cognitive functioning. Better reported physical health is associated with greater resilience and lower depression (Jeste et al., 2013). A recent study comparing older widows with married women noted no difference in daily and general well-being and comparable use of time between the groups, supporting the hypothesis of strong capacity to adapt to major life changes among older women (Hahn, Cichy, Almeida, & Haley, 2011). Older adults, in general, have a greater match between their aspirations and their achievements than younger groups, and the level of subjective well-being increases with age. Consistent with greater advantage, in late life, men are more content with their successes and report greater happiness than women, and White older adults report greater life satisfaction than Black and Hispanic older adults (George, 2010).

Depression

Depression is a common, and often underrecognized and undertreated, mental health condition in late life. Women are more likely than men to report depressive symptoms, and health disparities in depression between Black and White older women are associated with both lower socioeconomic status and physical health (Spence, Adkins, & Dupre, 2011). Depression is frequently accompanied by other physical health conditions, functional disabilities, and higher health-care utilization (Barry, Allore, Guo, Bruce, & Gill, 2008; Barry, Soulos, Murphy, Kasl, & Gill, 2013), and, for women in particular, it is also associated with poor health in a partner (Ayotte, Yang, & Jones, 2010). A number of interacting risk factors are associated with late-life depression, including genetics, neurobiological changes, stress, insomnia, chronic illness, and functional decline. Protective factors also come into play, including education and higher socioeconomic status, social engagement, and spirituality. Depression prevention is a cornerstone in comprehensive health promotion for older women, through screening, education, building problem-solving skills, engaging in group support, life review, and behavioral activation. A variety of treatments, alone or in combination, are effective, yet often underused. Therapies that have demonstrated efficacy and effectiveness include behavioral, cognitive–behavioral, problem solving, brief psychodynamic, and life review approaches (Fiske, Wetherell, & Gatz, 2009).

Anxiety

Anxiety is another underrecognized condition that can have an important role in the ability of an older woman to engage socially, manage chronic illness, and optimize function. In a recent systematic review, the authors identified the prevalence of anxiety between 1.2% and 15% in community samples and up to 28% in clinical settings. Importantly, the prevalence of anxiety symptoms (feeling fearful, tense, or shaky/nervous) is considerably higher, from 15% to over 50%, among both community and clinical samples (Bryant, Jackson, & Ames, 2008). Anxiety can occur as part of a symptom cluster, along with depression, pain, and fatigue. Cognitive–behavioral therapy and relaxation training are the most effective approaches for treating generalized anxiety disorders (Ayers, Sorrell, Thorp, & Wetherell, 2007).

The stereotype of **loneliness** in old age oversimplifies the issues of social connectedness and isolation. With increasing age, social roles change and networks shift, with losses associated with the death of close family members and friends. At the same time, retirement brings the opportunity for greater social involvement and the possibility of new relationships and ties that matter. More important than the actual size of the social network is the older woman's perception of isolation, with loneliness very weakly correlated with number and frequency of social contacts. Older women with social connections who perceive that they have strong support report better health. However, social disconnectedness and perceived isolation are associated with poorer physical health, and perceived isolation is associated with poor mental health (Cornwell & Waite, 2009).

Cognitive Aging

Cognition usually refers to multiple domains of thinking, including attention, language, learning, memory, visuospatial skills, and executive functioning skills such as judgment, problem solving, decision making, goal-setting, planning, and judgment (Daviglus et al., 2010). Although some decrements in cognition-related skills, such as performance of complex tasks and memory, are associated with aging, these changes often do not affect daily functioning or even meet definitions of mild cognitive impairment (Segal, Qualls, & Smyer, 2011). In fact, many older women have sufficient cognitive reserve, resilience, and capacity to compensate for these changes, such that neither mild cognitive impairment (MCI) nor dementia is considered a part of normal aging (Daviglus et al., 2010).

By definition, MCI is an age-related condition associated with measurable and noticeable change in at least one domain of thinking, but without impact on daily activities (Alzheimer's Association, 2013). In some cases, MCI will progress to Alzheimer disease (AD) or other dementias, but the majority of MCI cases have relatively stable trajectories over time (Xie, Mayo, & Koski, 2011) and warrant careful evaluation for possible treatable causes.

Delirium is an acute and usually reversible cognitive condition, which may include symptoms of confusion, lethargy, aggression, or hallucinations. This condition occurs in between 10% and 50% of hospitalized older adults, and is an emergency associated with increased mortality and morbidity. Common risk factors include restraints, medications, pain, malnutrition, constipation, and iatrogenic events. Treatment involves identifying and addressing the underlying cause.

Age-related dementias in older persons are of four main types—AD, vascular, frontotemporal, and dementia with Lewy bodies. AD, the most common dementia, is characterized by progressive decline in cognitive function over multiple domains, including memory and at least one additional area of learning, orientation, language, comprehension, and judgment. In addition, this deterioration in cognitive function with AD is severe enough to interfere with daily life (Daviglus et al., 2010). Women's lifetime risk of AD at age 65 has been estimated to be nearly one in five (17.2%), and risk increases dramatically with age. Rates of AD in women are twice as high as those in men, but these differences are largely due to women's longer life expectancy (Alzheimer's Association, 2013). A complete geriatric and neuropsychiatric evaluation is indicated with suspected dementia to rule out preventable causes of cognitive change and, if dementia is diagnosed, to identify the type and treatment options.

The progressive deterioration of cognitive functioning in AD and its profound impact on morbidity and mortality prompted a recent consensus development conference at the National Institutes of Health to identify the state of the science on preventing AD and cognitive decline (Daviglus et al., 2010). Although the scientists concluded that there is insufficient evidence for clear modifiable risk factors, medications, or dietary therapy to prevent or slow this decline, research is planned or in progress on such promising therapies as antihypertensive medications, omega-3 fatty acids, physical activity, and cognitive engagement activities. Similarly, although no AD treatments available today slow or stop brain cell death and neuronal malfunction, studies of both pharmacological and nonpharmacological therapies are underway (Alzheimer's Association, 2013), and evidence-based interventions for behavioral symptoms of the disease (acetylcholinesterase inhibitors, memantine, caregiver education and support) are available. At this time, effective management of AD includes judicious use of currently available therapies, management of comorbidities, access to and participation in ongoing activities and programs, and appropriate training and coordination of the interprofessional health-care team and involved informal caregivers (Alzheimer's Association, 2013; Gies & Lessick, 2009; Teri, Logsdon, & McCurry, 2005).

Physical Health

Postmenopausal Health

Postmenopausal health concerns in older women generally focus on major causes of morbidity and mortality rather than gynecological or genitourinary concerns. Past notions of restoring premenopausal levels of circulating estrogens long-term to prevent cardiovascular and other chronic diseases and maintain gynecological health have been largely abandoned since findings from the landmark Women's Health Initiative Hormone Therapy Trials failed to support the use of hormone (replacement) therapy in disease prevention (Manson et al., 2013). Genitourinary health, however, remains an important consideration in older women's lives.

Although not a disease, urinary incontinence (UI), which is much more prevalent in older women than older men, is considered a common geriatric syndrome that is associated with significant functional and quality of life concerns, falls, social isolation, and admission to long-term care facilities (Goode, Burgio, Richter, & Markland, 2010; Hawkins et al., 2011). Depending on how it is defined, diagnosed or undiagnosed UI may be prevalent in well over 60% of older women, who may experience stress (the most common type, defined as urine leakage on exertion, such as coughing, sneezing, lifting, or laughing), urge (unable to get to the toilet in time, associated with overactive bladder syndrome), mixed, or other types of UI (Minassian, Devore, Hagan, & Grodstein, 2013; Wallner et al., 2009). In addition to risk factors such as age, race/ethnicity (higher risk in White women than in African Americans or Asians), parity, hysterectomy, and menopause, modifiable risk factors for UI include certain drugs (e.g., systemic hormone therapy, diuretics, angiotensin-converting enzyme inhibitors, sedatives, caffeine), obesity, poor control of diabetes, mobility impairment, constipation, frequent urinary tract infections, and sleep apnea (Goode et al., 2010). Treatment of UI, therefore, involves addressing these modifiable factors, as well as behavioral therapies (e.g., pelvic floor training with Kegel exercises, bladder training with voiding schedules), lifestyle changes (e.g., decreased caffeine intake, fluid management, and weight management), pharmacological treatments (antimuscarinic agents such as oxybutynin and possibly vaginal estrogen at low doses), pessaries, and surgery.

Cardiovascular Health

In the past, cardiovascular disease (CVD) was considered a disease of older men, and our knowledge of CVD risk factors, prevention strategies, and treatments was based on research primarily with men. However, over two decades of rigorous CVD research with women has now provided an evidence base for CVD health guidelines for women. For example, we now know that even with observational study findings to the contrary, randomized controlled clinical trials of postmenopausal hormone therapy do not support its use in preventing CVD in women, and may even increase their risk of stroke (Manson et al., 2013). In addition, annual "red dress" campaigns, such as the American Heart Association's "Go Red for Women" and the National Heart, Lung, and Blood Institute's "The Heart Truth" initiatives have resulted in a near-doubling in the rate of awareness of CVD as the leading cause of death in women from 1997 to 2012, a profound reversal from the notion in 1997 that breast cancer was the leading cause of death (Mosca et al., 2013). Cardiovascular mortality rates in both women and men have decreased steadily since 2000—a decline attributed to greater utilization of evidence-based medical therapies and lifestyle and environmental changes in risk factors—but rates have been higher in women than in men since the mid-1980s (Go et al., 2013). Women have their first CVD event, typically angina, approximately 10 years later than men. Women's older age and accompanying complex comorbidity at that first event undoubtedly contribute to their increased early death rates from myocardial infarction compared with men (Go et al., 2013).

Risk factors for coronary heart disease (age, family history, hypertension, diabetes, smoking, abdominal aortic aneurysm, chronic kidney disease, hypercholesterolemia) are very similar in women and men, although diabetes confers a greater risk for women, essentially negating the 10-year advantage in CVD development (Mosca, Barrett-Connor, & Wenger, 2011; Mosca, Benjamin, et al., 2011). Cigarette smoking rates remain lower in women than men, and physical activity rates are higher, but physical activity rates in both men and women have shown a decline over the last two decades, probably related in part to increasing rates of overweight and obesity. A history of certain pregnancy-related factors, such as preeclampsia, gestational diabetes, and pregnancy-induced hypertension, also increase women's risk for later CVD (Mosca, Benjamin, et al., 2011). Detailed evidence-based guidelines for prevention of heart disease in women are now based on a careful evaluation of their risk and very specific risk categories that address various risk factors (Hsia et al., 2010; Mosca, Benjamin, et al., 2011).

When women experience a myocardial infarction, they often have what are described as atypical symptoms (unusual fatigue, shortness of breath, weakness, jaw ache), sometimes occurring a month or more before the acute event, but the more typical chest discomfort is the most frequent acute symptom in both women and men (DeVon, Ryan, Ochs, & Shapiro, 2008; McSweeney et al., 2013). Of particular importance, women's delay in obtaining diagnosis and treatment of symptoms of coronary heart disease—including failure to contact emergency medical services for transportation—can both limit treatment options and increase adverse outcomes, such as heart failure and limited activity tolerance (Go et al., 2013; Sullivan et al., 2014).

More women than men have strokes each year, and women have a higher lifetime risk of stroke than men, but this difference is due largely to women's longer life expectancy and the increased risk of stroke with age (Bushnell et al., 2014; Go et al., 2013). Although incidence rates of stroke have declined in both women and men, this decline may be smaller in women. Awareness of stroke risk factors (e.g., hypertension, hypercholesterolemia, diabetes, migraine with aura, atrial fibrillation, history of pregnancy-related complications, oral contraceptive or postmenopausal hormone therapy, smoking, physical inactivity, obesity) and warning symptoms (facial drooping, arm weakness, difficulty with speech, numbness, problems with dizziness or balance, vision symptoms, and severe headache) is limited in both women and men, particularly in racial/ethnic minorities (Bushnell et al., 2014). Findings that only about 50% to 60% of women or men know at least one risk factor or one symptom and an undoubtedly related 16-hour median delay from symptom onset to hospital arrival puts most women well outside the 3-hour eligibility window for thrombolytic treatment and increases risk of adverse outcomes (Bushnell et al., 2014). Stroke is a leading cause of profound, long-term disability, and although more research is needed on stroke in women, population-based and individual efforts to increase awareness of stroke prevention and recognition in women can have an important impact on health and health-care costs. Prevention strategies, such as blood pressure and diabetes management, improved lifestyle habits, low-dose aspirin, and judicious use of anticoagulants for atrial fibrillation, are important points to discuss in health-care encounters.

Hypertension, an important risk factor for coronary heart disease and stroke, is more prevalent in men than women up to age 55, but the prevalence is greater in women 65 years of age and older, with the highest rates among African American women (Mosca et al., 2011). In fact, rates of hypertension among African American women are increasing, and mortality rates in this population are well over twice those in White women. Among individuals with hypertension, over 80% are aware of their diagnosis, and 75% are taking antihypertensives, but rates of controlled hypertension are somewhat lower (Go et al., 2013).

The United States Preventive Services Task Force (USPSTF) recommends aspirin prophylaxis according to the following guideline: women ages 55 to 79 years old when the potential benefit of a reduction in ischemic stroke outweighs the potential harm of an increase in gastrointestinal hemorrhage. They concluded that there is insufficient evidence to support aspirin prophylaxis for women over age 80 (US Preventive Services Task Force, 2009).

Bone Health

An important clinical concern for older women is bone health—preventing and treating bone loss, joint immobility, bone-related pain, falls, and fractures. In fact, osteoporosis, fall prevention, and arthritis are basic considerations during any clinical or home-based health-care encounter with older women.

Osteoporosis (decreased bone mass and deterioration of bone matrix) and osteopenia (low bone mass that does not meet criteria for osteoporosis) are nearly twice as prevalent in older women compared with older men, in part related to decreased postmenopause estrogen, which has a role in preventing bone resorption (breakdown of bone) and bone formation (Office of Research on Women's Health in Collaboration with the NIH Coordinating Committee on Research on Women's Health, 2010). Osteoporosis itself is not generally associated with symptoms or health decline, but the bone loss does increase risk for fractures from vertebral compression and falls. Appropriate care to promote bone health in older women includes identifying risk for fracture and reducing modifiable risk factors through diet, lifestyle, and, if indicated, pharmacological therapy (North American Menopause Society, 2010). Adequate nutritional calcium (1,200 mg daily) and vitamin D (800–1,000 IU daily), with supplementation as needed, are recommended for all older women to prevent osteoporosis (National Osteoporosis Foundation, 2013). For prevention and treatment, bisphosphonates (e.g., alendronate, ibandronate, risedronate) are now commonly prescribed. These preparations have convenient dosing schedules (daily to monthly) and fewer disease risks compared with postmenopausal estrogen therapy (Manson et al., 2013), an earlier mainstay of osteoporosis treatment.

At age 50, one in three women will have a hip fracture in their remaining years (National Osteoporosis Foundation, 2013). These fractures, usually related to falls with low bone density, are associated with an increased risk of repeat fracture, morbidity, and mortality in older women. Only about 40% of women with hip fracture will return to their prefracture level of independence, a finding that helps explain why fall prevention in older adults has become such an important health promotion priority (National Osteoporosis Foundation, 2013). Because of pain, decreased height, and kyphosis, vertebral fractures may be even more common than hip fractures in older women and can have a marked impact on their functional health, particularly activities that involve bending and reaching.

Prevention of falls is a high-priority health promotion strategy related to bone health in older women. Fractures that result from falls increase a woman's risk for further decline. A comprehensive evaluation of risk factors for falls, including previous falls, fear of falling, a hazardous home environment, medications with psychotropic side effects, low bone density, and decreased vitamin D, can be carried out by various health-care professionals in multiple settings. The National Council on Aging, as well as other federal, professional, and lay organizations, have sponsored or supported a National Fall Prevention Awareness Day on the first day of fall each year to promote public awareness of their risk of falls and strategies for minimizing this risk.

Arthritis is reported by more women than men ages 65 and older (56% compared with 45%, respectively) and may include nearly 100 different medical conditions (Federal Interagency Forum on Aging-Related Statistics, 2012). Osteoarthritis, also described as degenerative joint disease, is the most common of these conditions and involves deterioration in joint cartilage with associated stiffness and pain. Estrogen is known to play a role in joint health, consistent with the higher prevalence of osteoarthritis among women in their postmenopausal years (Tanamas et al., 2011). Medications such as nonsteroidal anti-inflammatory drugs, surgery, and a variety of complementary and alternative medicine strategies can address some of the pain associated with arthritis, but weight loss and judicious physical activity remain important interventions for its symptoms.

Cancer

Cancer is the second leading cause of death in individuals 65 years and over (Federal Interagency Forum on Aging-Related Statistics, 2012). The incidence of cancer increases by age, such that about 77% of all cancers are diagnosed in individuals age 55 years or over (American Cancer Society, 2014). The lifetime risk of cancer in women is approximately one in three, with the risk of breast cancer higher than that of any other type of cancer. Lung cancer remains the leading cause of cancer death in women, and although mortality rates have started to decline, the start of this decline is much more recent in women than in men (2003 versus 1991, respectively), probably because of differences in smoking patterns over the past several decades (American Cancer Society, 2014). Besides lung and breast cancer, which account for approximately 41% of all cancer deaths in women, the

American Cancer Society estimates other leading causes of cancer death in women to be colorectal, pancreatic, and ovarian cancer. Screening patterns for cancer in older women differ somewhat from those in younger women, in part because of age-related increased risks (with more frequent screening), but also—as women approach ages 85 and older—because the risks and benefits of screening may change.

At older ages, the workup of false-positive findings can be unnecessarily disruptive, whereas true-positive findings can raise questions about the utility of undergoing treatments that may negatively impact the quality of a woman's remaining years (American Cancer Society, 2013). Although screening recommendations for older women are often identified, the choice to screen should be made carefully between an individual woman and her health-care provider, taking into consideration her cancer risk factors, quality of life, and individualized goals and priorities.

Strategies for preventing cancer in older women include a lifestyle focus on healthy eating, physical activity, weight management, smoking cessation, and sun protection (American Cancer Society, 2013). Cancer is now a chronic disease, in that cancer survivorship—even in older women—is often an achievable treatment goal. An important priority for meeting survivorship goals in older women is to ensure that health disparities in access to cancer treatment and follow-up by racial/ethnic minority women are minimized (Bhargava & Du, 2009).

Immune System

Changes in both cell-mediated and humoral immunity are considered a normal, age-related change. A normal decrease in T cells is associated with decreased interleukin-2 production and reduced response to novel antigens. At the same time, there is an increase in memory T cells, which results in greater secretion of interleukin-10, leading to a suppressed cellular immunity response. In the humoral immune system, B cells are also affected by age, with less activation and proliferation leading to less ability to prevent infection due to slowed antibody production. These normal changes with age are exacerbated by environmental factors and by psychological stress. There is growing recognition of the autonomic and neuroendocrine pathways that link stress to reduced immunity (Hawkley & Cacioppo, 2004). Important observations have linked loneliness, grief, and the chronic stress of caregiving to reductions in immune function by accelerating changes typically associated with age. At the same time, the ability to manage stress and to restore function through adequate high-quality sleep can offset these detriments.

Sensory Changes (Vision/Hearing/Taste)

Sensory loss with age is a common experience and has significant implications for social interaction, geographic reach, and mental health. Women are generally less affected by hearing changes than men, yet 17% of women between the ages of 60 and 69 have bilateral hearing loss, with prevalence doubling with each ensuing decade of life. The most common cause of severe hearing loss is a history of occupational exposure to a noisy environment (Gopinath et al., 2009). Vision impairment follows a similar pattern, with 18% of adults over 70 reporting some impairment, and the prevalence increasing to almost 40% by age 90 and older. Cataracts are the leading cause of low vision at 50%. There are health disparities in causes of blindness, with macular degeneration accounting for 54% of the cases among Whites, and cataracts and glaucoma accounting for over 60% of blindness cases among Blacks (Eye Diseases Prevalence Research Group, 2004).

It is important to screen for both vision and hearing impairment, as early detection and treatment can be very effective in minimizing implications for function for a number of sensory conditions. Many visual acuity changes can be treated with corrective lenses. Several approaches can improve hearing, including hearing aids, amplifiers, assistive telephone attachments, computer-assisted communication, and decoders that allow for viewing closed caption television. A number of age-related conditions influence vision, including cataracts, glaucoma, macular degeneration, and diabetic retinopathy. Early identification can target prevention and treatment, such as glycemic control for diabetics, treating intraocular pressure for persons with glaucoma, and completing cataract surgery to remove and replace diseased lenses. (Wallhagen, Strawbridge, Shema, Kurata, & Kaplan, 2001).

Women are often affected by the sensory losses of partners. A recent study revealed that women whose husbands had hearing impairment suffered greater threats to physical, psychological, and social well-being than for men with wives with hearing loss (Wallhagen, Strawbridge, Shema, & Kaplan, 2004). This highlights the social and functional implications of changes in the health of a partner, and recognizes the ripple effect of disability on the family.

Changes in taste and chemosensory perception are also common with age, particularly the ability to identify sour (citric acid) and bitter (quinine-hydrochloride) compared with younger adults. The ability to taste sweet and salt remains similar across the life span. In addition to physiological changes, certain medications can have an effect, such as by introducing a metallic taste. These changes have implications for appetite and enjoyment of food, potentially leading to less dietary variation, weight loss, and poorer nutrition (Nordin et al., 2007).

Functional Health

Functional status becomes increasingly relevant with age, including the ability to manage both basic activities of daily living (e.g., bathing, dressing, toileting) and instrumental activities of daily living (e.g., housework, meal preparation, medications, finances). Illnesses and injuries can have both temporary and permanent implications for function, and home environments can provide both supports for function (single level, accessible bathrooms) and can pose challenges for independent living (high maintenance requirements, unsafe conditions). The ability to care for oneself and manage one's home is an aggregation of functional abilities, and significant impairments in being able to manage can lead to the need for additional help in the home or might necessitate a move to another setting such as to join other family or to a retirement or assisted living community.

For the past several decades, both longevity and prevalence of disability among older adults have improved. While the oldest old (> 80 years old) women are continuing to improve in overall functional status, there is evidence that the positive trend for improvement over the entire older population is reversing, according to recent comparative data on the prevalence of disability in the United States. Older adults over 80 continue to show lower levels of disability than previous cohorts; those between 70 and 79 are holding at previous rates; and for the first time, younger older adults (age 60–69) are experiencing higher rates of disability. Older persons of color and those who are overweight/obese are at particular risk for faster declines in functional status (Seeman, Merkin, Crimmins, & Karlamangla, 2010). Related trends also raise important issues for health promotion—along with greater functional decline, the prevalence of overweight/obesity and the number of chronic diseases have increased, and the amount of physical activity has significantly decreased when comparing age-similar populations of older adults between 1988 and 1994 with those between 1999 and 2004.

Functional status can be affected by pain, which can limit mobility, energy, and motivation. In a community sample of older adults, 28% reported having pain, and 17% reported limitations in function as a result of pain. Health disparities in pain experience and treatment exist, both by gender and ethnicity—older women reported more pain than men, and Blacks and Hispanics were at higher risk for severe pain than Whites. Pain is also associated with having more chronic conditions, psychological distress, and lower socioeconomic status (Reyes-Gibby, Aday, Todd, Cleeland, & Anderson, 2007). These findings support the need for comprehensive assessment of pain, particularly in association with mental health and function to assure appropriate prevention and proactive management of chronic conditions.

Promoting Healthy Behaviors

The concepts of successful aging and healthy aging have gained much greater attention in the past decade, and there are many definitions of these terms. Pruchno, Wilson-Genderson, and Cartwright (2010) have proposed a working definition that includes both objective and subjective aspects. The objective component includes having few chronic diseases, possessing functional ability, and having little or no pain. The subjective component is the older adult's perspective on how well he or she is aging and their view of their life as positive (Pruchno et al., 2010). Healthy aging is both a goal and a process that optimizes well-being and function and effectively manages chronic conditions. There are many opportunities for health promotion throughout the life span to contribute to health in late life, and efforts to improve health can yield results whenever they begin. A recent survey identified a number of goals shared by older adults—to live independently, spend time with family, get in shape, pursue hobbies, travel, and deepen friendships (AARP, 2011). These aspirations are supported by effective health promotion, optimizing function, and managing chronic conditions. Chronic diseases are highly modifiable with adjustments in lifestyle that increase physical activity, improve nutrition, enhance safety, and minimize risks.

Increasingly, older adults are turning to online resources to manage their health, with over half of adults between 65 and 74 and over 30% of those over 75 using the Internet, and 68% of these actively seeking health information at this source (Pew Research Center, 2012). Cohort trends indicate a growing desire to take control of one's health and to participate more actively in health-care decisions. Health-care professionals play a vital role in assisting the older woman to synthesize and interpret the vast amount of data available on health conditions, and to engage her in using relevant information to make appropriate health-care and behavioral choices. Core healthy behaviors, such as improving strength, endurance, balance, and nutrition while limiting negative behaviors, contribute to improvements in many chronic conditions and can significantly delay or mitigate functional and cognitive decline.

Physical Activity

The benefits of physical activity are well known to outweigh the risks in most individuals. Several positive health effects are evident, including improved quality of life, well-being, strength, flexibility, endurance, and chronic disease management. The regularity of exercise is more important than the type of exercise. Certain exercise approaches yield specific benefits, for example, Tai Chi improves balance and functional mobility, and reduces fear of falling, while elastic resistance bands can increase strength. Longitudinal studies over a decade of observation have substantiated the positive effects of physical activity on mortality, lowering risk from all causes, independent of age, smoking, comorbid conditions, body mass index, and baseline activity level (Wolin, Glynn, Colditz, Lee, & Kawachi, 2007). This effect was lessened for women over 75 and in poor health at baseline (Gregg et al., 2003).

Even though benefits of physical activity are well understood, the vast majority of older women do not engage in regular exercise of any kind. An important health promotion intervention involves motivating and coaching older women to adopt healthy patterns of activity. In particular, approaches that explore motivation, facilitating factors, and barriers can be useful in promoting action. Physical activity guidelines for older women are similar to those for younger populations, taking into account aerobic fitness and targeting moderate-intensity aerobic activity at 150 minutes per week, muscle strengthening, reducing sedentary behavior, and managing risk (Nelson et al., 2007).

Healthy Eating

A healthy diet for older women follows the same principles as in the case of other populations. Specifically, including a variety of fruits, vegetables, grains, low-fat or nonfat dairy, fish, legumes, poultry, and lean meats. Weight control remains an issue in late life, with optimal health occurring when energy intake matches energy needs, including regular physical activity. Certain foods should be limited, including those with high saturated fat and cholesterol, and excessive salt and alcohol (Krauss et al., 2000). Multivitamins are generally not indicated unless nutritional intake and dietary variety is inadequate. Oral health can influence nutritional status, so preventive dental care is important into late life, including removing plaque and bacteria daily with regular removal of calcified plaque. Dry mouth can be a side effect of medications and an age-related change that affects taste and enjoyment of food. Saliva stimulants can improve this condition. More detailed information on oral health is presented in Chapter 9.

Food is a social experience as well as a nutritional effort. Older women living alone are at risk for nutritional compromise when they limit preparation of complete meals and reduce dietary variety. Preventive efforts can include pursuing opportunities to share meals with others to improve appetite and enjoyment, and increase exposure to menu options.

Substance Issues

Moderate alcohol use in women is considered to be about 15 g of alcohol per day, approximately one drink. Longitudinal study of moderate drinking has established that moderate drinkers have better mean cognitive scores than nondrinkers and no significant associations between higher levels of drinking and increased cognitive decline (Stampfer, Kang, Chen, Cherry, & Grodstein, 2005). At the same time, excessive alcohol use among older women is a relatively hidden issue with underdetection by providers, with estimates of 12% of older women exceeding recommended guidelines (Blow, 2000). When combined with medications that interact with alcohol and/or affect cognition and balance, alcohol intake can pose additional risks. Excessive intake can exacerbate chronic illnesses and increase depression and the likelihood of accidents or injuries. Routine annual screening for alcohol use is recommended (Blow, 2000).

A growing issue among older women is misuse and abuse of prescription drugs and nonmedical use of prescription drugs, including opioids and other psychoactive medications. In general, approximately one quarter of older adults use psychoactive medications with abuse potential. Estimates suggest that up to 11% of older women misuse drugs, and those who are socially isolated, have a history of mental health problems or substance abuse, and have access to prescription drugs are more likely to misuse or abuse medications (Simoni-Wastila & Yang, 2006). Both screening and treatment are currently insufficient for older women, yet this is a problem that is likely to become more prevalent in the future, with the aging of the baby boom population. This increase is partly attributable to the larger number of older adults in coming years, but also to the relatively greater exposure to and tolerance of alcohol and drugs in this generation. Projections of future demand for substance abuse treatment suggests a fourfold increase over two decades, from 1.7 million in 2000 to 4.4 million in 2020 (Gfroerera, Penneb, Pembertonb, & Folsomb, 2003). This upcoming public health issue will require improved approaches to both screening and treatment for older women.

Medication Management

Prescription drugs are a major element of managing chronic illnesses, and older women consume the majority of prescription medications. With each additional chronic condition, the size and complexity of the medication regimen can increase, amplifying the potential for drug interactions and side effects from these therapeutic agents. In a recent study of drug use among community-dwelling older adults, 81% were taking at least one prescription medication, 42% took at least one over-the-counter (OTC) medication, and 49% used a dietary supplement. Importantly, 29% took at least five prescription medications, and more than half concurrently took more than five prescription, OTC, and dietary supplements. The number of medications increased with age, and women took more than men overall. In analyzing the potential for major drug–drug interactions, about 4% were at risk for this problem, half involving nonprescription medications (Qato et al., 2008).

In addition to taking more medications than younger populations, older adults also experience changes in pharmacokinetics and pharmacodynamics that alter drug metabolism and increase the probability of an adverse drug reaction. While adverse drug reactions can result in exacerbations of illness, disability, and higher health-care utilization, they are also the most preventable of all iatrogenic illnesses (Kane, Ouslander, & Abrass, 2003). The chance of an adverse drug reaction increases when multiple prescribers are involved and when the older woman has an inadequate understanding of the drug indications, administration guidelines, and side effects. Adverse drug events are also a significant cause of hospitalization, estimated to result in almost 100,000 hospitalizations annually, most commonly unintentional overdoses of four major medication classes: warfarin, insulin, oral antiplatelet agents, and oral hypoglycemic agents (Budnitz, Lovegrove, Shehab, & Richards, 2011). Given the frequency of a few commonly occurring problems, health promotion efforts among older adults can be targeted to improve outcomes related to the medications of highest risk to older women.

Most of the emphasis in medication management has been on managing polypharmacy, with efforts to reduce the number and interactions among medications. Another important issue is the potential for undertreatment of older adults according to evidence-based guidelines, where the full benefits of medications are not adequately deployed in managing chronic conditions, particularly among the oldest old (Simon et al., 2005). This issue is compounded when the older woman has multiple comorbidities, with each disease carrying evidence-based guidelines that need to be reconciled with one another to determine the optimum regimen to manage her simultaneous conditions holistically (McCormick & Boling, 2005).

Medication safety also involves having system supports such as legible labels, clear instructions, and, when needed, assistive devices/technologies to remind and track taking medications. While greater financial support is now available for medications for older adults, financial considerations can still contribute to difficulty adhering to medication recommendations, and warrant exploration at the level of prescribing and care coordination. Optimal medication management involves assuring appropriate prescribing that considers the older woman's goals, her comorbid conditions, age-related changes, relevant evidence-based guidelines, and potential drug interactions, while attempting to minimize the total medication burden. While this is no easy task, it is a crucial health promotion and prevention activity.

Cognitive and Social Engagement

Cognitive health and function involves a variety of elements, including memory, the ability to make decisions, emotional engagement, motivation, and creativity. A longitudinal population-based study of older adults revealed that intellectual stimulation in the form of cognitive activity and social engagement provides a protective effect for developing dementia (Wang, Karp, Winblad, & Fratiglioni, 2002). Among women, in particular, friendships form a vital source of support that enhances and promotes health (Aday, Kehoe, & Farney, 2006). More extensive detail on the importance of healthy relationships is presented in Chapter 16. The strongest predictor of positive subjective well-being in late life is perceived social support—being confident that if one needed emotional or instrumental support, it would be there. Having a partner is most strongly associated with greater subjective well-being, followed by relationships with friends. Interestingly, interactions with adult children have a weak relationship with subjective well-being (George, 2010).

Older adults are increasingly using computers and engaging in Internet activities. With the aging of baby boomers, this trend is likely to continue at a faster pace. Online opportunities abound for information-seeking and connecting with others, and can be a useful resource when mobility is more limited. A growing body of research is examining utilization and outcomes of technology for older adults. In general, researchers have noted a variety of positive effects of technology, including enhancing independence, building social networks, improving psychological well-being, and empowering older adults (Xie, 2003).

Philosophers and scientists have long recognized the importance of meaning in life, and have connected a sense of purpose and personal value to mental health. Making meaning is a highly personal endeavor and can include spirituality, a sense of belonging, making contributions to one's network and community, and many other expressions. Meaningful involvement is associated with happiness, physical and cognitive function, and reduced mortality (Menec, 2003). The ability to interpret one's experiences in the context of broader meaning is associated with better mental health and can reduce the impact of traumatic experiences (Krause, 2007). Organizations such as AARP recognize the importance of ongoing engagement in defining one's own future according to one's values and preferences, and provide resources to guide thinking in this area. For example, the AARP website provides an interactive opportunity to look at "Life Reimagined," facilitating self-assessment and identification of options to increase engagement and satisfaction with one's life (AARP, 2013).

Health-Care and Living Situation Planning/Advance Directives

Older women face a number of potentially life-altering situations, including transitions in health, ability to care for oneself, loss of partner and close friends, and relocation of family members. Thoughtful planning for one's potential health trajectory and changes in social network can obviate a crisis when conditions suddenly change. Because health, living situation, and available supports are inextricably linked in determining optimal decisions, it is useful to view these discussions as a series of conversations with relevant parties, including health-care providers, family, and friends.

Health-care providers can facilitate and encourage the necessary conversations and make referrals to appropriate resources. Discussions about health-care and living situation preferences typically take place over a long period, as new information becomes available and values and preferences come to the fore. It is useful to begin with a conversation about the older woman's likely health trajectory, given her current health and functional status, presence of chronic conditions, and risk factors. At the same time, exploring values and preferences about decision making, living situation, and health-care interventions can provide a framework for thinking through options at a later time. It is helpful to identify relevant family and friends and suggest that she discuss her preferences and expectations with those whom she wants involved in her health and care. Health-care decisions and preferences should be documented in the form of a health-care advance directive and both a health-care and financial durable power of attorney, a vehicle that authorizes another person to make decisions should the older woman become incapacitated. These forms can be prepared using state-appropriate forms available on the Internet, notarized, and copies distributed to those who need to know the decisions. A helpful resource in considering and communicating one's care preferences is the Five Wishes document, available from http://www.agingwithdignity.org/ Aging with Dignity (2013).

Once the older woman has a sense of possible future needs and has identified her values and priorities, it is helpful to explore community resources to meet those needs. For example, if she desires to stay in her own home as long as possible, it would be useful to identify resources in such areas as transportation, home repair, and personal assistance in the home. Should she be considering a move to a retirement community, it is helpful to visit local possibilities and determine which one is the best fit, as waiting lists are long and having a deposit on file expedites the move should circumstances change. Often, those who plan to move delay the decision because of logistical barriers, such as the energy it takes to sort and pack; such logistics can be handled by companies that specialize in assisting with moves for older adults. Helpful sources of information about community resources include the Area Agency on Aging, in every county, providing senior information and referral, and also AARP, providing a wide array of guides and information to assist with planning. Geriatric case managers are valuable resources available to assess needs, identify potential resources, and facilitate accessing appropriate supports. They can be hired for consultation or for ongoing care management, and can be located through the national membership organization, the National Association of Professional Geriatric Care Managers (http://www.caremanager.org/).

Screening/Vaccinations

Older women are a heterogeneous group when it comes to health, with varied chronic conditions and functional abilities. With multiple comorbidities, guidelines for

TABLE 6.1	Vaccination Recommendations for Older Women
Recommendation	Frequency
Influenza vaccine	Annually
Pneumococcal vaccine	Once after 65
Tetanus, diphtheria, acellular pertussis (TDAP)	Once
Tetanus–diptheria booster	Every 10 years
Herpes zoster	Once after 60

Data from American Geriatrics Society. (2014). Clinical guidelines and recommendations. *GeriatricsCareOnline. Org.* Retrieved from http://www.geriatricscareonline.org/ProductStore/clinical-guidelines-recommendations/8/

screening and treatment become more complex. Primary care providers are in a unique position to create a plan to approach care that incorporates health promotion, monitoring, prevention, and management of chronic and acute conditions. Both general and condition-specific guidelines for care of older adults can be readily accessed at the www. GeriatricsCareOnline.org website, sponsored by the American Geriatrics Society. This valuable resource provides a synthesis of current recommendations for older women. Federal websites provide detailed information about coverage under Medicare and eligibility for preventive services (see http://www.medicare.gov and http://www.healthcare. gov). Selected resources are provided in Tables 6.1 through 6.3. Table 6.1 summarizes vaccination recommendations. Table 6.2 addresses preventive services available through Medicare for older women. Table 6.3 highlights areas for screening that are specific for older adults and provide a guide for risk assessment and identifying opportunities for education and further evaluation.

TABLE 6.2	Screening and Preventive Services for Older Women under Medicare Coverage	
Preventive Service	What Is Covered	Who Medicare Covers
Alcohol misuse counseling	Screening and up to four face-to-face counseling sessions/year	All who are not alcohol-dependent
Breast cancer	Breast examinations, mammograms, digital technology	Over 40
Cardiovascular screening	Cholesterol, lipid, triglyceride	All
Cervical and vaginal cancer	Pap tests with pelvic examinations	All women
Colorectal cancer	Fecal occult blood, flexible sigmoidoscopy, screening colonoscopy	Over 50
Depression screening	One per year	All
Diabetes screening	Fasting blood glucose	At risk

TABLE 6.2	USPSTF Grade A B Recommendations for Adolescents and Women *(continued)*	
Preventive Service	**What Is Covered**	**Who Medicare Covers**
HIV screening	HIV test	At risk
Obesity screening/ counseling	Screening and face-to-face counseling	BMI >30
Osteoporosis	**Bone de**nsity test	At risk
Tobacco use cessation	Up to eight face-to-face counseling sessions/year	Use tobacco, not diagnosed with illness caused by tobacco
Vaccinations	Flu/pneumococcal/hepatitis B	All flu/pneumococcal/at risk for hepatitis B

Data from Centers for Medicare & Medicaid Services. (2014). What medicare covers. Retrieved from http:// www.medicare.gov/what-medicare-covers/index.html

TABLE 6.3	Screening for Geriatric Health Issues
Recommendation	**Frequency**
Falls	Annually
Incontinence	Annually
Cognitive status	If symptomatic
Depression	Annually
Vision	Annually
Hearing	Annually
Nutrition	Obtain weight each visit and height annually; calculate BMI
Mistreatment	Question with clinical suspicion
Safety and pre-venting injury	Check smoke detectors and carbon monoxide detectors, check water heater temperature, use sun protection, test driving skills, wear seat belts, complete advance directives, and determine health-care proxy

Data from American Geriatrics Society. (2014). Clinical guidelines and recommendations. GeriatricsCareOnline. Org. Retrieved from http://www.geriatricscareonline.org/ProductStore/clinical-guidelines-recommendations/8/

Promoting Healthy Body Image, Self-Esteem, and Relationships

Aging and Body Image

Aging in Western society is fraught with negative stereotypes about changes in appearance. A scan of women's magazines in the popular press reveals positive images of youth and vibrancy, and the availability of many products to disguise or fight the effects of age on hair color, skin tone, body shape, and general appearance. In the United States, plastic surgery is readily available, and in 2012, Americans spent over $11 billion on cosmetic surgeries and minimally invasive cosmetic procedures such as Botox injections. Among adults over 55, there were over 360,000 cosmetic surgical procedures (including face-lifts, breast augmentation) and over 3.6 million cosmetic procedures (such as chemical peels, laser varicose vein removal) (American Society of Plastic Surgeons, 2014).

Indeed, older women share a common concern about body appearance with younger women, a dissatisfaction that remains stable across the life span until one reaches advanced age. Yet older women place less and less importance on body shape, weight, and appearance as they age, becoming less troubled by issues of body image (Tiggeman, 2004). Into late life, approximately 80% of women continue to control their weight and a similar proportion (about 4%) as younger women meet criteria for eating disorders (Mangweth-Matzek et al., 2006).

Self-esteem is a complex reflection of how one sees oneself, including one's physical, emotional, and cognitive capacity, in relation to others and to societal expectations. A large cohort study of over 3,600 individuals aged 25 to 104 revealed that self-esteem increases during young and middle adulthood, peaks around 60 years of age, and then declines in the following decades (Orth, Trzesniewski, & Robins, 2010). While women had lower self-esteem than men early in life, this difference disappears with age. Across ethnic groups, Whites and Blacks had similar trajectories in the first half of life, with greater declines in late life among Blacks. Overall self-esteem was higher for those with more education, but trajectories were similar over the life span. The greatest threats to self-esteem for older women are changes in socioeconomic status and physical health.

Sexuality

Sexuality, intimacy, and the desire for loving relationships remain a life force for many older women. The most important predictor of sexual activity for older women is the availability of a sexual partner, a challenge that many face when they outlive a spouse or partner. A number of additional factors influence the expression of sexuality in late life, including past sexuality and preferences, relationship quality, physical health, the presence of chronic conditions, medications, self-esteem, life stressors, and emotional well-being. Normal changes with age generally do not affect sexuality, and the ability to experience an orgasm is unchanged with age. Physiological changes associated with lowered estrogen affecting vaginal blood flow can make intercourse uncomfortable. The prevalence of sexual activity declines with age from over 60% of older women between 57 and 64, to 40% among those between 65 and 74, to less than 20% for women between 75 and 85. Among women who are sexually active, approximately half report a problem that is bothersome to them, most commonly low desire (43%), difficulty with vaginal lubrication, (39%), and inability to have an orgasm (34%). These concerns are more likely among women with chronic health conditions (Lindau et al., 2007). Despite the presence of these issues, this study reported that only 22% of women over 50 have discussed sex with their physician. Because several troublesome issues are reversible, it is important to complete a thorough sexual history to guide possible treatments, such as estrogen cream or lubricants. Other issues that affect sexuality, such as relationship quality, could be addressed in other ways, potentially including counseling.

Promoting Healthy Relationships

Social engagement is a fundamental element of healthy aging. With age, the social circle changes, with losses to the social network and the opportunity to form new relationships. Older women experience several phases in their lives, moving in late life through transitions of retirement, changing family demands, and living situation. With greater longevity, there are opportunities for reinvention and developing new interests and relationships, adding new members to the network, even at a time of losses of partners and long-standing friends. Women have a gender advantage in forming and maintaining relationships, with skills and abilities to nurture meaningful connections across the life span. Women are commonly at the center of nurturing family connectivity, and seek and maintain friendships over longer periods of time than men do, forming close relationships and actively engaging in friendships through life.

Relationships take on new meaning with age, as one becomes more dependent on others for assistance. Family and friends can contribute in different ways to the social network. For example, friends may be able to provide greater social support and intimacy, while families contribute to mental health by providing instrumental support (Siu & Phillips, 2002). For older women, despite loss of friends due to death and moving, friendships remain relevant and active, even among the very old. A study of late-life friendship revealed that older women had regular interaction with at least one friend at least weekly, with half having contact daily. The average social network size for these older women was 11.8, with African American women identifying 13.5 friends, and White women naming 10.2. Most (60%) had recently made a new close friend. Compared with earlier in their lives, over half had made younger (> 25 years), cross-generational friends, and several reported their first cross-ethnic friendships (Armstrong, 2000).

Living Situation

Older women commonly experience transitions in family and their living situation as they survive partners and have greater longevity. Older women have a greater likelihood of becoming widows than older men, particularly by the time they reach the ninth decade. Among those over 85, 35% of men are widowed compared with 78% of women (He, Sengupta, Velkoff, & DeBarros, 2005). While some women live with family or in communal settings, about 40% live alone, compared with 19% of older men (He et al., 2005). Projections suggest that this trend will only increase so that by 2020, 85% of those living alone will be women, with approximately 50% of this group aged 75 years or older. This pattern holds across ethnic and racial groups; however, women who are non-Hispanic White or African American are more likely to live alone, while older Hispanic or Asian women are more likely to reside with other relatives (He et al., 2005).

While most women overcome the social isolation that living alone can bring through other relationships, the economic consequences of early widowhood can be significant. In general, older women have not accrued the same level of pension and social security benefits that their male counterparts have in late life. The death of a spouse can significantly reduce household income and net worth. This is particularly true for minority women, with African American and Hispanic women having a substantially higher risk of poverty in late life (Angel, Jimenez, & Angel, 2007). Thus, financial planning and promotion of both education and work experience for women across the life span is crucial for economic security in late life. Older women are commonly the source of support and assistance for others, yet are more likely to be alone without available support in late life. It is ironic that women commonly provide care to others across the life span, but are more likely to have to pay for their own care when they need assistance as they grow older (Weitz & Estes, 2001).

In general, the majority of older adults state a preference to live in their own homes throughout their lives, yet in fact about 98% of older women live in community settings (Federal Interagency Forum on Aging-Related Statistics, 2012). The ability to remain in one's home depends on a number of factors, including availability of the necessary human, physical, and financial resources to maintain a household and to support function and health. Homes appropriate for a growing family may no longer support aging in place, particularly if housekeeping and maintenance demands are high, accessible transportation is not readily available, and neighborhood safety is a concern. The ability to live independently throughout life is frequently enabled by external supports, such as meals, personal care, and transportation. Adult day health or adult day care can augment and provide necessary supports in the form of meals, activities, and the opportunity for social connection. Coordination of such resources requires effort, contributed by the older woman herself, family or friends, or formal care coordinators. Planning ahead is crucial to enacting aspirations to live in one's home.

For those who are interested in alternate living situations, many are available in communities across the country, ranging from retirement housing with multiple levels of care, to freestanding senior apartments or assisted living, to cohousing. With the growing numbers of options, it is helpful to begin with a sense of what is needed/desired, a projection of likely needs in the coming years, and an assessment of financial resources and need. For older women in need of financial support for housing and services, county area agencies on aging are a good resource for establishing eligibility and identifying local options. The search for housing can be daunting, but can be simplified by developing the criteria of importance to the older woman and then comparison shopping with local options, including spending some time at meals or activities in the settings under review. Once an alternative is identified, it is helpful to get on the waiting list to assure availability.

Assisted living is the fastest growing sector of housing for older adults, and differs across states in the degree of health care provided. Nursing homes are increasingly providing specialized and often time-limited care, such as for rehabilitation after a hospitalization or advanced dementia care. While fewer than 5% of older adults live in nursing homes, there is about a one in five chance that each of us will spend some time in a nursing home at some time in late life (Federal Interagency Forum on Aging-Related Statistics, 2012). The likelihood of nursing home residence is higher among White older women, as Black, Hispanic, and Asian women more commonly live in the community or with relatives. Certain conditions, such as dementia and severe functional impairment, increase the likelihood of admission to either assisted living or a nursing home.

Lesbian, Gay, Bisexual, Transgender, Queer (LGBTQ Issues)

The population of older lesbian, bisexual, and transgender women is growing, and health disparities exist among this population (Institute of Medicine, 2011). Research with older lesbian women is sparse, with even less attention to the issues and concerns of older bisexual or transgender women. Older lesbians remain relatively invisible and underserved within the health-care system (Brotman, Ryan, & Cormier, 2003). Among older women today, there is a range of visibility within the lesbian community, from those who have not revealed their orientation to those who are "out." Recent state laws have been expanding opportunities for same-sex couples to benefit from the privileges of other citizens, yet full participation in benefits and decision making is not the norm across the nation. Financial security is of particular concern for older women in general, and for older lesbian women, as access to the social security of a partner remains a barrier to late-life financial health.

Because societal intolerance for same-sex relationships remains a force in many health systems, older lesbians can face particular challenges in advocating for and participating in decision making for their partners during acute and chronic illness episodes, as well as accessing partner health benefits for their own health care. In cities with a critical mass of older LGBTQ members, retirement housing and other services specific to this population are growing, yet many communities have not achieved widespread access, creating a sense of invisibility and assumed heterosexuality for older LGBTQ women. Because of the unwelcoming nature of some congregate housing environments, older women may become more circumspect about their preferences when they leave the privacy of home.

Older LGBTQ women share many of the same health concerns as other older women, but experience their care through the lens of a system that is not geared to their needs. For this population, mental health poses a particular risk, with higher prevalence of depression, suicidal behavior, substance misuse, and dependence than among heterosexual older women (Ward, Pugh, & Price, 2010). These findings point to the importance of training for health-care providers and attention to inclusiveness in services. LGBTQ older women identified greatest needs for LGBTQ-oriented/friendly legal advice, social events, grief and loss counseling, social workers, and assisted living (Smith, McCaslin, Chang, Martinez, & McGrew, 2012). Both older LGBTQ adults and health-care providers lack knowledge to engage in effective end-of-life planning, including legal rights and assuring designated decision makers such as durable powers of attorney (Cartwright, Hughes, & Lienert, 2012). Education about these important matters is critical to assuring equal treatment at the end of life. LGBTQ issues are relevant across the life span, and more discussion is included in Chapter 7. Women in special populations is presented in Chapter 7.

Caregiving

For the first time in history, there are three generations of women over the age of 65. Given the many roles women play in the lives of families, it is not surprising that older women are often caregivers, of partners, parents, friends, other relatives, and children with special needs. In fact, across the United States, over a third of households are engaged in caregiving, and women comprise 66% of active caregivers (National Alliance for Caregiving, 2009). One third are caring for more than one person, and one third provide care for over five years. The role is varied and includes personal care, doing complex medical and nursing tasks, financial and instrumental assistance, and providing emotional and social support.

Most older women will be caregivers at some time, participating in an experience that brings both rewards and strains. For many, its meaning is the enactment of family obligations and an opportunity to express love and concern. This can be mixed with a variety of responses of emotional stress, guilt that it is never enough, and exhaustion from the unrelenting demands. Caregiving can have financial implications, in terms of both missed work and also additional costs to deploy the necessary help. The impact of caregiving varies across older women, depending on the characteristics of the situation and the needs of the care recipient, their perspective of the demands, their vulnerability and resources, available social supports, the quality of the relationship, and their own needs for support (Young, 2003). Particularly when providing care over a period of many years, such as when caring for a person with dementia, the physical and emotional demands can lead to negative health outcomes, including increased morbidity and mortality (Vitaliano, Young, & Zhang, 2004). A variety of supports are available to caregivers, through resources such as the National Alliance for Caregiving (http://www.caregiving.org), AARP (www.aarp.org), and the Alzheimer's Association (www.alz.org).

Health-Care Systems for Older Women

In late life, a variety of health-care systems are relevant, including acute care, ambulatory care, long-term care, and community-based services. Depending on need, older women may access some or all of the above possibilities, often in conjunction with one another. For example, an acute illness or injury might result in a hospitalization, followed by a short stay in a nursing home for intensive rehabilitation, then discharge to home with home health supports, followed by community services to provide transportation and meals. Under the current financial model, each of these segments possesses particular eligibility criteria and mechanisms for reimbursement. With the Affordable Care Act of 2010, there is movement toward bundling services and payment across trajectories of health and illness, to incentivize collaboration among providers across settings, and to bring greater value to the person and family. For example, Transitional Care Management Services have been recently authorized to reimburse activities that promote continuity of care for older adults discharged from hospital with complex health conditions.

Many older women and health-care providers are unaware of the limits and benefits of Medicare and Medicaid, both of which continue to evolve. Understanding available benefits is crucial to navigating both acute and chronic illness in the most effective way possible. Extensive information is available for consumers at the Medicare website (http://www.medicare.gov/) and for health-care providers at the Centers for Medicare and Medicaid Service website (http://www.cms.gov/). Table 6.4 summarizes Medicare coverage for annual wellness visits. In addition, Area Agencies on Aging are federally funded programs in each county in the United States, with resources for information and referral for older adults and their families.

Self-Management of Chronic Conditions

The public health burden of multiple chronic conditions is substantial. More than 75% of US health-care dollars are spent on persons with chronic diseases, and these diseases limit

TABLE 6.4	Annual Wellness Visit Covered by Medicare (as of 2012)
Covered Services	
Routine measurements (height, weight, blood pressure, BMI)	
Review of individual medical and family history	
Review of current medications, supplements, and vitamins	
Discussion of care currently being received from other providers	
Review of functional ability and level of safety (e.g., fall risk), including cognitive impairment, screening for depression	
Discussion of personalized health advice, taking into account risk factors and specific health conditions or needs (e.g., weight loss, physical activity, smoking cessation, fall prevention, nutrition)	
Discussion of referrals to appropriate health education or preventive counseling services that may help minimize or treat potential health risks	
Planning a schedule for Medicare screening and preventive services that will be needed over the next 5 to 10 years	

Data from Centers for Medicare & Medicaid Services. (2014). What medicare covers. Retrieved from http://www.medicare.gov/what-medicare-covers/index.html

daily activities for about one quarter of those affected (Anderson, 2004). The incidence of chronic diseases has continued despite advances in medical technology, diagnostics, and interventions. In particular, the incidence of diabetes and obesity, labeled as twin epidemics by the Centers for Disease Control and Prevention, is soaring, and the prevalence of hypertension is substantial, afflicting one in three adults. Depression is a frequent comorbidity with other chronic diseases, with between 9% and 23% of individuals with one or more chronic condition having comorbid depression (Moussavi et al., 2007). As is the case with diabetes, comorbid depression exacerbates morbidity and negatively impacts the outcome of many other chronic illnesses, such as heart and lung disease, obesity, cancer, inflammatory and immune diseases, and dementia (Bremmer et al., 2008; Steffens & Potter, 2008). Comorbid depression occurs in between 21% and 36% of patients with heart failure, and is associated with poorer quality of life, poorer adherence to medication regimens, worse outcomes in functional status, physical activity and hospital readmission, and increased mortality (May et al., 2009). Importantly, many of these chronic diseases share common risk factors related to lifestyle choices and unhealthy behaviors (unhealthy diet, lack of physical activity, obesity, use of alcohol and tobacco). For example, poor diet/nutrition, lack of physical activity, obesity, and alcohol and tobacco use are risk factors for diabetes, heart and lung disease, and depression.

Improvements in health behaviors have the potential to improve general health and quality of life by reducing the negative impact of chronic diseases. To address the staggering escalation of chronic diseases, it is crucial to include treatment modalities that address lifestyle and behavioral modification and increase the capacity of older women to engage in self-management of their chronic conditions. Lorig and Holman (2003) developed and tested a practical and useful community-based approach to increasing self-management of chronic conditions, recognizing that self-management is problem-focused and hinges on the person's perceptions of priorities to address. This comprehensive approach builds skills in six main areas: problem solving, decision making, resource utilization, the formation of a patient–provider partnership, action planning, and self-tailoring (Lorig & Holman, 2003). A variety of strategies are essential to promoting health, including assessment of health literacy, engaging the older woman in identifying her personal goals and priorities, providing educational and motivational supports, and addressing access to appropriate services to promote health. With the advent of enabling technologies, new possibilities exist in mHealth and telehealth to advance health and improve individual and family capacity to navigate complex conditions (Young et al., 2014). To promote optimal health for older women, health-care professionals must also expand the repertoire to include a broader approach that emphasizes partnership between the woman and her health-care provider.

References

AARP. (2011). *Voices of 50+ America: Dreams & Challenges.* Retrieved from http://www.aarp.org/personal-growth/transitions/info-02-2011/voices-america-dreams-challenges.html

AARP. (2013). *Life reimagined.* Retrieved from www.aarp.org

Aday, R. H., Kehoe, G. C., & Farney, L. A. (2006). Impact of senior center friendships on aging women who live alone. *Journal of Women and Aging, 18*(1), 57–73.

Aging with Dignity. (2013). *Five wishes.* Retrieved from http://www.agingwithdignity.org/

Alzheimer's Association. (2013). 2013 Alzheimer's disease factors and figures. *Alzheimer's & Dementia, 9*(2), 208–245.

American Cancer Society. (2013). *Cancer prevention & early detection facts & figures 2013.* Atlanta, GA: Author.

American Cancer Society. (2014). *Cancer facts & figures 2014.* Atlanta, GA: Author.

American Geriatrics Society. (2014). *Clinical guidelines and recommendations.* GeriatricsCareOnline.Org. Retrieved from http://www.geriatricscareonline.org/ProductStore/clinical-guidelines-recommendations/8/

American Society of Plastic Surgeons. (2014). *2012 Plastic surgery statistics report.* Retrieved from http://www.plasticsurgery.org/Documents/news-resources/statistics/2012-Plastic-Surgery-Statistics/cosmetic-procedures-ages-55-over.pdf

Anderson, G. (2004). *Chronic conditions: Making the case for ongoing care.* Baltimore, MD: John Hopkins University.

Angel, J. L., Jimenez, M. A., & Angel, R. A. (2007). The economic consequences of widowhood for older minority women. *Gerontologist, 47*(2), 224–234.

Armstrong, M. J. (2000). Older women's organization of friendship support networks: An African American-White American comparison. *Journal of Women & Aging, 12*(1/2), 93–108.

Ayers, C. R., Sorrell, J. T., Thorp, S. R., & Wetherell, J. L. (2007). Evidence-based psychological treatments for late-life anxiety. *Psychology and Aging, 22*(1), 8–17.

Ayotte, B. J., Yang, F. M., & Jones, R. N. (2010). Physical health and depression: A dyadic study of chronic health conditions and depressive symptomatology in older adult couples. *Journals of Gerontology. Series B, Psychological Sciences and Social Sciences, 65B*(4), 438–448.

Barry, L. C., Allore, H. G., Guo, Z., Bruce, M. L., & Gill, T. M. (2008). Higher burden of depression among older women: The effect of onset, persistence, and mortality over time *JAMA Psychiatry, 65*(2), 172–178.

Barry, L. C., Soulos, P. R., Murphy, T. E., Kasl, S. V., & Gill, T. M. (2013). Association between indicators of disability burden and subsequent depression among older persons. *Journals of Gerontology. Series A, Biological Sciences and Medical Sciences, 68*(3), 286–292.

Bhargava, A., & Du, X. L. (2009). Racial and socioeconomic disparities in adjuvant chemotherapy for older women with lymph node-positive, operable breast cancer. *Cancer, 115*(13), 2999–3008. doi:10.1002/cncr.24363

Blow, F. C. (2000). Treatment of older women with alcohol problems: Meeting the challenge for a special population. *Alcohol Clinical and Experimental Research, 24*(8), 1257–1266.

Bremmer, M. A., Beekman, A. T. F., Deeg, D. J. H., Penninx, B. W. J. H., Dik, M. G., Hack, C. E., & Hoogendijk, W. J. G. (2008). Inflammatory markers in late-life depression: Results from a population-based study. *Journal of Affective Disorders, 106*(3), 249–255.

Brotman, S., Ryan, B., & Cormier, R. (2003). The health and social service needs of gay and lesbian elders and their families in Canada. *Gerontologist, 43*(2), 192–202.

Bryant, C., Jackson, H., & Ames, D. (2008). The prevalence of anxiety in older adults: Methodological issues and a review of the literature. *Journal of Affective Disorders, 109*(3), 233–250.

Budnitz, D. S., Lovegrove, M. C., Shehab, N., & Richards, C. L. (2011). Emergency hospitalizations for adverse drug events in older Americans. *New England Journal of Medicine, 365*, 2002–2012.

Bushnell, C., McCullough, L. D., Awad, I. A., Chireau, M. V., Fedder, W. N., Furie, K. L., … Walters, M. R.; American Heart Association Stroke Council, Council on Cardiovascular and Stroke Nursing, Council on Clinical Cardiology, Council on Epidemiology and Prevention, and Council for High Blood Pressure Research. (2014). Guidelines for the prevention of stroke in women: A statement for healthcare professionals from the American Heart Association/American Stroke Association. *Stroke, 45*(5), 1545–1588. Retrieved from http://stroke.ahajournals.org/content/early/2014/02/06/01. str.0000442009.06663.48

Cartwright, C., Hughes, M., & Lienert, T. (2012). End-of-life care for gay, lesbian, bisexual and transgender people. *Culture, Health & Sexuality: An International Journal for Research, Intervention and Care, 14*(5), 537–548.

Centers for Medicare & Medicaid Services. (2014). *What medicare covers.* Retrieved from http://www.medicare.gov/what-medicare-covers/index.html

Cornwell, E. Y., & Waite, L. J. (2009). Social disconnectedness, perceived isolation, and health among older adults. *Journal of Health and Social Behavior, 50*(1), 31–48.

Daviglus, M. L., Bell, C. C., Berrettini, W., Bowen, P. E., Connolly, E. S., Cox, N. J., … Trevisan, M. (2010). National Institutes of Health State-of-the-Science Conference statement: Preventing Alzheimer's disease and cognitive decline. *Annals of Internal Medicine, 153*(3), 176–181.

DeVon, H. A., Ryan, C. J., Ochs, A. L., & Shapiro, M. (2008). Symptoms across the continuum of acute coronary syndromes: Differences between women and men. *American Journal of Critical Care, 17,* 14–24.

Eye Diseases Prevalence Research Group. (2004). Causes and prevalence of visual impairment among adults in the United States. *Archives of Ophthalmology, 122*(4), 477–485.

Federal Interagency Forum on Aging-Related Statistics. (2012). *Older Americans 2012: Key indicators of well-being.* Washington, DC: US Government Printing Office.

Fiske, A., Wetherell, J. L., & Gatz, M. (2009). Depression in older adults. *Annual Review Clinical Psychology*, 5, 363–389.

George, L. K. (2010). Still happy after all these years: Research frontiers on subjective well-being in later life. *Journals of Gerontology. Series B, Psychological Sciences and Social Sciences*, 65B(3), 331–339.

Gfroerera, J., Penneb, M., Pembertonb, M., & Folsomb, R. (2003). Substance abuse treatment need among older adults in 2020: The impact of the aging baby-boom cohort. *Drug and Alcohol Dependence*, 69(2), 127–135.

Gies, C., & Lessick, M. (2009). Alzheimer disease in women: A clinical and genetics perspective. *Nursing for Women's Health*, 13(4), 312–323; quiz 324. doi:10.1111/j.1751-486X.2009.01441.x

Go, S., Mozaffarian, D., Roger, V. L., Benjamin, E. J., Berry, J. D., Blaha, M. J., ... Turner, M. B.; American Heart Association Statistics Committee and Stroke Statistics Committee. (2013). Heart disease and stroke statistics—2014 update: A report from the American Heart Association. *Circulation*, 129, e28–e292.

Goode, P. S., Burgio, K. L., Richter, H. E., & Markland, A. D. (2010). Incontinence in older women. *Journal of the American Medical Association*, 303(21), 2172–2181. doi:10.1001/jama.2010.749

Gopinath, B., Rochtchina, E., Wang, J. J., Schneider, J., Leeder, S. R., & Mitchell, P. (2009). Prevalence of age-related hearing loss in older adults: Blue Mountains Study. *Archives of Internal Medicine*, 169(9), 415–418.

Gregg, E. W., Cauley, J. A., Stone, K., Thompson, T. J., Bauer, D. C., & Cummings, S. R.; Study of Osteoporotic Fractures Research Group. (2003). Relationship of changes in physical activity and mortality among older women. *Journal of the American Medical Association*, 289(18), 2379–2386.

Hahn, E. A., Cichy, K. E., Almeida, D. M., & Haley, W. E. (2011). Time use and well-being in older widows: Adaptation and resilience. *Journal of Women & Aging*, 23(2), 149–159.

Hawkins, K., Pernarelli, J., Ozminkowski, R. J., Bai, M., Gaston, S. J., Hommer, C., ... Yeh, C. S. (2011). The prevalence of urinary incontinence and its burden on the quality of life among older adults with medicare supplement insurance. *Quality of Life Research: An International Journal of Quality of Life Aspects of Treatment, Care & Rehabilitation*, 20(5), 723–732. doi:10.1007/s11136-010-9808-0

Hawkley, L. C., & Cacioppo, J. T. (2004). Stress and the aging immune system. *Brain, Behavior, and Immunity*, 18(2), 114–119.

He, W., Sengupta, M., Velkoff, V. A., & DeBarros, K. A. (2005). *US Census Bureau, Current Population Reports, 65+ in the United States: 2005* (pp. 23–209). Washington, DC: US Government Printing Office.

Hsia, J., Rodabough, R. J., Manson, J. E., Liu, S., Freiberg, M. S., Graettinger, W., ... Howard, B. V.; Women's Health Initiative Research. (2010). Evaluation of the American Heart Association cardiovascular disease prevention guideline for women. *Circulation: Cardiovascular Quality and Outcomes*, 3, 128–134.

Institute of Medicine. (2011). *The health of lesbian, gay, bisexual, and transgender people: Building a foundation for better understanding*.

Jeste, D. V., Savla, G. N., Thompson, W. K., Vahia, I. V., Glorioso, D. K., Martin, A. S., ... Depp, C. A. (2013). Association between older age and more successful aging: Critical role of resilience and depression. *American Journal of Psychiatry*, 170(2), 188–196.

Kane, R., Ouslander, J., & Abrass, I. (2003). *Essentials of clinical geriatrics* (5th ed.). New York, NY: McGraw-Hill.

Krause, N. (2007). Evaluating the stress-buffering function of meaning in life among older people. *Journal of Aging and Health*, 19(5), 792–812.

Krauss, R. M., Eckel, R. H., Howard, B., Appel, L. J., Daniels, S. R., Deckelbaum, R. J., ... Bazzarre, T. L. (2000). AHA Dietary Guidelines Revision 2000: A statement for healthcare professionals from the Nutrition Committee of the American Heart Association. *Circulation*, 102, 2289–2299.

Lindau, S. T., Schumm, L. P., Laumann, E. O., Levinson, W., O'Muircheartaigh, C. A., & Waite, L. J. (2007). A study of sexuality and health among older adults in the United States. *New England Journal of Medicine*, 357, 762–774.

Lorig, K. R., & Holman, H. R. (2003). Self-management education: History, definition, outcomes, and mechanisms. *Annals of Behavioral Medicine*, 26(1), 1–7.

Mangweth-Matzek, B., Rupp, C. I., Hausmann, A., Assmayr, K., Mariacher, E., Kemmler, G., ... Biebl, W. (2006). Never too old for eating disorders or body dissatisfaction: A community study of elderly women. *International Journal of Eating Disorders*, 39(7), 583–586.

Manson, J. E., Chlebowski, R. T., Stefanick, M. L., Aragaki, A., Rossouw, J. E., Prentice, R. L., ... Wallace, R. B. (2013). Menopausal hormone therapy and health outcomes during the intervention and extended poststopping phases of the Women's Health Initiative randomized trials. *New England Journal of Medicine*, 310(13), 1353–1368. doi:10.1001/jama.2013.278040

May, H. T., Horne, B. D., Carlquist, J. F., Sheng, X., Joy, E., & Catinella A. P. (2009). Depression after coronary artery disease is associated with heart failure. *Journal of the American College of Cardiology,* *53*(16), 1440–1447.

McCormick, W. C., & Boling, P. (2005). Multi-morbidity and a comprehensive Medicare care-coordination benefit. *Journal of the American Geriatrics Society, 53,* 2227–2228.

McSweeney, J., Cleves, M. A., Fischer, E. P., Moser, D. K., Wei, J., Pettey, C., ... Armbya, N. (2013). Predicting coronary heart disease events in women: A longitudinal cohort study. *Journal of Cardiovascular Nursing.* doi:10.1097/JCN.0b013e3182a409cc

Meleis, A. I., Sawyer, L. M., Im, E.-O., Messias, D. K. H., & Schumacher, K. L. (2010). Experiencing transitions: An emerging middle-range Theory. *Transition theory* (pp. 52–65). New York, NY: Springer.

Menec, V. H. (2003). The relation between everyday activities and successful aging: A 6-year longitudinal study. *Journal of Gerontology: Social Sciences, 58B*(2), S74–S82.

Minassian, V. A., Devore, E., Hagan, K., & Grodstein, F. (2013). Severity of urinary incontinence and effect on quality of life in women by incontinence type. *Obstetrics and Gynecology, 121*(5), 1083–1090. doi:10.1097/AOG.0b013e31828ca761

Mosca, L., Barrett-Connor, E. L., & Wenger, N. K. (2011). Sex/gender differences in cardiovascular disease prevention: What a difference a decade makes. *Circulation, 124,* 2145–2154.

Mosca, L., Benjamin, E. J., Berra, K., Bezanson, J. L., Dolor, R. J., Lloyd-Jones, D. M., ... Wenger, N. K. (2011). Effectiveness-based guidelines for the prevention of cardiovascular disease in women: 2011 update: A guideline from the American Heart Association. *Circulation, 123,* 1243–1262.

Mosca, L., Hammond, G., Mochari-Greenberger, H., Towfighi, A., Albert, M. A.; American Heart Association Special Report (2013). Fifteen-year trends in awareness of heart disease in women: Results of a 2012 American Heart Association national survey. *Circulation, 127*(11), 1254–1263, e1251–e1229. doi:10.1161/CIR.0b013e318287cf2f

Moussavi, S., Chatterji, S., Verdes, E., Tandon, A., Patel, V., & Ustun, B. (2007). Depression, chronic diseases, and decrements in health: Results from the World Health Surveys. *Lancet, 370*(9590), 851–858.

National Alliance for Caregiving. (2009). Caregiving in the US: 2009. Retrieved from http://www.caregiving.org/data/Caregiving_in_the_US_2009_full_report.pdf

National Osteoporosis Foundation. (2013). *Clinician's guide to prevention and treatment of osteoporosis.* Washington, DC: Author.

Nelson, M. E., Rejeski, W. J., Blair, S. N., Duncan, P. W., Judge, J. O., & King, A. C. (2007). Physical activity and public health in older adults: Recommendation from the American College of Sports Medicine and the American Heart Association. *Circulation, 116*(9), 1094–1105.

Nordin, S., Brämerson, A., Bringlöv, E., Kobal, G., Hummel, T., & Bende, M. (2007). Substance and tongue-region specific loss in basic taste-quality identification in elderly adults. *European Archives of Oto-Rhino-Laryngology, 264*(3), 285–289.

North American Menopause Society. (2010). Management of osteoporosis in postmenopausal women: 2010 Position statement of The North American Menopause Society. *Menopause, 17*(1), 25–54.

Office of Research on Women's Health in Collaboration with the NIH Coordinating Committee on Research on Women's Health. (2010). *Highlights of NIH women's health and sex differences research 1990–2010* (NIH Publication No. 10-7606-D). Bethesda, MD: National Institutes of Health.

Orth, U., Trzesniewski, K. H., & Robins, R. W. (2010). Self-esteem development from young adulthood to old age: A cohort-sequential longitudinal study. *Journal of Personality and Social Psychology, 98*(4), 645–658.

Pew Research Center. (2012). *Older adults and internet use.* Retrieved from http://www.pewinternet.org/Topics/Demographics/Seniors.aspx?typeFilter=5

Pruchno, R. A., Wilson-Genderson, N., & Cartwright, F. (2010). A two-factor model of successful aging. *Journals of Gerontology. Series B, Psychological Sciences and Social Sciences 65B*(6), 671–679.

Qato, D. M., Alexander, G. C., Conti, R. M., Johnson, M., Schumm, P., & Lindau, S. T. (2008). Use of prescription and over-the-counter medications and dietary supplements among older adults in the United States. *Journal of the American Medical Association, 300*(24), 2867–2878.

Reyes-Gibby, C. C., Aday, L. A., Todd, K. H., Cleeland, C. S., & Anderson, K. O. (2007). Pain in aging community-dwelling adults in the United States: Non-Hispanic Whites, Non-Hispanic Blacks, and Hispanics. *Journal of Pain, 8*(1), 75–84.

Seeman, T. E., Merkin, S. S., Crimmins, E. M., & Karlamangla, A. S. (2010). Disability trends among older Americans: National Health and Nutrition Examination Surveys, 1988–1994 and 1999–2004. *American Journal of Public Health, 100,* 100–107.

Segal, D. L., Qualls, S. H., & Smyer, M. A. (2011). *Aging and mental health* (2nd ed.). Malden, MA: Wiley-Blackwell.

Simon, S. R., Chan, K. A., Soumerai, S. B., Wagner, A. K., Andrade, S. E., Feldstein, A. C., & Gurwitz, J. H. (2005). Potentially inappropriate medication use by elderly persons in the US Health Maintenance Organizations. *Journal of the American Geriatrics Society, 53*(2), 227–232.

Simoni-Wastila, L., & Yang, H. K. (2006). Psychoactive drug abuse in older adults. *American Journal of Geriatric Pharmacotherapy, 4*(4), 380–394.

Siu, O. L., & Phillips, D. R. (2002). A study of family support, friendship, and psychological well-being among older women in Hong Kong. *International Journal of Aging and Human Development, 55*(4), 299–319.

Smith, L. A., McCaslin, R., Chang, J., Martinez, P., & McGrew, P. (2012). Assessing the needs of older gay, lesbian, bisexual, and transgender people: A service-learning and agency partnership approach. *Journal of Gerontological Social Work, 53*(5), 387–401.

Spence, N. J., Adkins, D. E., & Dupre, M. E. (2011). Racial differences in depression trajectories among older women socioeconomic, family, and health Influences. *Journal of Health and Social Behavior, 52*(4), 444–459.

Stampfer, M. J., Kang, J. H., Chen, J., Cherry, R., & Grodstein, F. (2005). Effects of moderate alcohol consumption on cognitive function in women. *New England Journal of Medicine, 352,* 245–253.

Steffens, D. C., & Potter, G. G. (2008). Geriatric depression and cognitive impairment. *Psychological medicine, 38*(02), 163–175.

Sullivan, A. L., Beshansky, J. R., Ruthazer, R., Murman, D. H., Mader, T. J., & Selker, H. P. (2014). Factors associated with longer time to treatment for patients with suspected acute coronary syndromes: A cohort study. *Circulation: Cardiovascular and Quality Outcomes, 7,* 86–94.

Tanamas, S. K., Wijethilake, P., Wluka, A. E., Davies-Tuck, M. L., Urquhart, D. M., Wang, Y., & Cicuttini, F. M. (2011). Sex hormones and structural changes in osteoarthritis: A systematic review. *Maturitas, 69,* 141–156.

Teri, L., Logsdon, R. G., & McCurry, S. M. (2005). The Seattle protocols: Advances in behavioral treatment of Alzheimer's disease. In B. Vellas, M. Grundman, H. Feldman, L. J. Fitten, B. Winblad & E. Giacobini (Eds.), *Research and practice in Alzheimer's disease and cognitive decline* (pp. 153–158). New York, NY: Springer.

Tiggeman, M. (2004). Body image across the adult life span: Stability and change. *Body Image, 1*(1), 29–41.

US Census. (2011). *The older population: 2010.* US Department of Commerce, Economics and Statistics Administration, US Census Bureau.

US Preventive Services Task Force. (2009). Aspirin for the prevention of cardiovascular disease: US Preventive Services Task Force recommendation statement. *Annals of Internal Medicine, 150*(6), 396.

Vitaliano, P. P., Young, H. M., & Zhang, J. (2004). Is caregiving a risk factor for illness? *Current Directions in Psychological Science, 13*(1), 13–16.

Wallhagen, M. I., Strawbridge, W. J., Shema, S. J., & Kaplan, G. A. (2004). Impact of self-assessed hearing loss on a spouse: A longitudinal analysis of couples. *Journals of Gerontology. Series B, Psychological Sciences and Social Sciences, 59*(3), S190–S196.

Wallhagen, M. I., Strawbridge, W. J., Shema, S. J., Kurata, J., & Kaplan, G. A. (2001). Comparative impact of hearing and vision impairment on subsequent functioning. *Journal of the American Geriatrics Society, 49*(8), 1086–1092.

Wallner, L. P., Porten, S., Meenan, R. T., O'Keefe Rosetti, M. C., Calhoun, E. A., & Sarma, A. V. (2009). Prevalence and severity of undiagnosed urinary incontinence in women. *American Journal of Medicine, 122*(11), 1037–1042. doi:10.1016/j.amjmed.2009.05.016

Wang, H.-X., Karp, A., Winblad, B., & Fratiglioni, L. (2002). Late-life engagement in social and leisure activities is associated with a decreased risk of dementia: A longitudinal study from the Kungsholmen Project. *American Journal of Epidemiology, 155*(12), 1081–1087.

Ward, R., Pugh, S., & Price, E. (2010). *Don't look back? Improving health and social care service delivery for older LGB users.* Manchester, UK: Equality and Human Rights Commission.

Weitz, T. & Estes, C.L. (2001). Adding aging and gender to the women's health agenda. *Journal of Women and Aging, 13*(2), 3-20.

Wolin, K. Y., Glynn, R. J., Colditz, G. A., Lee, I.-M., & Kawachi, I. (2007). Long-term physical activity patterns and health-related quality of life in US women. *American Journal of Preventive Medicine, 32*(6), 490–499.

Xie, B. (2003). Older adults, computers, and the Internet: Future directions. *Gerontechnology, 2*(4), 289–305.

Xie, H., Mayo, N., & Koski, L. (2011). Identifying and characterizing trajectories of cognitive change in older persons with mild cognitive impairment. *Dementia and Geriatric Cognitive Disorders, 31*(2), 165–172. doi:10.1159/000323568

Young, H. (2003). Challenges and solutions for care of frail older adults. *Online Journal of Issues in Nursing, 8*(2), Manuscript 4.

Young, H. M., Miyamoto, S., Ward, D., Dharmar, M., Tang-Feldman, Y., & Berglund, L. (2014). Sustained effects of a nurse coaching intervention via telehealth to improve health behavior change in diabetes. *Telemedicine Journal and E-Health* published on-line ahead of print July 25, 2014.

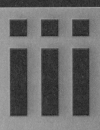
Promoting Women's Wellness across the Life Span

Chapter **7** Wellness for Special Populations of Women

Chapter **8** Body Composition: Enhancing Health through Exercise and Nutrition

Chapter **9** Oral Health

Chapter **10** Resilience in Women

Chapter **11** Self-Care: Healing Energy and Other Complementary Therapies

Chapter **12** Women and Herbal Medicine

Chapter **13** Pharmacologic Approaches to Wellness and Disease Prevention in Women over the Life span

Chapter **14** Healing Arts: Movement in the Form of Pilates

Chapter **15** Healing Environments

Chapter **16** Healing Relationships

Chapter **17** Promoting Healthy Sleep

Chapter **18** Peaceful Dying

Chapter 7

Wellness for Special Populations of Women

Ellen F. Olshansky and Robynn Zender

There are specific populations of women who have unique health-care needs and deserve mention, particularly in a book that is focused on health and wellness. These women have special challenges that must be addressed in order for them to attain their own optimum level of wellness. Health-care providers must be aware of and sensitive to these issues and integrate this awareness and sensitivity into their care. This chapter presents health-care issues related to women in the military and veterans; women immigrants; women in poverty; lesbian, gay, bisexual, transgender (LGBT) women; women with disabilities; and women recovering from trauma (interpersonal violence, abuse, substance abuse).

Women in the Military and Veterans

Women have always had an important role in the military, as evidenced by the Women's Army Corps (WACs) and the women at Bataan in the Philippines, who were US Army and Navy nurses. Approximately 15% of active duty military personnel are women (Haskell et al., 2011; Lehavot, Hoerster, Nelson, Jakupcak, & Simpson, 2012), 17% of the National Guard Reserves are women, and 20% of new recruits to the military are women (Haskell et al., 2011). Active military women and veterans exhibit significant health concerns. Lehavot and colleagues noted that women veterans engage in more risky lifestyle behaviors including tobacco use and lack of exercise, compared with civilian women. In addition, they experience more depression and anxiety and are more overweight with a higher incidence of cardiovascular disease compared with civilian women. Women in active military duty actually have better access to health care, including having had recent Pap smears and breast examinations, and they are in better physical condition than civilian women. These findings lead one to question the consequences to women's health after a tour of duty, when women are no longer on active duty. It is striking that women veterans are at a significantly (3 to 4 times) higher risk of becoming homeless than their civilian counterparts (Washington et al., 2010).

Despite the reports of better access to health care for women while on active duty, data also show that women on active duty experience sexual trauma, with evidence that such trauma leads to an increased risk after deployment of depression, substance abuse, and other health conditions (Haskell et al., 2011). Kelly and colleagues (Kelly, Skelton, Patel, & Bradley, 2011) stated that military sexual trauma (MST), which is a term used in the military to describe both actual sexual assaults and sexual harassment while in the military, was reported by women veterans to have occurred during their active military duty. These authors also noted that posttraumatic stress disorder (PTSD) often accompanied MST. One study found that in women who had PTSD, 31% also had a history of MST, which is very different from the case of men, where 1% of men who had PTSD also had a history of MST (Maguen et al., 2012). PTSD is significant because women veterans with PTSD were found to have 7.0 medical conditions when compared with women veterans without PTSD, who had a median number of 4.5 medical conditions. Male veterans with PTSD had 5.0 medical conditions as compared with male veterans without PTSD, who had a median of 4.0 medical conditions (Frayne et al., 2011).

From a wellness perspective, it is imperative that integrated, comprehensive health-care services be available consistently to women veterans. These services must be sensitive to the stresses experienced by these women while in combat, many of whom continue to suffer from PTSD. A longitudinal study by Friedman and colleagues (Friedman et al., 2011) found a significant increase in the use of Veterans Health Administration (VHA) services by women veterans. Many were new patients to the VHA, with 40% of the new women patients seeking care for mental health problems, and 20% seeking repeated care for mental health problems. Therefore, primary care services for women veterans should include a focus on mental health issues, including referring for more extensive care when appropriate.

Immigrant Women

Immigrant women experience many challenges related to their health. There are many and varied reasons that women immigrate to the United States, and the transitions they confront are related to adapting to new environments, new cultures, lifestyles, languages. Often, they must adapt to different eating habits, particularly those immigrants from non-Westernized cultures who come to the United States, where it is more common to eat processed foods. Health consequences of these changes can include increased stress, hypertension, obesity, and diabetes (Rosenthal, 2014).

These health consequences vary among various cultural groups who experience different situations as they go through the process of immigration. In addition, their former conditions (in the countries from which they emigrated) influence their current health. Rosenthal's (2014) review presented an overview of various health conditions faced by immigrants from many different countries. For example, citizens from the Former Soviet Union (FSU) often came from a culture in which it was common to smoke and drink alcohol with scant attention to preventive health measures. Rosenthal (2014) noted that Russians had the highest death rate from heart disease as compared with people from other countries. When these immigrants came to the United States, it was very common for them to have hypertension. In a group of 30,000 immigrants from the FSU to Denver in 2001, 56% had hypertension compared with 25% of adults across the United States. Also, Russian immigrants experienced difficulty in acculturating to their new environment, especially because of disappointment in not meeting their expectations, particularly in having to take lower-status employment. Mental health issues are prevalent due to stresses in relationships, acculturation, and reduced expectations.

Rosenthal (2014) reported that Chinese Americans had a high prevalence of cardiovascular disease risk factors despite having lower body mass index (BMI) and smaller waist circumference. One postulated reason is lack of adherence to blood pressure medications (Hsu, Mao, & Wey, 2010; Li, Wallhagen, & Froelicher, 2010). In addition, in the process of acculturating to the United States, many Asians may have substituted their traditional diets with more processed, high fat, and sugary foods (Wong, Beth Dixon, Gilbride, Chin, & Kwan, 2011). Korean Americans were also found to have significant levels of hypertension, high cholesterol, obesity, and diabetes, and to engage in smoking and sedentary lifestyle behaviors (Kim, Lee, Ahn, & Lee, 2011). Filipinos have also been found to have significantly high levels of hypertension (dela Cruz & Galang, 2008). Japanese Americans were found to have higher levels of diabetes as compared with Japanese in Tokyo (Fujimoto et al., 2012), as evidenced by 16% of Japanese American women and 20% of Japanese American men in Seattle having diabetes versus 4% to 5% of Japanese in Tokyo. Another group of immigrants, South Asian Indians, have been found to have a high prevalence of oral cancer on account of using smokeless tobacco (Changrani, Gany, Cruz, Kerr, & Katz, 2006) and of type 2 diabetes (Venkatesh, Weatherspoon, Kaplowitz, & Song, 2013). Appel, Huang, Ai, and Lin (2011) noted that, in general, Asian Americans sought more help for their health problems as compared with European Americans.

Hispanic women in the United States have the highest rates of cervical cancer among all women, and a greater risk of mortality due to cervical cancer as compared with non-Hispanic White women. This disparity is believed to be due to lack of routine screening via Pap smears and HPV testing (Women'sHealth.gov, 2010), which may be due to complex reasons for not receiving such screening.

Approximately 2.1 million children have immigrated to the United States, comprising almost 19% of the total undocumented population (Gonzales, Suarez-Orozco, & Dedios-Sanguinetti, 2013). While guaranteed a K-through-12 education, these children and eventual adults are precluded from legally working, voting, securing financial aid, or driving in many states. They also face the possibility of deportation. The stress of their status as being part of the "1.5 generation" (not really first generation or second generation) can have negative health consequences, particularly because of stress and lack of adequate health care.

Although many of the studies reported in this chapter include both men and women, women are significantly affected. Clearly, more research is needed that focuses specifically on women and immigration.

Women in Poverty

The American Psychological Association (APA) notes that women in poverty have generally higher rates of mental illness, including depression, anxiety, PTSD, panic disorders, and other serious conditions such as bipolar disease and schizophrenia (APA, 2014). Women in poverty often cannot afford healthy fresh foods, resorting to processed fast foods. In addition, they often have so many responsibilities that they cannot devote time to healthy behaviors such as exercise. Interestingly, obesity in men does not differ by income or education, but among women, both lower income and lower education are associated with an increased risk of being obese (Ogden, Lamb, Carroll, & Flegal, 2010).

Cardiovascular disease, diabetes, and some cancers are also more prevalent in women with a lower socioeconomic status (SES) (Beckles & Chou, 2013; Daviglus et al., 2012; de

Martel, Forman, & Plummer, 2013; DeSantis, Siegel, Bandi, & Jemal, 2011; Li, Du, Reitzel, Xu, & Sturgis, 2013). Colonoscopy use generally decreases with increasing levels of poverty (Steele, Rim, Joseph, King, & Seeff, 2013), and little to no changes have been seen in smoking prevalence for those below the Federal Poverty Level (Garrett, Dube, Winder, & Caraballo, 2013). Low SES in childhood is associated with a higher prevalence of metabolic syndrome at midlife; however, many children raised in low-SES households do not develop metabolic syndrome as adults. Interestingly, high levels of maternal nurturance may offset the metabolic consequences of childhood disadvantage (Miller et al., 2011).

Reproductive health services are also used less by younger and socially disadvantaged women than by women with greater means, which may be one factor in the poor and disparate reproductive outcomes seen in these women (Hall, Moreau, & Trussell, 2012). Likewise, poor women are five times more likely to suffer intimate partner violence (IPV) (Aizer, 2010). Women who live in poverty are also more likely to be a racial minority, less educated, and engage in risky behavior. Pregnant women of low SES are more likely to be admitted to a hospital for assault while pregnant. Severe violence during pregnancy has been shown to reduce neonatal birth weight by 163 g (5.7 ounces), with larger effects associated with violence earlier in the pregnancy. These effects are similar to the estimated impact of smoking during pregnancy on birth weight (Aizer, 2010).

LGBT Women

Chapter 6 describes the challenges faced by LGBT women. Gates (2011) noted that 3.5% of US adults describe themselves as lesbian, gay, or bisexual, with 0.3% referring to themselves as transgendered. As noted by Gates (2011), these percentages translate into 9 million people identifying as LGBT, approximately the population of New Jersey. LGBT women have unique health challenges due to differences in sexual behaviors, and social inequality, including barriers to health care, in addition to the usual risk factors of age, education, and race. They are at increased risk for IPV, poor mental health, and substance abuse (US Department of Health and Human Services, Health Resources and Services Administration, Maternal and Child Health Bureau 2013). LGBT women are less likely to have received a Pap smear in the past 12 months (44% compared with 66% of heterosexual women), more likely to be obese (34% compared with 31%, with 43% of bisexual women being obese), to smoke (38% compared with 26%, with 56% of bisexual women smoking), and to binge drink (31% compared with 12%) (Chandra, Mosher, Copen, & Sionean, 2011).

Lesbian teenage girls experience mental health problems, such as depression and suicide, and substance abuse, at a higher rate than their heterosexual counterparts (Marshal et al., 2013). McNair and Brown (2013) reported that lesbian and bisexual adult women take a more permissive approach to drinking alcohol than do their heterosexual counterparts. IPV exists to a similar degree among LGBT women as among heterosexual women, but LGBT women are rarely screened for it. Transgender individuals have unique health challenges owing to the inexperience or transphobia of providers, delaying care due to gender identity, and lack of IPV services, where transgender women may be denied access, though depression, inactivity, drinking, smoking, overweight, and asthma occur to about the same degree as in heterosexual women (Reisner, Gamarel, Dunham, Hopwood, & Hwahng, 2013).

LGBT individuals often feel stigmatized, and this sometimes results in reluctance to seek routine health care. Health-care providers must learn to be open and nonjudgmental, never assuming that their patients are heterosexual, but instead routinely asking, "If you are sexually active, do you have sex with men, women, or both men and women?"

Women with Disabilities

About 27 million women in the United States have disabilities, and this number is rising (Centers for Disease Control and Prevention [CDC], 2012). The World Bank (2009) reports that women with disabilities make up at least 10% of all women globally, comprise three quarters of all disabled people in low and middle-income countries, and women are generally more likely than men to become disabled owing to poorer working conditions, poor access to quality health care, and gender-based violence.

Having a disability often creates barriers to health promotion and disease prevention activities and services. Adults with mobility limitations have worse health than those with cognitive or no limitations, rate their health as worse, are more likely to have poor health behaviors, are less likely to receive preventive cancer and heart disease screenings, and have a greater number of cardiovascular disease risk factors (Reichard, Stolzle, & Fox, 2011). Disabled individuals have a greater prevalence of obesity, and report 13 secondary health conditions per person, on average (Nosek et al., 2006). A greater degree of mobility limitation is associated with a higher number of secondary conditions, including pain, fatigue, spasticity, weakness, sleep problems, vision impairment, circulatory problems, hypertension, and periodontal disease, to name a few.

The life span of people with severe mental illness (SMI), including schizophrenia, bipolar disorder, schizoaffective disorder, and major depressive disorder, is shorter compared with the general population at a magnitude of two or three times that of the general population. This mortality gap translates to a 13- to 30-year shortened life expectancy in SMI patients. About 60% of this excess mortality is due to physical illness, primarily nutritional and metabolic diseases, cardiovascular diseases, viral diseases, respiratory tract diseases, musculoskeletal diseases, sexual problems, pregnancy complications, stomatognathic (jaw and mouth) diseases, and possibly obesity-related cancers. Increased morbidity and mortality seen in this population are largely due to a higher prevalence of modifiable risk factors, many of which are related to individual lifestyle choices. However, the somatic well-being of people with a (severe) mental illness has also been neglected, with people with SMI being less likely to receive standard levels of care for most physical diseases (De Hert et al., 2011).

Women in Recovery

Women in recovery from substance abuse and the trauma of IPV have special healthcare needs. Women recovering from opioid abuse suffer substantial morbidity and mortality, and their overall health is poorer than that of the general population. Substance abuse and suffering IPV often coexist, are highly prevalent among impoverished urban women, and increase the risk for a myriad of diseases and disorders.

Substance Abuse

In addition to the well-known risks of contracting blood-borne viral infections such as hepatitis C and human immunodeficiency virus, and mental health problems, a broader range of general health problems often exist among substance abusers and women recovering from abuse. Such problems include liver fibrosis and cirrhosis, obesity-related diseases, cardiac health issues, chronic obstructive pulmonary disease, sexual dysfunctions (Islam, Taylor, Smyth, & Day, 2013), and severe pain (Cicero, Surratt, Kurtz, Ellis, & Inciardi, 2012). These issues are often exacerbated by poor nutrition and high rates of tobacco and alcohol use, and are likely to impact the degree to which recovery goals are achieved. Drug dependence and low SES often relegate the seeking of health-care services to low priority, and nonurgent health problems may remain unknown until the condition becomes severe.

Women in treatment are also more likely to have unintended pregnancies, with almost 30% of women in one study reporting having had six or more pregnancies: only 55% of sexually active women who did not want to get pregnant used contraception (Black, Stephens, Haber, & Lintzeris, 2012). Recovering women also have high rates of adverse pregnancy outcomes (miscarriage, termination, and stillbirth) compared with national data.

Women who inject drugs face multiple gender-specific health risks. Although the prevalence of women who inject drugs is difficult to quantify, limited evidence suggests that large populations of women who inject drugs exist, and are in need of improved health services (Pinkham, Stoicescu, & Myers, 2012). Effective interventions tailored for women who inject drugs suggest that HIV risk practices must be addressed within the larger context of women's lives. Multifaceted interventions that target personal relationships, housing, employment, and children's needs may more successfully reduce risky practices than interventions focused exclusively on injecting practices and condom use (Pinkham et al., 2012).

Intimate Partner Violence

IPV is a public health concern that exists around the world, affecting predominantly women of reproductive age. The CDC defines IPV as "physical violence, sexual violence, threats of physical/sexual violence, and psychological/emotional abuse perpetrated by a current or former spouse, common-law spouse, nonmarital dating partners, or boyfriends/girlfriends of the same or opposite sex" (Saltzman, Fanslow, McMahon, & Shelley, 1999, p. 11). Violence perpetrated by an intimate partner has been linked with numerous health sequelae, including injury, physical disability, chronic pain, arthritis, headaches, gastrointestinal disorders, sexually transmitted infections, substance use and abuse, social dysfunction, insomnia, PTSD, anxiety, depression, and suicidal ideation (Bradley, Schwartz, & Kaslow, 2005; Campbell, 2002; Dutton et al., 2006). IPV also increases the risk for postpartum depression (Beydoun, Al-Sahab, Beydoun, & Tamim, 2010).

Substance abuse, violence, and HIV/AIDS have been identified as conditions that co-occur and act synergistically to impact women's health. The SAVA syndemic—synergistic epidemics of substance abuse, violence, and HIV/AIDS—exists largely in populations of urban-dwelling women who are socially and economically disadvantaged. Violence and victimization are intertwined with poor decision making, increased risk taking, and poor health, particularly in the context of substance abuse. Incorporation of violence prevention and victimization management to target this vulnerable group of women is urgently needed (Meyer, Springer, & Altice, 2011).

Recent experiences of violence predict the risk of homelessness and substance abuse for women (Stein, Leslie, & Nyamathi, 2002). One study of homeless individuals with co-occurring substance abuse and mental health disorders reported an unheard of 100% of women having experienced physical or sexual abuse (Christensen et al., 2005). Women often use and abuse recreational drugs to cope with such trauma (Yeater, Austin, Green, & Smith, 2010). Ponce, Lawless, and Rowe (2014) suggest recommendations for health-care providers working with women recovering from IPV; however, their recommendations likely apply to a wide variety of practice settings: "Taking a Nonjudgmental Approach" entails the skilled use of counseling and instinct to support a woman to act autonomously, while at the same time not giving her the impression that the provider approves of a choice to remain with an abusive partner. It is thought that an effective approach may include exploring the benefits she receives by staying with this partner, as well as referring the partner to services for his or her own benefit. "Employing Staff of Same Gender and Experiences" may smooth developing relationships between clients and providers from a "women helping women" perspective. "Utilizing Principles and Practices of Mental Health Outreach" means going to where the client is, both physically and existentially (recognizing marginalization, case-specific contexts, understanding the possibility of general mistrust of caseworkers). Specific training in outreach principles is imperative. "Utilizing Peer Engagement" capitalizes on the unique ability of peers to engage with and motivate women with similar experiences toward treatment. "Providing Staff Training in Understanding and Addressing Trauma" can develop sensitivity and appreciation for the vulnerabilities of this population, such as grief, fear, shame, and the potential conflicting consequences of accepting help. "Offering Multiple Meeting Sites" may increase utilization of services, as well as provide options for women whose partners know about certain locations, but not others, which will help increase attention to safety concerns. "Attending to Staff Needs and Mental Well-being" may mitigate the effects of vicarious trauma experienced by service providers through learning about or witnessing the trauma of others. Attention paid to managing staff identification with clients, supporting burned-out staff, and triggers of personal trauma are essential to building effective teams and successful interventions.

Summary

Nurses and other health-care providers who care for women must be attuned and sensitive to various populations of women. As discussed in this chapter, women in various groups are at risk for certain health conditions. Understanding these risks is imperative, and assisting women to achieve their optimal wellness despite these risks is of key concern to all health-care providers.

References

Aizer, A. (2010). The gender wage gap and domestic violence. *The American Economic Review, 100*(4), 1847-1859.

American Psychological Association. (2014). Poverty's impact on women's mental health. Retrieved from http://www.apa.org/pi/women/programs/poverty/

Appel, H. B., Huang, B., Ai, A. L., & Lin, C. J. (2011). Physical, behavioral, and mental health issues in Asian American women: Results from the National Latino Asian American Study. *Journal of Women's Health (Larchmt), 20*, 1703–1711.

Beckles, G.L. & Chou, C.F. (2013). Diabetes: United States 2006 and 2010, Centers for Disease Control and Prevention, Morbidity and Mortality Weekly Reports, *supplement 3*, 99-104.

Beydoun, H. A., Al-Sahab, B., Beydoun, M. A., & Tamim, H. (2010). Intimate partner violence as a risk factor for postpartum depression among Canadian women in the Maternity Experience Survey. *Annals of Epidemiology, 20*(8), 575–583.

Black, K. I., Stephens, C., Haber, P. S., & Lintzeris, N. (2012). Unplanned pregnancy and contraceptive use in women attending drug treatment services. *Australian and New Zealand Journal of Obstetrics and Gynaecology, 52*(2), 146–150.

Bradley, R., Schwartz, A. C., & Kaslow, N. J. (2005). Posttraumatic stress disorder symptoms among low-income, African American women with a history of intimate partner violence and suicidal behaviors: Self-esteem, social support, and religious coping. *Journal of Trauma and Stress, 18*, 685–696.

Campbell, J. C. (2002). Health consequences of intimate partner violence. *Lancet, 359*, 1331–1336.

Centers for Disease Control and Prevention. (2012). Retrieved from http://www.cdc.gov/ncbddd/disabilityandhealth/women.html

Chandra, A., Mosher, W. D., Copen, C., & Sionean, C. (2011). Sexual behavior, sexual attraction, and sexual identity in the United States: Data from the 2006–2008 National Survey of Family Growth. *National Health Statistics Reports* (No. 36). Hyattsville, MD: National Center for Health Statistics.

Changrani, J., Gany, F. M., Cruz, G., Kerr, R., & Katz, R. (2006). Paan and Gutka use in the United States: A pilot study in Bangladeshi and Indian-Gujarati immigrants in New York City. *Journal of Immigration and Refugee Studies, 4,* 99–110.

Christensen, R. C., Hodgkins, C. C., Garces, L., Estlund, K. L., Miller, M. D., & Touchton, R. (2005). Homeless, mentally ill and addicted: The need for abuse and trauma services. *Journal of Health Care for the Poor and Underserved, 16*(4), 615–622.

Cicero, T. J., Surratt, H. L., Kurtz, S., Ellis, M. S., & Inciardi, J. A. (2012). Patterns of prescription opioid abuse and comorbidity in an aging treatment population. *Journal of Substance Abuse Treatment, 42*(1), 87–94.

Daviglus, M.L., Talavera, G.A., Aviles-Santa, M.L., Allison, M., Cai, J., Criqui, M.H., ... Stamler, J. (2012). Prevalance of major cardiovascular risk factors and cardiovascular diseases among Hispanic/Latino individuals of diverse backgrounds in the United States. *Journal of the American Medical Association, 308*(17), 1775–1784.

DeHert, M., Cohen, D., Bobes, J., Cetkovich-Bakmas, M., Leucht, S., Ndetei, D.M., ... Correll, C.U. (2011). Physical illness in patients with severe mental disorders. II. Barriers to care, monitoriing and treatment guidelines, plus recommendations at the system and individual level. *World Psychiatry, 10*(2), 138.

deMartel, C., Forman, D., & Plummer, M. (2013). Gastric cancer: Epidemiology and risk factors. *Gastroenterology Clinics of North America, 42*(2), 219–240.

dela Cruz, F. A., & Galang, C. B. (2008). The illness beliefs, perceptions, and practices of Filipino Americans with hypertension. *Journal of the American Academy of Nurse Practitioners, 20,* 118–127.

DeSantis, C., Siegel, R., Bandi, P., & Jemal, A. (2011). Breast cancer statistics, 2011. *Cancer: A Journal for Clinicians, 61*(6), 408–418.

Dutton, M. A., Green, B. L., Kaltman, S. I., Roesch, D. M., Zeffiro, T. A., & Krause, E. D. (2006). Intimate partner violence, PTSD, and adverse health outcomes. *Journal of Interpersonal Violence, 21,* 955–968.

Frayne, S. M., Chiu, V. Y., Iqbal, S., Berg, E. A., Laungani, K. J., Cronkite, R. C., & Kimerling, R. (2011). Medical care needs of returning veterans with posttraumatic stress disorder: Their other burden. *Journal of General Internal Medicine, 26*(1), 33–39.

Friedman, S. A., Phibbs, C. S., Schmitt, S. K., Hayes, P. M., Herrera, L., & Frayne, S. M. (2011). New women veterans in the Veterans Health Administration: A longitudinal profile. *Women's Health Issues, 21*(4), S103–S111.

Fujimoto, W. Y., Boyko, E. J., Hayashi, T., Kahn, S. E., Leonetti, D. L., & McNeely, M. J. (2012). Risk factors for type 2 diabetes: Lessons learned from Japanese Americans in Seattle. *Journal of Diabetes Investigations, 3,* 212–224.

Garrett, B.E., Dube, S.R., Winder, C., & Caraballo, R.S. (2013). Cigarette smoking: United States, 2006-2008 and 2009-2010. *CDC Health Disparities and Inequalities Report - United States, 2013, 62*(3), 81.

Gates, G.J. (2011). How many people are lesbian, gay, bisexual and transgender? *The Williams Institute.* University of California e-scholarshiip. https://escholarship.org/uc/item/09h684x2. doi:10.1007/s10597-014-9712-0

Gonzales, R.G., Suarez-Orozco, C., & Dedios-Sanguineti, M.C. (2013). No place to belong: Contextualizing concepts of mental health among undocumented immigrant youth in the United States. *American Behavioral Scientist, 57* (8), 1174. 0002764213487349

Hall, K.S., Moreau, C., & Trussell, J. (2012). Determinants of and disparities in reproductive health service use among adolescent and young adult women in the United States, 2002-2008. *American Journal of Public Health, 102*(2), 359–367.

Haskell, S. G., Mattocks, K., Goulet, J. L., Krebs, E. E., Skanderson, M., Leslie, D., & Brandt, C. (2011). The burden of illness in the first year home: Do male and female Veterans Administration users differ in health conditions and healthcare utilization? *Women's Health Issues, 21*(1), 92–97.

Hsu, Y. H., Mao, C. L., & Wey, M. (2010). Antihypertensive medication adherence among elderly Chinese Americans. *Journal of Transcultural Nursing, 21,* 297–305.

Islam, M. M., Taylor, A., Smyth, C., & Day, C. A. (2013). General health of opioid substitution therapy clients. *Internal Medicine Journal, 43*(12), 1335–1338.

Kelly, U. A., Skelton, K., Patel, M., & Bradley, B. (2011). More than military sexual trauma: Interpersonal violence, posttraumatic stress disorder, and mental health in women veterans. *Research in Nursing and Health, 34*(6), 457–467.

Kim, M. J., Lee, S. J., Ahn, Y. H., & Lee, H. (2011). Lifestyle advice for Korean Americans and native Koreans with hypertension. *Journal of Advanced Nursing, 67,* 531–539.

Lehavot, K., Hoerster, K. D., Nelson, K. M., Jakupcak, M., & Simpson, T. L. (2012). Health indicators for military, veteran, and civilian women. *American Journal of Preventive Medicine, 42*(5), 473–480.

Li, N., Du, X.L., Reitzel, L.R., Xu, L., & Sturgis, E.M. (2013). Impact of enhanced detection on the increase in thyroid cancer incidence in the United States: Review of incidence trends by socioeconomic status within the surveillance, epidemiology, and end results registry, 1980-2008. *Thyroid, 23*(1), 103-110.

Li, W. W., Wallhagen, M. I., & Froelicher, E. S. (2010). Factors predicting blood pressure control in older Chinese immigrants to the United States of America. *Journal of Advanced Nursing, 66,* 2202–2212.

Maguen, S., Cohen, B., Ren, L., Bosch, J., Kimerling, R., & Seal, K. (2012). Gender differences in military sexual trauma and mental health diagnoses among Iraq and Afghanistan veterans with posttraumatic stress disorder. *Women's Health Issues, 22*(1), e61–e66.

Marshal, M. P., Dermody, S. S., Shultz, M. L., Sucato, G. S., Stepp, S. D., Chung, T., & Hipwell, A. E. (2013). Mental health and substance use disparities among urban adolescent lesbian and bisexual girls. *Journal of the American Psychiatric Nurses Association, 19*(5), 271–279.

McNair, R., & Brown, R. (2013). Clinical translation of the research article titled "the influence of early drinking contexts on current drinking among adult lesbian and bisexual women." *Journal of the American Psychiatric Nurses Association, 19*(5), 255–258.

Meyer, J. P., Springer, S. A., & Altice, F. L. (2011). Substance abuse, violence, and HIV in women: A literature review of the syndemic. *Journal of Women's Health, 20*(7), 991–1006.

Miller, G.E., Lachman, M.E., Chen, E., Gruenewald, T.L., Karlamangla, A.S., & Seeman, T.E. (2011). Pathways to resilience: Maternal nurturance as a buffer against the effects of childhood poverty on metabolic syndrome at midlife. *Psychological Science, 22*(12), 1591–1599.

Nosek, M. A., Hughes, R. B., Petersen, N. J., Taylor, H. B., Robinson-Whelen, S., Byrne, M., & Morgan, R. (2006). Secondary conditions in a community-based sample of women with physical disabilities over a 1-year period. *Archives of Physical Medicine and Rehabilitation, 87*(3), 320–327.

Ogden, C.L., Lamb, M.M., Carroll, M.D., Flegal, K.M. (2010). Obesity and socioeconomic status in adults: United States 1988–1994 and 2005–2008. NCHS Data Brief No. 50, Hyattsville, MD: National Center for Health Statistics.

Pinkham, S., Stoicescu, C., & Myers, B. (2012). Developing effective health interventions for women who inject drugs: Key areas and recommendations for program development and policy. *Advances in Preventive Medicine, 2012.*

Ponce, A. N., Lawless, M. S., & Rowe, M. (2014). Homelessness, behavioral health disorders and intimate partner violence: Barriers to services for women. *Community Mental Health Journal,* 1–10.doi: 10.1007/s10597-014-9712-0

Reichard, A., Stolzle, H., Fox, M.H. (2011). Health disparities among adults with physical disabilities or cognitive limitations compared to individuals with no disabilities in the United States. *Disability and Health Journal, 4*(2), 59-67.

Reisner, S. L., Gamarel, K. E., Dunham, E., Hopwood, R., & Hwahng, S. (2013). Female-to-male transmasculine adult health a mixed-methods community-based needs assessment. *Journal of the American Psychiatric Nurses Association, 19*(5), 293–303.

Rosenthal, T. (2014). The effect of migration on hypertension and other cardiovascular risk factors: A review. *Journal of the American Society of Hypertension, 8*(3), 171–191.

Saltzman, L.E., Fanslow, J., McMahon, P., & Shelley, G. (1999). *Intimate partner violence surveillance: Uniform definitions and recommended data elements, Version 1.0,* Atlanta, GA: National Center for Injury Prevention and Control, Centers for Disease Control and Prevention.

Steele, C.B., Rim, S.H., Joseph, D.A., King, J.B., & Seeff, L.C. (2013). Colorectal cancer incidence and screening: United States, 2008 and 2010. *CDC Health Disparities and Inequalities Report - United States, 2013, 62*(3), 53.

Stein, J. A., Leslie, M. B., & Nyamathi, A. (2002). Relative contributions of parent substance use and childhood maltreatment to chronic homelessness, depression, and substance abuse problems among homeless women: Mediating roles of self-esteem and abuse in adulthood. *Child Abuse and Neglect, 26*(10), 1011–1027.

US Department of Health and Human Services, Health Resources and Services Administration, Maternal and Child Health Bureau. (2013). *Women's Health USA 2013.* Rockville, MD: US Department of Health and Human Services.

Venkatesh, S., Weatherspoon, L. J., Kaplowitz, S. A., & Song, W. O. (2013). Acculturation and glycemic control of Asian Indian adults with type 2 diabetes. *Journal of Community Health, 38,* 78–85. Retrieved from http://dx.doi.org/10.1007/s10900-012-9584-6

Washington, D. L., Yano, E. M., McGuire, J., Hines, V., Lee, M., & Gelberg, L. (2010). Risk factors for homelessness among women veterans. *Journal of Health Care for the Poor and Underserved, 21*(1), 82–91.

Women'sHealth.gov. (2010). Minority women's health: Cervical cancer. Retrieved from http://womenshealth.gov/minority-health/latinas/cervical-cancer.html

Wong, S. S., Beth Dixon, L., Gilbride, J. A., Chin, W. W., & Kwan, T. W. (2011). Diet, physical activity, and cardiovascular disease risk factors among older Chinese Americans living in New York City. *Journal of Community Health, 36,* 446–455.

World Bank. (2009). Retrieved from http://web.worldbank.org/WBSITE/EXTERNAL/TOPICS/EXTSOCIALPROTECTION/EXTDISABILITY/0,contentMDK:20193528~menuPK:418895~pagePK:148956~piPK:216618~theSitePK:282699,00.html

Yeater, E. A., Austin, J. L., Green, M. J., & Smith, J. (2010). Coping mediates the relationship between posttraumatic stress disorder (PTSD) symptoms and alcohol use in homeless, ethnically diverse women: A preliminary study. *Psychological Trauma: Theory, Research, Practice, and Policy, 2*(4), 307–310.

Chapter 8

Body Composition: Enhancing Health through Exercise and Nutrition

Robynn Zender

Introduction

The concept of body composition is intimately tied with that of body weight, obesity, and health, and is therefore a key aspect of women's health and wellness. This chapter presents this information related to human wellness, while including a specific focus on women. This chapter emphasizes how women can enhance their own wellness at various stages of their lives by improving their body composition through exercise and nutrition. Information presented includes the definition of body composition and its measurement in terms of practical applications to health; epidemiological patterns that exist across ethnic, racial, gender, and age variables; metabolic actions of the primary compositional tissues: adipose, skeletal, and muscle; and behavioral and environmental influences that optimize body composition toward wellness within the constraints imposed by genetic inheritance.

The study of the human body has traditionally been divided into compartments or systems, such as skeletal, muscular, nervous, glandular, adipose, respiratory, cardiovascular systems, and others, in order to simplify the task of understanding these compartmental structures and functions. Recent discoveries of the metabolic cross talk that occurs between and among various compartments, however, has required a shift toward viewing the body as an integrated system where most tissues are now known to exert metabolic influences that impact the entire organism. Some of the most recent advances include the understanding of the metabolic activity of adipose tissue, and the differing actions adipose tissue exhibit depending on its distribution within the body. Environmental influences, such as nutrition and exercise, on the metabolic activity of adipose tissue, and the metabolism of sugars and fats within the body, are also among the exciting discoveries of current body composition research.

Body Composition Defined and Measured

Body composition can be divided into five levels of analysis: atomic, molecular, cellular, tissue–organ, and whole body (Shen, St. Onge, Wang, & Heymsfield, 2005). Measuring body composition to predict individual health and wellness can be simplified into understanding a person's fat-free mass (FFM) in relation to total fat mass (FM). However, determining FM distribution within various parts of the body, including visceral, subcutaneous, intramuscular, and osseous deposits provides even greater accuracy in gauging health risks. What makes fat distribution important is the metabolic activity of adipose tissue as it inhabits different areas of the body.

The study of body composition has exploded in recent years, as modifiable behavioral risk factors (i.e., smoking, physical activity [PA], diet, and weight status) have become the primary causes of mortality in the United States for both women and men (Mokdad, Marks, Stroup, & Gerberding, 2004). The determination of one's body composition is aimed at discerning various aspects of adipose tissue in relation to that of all other tissues. The most accurate methods of measuring body composition include dual-energy X-ray absorption (DXA), underwater weighing, air displacement, computed tomography, and bioelectrical impedance. DXA and bioelectrical impedance analysis (BIA) have become the instruments of choice for measuring percent body fat (PBF) in research. DXA uses low-level X-rays to discern FM, and is considered the gold standard for determining PBF, and regional adipose deposition patterns. BIA, a measurement of the resistance to an electrical signal that is found in muscle and fat tissue as it travels through water, is also a valid method for determining PBF and regional FM. These technologies, however, are often too expensive, cumbersome, time-consuming, labor-intensive, not always readily available, and require highly trained personnel. Many of these methods can also be difficult to standardize across observers or machines, which complicate comparisons across time periods. Anthropometric measurements of body composition provide more cost-effective and clinically accessible information, but the use of these measures for predicting health risks is the subject of much research and debate. The goal of various measures is to determine an individual's PBF, the distribution patterns of fat tissue, and health risks associated with fat distribution patterns.

Percent Body Fat

PBF is the amount of fat tissue in the body in relation to FFM. Because average PBF differs significantly according to gender, age, and ethnicity, there are no universal cutoff points. PBF can be measured directly using DXA or BIA, or indirectly using one of many formulas found online that incorporate any of a number of the following data points: gender; age; height; weight; waist, hip, neck, wrist, thigh, and/or forearm circumference.

BIA is a valid method of measuring PBF, as it correlates highly with DXA. BIA measures the impedance or resistance to an electrical signal that is found in muscle and fat as it travels through water. The more muscle a person has, the more water their body can hold. The greater the amount of water in a person's body, the easier it is for the current to pass through it. The more fat, the more resistance to the current. BIA may become a more accessible measurement tool clinically as, despite the device's expense (between $2,000 and $3,000 per unit), it is easy to use, has a high inter- and intra-rater reliability, high sensitivity and specificity, and is portable. BIA is safe, and the electrical signal cannot be felt by the person being measured (Bell, McClure, Hill, & Davies, 1998; Roubenoff, 1996). Accuracy of BIA fluctuates based on the body's hydration level, the timing and constituents of the last meal and drink, menstrual cycle, and skin temperature. Box 8.1 presents healthy body fat percentage ranges.

Box 8.1 Healthy Body Fat Percentage Range

Age (Years)	Healthy Range of Body Fat for Females (%)	Healthy Range of Body Fat for Males (%)
18–39	21–33	8–20
40–59	23–34	11–22
60–79	24–36	13–25

Anthropomometry

Body mass index (BMI) is the default measurement of body composition that has prevailed for the past 50 years. It was developed in the mid-1800s by a Belgian scientist, Adolphe Quetelet. BMI is defined as body mass divided by the square of one's height, as presented in Box 8.2.

BMI does not, however, accurately indicate health-related risks because it does not account for important structural factors such as frame size, muscularity, differential deposition patterns of adipose tissue, or varying proportions of body constituents such as bone, muscle, water, and fat. Its development was originally intended for use in population studies, rather than as a diagnostic tool to determine health risks of individuals. Although more accurate and useful measures of body composition are gaining in use, BMI remains the predominant evaluation tool of the Centers for Disease Control and Prevention (CDC) as a way of screening for potential health problems that could occur due to weight (http://www.cdc.gov/healthyweight/assessing/bmi/index.html). Donini et al. (2013) found, however, that BMI performed similarly to a "coin flip" at estimating PBF when evaluated by predictive value analysis, confirming results that other anthropometric and biochemical measurements explained a greater amount of the variance in estimating FM when BMI was not included in the model.

Waist-to-hip ratio and waist-to-height ratios are measured simply with a tape measure: waist circumference at the level of the navel, or slightly above the navel; and hip circumference (HC) at the widest point of the hip, usually around the level of the femoral greater trochanters. For clinical utility (Petursson, Sigurdsson, Bengtsson, Nilsen, &

Box 8.2 BMI Calculation and Classifications

$$BMI = \frac{(mass\ (kg))}{(height\ (m))^2} \text{ or } BMI = \frac{(mass\ (lb))}{(height\ (inches))^2} \times 703$$

BMI-based weight classification
- Underweight = <18.5
- Normal weight = 18.5–24.9
- Overweight = 25–29.9
- Obese (Grade I) = 30–34.9
- Obese (Grade II) = 35–39.9
- Obese (Grade III) = >40

Box 8.3 Anthropometric-Based Weight and Health-Risk Categorizations

Waist Circumference	Waist-to-Hip Ratio
Obesity defined as Men > 40 in (102 cm) Women > 35 in (88 cm)	Obesity defined as Men > 0.9 Women > 0.85

Waist-to-Hip Ratio Risk Chart

Male	Female	Health Risk Based Solely on WHR
0.95 or below	0.80 or below	Low risk
0.96–1.0	0.81–0.85	Moderate risk
1.0+	0.85+	High risk

Waist-to-Height–Based Weight Classification

Male:	Female:
<0.35 abnormally slim	<0.35 abnormally slim
0.35–0.43 very slim	0.35–0.42 very slim
0.43–0.46 slender	0.42–0.46 slender
0.46–0.54 normal	0.46–0.49 normal
0.54–0.58 overweight	0.49–0.54 overweight
0.58–0.63 obese	0.54–0.58 obese
0.63+highly obese	0.58+highly obese

Getz, 2011), waist-to-hip ratio is recommended as the primary measure of body composition and obesity. However, a review by Ashwell, Gunn, and Gibson (2012) found waist-to-height ratio to be a better screening tool for cardiometabolic risk factors among more than 300,000 adult men and women across several ethnic groups as compared with either waist circumference or BMI. The same measure, waist-to-height ratio, has also emerged as the best indicator for undiagnosed or future development of type 2 diabetes (specifically, a weight-to-height ratio of >0.5) (Kodama et al., 2012; Xu, Qi, Dahl, & Xu, 2013). Box 8.3 presents various anthropometric-based weight and health-risk categorizations.

Inter- and intra-rater reliability of anthropometric techniques, including waist, height, and waist and HC measures, is generally high, with the lowest reliability seen in inter-rater measurement of HC (reliability coefficient = 0.89), and highest reliability in inter-rater measures of height (reliability coefficient = 0.99) (Ulijaszek & Kerr, 1999).

Compositional Tissues

Compositional tissues refer to the main bodily tissues that interact through systemic metabolic pathways to impact health. Tissues that exert these metabolic effects are primarily adipose, muscle, and bone. Chief among these is adipose tissue, which exists as white, brown, or beige adipocytes (fat cells). Adipose tissue is described in the next section.

Adipose Tissue

Adipose tissue is divided into regional deposits, each of which differs with regard to structural organization, cell size, and biological function, and is tightly regulated through systemic hormonal (insulin) and sympathetic (andrenergic) stimulation (Bjørndal, Burri, Staalesen, Skorve, & Berge, 2011). Adipose tissue is a complex and active endocrine organ that is important in managing energy homeostasis; it produces hormones, such as adiponectin and leptin, which regulate energy balance through feedback loops with the pituitary and pancreatic glands.

White adipose tissue is found subcutaneously and around visceral organs. Visceral fat can be deposited within the following compartments: omental (upper abdominal viscera; stomach, spleen), mesenteric (lower abdominal viscera; intestines), retroperitoneal (surrounding kidneys), gonadal (around uterus/ovaries, or epididymis/testes), and pericardial (around the heart). White adipose tissue is also deposited intramuscularly, and within bone tissue. Subcutaneous fat can be distributed superficially or deep, is divided anatomically by a fascia layer, and is histologically distinct depending on whether the cells reside superficially or deep. Superficial subcutaneous adipose tissue (SAT) is distributed beneath the skin throughout the body, with greater deposits in the gluteofemoral (GF) and abdominal regions. Obesity characterized by greater GF fat deposition in conjunction with low abdominal fat is termed "gynoid obesity." On the other hand, "android obesity" is characterized by fat deposition patterns that consist of fat deposition to a greater degree abdominally than in the GF compartment. These two fat distribution patterns are referred to, colloquially, as "pear" versus "apple" patterns respectively.

White adipose tissue stores excess dietary fat in the form of triglycerides, and mobilizes free fatty acids through lipolysis when energy is in demand. Intercellular lipolytic activity is dependent upon the number of mitochondria present within the cell. Adipocytes located subcutaneously have fewer mitochondria than do viscerally-deposited adipocytes. As a result, visceral fat deposits are more lipolytically active than are subcutaneous adipocytes, and so contribute more to circulating blood fat levels. SAT demonstrates greater short- and long-term energy storage capacity, because it is less metabolically active. GF adipose tissue accumulates recycled fat, rather than dietary fat, and is therefore active in the long-term sequestering of fatty acids. Because GF adipose tissue is more metabolically inert than both visceral and abdominal SAT, it is protective against unfavorable lipid, insulin, and glucose profiles, and metabolic and cardiovascular diseases (CVDs) (Manolopoulos, Karpe, & Frayn, 2010; Sood & Dixon, 2013). Deep SAT functions more like viscerally deposited fats in that a high correlation exists between deep SAT and circulating levels of insulin and insulin utilization. Gynoid obesity is characterized by adipocyte hyperplasia, as opposed to hypertrophy (Sood & Dixon, 2013).

Adipocyte hypertrophy (cell expansion) is associated with chronic overfeeding, metabolic abnormalities, lipolysis from fat cells, and increased insulin production (Bays, 2009), whereas adipocyte hyperplasia (increase cell number) poses less risk for chronic diseases due to its greater metabolic stability (Drolet et al., 2008).

Intermuscular adipose fat tissue is considered white adipose tissue, and appears to increase health risks for obesity-related diseases. It is associated with inactivity and greater accumulation with age, similar to that of visceral adipose tissue (VAT).

Brown adipose tissue, named for its high concentration of iron-containing mitochondria, exists in greater proportions in newborns, and in small quantities in adults, mostly between the scapulae and in the supraclavicular anterior neck area. This tissue arises from a different cellular lineage (skeletal muscle) from white adipose tissue, and contains high numbers of mitochondria, but fewer lipid droplets than white adipose tissue. Brown adipose tissue mobilizes fatty acids for use within mitochondria to produce heat, termed nonshivering thermogenesis, during cold temperatures. Chronic cold exposure stimulates expansion and activation of brown adipose tissue.

A newly isolated cell type, beige adipocytes, are adipocytes that emerge from the same stem cell origin as white adipose tissue (Wu, Cohen, & Spiegelman, 2013). Beige adipose tissue appears to have even greater metabolic influence through endocrine function than brown adipose tissue, and is inducible (preadipocytes can be induced toward beige development stimulated by cAMP signal transduction) in both white and brown adipose fat deposits. Thermogenic activity of both brown and beige adipose tissue increases whole-body energy expenditure, which maintains a stable body weight and inhibits weight gain. A reduced amount and thermogenic capacity of brown adipose tissue correlates with lower energy expenditure, greater insulin resistance, and excess weight gain (Rahman et al., 2013). Both brown and beige adipose tissues are under intense scrutiny as targets for treatments related to obesity and diabetes.

Adipose deposition in the bone. *Adipose deposition* in the bone has been discovered to be significant like adipose tissue, bone tissue has long been viewed as metabolically inert and separate from other tissues. Recently, adipose tissue existing within bone marrow and bony tissue has been discovered to have significant interaction with bone tissue and to affect endocrine function. In fact, evidence suggests that adipose tissue in bone marrow is bidirectionally linked to systemic energy metabolism, as well as local mineralization activity, where bone marrow adipocytes and osteocytes (bone cells) interact inversely via local and systemic means. Adipokines, produced locally from adipocytes within bone marrow, inhibit the function and survival of osteoblasts such that osteocalcin production, bone formation, and differentiation of marrow stem cells (called mesenchymal cells) toward osteoblasts (as opposed to adipocytes) are reduced. Bone marrow fat also stimulates osteoclast differentiation and functions to reduce bone density (Elia, 2012). Bone marrow containing hematopoietic tissue (blood-forming tissue) fosters bone formation, whereas replacement of red marrow with yellow fat as people age reduces mineralization and promotes more fat to form in bone marrow.

Systemically, bone cells respond to circulating insulin through insulin receptors that exist on osteoblasts (Elia, 2012). This insulin signaling inhibits osteoblasts from producing and releasing into circulation osteocalcin, which, in turn, inhibits leptin and insulin secretion. Reduced insulin and leptin production promotes insulin resistance, poor glucose homeostasis, and greater peripheral (extra-osseous) adiposity. Extraosseous fat tissue that is more metabolically active (VAT), as opposed to SAT, promotes greater amounts of leptin to be released into circulation. This, in turn, stimulates insulin production, which, in terms of bone cell function, reduces osteocalcin production that furthers both local and systemic action. Bone tissue and the pancreas engage in a feedback loop where insulin signals osteoblast differentiation and osteocalcin production, which, in turn, regulates insulin sensitivity and pancreatic insulin production (Fulzele et al., 2010).

Because bone tissue is highly interactive with other metabolic tissues, it is important to engage in activities and diets that improve bone health, especially for women, who have a greater risk for osteoporosis (OP) and bone fractures (Sheu & Cauley, 2011). Resistance training that improves muscle health and adipose tissue function may also benefit bone health independent of mechanically-stimulated bone formation.

Skeletal Muscle/Lean Muscle Mass

Much like the study of bone has identified bone tissue as endocrinologically active, so has the study of muscle biology revealed muscle tissue to function locally and systemically. The understanding of muscle tissue as being secretory with metabolic functions is a very recent discovery but, in hindsight, not a surprising one. Skeletal muscle is the largest internal organ in the body and, given its great demand for glucose, and essential mechanical action upon bone, it may be that skeletal muscle participates in energy regulation and bone formation via paracrine and endocrine signaling pathways (Hamrick, 2011). It is well known that contracting skeletal muscle increases glucose uptake, which corresponds to glucose production in the liver in order to maintain glucose homeostasis. Likewise, adipose tissue releases fatty acids into circulation in response to exercise, but detailed knowledge of physiological interactions among muscle, fat, and bone tissue is minimal.

Whereas adipocytes release adipokines (metabolically active hormones) and osteoblasts secrete osteocalcin, myocytes secrete myokines. Myokines that are important in terms of body composition include IL-6, IL-15, and irisin. IL-6 is a proinflammatory cytokine that is active in immune responses to infection and injury. Initially, the IL-6 response to exercise was assumed to be related to muscle damage sustained during PA. However, IL-6 is now known to be released by contracting muscle tissue, and has numerous biological effects, including glucose and fat metabolism (Pedersen, 2013). IL-15, a cytokine that supports lymphocyte proliferation, is also expressed in skeletal muscle following strength training. In addition to its anabolic effects on skeletal muscles (using energy to build tissue mass), IL-15 also reduces adipose tissue mass, and decreases lipid deposition in preadipocytes, thereby playing a role in muscle–fat cross talk (Pedersen, 2013). Irisin, also released into circulation during exercise, drives white fat cells into a brown fat–like phenotype called "brite" cells. Brite fat increases total body energy expenditure through heat generation from mitochondrial activation, and also improves glucose tolerance. Pedersen (2013) makes a strong case for the detrimental effects of muscular disuse, and salutary effects of PA not only in terms of mechanical changes in strength and coordination, but also in impacting endocrine function that is key to metabolic health.

Body Composition and Health

The quality of health of an individual is directly linked to body composition. "The distribution of fat between these depots seems to be more important than the total adipose tissue mass for the risk of developing obesity-related diseases" (Bjørndal et al., 2011, p. 1). Android and gynoid patterns of fat deposition are associated differentially with health risks. GF body fat (gynoid distribution) is protective against many disorders, because it is less metabolically active, entraps fatty acids long term, improves adipokine and leptin profiles, and reduces inflammatory cytokines (Manolopoulos et al., 2010).

The relationship between weight and health risk is often thought of as linear: that with increasing weight, health risks increase equally. What many studies report, however, is no increased risk of certain health conditions, or even protective effects, of overweight and mild obesity (class I). Concomitantly, up to 40% of individuals with a normal BMI demonstrate some degree of metabolic or cardiovascular evidence of disease (Weiss, Bremer, & Lustig, 2013), such as insulin resistance, high blood pressure, hyperlipidemia, prediabetes, or type 2 diabetes, in addition to an excess risk of all-cause mortality (Flegal, Kit, Orpana, & Graubard, 2013; Kahn, Bullard, Barker, & Imperatore, 2012). This conundrum has been termed the "obesity paradox" (Kahn et al., 2012). What is clear is that in the highest classifications of obesity (class II and III), excess risks of morbidity and mortality exist. This "bookend" effect of increased health risks in low/normal weight, and high obesity, with lowest risks existing in the middle weight range of overweight and class I obesity, suggests factors beyond BMI are involved.

Lavie, De Schutter, and Milani (2013) explained some of this "overweight paradox." They found that individuals with both low BMI and low PBF have the highest CVD mortality rates, even with underweight persons excluded from analysis. Furthermore, when PBF and FFM were considered, the highest mortality occurs in individuals with low PBF and low FFM, with the lowest mortality seen in those with high PBF and high FFM. Having a lower FFM contributed to mortality more than measures of PBF. Additional work by this group has revealed the impact of cardiorespiratory fitness (CRF) in relation to PBF and FFM on CVD prognosis and mortality risks. High CRF demonstrated lower mortality rates and no obesity paradox, regardless of method of defining obesity (BMI, PBF, or waist circumference), suggesting that CRF modifies the effects of BMI on survival. This result has been confirmed in many studies (Barry et al., 2014; Lee, Artero, Sui, & Blair, 2010; Lee, Sui, Artero, et al. 2011; Lee, Sui, Ortega, et al., 2011).

Morbidity and Mortality

Morbidity and mortality show direct correlations with differential patterns of adipose tissue deposition. Because measurements of waist and HC distinguish abdominal fat deposits relative to GF fat accumulation, these measurements are often used in conjunction with BMI to understand health risks of distinct fat deposits. Waist-to-hip ratios and waist-to-height ratios are both strong predictors of all-cause mortality, whereas BMI has a weaker association with mortality (Petursson et al., 2011). Petursson et al. (2011) found waist-to-hip ratio offers the greatest discrimination to prediction models for mortality and, in particular, CVD mortality, followed by waist-to-height, and then waist circumference.

All-cause and CVD mortality is lower in people with high BMI and high CRF, in comparison with those with normal BMI and low CRF, even though having a high BMI, with high CRF, does not attenuate the risk of diabetes or CVD morbidity (Fogelholm, 2010). Waist circumference has been positively associated with all-cause mortality within all BMI categories, with the highest category (BMI ≥ 30) demonstrating the highest mortality risk (Jacobs et al., 2010). Cameron, Magliano, and Söderberg (2013) discussed the importance of including HC measurements in conjunction with waist circumference in all morbidity and mortality studies, since HC accounts for the protective effect of gynoid adipose distribution patterns. Without HC, mortality risks may be significantly underestimated.

Metabolic Syndrome

Metabolic syndrome is characterized as having three or more indicators of metabolic dysregulation: central obesity, high triglycerides, low high-density lipoprotein (HDL) concentrations, high blood pressure, or high fasting blood glucose (Alberti et al., 2009). Metabolic dysregulation occurs when the action of hormones, such as insulin and leptin, is impaired such that fat cells disallow blood glucose from entering fat cells, and insulin continues to be secreted into circulation, inhibiting the hypothalamus from receiving leptin signals from fat cells, increasing appetite, and demotivating PA. Because adipose tissue is highly metabolically active and is responsible for supplying short and long-term energy needs, dysfunctional adipose tissue results in dysfunctional metabolism regulation. Lipotoxicity (excess fatty acids in circulation), is an important step in the development of metabolic syndrome, as it initiates a state of systemic inflammation, as measured by serum C-reactive protein (CRP), a commonly used biomarker of systemic inflammation. As adipose tissue reaches its maximum storage capacity, excess blood fat is deposited in visceral organs and muscle, and inhibits normal organ function. Excessive blood fat impairs the functions of organ and adipose tissue, insulin and leptin utilization, and increases systemic inflammation (Bays et al., 2013; Frigerio et al., 2010; McLaughlin, 2012; Phillips & Perry, 2013). Furthermore, as fat cells distend to their maximum capacity, they can burst and initiate an inflammatory response by the immune system that recruits phagocytes to the site to clear the apoptotic cell.

Metabolic dysregulation increases an individual's risk of obesity, type 2 diabetes, insulin resistance, kidney disease, CVD, nonalcoholic fatty liver disease (NAFLD), polycystic ovarian syndrome, and certain cancers (Grundy, 2011). Importantly, there is a difference between being fat and being sick: our risk for disease is increasing faster than the incidence of obesity, and 20% of morbidly obese (BMI > 30) individuals are metabolically healthy (Weiss et al., 2013). Furthermore, as much as 40% of normal-weight individuals are insulin-resistant or have metabolic syndrome, the so-called metabolically-obese, normal-weight (MONW). Of these, 20% have fatty liver disease, which is a primary risk factor for diabetes (Smith & Adams, 2011). Individuals with a high PBF and normal weight are at higher risk for cardiometabolic disease (hypertension, vascular dysfunction, type 2 diabetes) (Shea, King, Gullivere, & Sun, 2012), with vascular endothelial function impairment seen among healthy people with modest weight gains, even without noticeable changes in blood pressure. Impairments in endothelial function may resolve with subsequent weight loss (Romero-Corral et al., 2010). Gomez-Ambrosi et al. (2011) found an increased risk of type 2 diabetes with increased body fat, but within a normal BMI. The "thin-on-the-outside, fat-on-the-inside" phenotype, or TOFI, shows many lean men and women with more VAT than overweight or obese persons (Thomas, Frost, Taylor-Robinson, & Bell, 2012). Fat deposition tendencies also have a strong genetic component: even after controlling for BMI, heritability of fat deposit distribution is estimated to be between 22% and 61% (Heid et al., 2010), with up to 55% of the variance in visceral FM being genetically determined (Crowther & Ferris, 2010). The great variability in physical and metabolic adaptability seen in lean individuals suggests a more dynamic phenotyping of metabolically healthy versus pathologic body type may improve our understanding of the complex nature and trajectory of obesity and its related disorders (Dulloo, Jacquet, Solinas, Montani, & Schutz, 2010).

Bone Health

OP and osteopenia are the most prevalent bone disorders (http://www.ncbi.nlm.nih.gov/pubmedhealth/PMH0001400/), with approximately one third of women and one fifth of men over the age of 50 qualifying for treatment in the US population (Dawson-Hughes et al., 2010). Body composition impacts bone health through mechanical and metabolic pathways involving adipose, muscle, and bone tissue interaction. Excess weight has long been thought to improve bone density owing to increased weight loads on bone tissue (Gnudi, Sitta, & Fiumi, 2007). OP, however, is now thought of as "the obesity of bone," with lipotoxicity driving bone loss in old age (Griffith et al., 2012).

SAT and VAT demonstrate opposing effects on bone structure and strength in young women (Gilsanz et al., 2009). Subcutaneous, beige, and brown adipose tissues appear to benefit bone structure and strength (Rahman et al., 2013), whereas visceral fat is pathogenic to bone health (Gilsanz et al., 2009).

Diabetes is also closely linked with bone health owing to the interactions between metabolism, fat tissue, and insulin functions. Those with both type 1 and type 2 diabetes suffer a greater risk of fractures to the extent that a diabetes diagnosis is now included in the formula for clinically determining fracture risk (de Paula, Horowitz, & Rosen, 2010). Furthermore, a greater decrease in bone mass is seen in individuals with one cardiometabolic risk factor (CRF), and individuals having greater than two CRFs demonstrate greater visceral fat deposition, lower HDL concentrations, and increased insulin resistance (Pollock et al., 2011). Clearly, the subject of bone health cannot be separated from the health status of one's adipose, muscle, and endocrine systems.

Sarcopenia

Sarcopenia is the natural loss of muscle mass over time, but this loss is accelerated in overweight and obese individuals. In healthy people, muscle mass peaks through the mid-to late 20s, and by age 50, roughly 10% of muscle mass is lost. After age 60, sharp declines in muscle mass are seen, with just more than half of peak muscle mass remaining at age 80. Sarcopenia results from reduced sensitivity of muscle tissue to growth-promoting hormones, such as insulin, chronic systemic inflammation, and obesity. Coexistent muscle mass loss with increased FM within muscle tissue is termed "sarcobesity." With lipid accumulation of obesity, skeletal muscle is prevented from utilizing amino acid to synthesize proteins necessary to maintain muscle integrity (Parr, Coffey, & Hawley, 2013).

Dynapenia, the loss of muscle strength, denotes a reduction in muscle quality, as opposed to muscle atrophy seen in sarcopenia. Muscle strength is lost more rapidly over time than is muscle mass, at a rate of two to five times, and is a more consistent risk for morbidity and mortality (Mitchell et al., 2012). Taken together, sarcopenia, sarcobesity, and dynapenia reflect the synergistic action of natural loss of muscle mass and strength with the accelerative action of added adipose tissue to create functional impairments in mobility, and comorbidity with metabolic disorders.

Other Conditions

Other prevalent health conditions associated with a pathologic body composition include asthma, depression, and sleep apnea. An android body shape is associated with greater asthma risk in women more than men, perhaps through an inflammatory pathway (Sood & Dixon, 2013). Women with major depressive disorder have a 335% higher visceral fat content than nondepressed women (Greggersen et al., 2011). Sleep apnea is more prevalent among older, heavier individuals with greater upper body fat deposition (than lower body fat deposition), and epicardial fat quantity (cardiac adiposity) (Lubrano et al., 2012).

Body Composition across a Woman's Life Span

Women are affected by changes in body composition, having implications for their health and well-being, at various stages of their life spans. This section presents an overview of life span changes in women's body composition.

Prenatal and Infancy

The prenatal environment sets the phenotype for adult body composition and fat distribution patterns. Percent liver fat correlated positively with prepregnancy body mass in the mother, but not subcutaneous adiposity. Maternal diet may be modified to alter the offspring's adult disease risk (Blumfield et al., 2012). In a recent study, infants of obese mothers or mothers with gestational diabetes had a 68% increase in liver fat compared with babies born to mothers of a normal weight (Brumbaugh et al., 2013). Thin babies have a greater risk for cardiometabolic disease in adulthood, especially when the thinness results from reduced lean body mass (Hediger et al., 1998).

Childhood

Among both sexes, lean soft tissue and FFM were found to be lowest at the ages of 8 to 11 years (Borrud et al., 2010). Waist circumference and waist-to-height ratio have been shown to best predict risk of cardiometabolic disease in overweight children, with overweight being determined by BMI (Maffeis, Banzato, & Talamini, 2008). Greater FFM shows a positive correlation with bone mineralization in 6- to 18-year-old boys and girls, and Hispanic children demonstrate significantly greater bone mineral content than children from any other race or ethnicity (Dorsey, Thornton, Heymsfield, & Gallagher, 2010).

Adolescence

A large population–based study suggests the percentage of body fat is lowest in males at the ages of 16 to 19 years, and at the ages of 8 to 15 years for females (Borrud et al., 2010). Clinical measurement of insulin resistance in the adolescent population uses both waist circumference and PBF. Waist circumference predicted insulin resistance in obese children, and PBF better predicted insulin resistance in lean children (Wedin, Diaz-Gimenez, & Convit, 2012). Skeletal muscle insulin resistance is the earliest metabolic defect observable in young, lean, insulin-resistant children of parents with type 2 diabetes, and results from increased fat accumulation in muscle tissue (Petersen et al., 2012). In adolescents, both fat accumulation and insulin resistance by muscle tissue are reversible with modest weight loss.

Reproductive Phase and Older Women

Both fat- and lean-tissue mass increase during pregnancy and decline during the postpartum period in accordance with breast-feeding status: there is a slower decline of body mass loss as length of breast-feeding increases (Møller, viò Streym, Mosekilde, & Rejnmark, 2012). During pregnancy and breast-feeding, women lose a significant amount of bone density, but the loss is reversible once breast-feeding stops or, in the case of prolonged breast-feeding, returns to prepregnancy levels by 19 months postpartum (Møller et al., 2012). Pregnancy-related loss of bone density occurs irrespective of calcium and vitamin D intake.

Body composition in older women follows similar patterns to those of middle-aged women: greater visceral adiposity, lower lean body mass, greater fat deposition in muscle tissue correlates with a greater risk of cardiometabolic and skeletal disorders; GF subcutaneous fat imparts a protective effect against cardiometabolic risks; and physical exercise, particularly resistance training, reduces risk in every category (Peppa, Koliaki, & Dimitriadis, 2012; Shin, Panton, Dutton, & Ilich, 2011). The exception to following the pattern of younger adults relates to estrogen: the estrogen reduction of menopause amplifies health risks, and makes remediation more difficult and less effective (Abildgaard et al., 2013). Hormone therapy does appear to improve lean body mass and reduce fall risk in the first 3 years of use, although this benefit levels off after 6 years of use (Bea et al., 2011).

Bone marrow fat rises sharply in women aged 55 to 65, and correlates with extraosseous fat deposition changes from a gynoid pattern (thigh and gluteal deposition) to an android pattern of abdominal deposition (Griffith, 2012). The only consistent predictors of low bone density in healthy women between 40 and 60 years of age were having a low total body mass and postmenopausal status (Waugh et al., 2009). In this systematic review, fair evidence was found that no predictive risk of low bone density exists in relation to alcohol and caffeine intake, or reproductive history. Possible, but inconclusive, risks existed between low bone mass and a number of factors: calcium intake, PA, smoking, age at menarche, history of amenorrhea, family history of OP, race, and current age.

Respiratory function has been shown to be inversely associated with visceral fat and sarcopenia in a cohort of older women and men. Increased weight gain over a 5-year period was associated with more rapid declines in forced expiratory volume (FEV_1) and forced vital capacity (FVC) (Rossi et al., 2011).

Patterns of Body Composition in Women

In addition to life span considerations in body composition and women's health, there are specific patterns of body composition related to gender as well as race. Women may be at a higher risk for morbidity and mortality from living in an "obesogenic environment" (increased food availability, decreased mobility, and increased energy density combined with reduced nutritionally dense processed foods) than are men, given their innate tendency toward fat accumulation, and risks for deficiency disorders associated with nutrient-exhausting activities such as pregnancy and lactation (Shapira, 2013). Women have more adiposity than men, as seen by a higher percentage of body fat than males. After age 11, males have a higher lean tissue and FFM than females (Borrud et al., 2010). However, men have more visceral and hepatic adipose tissue, while women have more peripheral and SAT. Differences in sex hormones contribute to a more insulin-sensitive environment in women (Geer & Shen, 2009). Men generally have greater insulin resistance than women, as estrogen is thought to be protective for women because it increases insulin sensitivity (Cowther & Ferris, 2010). Women also possess more active brown/beige fat than do men, which appears to be linked to differential hormone profiles (Wu et al., 2013). The relationship between testosterone level and active brown/beige fat in men is as yet unknown.

It is also important to note that not only are there gender differences in body composition, but body composition varies by ethnic group, and appears to be driven by differential capacities for triglyceride accumulation between compartments of adipose deposits (Crowther & Ferris, 2010). Diet has been conjectured to interact with ancestral genetic admixture to produce the present day differences seen in fat storage among different populations such as Europeans, African Americans, and Hispanics (Casazza, 2011). Asians of many ethnicities demonstrate higher PBF in both men and women at each level of BMI (Dullo et al., 2010). Asians of Chinese origin have a higher PBF and trunk fat than whites within a given BMI, even though only trunk fat has been shown to account for increased metabolic risk (He & Zhang, 2013).

Caucasian males demonstrate greater FM than either Mexican Americans or African Americans, whereas African American women have greater FM than the other two populations of women (Crowther & Ferris, 2010). Mexican American males and females present with less lean soft tissue than either Caucasians or African Americans (Borrud et al., 2010).

Exercise and Nutrition to Enhance Body Composition

What has become apparent in recent years is the importance of metabolic functioning as the foundation for health in all bodily systems. A holistic approach, including bio-psychosocial, emotional and spiritual factors, and social determinants of health, must be incorporated into a healthy regimen. Metabolic action binds all systems together for whole organism functioning, adaptation, and growth. Because metabolism is systemic in nature, specific actions targeted at improving health must consider its impact on discrete systems as they relate to other systems, as well as to the organism in its entirety. Thus, weight-loss regimens must include muscle resistance training to prevent the loss of lean body mass and bone density while reproportioning the body toward a healthier composition overall.

The widely held belief that thinner is better is inaccurate if cardiorespiratory and muscular fitness is inadequate. Furthermore, chronic distress from long-term economic, relational, physical, medical, environmental, and social threats provokes inflammatory processes that are also systemic in nature. In fact, it is possible that inflammation constitutes the primary condition underlying most chronic diseases in industrialized nations, as biomarkers of inflammation correlate positively with morbidity and mortality from all-cause, cardiovascular, and non—cardiovascular diseases (Ahmadi-Abhari, Luben, Wareham, & Khaw, 2013). An increase in CRP showed increased risk estimates comparable to other risk factors for mortality, such as smoking, BMI, diabetes, cholesterol, and blood pressure. Excess biomarkers of inflammation also exist in individuals suffering chronically conflictual relationships (Kiecolt-Glaser, Gouin, & Hantsoo, 2010), social isolation (Eisenberger, 2012), social exclusion and rejection (Dickerson & Zoccola, 2013; Slavich, Way, Eisenberger, & Taylor, 2010), and social disadvantages, such as poverty and lack of education (Clark et al., 2012). Thus, in addition to cardiorespiratory and strengthening exercise, reducing systemic inflammation through stress reduction and therapeutic activity (relaxation, visualization, breath work, mindfulness training, psychotherapy, yoga, others), pharmacotherapy, and improving social and relationship issues may improve body composition through improved metabolic regulation and health.

Weight loss without strengthening can reduce muscle integrity and does not necessarily promote health in the long term (Heymsfield et al., 2011). Weight loss plus exercise results in additional improvements in function (as measured by strength and physical performance) as opposed to exercise alone in older adults, primarily due to the loss of body fat. Weight loss alone can facilitate lean muscle loss, in addition to the loss of FM, which may reduce functional status, and increase the risk of falls and fractures. Therefore, exercise along with weight loss is important to prevent concomitant loss of strength and performance (Parr et al., 2013; Santanasto et al., 2011). Weight loss without resistance training also reduces bone integrity, due to the dynamic interactions among bone, muscle, and adipose tissue.

Healthy Exercises

Exercise benefits women in innumerable ways. Exercise increases energy expenditure in brown and white adipose tissue (Wu et al., 2013). Reduced body fat with exercise increases cardiovascular fitness, increases Vo_2 max, and improves fasting glucose levels (Carrel et al., 2005). PA influences adipose tissue both acutely and in the long term. A single bout of PA stimulates blood flow to adipose tissue, and fat mobilization to deliver fatty acids to skeletal muscle. For a short time period following one bout of PA, fatty acids are directed away from adipose tissue and toward skeletal muscle, reducing storage of dietary fat. Chronic exercise training increases fat mobilization during acute exercise. PA contributes to metabolic health via beneficial dynamic changes in adipose tissue in response to each activity bout (Thompson, Karpe, Lafontan, & Frayn, 2012).

Maintaining skeletal integrity (bone density and strength) can be achieved through holding certain stretching poses a minimum of 8 seconds, up to 72 seconds, but no greater benefit is seen by holding a pose beyond 72 seconds (Fishman, 2009; Pead, Suswillo, Skerry, Vedi, & Lanyon, 1988; Rubin & Lanyon, 1984). Weight cycling (yo-yo dieting) has been associated with overall heavier weight, poorer metabolic profiles, and greater mortality than non–weight cyclers. However mortality risks may be confounded by health status (Casazza et al., 2013). Weight cyclers may benefit more than noncyclers in improvement of metabolic indices and body composition when adhering to a lifestyle intervention (Mason et al., 2013).

The thermogenic activity of brown and beige fat is inversely associated with weight, such that this tissue becomes more active in women undergoing bariatric surgery (Wu et al., 2013). White adipose tissue may be provoked into becoming beige tissue through active participation in one's environment (Cao et al., 2011), exercise, weight loss, lactation, and exposure to cold (Smorlesi, Frontini, Giordano, & Cinti, 2012). A quick reference for the benefits of exercise to improve a healthy body composition is provided in Table 8.1.

TABLE 8.1.	Exercise Types and Benefits	
Exercise Types	**Examples**	**Benefits**
Endurance training	Anything that increases heart rate for 30 minutes or more: walking, running, swimming, cycling, jump rope, aerobics, etc.	Increases thermal energy output Improves metabolic function Improves cardiorespiratory fitness Increases FFM Reduces visceral fat Increases brown fat tissue Strengthens muscle Recruits more muscle fibers Builds existing muscle fibers Reduces intramuscular fat deposits Reduces stress Reduces inflammation
Resistance exercise	Weight lifting Isometric exercises Pilates Swimming Exercise ball work	Increases thermal energy output Increases FFM Improves metabolic function Strengthens muscle Recruits more muscle fibers Builds existing muscle fibers Improves bone mineralization Reduces adipose deposits in bone marrow and muscle tissue Decreases bone resorption Reduces visceral fat Increases brown fat tissue Improves balance and coordination

TABLE 8.1.	Exercise Types and Benefits *(continued)*	
Exercise Types	**Examples**	**Benefits**
Interval training: Spurts of endurance activity at regular intervals	Sprint for 30 seconds every 5 minutes of a run (swim, walk, cycle)	Increases thermal energy output Increases FFM Improves metabolic function Strengthens muscle Recruits more muscle fibers Builds existing muscle fibers Improves bone mineralization Reduces adipose deposits in bone marrow and muscle tissue Decreases bone resorption Reduces visceral fat Increases brown fat tissue Improves cardiorespiratory fitness Reduces stress Reduces inflammation
High-impact exercise	Jump rope Running Aerobics	Increases thermal energy output Improves bone mineralization Reduces adipose deposits in bone marrow Decreases bone resorption
Stretching	Hold pose for 8–72 seconds Yoga	Reduces stress Improves bone mineralization Reduces adipose deposits in bone marrow Decreases bone resorption Increases thermal energy output Improves balance and coordination Reduces inflammation
Engage with your environment	Living in an enriched environment with complex physical and social stimulation (larger spaces, opportunities for exercise, regularly changing play and challenge activities)	Increases thermal energy output Increases amount of brown fat tissue Reduces stress Improves balance and coordination
Acute episode of PA Chronic exercise training	One 30-minute exercise session Regular exercise over time	Increase blood flow to adipose tissue Deliver fatty acids to muscles Direct fatty acids away from adipose tissue Increase responses to acute-episode PA in all areas (fatty acid mobilization, etc.) Improve cardiorespiratory fitness Improve metabolic function

Healthy Nutrition

Not surprisingly, diet also significantly impacts body composition. Eating to improve metabolic efficacy entails understanding qualitative differences in types of calories, protein, fat, and carbohydrate consumed, and how our bodies use these nutrients based on our metabolism. While every unit of fat, protein, and carbohydrate releases the same number of calories per gram, different types of fats, proteins, and carbohydrates are metabolized differently. For example, monounsaturated fats can reduce inflammation, while saturated fats can increase inflammation and cause heart and fatty liver disease (Nicholls et al., 2006). Egg protein can build muscle, while ground beef can increase insulin resistance (Hirabara, Curi, & Maechler, 2010). Fructose is almost exclusively metabolized directly into fat, while starch (glucose) is a food source that can be used for energy by every cell in the body (Samuel, 2011). Fiber is also critically important in our diet, even though it contributes no nutritional value in itself. Fiber slows the absorption of fats, glucose, and fructose by forming a gelatinous barrier between food and the intestinal wall and preventing reabsorption in the colon. Fiber keeps blood insulin levels low by slowing absorption of fats and carbohydrates. By delaying stomach emptying into the small intestine, fiber provides a sense of fullness and reduces excessive food intake. Soluble fiber binds bile acids in the intestine and prevents them from being reabsorbed, lowering blood levels of low-density lipoproteins (LDL). Fiber also improves beneficial gut flora and reduces pathogenic gut flora that can contribute to obesity (Brownlee, 2011).

Eating habits that promote metabolic health do so based on four main metabolic actions: reducing insulin load, reducing ghrelin (hunger hormone), increasing peptide YY (PYY) (satiety hormone), and reducing cortisol (Lustig, 2012). Insulin is reduced through ingesting fiber, low amounts of sugar, and exercise. Ghrelin is reduced through eating a protein-rich breakfast, not bingeing at nighttime, and getting sufficient sleep. PYY can be increased through portion control, waiting 20 minutes after eating before taking a second helping, and eating fiber. Cortisol is reduced through exercise and stress reduction. Food components that improve metabolic efficacy include negligible amounts of refined sugar, low omega-6 fats (found in meats and dairy), high omega-3 fats (found in nut, seed, olive, and fish oils), high fiber, and eating whole, unprocessed foods. A general guideline for a metabolically healthy diet is presented in Box 8.4, where foods considered "green light"

Box 8.4 Traffic Signal Dietary Guidelines for a Healthy Metabolism

Green Light	Yellow Light	Red Light
Whole fruits and vegetables	Pulverized (flour)-containing	Candy
Olive oil	products	Processed foods
Whole, rolled, steel cut,	Dairy	Anything with added
sprouted, hulled, and pearled	Meat	sugar, especially juice
grains		Juice, even without
Legumes		added sugar
Nuts and seeds		

Adapted from Lusting, R. H. (2013). Table 17.2: A "Real" versus "Processed" Food Shopping List. In Fat chance: Beating the odds against sugar, processed.

are healthy and should be encouraged, those considered "yellow light" eaten occasionally, and those considered "red light" should be avoided.

Not only does the quality of carbohydrates, fats, and proteins impact metabolism and body composition, but so does the proportion of these constituents consumed. Diets of proportionately greater protein content (27% of energy as protein, 44% as carbohydrate, and 29% as fat) than the average protein-containing diet (16% of energy as protein, 57% as carbohydrate, and 27% as fat) preserve total lean mass, reduce glycemic response, serum triglyceride levels, with no deleterious effects on markers of bone turnover, calcium excretion, or systolic blood pressure (Farnsworth et al., 2003; Krieger, Sitren, Daniels, & Langkamp-Henken, 2006). Furthermore, a high-protein diet in conjunction with cardiorespiratory and resistance exercise promotes greater weight loss than exercise with a high-carbohydrate diet, and maintains higher concentrations of HDL cholesterol (Layman et al., 2005). Layman et al. (2005) also noted that those consuming a high-carbohydrate diet had reductions in total cholesterol and LDL cholesterol, but did not share the improvement in triglycerides and HDL levels seen among those eating a high-protein diet.

One last comment on diet pertains to the consumption of alcoholic beverages. Moderate alcohol use (one drink per day for women, two for men) has been shown to provide a protective effect for a number of cardiovascular diseases CDSs (Rimm, Williams, Fosher, Criqui, & Stampfer, 1999; Ronksley, Brien, Turner, Mukamal, & Ghali, 2011). In fact, healthy cardiovascular biomarkers have been associated with moderate alcohol intake of any type (wine, beer, spirits): increased HDL, apolipoprotein A1, and adiponectin, and reduced circulating fibrinogen levels, but with no effect on triglyceride levels (Brien, Ronksley, Turner, Mukamal, & Ghali, 2011). However, greater than moderate alcohol intake immediately and steeply increases mortality and morbidity from a number of alcohol-related health conditions, such as liver cirrhosis ("Health risks and benefits of alcohol consumption," 2000).

Summary

Body composition is a complex with many health implications and implications for health-care providers who can suggest constructive lifestyle changes (exercise and nutrition) to their patients. The primary tissues important in body composition are adipose, bone, and skeletal muscle tissues. All three of these tissues have become fairly recently known for their endocrine action and impact on metabolic function. Partitioning of adipose tissue into distinct depots within the body dictates the metabolic activity of that tissue such that subcutaneous fat is less metabolically active and, therefore, protective against metabolic dysregulation; visceral, muscular, and ectopic fat are more metabolically active, contributing greatly to insulin resistance and systemic inflammation. Brown and beige fat function in opposition to white fat tissue in that it burns energy through thermogenic heat production, and is active primarily in infancy, but can be increased in amount and activity through exercise. Body composition differs by gender, race, and age. Impacting body composition toward a healthier dynamic balance is attained through cardiorespiratory and musculoskeletal fitness, diet, stress management, and moderate to minimal alcohol consumption. Ultimately, greater benefit is gained by improving metabolic balance through adipose tissue redistribution, bone remodeling, and increasing or maintaining muscle strength and quality than can be made with weight loss as the sole goal of lifestyle changes. A glossary of terms is included in Table 8.2.

TABLE 8.2.	Glossary

Adipocyte: fat cell

VAT: visceral adipose tissue

SAT: subcutaneous adipose tissue

Ectopic fat: lipid accumulation in nonadipose cells, such as liver, skeletal muscle, and pancreas

Adiponectin: hormone secreted by adipose tissue that regulates glucose utilization and fatty acid oxidation

Leptin: an adipokine released by fat cells when adequate energy has been stored (reduces appetite and motivates physical activity)

Insulin: pancreatic hormone released in proportion to a rise in blood glucose that transforms sugar into triglyceride, glycogen, or fat for storage within fat cells, the liver, or muscle tissue, respectively

Adipokine: metabolically active hormones produced by adipocytes such as leptin and cytokines such as TNF-α

White adipose tissue: the primary fat tissue within the body that functions to store energy and insulate against extreme body temperature changes. The metabolic activity (in this case, how readily the stored energy will release fat into the bloodstream) of white adipose tissue differs according to where in the body it is stored (i.e., subcutaneously, viscerally, or gluteo-femoral deposition)

Brown adipose tissue: energy-consuming fat tissue efficient in changing chemical energy into heat, exists in greatest concentrations in infants, brown in color due to the great number of mitochondria contained within the tissue

Beige adipose tissue: fat cells inducible toward thermogenic, brown-cell activity and derived from the same stem cell origin as white fat cells; activity enhanced by weight loss

Brite adipose tissue: white fat cells driven into a brown fat–like phenotype in response to exercise

Yellow adipose tissue: Found in bone marrow, demonstrates a distinct phenotype resembling both white and brown adipose tissue

Osteocyte: general term for bone cells

Osteoblast: bone cell type responsible for bone formation; produces and secretes osteocalcin

Osteoclast: bone cell type responsible for bone resorption

Osteocalcin: a hormone produced by osteoblasts that initiates bone formation; and promotes fat deposition and insulin secretion systemically

Mesenchymal stem cells: immature cells in bone marrow that can develop into a number of different cells, including osteoblasts, osteoclasts, adipocyctes, chondrocytes (collagen cells), and myocytes (muscle cells)

Hematopoietic: blood-forming

Extra-osseous fat tissue: adipose tissue in the body outside of the skeletal system

Myocyte: muscle cell

Myokine: metabolically active hormones and proteins produced by muscle tissue

TABLE 8.2.	Glossary *(continued)*

Paracrine: chemical signals that diffuse into the nearby area and interact with receptors on local cells

Endocrine: chemicals secreted into blood that travel to distant tissues and organs upon which they function

Metabolism: enzyme-catalyzed reactions for life-sustaining allostasis and activity; metabolic action can be system-wide (endocrine), local (paracrine), and autocrine (intracellular)

Metabolic syndrome: a combination of medical disorders (such as insulin resistance, glucose intolerance, hypertension, dyslipidemia, and central obesity) that, together, increase an individual's risk of cardiovascular disease and diabetes

Insulin resistance: inhibited insulin-mediated glucose uptake

MONW: metabolically-obese, normal-weight

Glucose intolerance: a prediabetic state of hyperglycemia

Type 1 diabetes: a form of diabetes mellitus resultant from autoimmune destruction of insulin-producing cells of the pancreas

Type 2 diabetes: metabolic disorder characterized by hyperglycemia, insulin resistance, and insulin deficiency. Differs from type 1 diabetes in that type 1 presents with an absolute deficiency of insulin from pancreatic islet cell destruction

Cardiovascular disease: another name for heart disease that encompasses a class of disorders of the heart and/or blood vessels

NAFLD: nonalcoholic fatty liver disease

CRP: C-reactive protein, a proinflammatory cytokine that functions as a biomarker of systemic inflammation

IL-6: interleukin-6, an immune system molecule secreted by many cell types in the body that is classified as a proinflammatory cytokine; important in glucose and fat metabolism, in addition to many other actions

IL-15: interleukin-15, an immune system molecule secreted by many cell types in the body that is important in innate and adaptive immunity; reduces adipose tissue mass, and decreases lipid deposition in preadipocytes, in addition to many other actions

Irisin: irisin is a hormone released into circulation by muscle tissue during exercise, and functions in inducing brown adipose cell phenotypes within white fat tissue

References

Abildgaard, J., Pedersen, A. T., Green, C. J., Harder-Lauridsen, N. M., Solomon, T. P., Thomsen, C., & Lindegaard, B. (2013). Menopause is associated with decreased whole body fat oxidation during exercise. *American Journal of Physiology-Endocrinology and Metabolism, 304*(11), E1227–E1236.

Ahmadi-Abhari, S., Luben, R. N., Wareham, N. J., & Khaw, K. T. (2013). Seventeen year risk of all-cause and cause-specific mortality associated with C-reactive protein, fibrinogen and leukocyte count in men and women: the EPIC-Norfolk study. *European Journal of Epidemiology, 28*(7), 541–550.

Alberti, K. G. M. M., Eckel, R. H., Grundy, S. M., Zimmet, P. Z., Cleeman, J. I., Donato, K. A., & Smith, S. C. (2009). Harmonizing the metabolic syndrome a joint interim statement of the International Diabetes Federation Task Force on Epidemiology and Prevention; National Heart, Lung, and Blood

Institute; American Heart Association; World Heart Federation; International Atherosclerosis Society; and International Association for the Study of Obesity. *Circulation, 120*(16), 1640–1645.

Ashwell, M., Gunn, P., & Gibson, S. (2012). Waist-to-height ratio is a better screening tool than waist circumference and BMI for adult cardiometabolic risk factors: A Systematic review and meta-analysis. *Obesity Reviews, 13*(3), 275–286.

Barry, V. W., Baruth, M., Beets, M. W., Durstine, J. L., Liu, J., & Blair, S. N. (2014). Fitness vs. fatness on all-cause mortality: A meta-analysis. *Progress in Cardiovascular Diseases, 56*(4), 382–390.

Bays, H. E. (2009). "Sick fat," metabolic disease, and atherosclerosis. *American Journal of Medicine, 122,* S26–S37.

Bays, H. E., Toth, P. P., Kris-Etherton, P. M., Abate, N., Aronne, L. J., Brown, W. V., … Samuel, V. T. (2013). Obesity, adiposity, and dyslipidemia: A consensus statement from the National Lipid Association. *Journal of Clinical Lipidology, 7*(4), 304–383.

Bea, J. W., Zhao, Q., Cauley, J. A., LaCroix, A. Z., Bassford, T., Lewis, C. E., & Chen, Z. (2011). Effect of hormone therapy on lean body mass, falls, and fractures: Six-year results from the Women's Health Initiative Hormone Trials. *Menopause, 18*(1), 44.

Bell, N. A., McClure, P. D., Hill, R. J., & Davies, P. S. (1998). Assessment of foot-to-foot bioelectrical impedance analysis for the prediction of total body water. *European Journal of Clinical Nutrition, 52*(11), 856–859.

Bjørndal, B., Burri, L., Staalesen, V., Skorve, J., & Berge, R. K. (2011). Different adipose depots: Their role in the development of metabolic syndrome and mitochondrial response to hypolipidemic agents. *Journal of Obesity*, Article ID 490650, 15 pages.

Blumfield, M. L., Hure, A. J., MacDonald-Wicks, L. K., Smith, R., Simpson, S. J., Giles, W. B., & Collins, C. E. (2012). Dietary balance during pregnancy is associated with fetal adiposity and fat distribution. *The American Journal of Clinical Nutrition, 96*(5), 1032–1041.

Borrud, L. G., Flegal, K. M., Looker, A. C., Everhart, J. E., Harris, T. B., & Shepherd, J. A. (2010). Body composition data for individuals 8 years of age and older: US population, 1999–2004. *Vital and Health Statistics. Series 11, Data from the National Health Survey, 250,* 1.

Brien, S. E., Ronksley, P. E., Turner, B. J., Mukamal, K. J., & Ghali, W. A. (2011). Effect of alcohol consumption on biological markers associated with risk of coronary heart disease: Systematic review and meta-analysis of interventional studies. *British Medical Journal, 342:d636.*

Brownlee, I. A. (2011). The physiological roles of dietary fibre. *Food Hydrocolloids, 25*(2), 238–250.

Brumbaugh, D. E., Tearse, P., Cree-Green, M., Fenton, L. Z., Brown, M., Scherzinger, A., & Barbour, L. A. (2013). Intrahepatic fat is increased in the neonatal offspring of obese women with gestational diabetes. *Journal of Pediatrics, 162*(5), 930–936.

Cameron, A. J., Magliano, D. J., & Söderberg, S. (2013). A systematic review of the impact of including both waist and hip circumference in risk models for cardiovascular diseases, diabetes and mortality. *Obesity Reviews, 14*(1), 86–94.

Cao, L., Choi, E. Y., Liu, X., Martin, A., Wang, C., Xu, X., & During, M. J. (2011). White to brown fat phenotypic switch induced by genetic and environmental activation of a hypothalamic-adipocyte axis. *Cell Metabolism, 14*(3), 324–338.

Carrel, A. L., Clark, R. R., Peterson, S. E., Nemeth, B. A., Sullivan, J., & Allen, D. B. (2005). Improvement of fitness, body composition, and insulin sensitivity in overweight children in a school-based exercise program: A randomized, controlled study. *Archives of Pediatrics & Adolescent Medicine, 159*(10), 963.

Casazza, K., Fontaine, K. R., Astrup, A., Birch, L. L., Brown, A. W., Bohan Brown, M. M., & Allison, D. B. (2013). Myths, presumptions, and facts about obesity. *New England Journal of Medicine, 368*(5), 446–454.

Clark, C. R., Ridker, P. M., Ommerborn, M. J., Huisingh, C. E., Coull, B., Buring, J. E., & Berkman, L. F. (2012). Cardiovascular inflammation in healthy women: multilevel associations with state-level prosperity, productivity and income inequality. *BMC Public Health, 12*(1), 211.

Crowther, N. J., & Ferris, W. F. (2010). The impact of insulin resistance, gender, genes, glucocorticoids and ethnicity on body fat distribution. *Journal of Endocrinology, Metabolism and Diabetes of South Africa, 15*(3), 115–120.

Dawson-Hughes, B., Looker, A. C., Tosteson, A. N. A., Johansson, H., Kanis, J. A., Melton, L. J., III. (2010). The potential impact of new National Osteoporosis Foundation guidance on treatment patterns. *Osteoporosis International, 21*(1), 41–52.

de Paula, F. J., Horowitz, M. C., & Rosen, C. J. (2010). Novel insights into the relationship between diabetes and osteoporosis. *Diabetes/Metabolism Research and Reviews, 26*(8), 622–630.

Dickerson, S. S., & Zoccola, P. M. (2013). Cortisol responses to social exclusion. In C. N. DeWall (Ed.), *Oxford handbook of social exclusion* (pp. 143–151). New York, NY: Oxford University Press.

Donini, L. M., Poggiogalle, E., del Balzo, V., Lubrano, C., Faliva, M., Opizzi, A., & Rondanelli, M. (2013). How to estimate fat mass in overweight and obese subjects. *International Journal of Endocrinology*, Article ID 285680, 9 pages.

Dorsey, K. B., Thornton, J. C., Heymsfield, S. B., & Gallagher, D. (2010). Research: Greater lean tissue and skeletal muscle mass are associated with higher bone mineral content in children. *Nutrition & Metabolism*, 7, 41.

Drolet, R., Richard, C., Sniderman, A. D., Mailloux, J., Fortier, M., Huot, C., & Tchernof, A. (2008). Hypertrophy and hyperplasia of abdominal adipose tissues in women. *International Journal of Obesity*, 32(2), 283–291.

Dulloo, A. G., Jacquet, J., Solinas, G., Montani, J. P., & Schutz, Y. (2010). Body composition phenotypes in pathways to obesity and the metabolic syndrome. *International Journal of Obesity*, 34, S4–S17.

Eisenberger, N. I. (2012). The pain of social disconnection: Examining the shared neural underpinnings of physical and social pain. *Nature Reviews Neuroscience*, 13(6), 421–434.

Elia, M. (2012). Mechanisms and implications of bone adipose tissue-mineral relationships. *European Journal of Clinical Nutrition*, 66(9), 979–982.

Farnsworth, E., Luscombe, N. D., Noakes, M., Wittert, G., Argyiou, E., & Clifton, P. M. (2003). Effect of a high-protein, energy-restricted diet on body composition, glycemic control, and lipid concentrations in overweight and obese hyperinsulinemic men and women. *American Journal of Clinical Nutrition*, 78(1), 31–39.

Fishman, L. M. (2009). Yoga for osteoporosis: A pilot study. *Topics in Geriatric Rehabilitation*, 25(3), 244–250.

Flegal, K. M., Kit, B. K., Orpana, H., & Graubard, B. I. (2013). Association of all-cause mortality with overweight and obesity using standard body mass index categories: A systematic review and meta-analysis. *Journal of the American Medical Association*, 309(1), 71–82.

Fogelholm, M. (2010). Physical activity, fitness and fatness: Relations to mortality, morbidity and disease risk factors. A systematic review. *Obesity Reviews*, 11(3), 202–221.

Frigerio, F., Brun, T., Bartley, C., Usardi, A., Bosco, D., Ravnskjaer, K., ... Maechler, P. (2010). Peroxisome proliferator-activated receptor α (PPARα) protects against oleate-induced INS-1E beta cell dysfunction by preserving carbohydrate metabolism. *Diabetologia*, 53(2), 331–340.

Fulzele, K., Riddle, R. C., DiGirolamo, D. J., Cao, X., Wan, C., Chen, D., & Clemens, T. L. (2010). Insulin receptor signaling in osteoblasts regulates postnatal bone acquisition and body composition. *Cell*, 142(2), 309–319.

Geer, E. B., & Shen, W. (2009). Gender differences in insulin resistance, body composition, and energy balance. *Gender Medicine*, 6, 60–75.

Gilsanz, V., Chalfant, J., Mo, A. O., Lee, D. C., Dorey, F. J., & Mittelman, S. D. (2009). Reciprocal relations of subcutaneous and visceral fat to bone structure and strength. *Journal of Clinical Endocrinology & Metabolism*, 94(9), 3387–3393.

Gnudi, S., Sitta, E., & Fiumi, N. (2007). Relationship between body composition and bone mineral density in women with and without osteoporosis: Relative contribution of lean and fat mass. *Journal of Bone and Mineral Metabolism*, 25(5), 326–332.

Gomez-Ambrosi, J., Sliva, C., Galofre, J.C., Escalada, J., Santos, S., Gil, M.J., ... Fruhbeck, G. (2011). Body adiposity and type 2 diabetes: Increased risk with a high body fat percentage even having a normal BMI. *Obesity*, 19(7), 1439–1444.

Greggersen, W., Rudolf, S., Fassbinder, E., Dibbelt, L., Stoeckelhuber, B. M., Hohagen, F., & Schweiger, U. (2011). Major depression, borderline personality disorder, and visceral fat content in women. *European Archives of Psychiatry and Clinical Neuroscience*, 261(8), 551–557.

Griffith, J. F., Yeung, D. K., Ma, H. T., Leung, J. C. S., Kwok, T. C., & Leung, P. C. (2012). Bone marrow fat content in the elderly: A reversal of sex difference seen in younger subjects. *Journal of Magnetic Resonance Imaging*, 36(1), 225–230.

Grundy, S. M. (2011). The metabolic syndrome. In *Atlas of atherosclerosis and metabolic syndrome* (pp. 1–26). New York, NY: Springer.

Hamrick, M. W. (2011). A role for myokines in muscle-bone interactions. *Exercise and Sport Sciences Reviews*, 39(1), 43–47.

Health Risks and Benefits of Alcohol Consumption. (2000). *Alcohol Research & Health*, 24, 5–11.

Hediger, M. L., Overpeck, M. D., Kuczmarski, R. J., McGlynn, A., Maurer, K. R., & Davis, W. W. (1998). Muscularity and fatness of infants and young children born small- or large-for-gestational-age. *Pediatrics*, 102, E60.

Heid, I. M., Jackson, A. U., Randall, J. C., Winkler, T. W., Qi, L., Steinthorsdottir, V., ... Yang, J. (2010). Meta-analysis identifies 13 new loci associated with waist-hip ratio and reveals sexual dimorphism in the genetic basis of fat distribution. *Nature Genetics*, 42(11), 949–960.

Heymsfield, S. B., Thomas, D., Nguyen, A. M., Peng, J. Z., Martin, C., Shen, W., ... Muller, M. J. (2011). Voluntary weight loss: Systematic review of early phase body composition changes. *Obesity Reviews*, 12(5), 348–361.

Hirabara, S. M., Curi, R., & Maechler, P. (2010). Saturated fatty acid-induced insulin resistance is associated with mitochondrial dysfunction in skeletal muscle cells. *Journal of Cellular Physiology*, 222(1), 187–194.

Jacobs, E.J., Newton, C.C., Wang, Y, Patel, A.V., McCullough, M.L., Campbell, P.T., ... Gapstur, S.M. (2010). Wasit circumference and all-cause mortality in a large US cohort. *Archives of Internal Medicine, 170*(15), 1293–1301.

Kahn, H. S., Bullard, K. M., Barker, L. E., & Imperatore, G. (2012). Differences between adiposity indicators for predicting all-cause mortality in a representative sample of United States non-elderly adults. *PLoS One*, 7(11), e50428.

Kiecolt-Glaser, J. K., Gouin, J. P., & Hantsoo, L. (2010). Close relationships, inflammation, and health. *Neuroscience & Biobehavioral Reviews*, 35(1), 33–38.

Kodama, S., Horikawa, C., Fujihara, K., Heianza, Y., Hirasawa, R., Yachi, Y., & Sone, H. (2012). Comparisons of the strength of associations with future type 2 diabetes risk among anthropometric obesity indicators, including waist-to-height ratio: A meta-analysis. *American Journal of Epidemiology*, 176(11), 959–969.

Krieger, J. W., Sitren, H. S., Daniels, M. J., & Langkamp-Henken, B. (2006). Effects of variation in protein and carbohydrate intake on body mass and composition during energy restriction: a meta-regression. *American Journal of Clinical Nutrition*, 83(2), 260–274.

Lavie, C. J., De Schutter, A., & Milani, R. V. (2013). Is there an obesity, overweight, or lean paradox in coronary heart disease? Getting to the 'fat'of the matter. *Heart*, 99(9), 596–598.

Layman, D. K., Evans, E., Baum, J. I., Seyler, J., Erickson, D. J., & Boileau, R. A. (2005). Dietary protein and exercise have additive effects on body composition during weight loss in adult women. *Journal of Nutrition*, 135(8), 1903–1910.

Lee, D. C., Artero, E. G., Sui, X., & Blair, S. N. (2010). Review: Mortality trends in the general population: The importance of cardiorespiratory fitness. *Journal of Psychopharmacology*, 24(4 Suppl.), 27–35.

Lee, D. C., Sui, X., Artero, E. G., Lee, I. M., Church, T. S., McAuley, P. A., & Blair, S. N. (2011). Long-term effects of changes in cardiorespiratory fitness and body mass index on all-cause and cardiovascular disease mortality in men clinical perspective: The Aerobics Center Longitudinal Study. *Circulation*, 124(23), 2483–2490.

Lee, D. C., Sui, X., Ortega, F. B., Kim, Y. S., Church, T. S., Winett, R. A., & Blair, S. N. (2011). Comparisons of leisure-time physical activity and cardiorespiratory fitness as predictors of all-cause mortality in men and women. *British Journal of Sports Medicine*, 45(6), 504–510.

Lubrano, C., Saponara, M., Barbaro, G., Specchia, P., Addessi, E., Costantini, D., & Gnessi, L. (2012). Relationships between body fat distribution, epicardial fat and obstructive sleep apnea in obese patients with and without metabolic syndrome. *PLoS One*, 7(10), e47059.

Lustig, R. H. (2012). *Fat chance: Beating the odds against sugar, processed food, obesity, and disease*. Penguin.com.

Maffeis, C., Banzato, C., & Talamini, G. (2008). Waist-to-height ratio, a useful index to identify high metabolic risk in overweight children. *Journal of Pediatrics*, 152(2), 207–213.

Manolopoulos, K. N., Karpe, F., & Frayn, K. N. (2010). Gluteofemoral body fat as a determinant of metabolic health. *International Journal of Obesity*, 34(6), 949–959.

Mason, C., Foster-Schubert, K. E., Imayama, I., Xiao, L., Kong, A., Campbell, K. L., & McTiernan, A. (2013). History of weight cycling does not impede future weight loss or metabolic improvements in postmenopausal women. *Metabolism*, 62(1), 127–136.

McLaughlin, T. (2012). Metabolic heterogeneity of obesity: Role of adipose tissue. *International Journal of Obesity Supplements*, 2, S8–S10.

Mitchell, W. K., Williams, J., Atherton, P., Larvin, M., Lund, J., & Narici, M. (2012). Sarcopenia, dynapenia, and the impact of advancing age on human skeletal muscle size and strength: A quantitative review. *Frontiers in Physiology*, 3, Article ID: 260.

Mokdad, A. H., Marks, J. S., Stroup, D. F., & Gerberding, J. L. (2004). Actual causes of death in the United States, 2000. *Journal of the American Medical Association*, 291(10), 1238–1245.

Møller, U. K., viò Streym, S., Mosekilde, L., & Rejnmark, L. (2012). Changes in bone mineral density and body composition during pregnancy and postpartum. A controlled cohort study. *Osteoporosis International*, 23(4), 1213–1223.

Nicholls, S. J., Lundman, P., Harmer, J. A., Cutri, B., Griffiths, K. A., Rye, K. A., & Celermajer, D. S. (2006). Consumption of saturated fat impairs the anti-inflammatory properties of high-density lipoproteins and endothelial function. *Journal of the American College of Cardiology*, 48(4), 715–720.

Parr, E. B., Coffey, V. G., & Hawley, J. A. (2013). 'Sarcobesity': A metabolic conundrum. *Maturitas*, 74(2), 109–113.

Pead, M. J., Suswillo, R., Skerry, T. M., Vedi, S., & Lanyon, L. E. (1988). Increased 3H-uridine levels in osteocytes following a single short period of dynamic bone loading in vivo. *Calcified Tissue International*, 43(2), 92–96.

Pedersen, B. K. (2013). Muscle as a secretory organ. *Comprehensive Physiology*, 3(3), 1337–1362.

Peppa, M., Koliaki, C., & Dimitriadis, G. (2012). Body composition as an important determinant of metabolic syndrome in postmenopausal women. *Endocrinology Metabolism Syndrome*, 2161–1017 S1:009. doi: 10.4172/2161-1017.

Petersen, K. F., Dufour, S., Morino, K., Yoo, P. S., Cline, G. W., & Shulman, G. I. (2012). Reversal of muscle insulin resistance by weight reduction in young, lean, insulin-resistant offspring of parents with type 2 diabetes. *Proceedings of the National Academy of Sciences*, 109(21), 8236–8240.

Petursson, H., Sigurdsson, J. A., Bengtsson, C., Nilsen, T. I., & Getz, L. (2011). Body configuration as a predictor of mortality: Comparison of five anthropometric measures in a 12 year follow-up of the Norwegian HUNT 2 study. *PLoS One*, 6(10), e26621.

Phillips, C. M., & Perry, I. J. (2013). Does inflammation determine metabolic health status in obese and nonobese adults? *Journal of Clinical Endocrinology & Metabolism*, 98(10), E1610–E1619.

Pollock, N. K., Bernard, P. J., Gutin, B., Davis, C. L., Zhu, H., & Dong, Y. (2011). Adolescent obesity, bone mass, and cardiometabolic risk factors. *Journal of Pediatrics*, 158(5), 727–734.

Rahman, S., Lu, Y., Czernik, P. J., Rosen, C. J., Enerback, S., & Lecka-Czernik, B. (2013). Inducible brown adipose tissue, or beige fat, is anabolic for the skeleton. *Endocrinology*, 154(8), 2687–2701.

Rimm, E. B., Williams, P., Fosher, K., Criqui, M., & Stampfer, M. J. (1999). Moderate alcohol intake and lower risk of coronary heart disease: Meta-analysis of effects on lipids and haemostatic factors. *British Medical Journal*, 319, 1523–1528.

Romero-Corral, A., Sert-Kuniyoshi, F.H., Sierra-Johnson, J., Orban, M., Gami, A., Davison, D., ... Somers, V.K. (2010). Modest Visceral Fat Gain Causes Endothelial Dysfunction in Healthy Humans. *Journal of the American College of Cardiology*, 56(8), 662–666.

Ronksley, P. E., Brien, S. E., Turner, B. J., Mukamal, K. J., & Ghali, W. A. (2011). Association of alcohol consumption with selected cardiovascular disease outcomes: A systematic review and meta-analysis. *British Medical Journal*, 342:d671.

Rossi, A. P., Watson, N. L., Newman, A. B., Harris, T. B., Kritchevsky, S. B., Bauer, D. C., & Zamboni, M. (2011). Effects of body composition and adipose tissue distribution on respiratory function in elderly men and women: The health, aging, and body composition study. *Journals of Gerontology Series A: Biological Sciences and Medical Sciences*, 66(7), 801–808.

Roubenoff, R. (1996). Applications of bioelectrical impedance analysis for body composition to epidemiologic studies. *American Journal of Clinical Nutrition*, 64(3), 459S–462S.

Rubin, C. T., & Lanyon, L. E. (1984). Regulation of bone formation by applied dynamic loads. *Journal of Bone and Joint Surgery. American Volume*, 66(3), 397–402.

Samuel, V. T. (2011). Fructose induced lipogenesis: From sugar to fat to insulin resistance. *Trends in Endocrinology & Metabolism*, 22(2), 60–65.

Santanasto, A. J., Glynn, N. W., Newman, M. A., Taylor, C. A., Brooks, M. M., Goodpaster, B. H., & Newman, A. B. (2011). Impact of weight loss on physical function with changes in strength, muscle mass, and muscle fat infiltration in overweight to moderately obese older adults: A randomized clinical trial. *Journal of Obesity*, Article ID 516576, 10 pages.

Shapira, N. (2013). Women's higher health risks in the obesogenic environment: A gender nutrition approach to metabolic dimorphism with predictive, preventive, and personalised medicine. *The EPMA Journal*, 4(1), 1–12.

Shea, J.L., King, M.T.C., Yi, Y., Gulliver, W., & Sun, G. (2012). Body fat percentage is associated with cardiometabolic dysregulation in BMI-defined normal weight subjects. *Nutrition, Metabolism and Cardiovascular Diseases*, 22(9), 741–747.

Shen, W., St. Onge, M. P., Wang, Z., & Heymsfield, S. B. (2005). Study of body composition: An overview. In S. B. Heymsfield, T. G. Lohman, Z. Wang & S. B. Going (Eds.), *Human body composition* (pp. 3–14). Champaign, IL: Human Kinetics.

Sheu, Y., & Cauley, J. A. (2011). The role of bone marrow and visceral fat on bone metabolism. *Current Osteoporosis Reports*, 9(2), 67–75.

Shin, H., Panton, L. B., Dutton, G. R., & Ilich, J. Z. (2011). Relationship of physical performance with body composition and bone mineral density in individuals over 60 years of age: A systematic review. *Journal of Aging Research*, Article ID 191896, 14 pages.

Slavich, G. M., Way, B. M., Eisenberger, N. I., & Taylor, S. E. (2010). Neural sensitivity to social rejection is associated with inflammatory responses to social stress. *Proceedings of the National Academy of Sciences*, 107(33), 14817–14822.

Smith, B. W., & Adams, L. A. (2011). Nonalcoholic fatty liver disease and diabetes mellitus: Pathogenesis and treatment. *Nature Reviews Endocrinology*, 7(8), 456–465.

Smorlesi, A., Frontini, A., Giordano, A., & Cinti, S. (2012). The adipose organ: White-brown adipocyte plasticity and metabolic inflammation. *Obesity Reviews*, 13(S2), 83–96.

Sood, A., & Dixon, A. E. (2013). Effect of obesity on the development and clinical presentation of asthma. In A. E. Dixon & E. M. Clerisme-Beaty (Eds.), *Obesity and lung disease* (pp. 119–138). New York, NY: Humana Press.

Thomas, E.L., Frost, G., Taylor-Robinson, S.D., & Bell, J.D. (2012). Excess body fat in obese and normal-weight subjects. *Nutrition Research Reviews*, 25(1), 150–161.

Thompson, D., Karpe, F., Lafontan, M., & Frayn, K. (2012). Physical activity and exercise in the regulation of human adipose tissue physiology. *Physiological Reviews*, 92(1), 157–191.

Ulijaszek, S. J., & Kerr, D. A. (1999). Anthropometric measurement error and the assessment of nutritional status. *British Journal of Nursing*, 82(3), 165–177.

Waugh, E., Lam, M.-A., Hawker, G., McGowan, J., Papaioannou, A., Cheung, A., … Jamal, S. (2009). Risk factors for low bone mass in healthy 40–60 year old women: A systematic review of the literature. *Osteoporosis International*, 20(1), 1–21.

Wedin, W. K., Diaz-Gimenez, L., & Convit, A. J. (2012). Prediction of insulin resistance with anthropometric measures: Lessons from a large adolescent population. *Diabetes, Metabolic Syndrome and Obesity: Targets and Therapy*, 5, 219.

Weiss, R., Bremer, A. A., & Lustig, R. H. (2013). What is metabolic syndrome, and why are children getting it? *Annals of the New York Academy of Sciences*, 1281(1), 123–140.

Wu, J., Cohen, P., & Spiegelman, B. M. (2013). Adaptive thermogenesis in adipocytes: Is beige the new brown? *Genes & Development*, 27(3), 234–250.

Xu, Z., Qi, X., Dahl, A. K., & Xu, W. (2013). Waist-to-height ratio is the best indicator for undiagnosed Type 2 diabetes. *Diabetic Medicine*, 30(6), e201–e207.

Chapter 9

Oral Health

Madeleine M. Lloyd and
Julia Lange Kessler

Introduction

Oral health has a significant impact on the overall health and well-being of the nation's population. The Surgeon General's key message in 2000 was that oral health is integral to overall health and that one's mouth is a mirror that reflects general health and well-being (Satcher, 2000). One of the leading national health goals in the US Department of Health and Human Services (2011) document, Healthy People 2020, is to prevent and control oral and craniofacial diseases, conditions, and injuries, and improve access to preventive services and dental care. In addition, oral health reports by the Institute of Medicine (2011a, 2011b), Oral Health During Pregnancy Expert Workgroup (2012), and the American Academy of Pediatrics Children's Oral Health (2011), project support the importance of improving the training of all health professionals about oral health and increasing access to oral health across the life span.

This chapter focuses on the unique oral health needs of women across the life span as oral health must be perceived and promoted as an essential element for achieving good overall systemic health (Niessen, Gibson, & Kinnunen, 2013). Chapter 9 is divided into three sections. First, oral and dental anatomy is described followed by how to perform an oral health examination. Second, an overview of the female hormonal changes that occur throughout the various life stages and the consequential oral health manifestations noted on examination are presented. Third, specific systemic health conditions that are correlated with oral health status are described. A brief discussion of the promotion of oral health and disease prevention through team-based collaboration and implications for health-care professionals conclude this chapter.

The health of a woman's mouth serves as a window into her body, reflecting her overall health (Satcher, 2000). Over the past decades, the scientific evidence for the connection between oral and systemic health has strengthened (Niessen et al., 2013). It is time to proactively address this bidirectional relationship by engaging in interprofessional collaboration to ultimately increase health-care access for every woman, decrease barriers to comprehensive care, and improve clinical health outcomes globally.

Performing the Oral Health Examination

Every health-care encounter provides the opportunity to screen for oral cancer, tooth decay, and consider any necessary health-care referrals (Fulmer & Cabrera, 2012). Performing an oral exam takes less than 2 minutes and is easily incorporated into the examination of the head, ears, eyes, nose, and throat (HEENT), which is a crucial part of any physical examination. It has been suggested that the acronym HEENT would be more useful if it were to read head, ears, eyes, nose, oral cavity, and throat (HEENOT) so that the provider does *not* forget the oral examination (Haber et al., unpublished - n.d.).

Oral and Dental Anatomy

In order to incorporate the oral examination into all physical examinations, an understanding of basic dental anatomy and dental terms is required. Descriptions of these parts are included below.

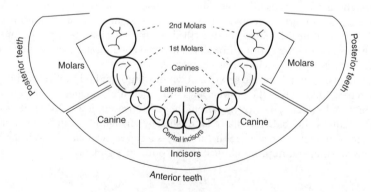

FIGURE 9.1 Anatomy of the mouth. Reprinted with permission from Scheid, R. C., & Weiss, G. (2011). *Woelfel's dental anatomy: Its relevance to dentistry* (8th ed.). Philadelphia, PA: LWW.

Mandibular is the lower jaw or mandible. Maxillary refers to the upper jaw or maxilla. Baby teeth are primary teeth or deciduous. Permanent teeth are succedaneous. Labial refers to lips and buccal refers to cheeks. Facial is both labial and buccal collectively. Lingual refers to the tongue. Mesial is the vertical tooth surface toward the front of the jaw and midline. Occlusal is the premolar and molar surfaces that come in contact with the teeth in the opposite jaw during closure. Incisal is the surface of incisors and canines that come in contact with the teeth in the opposite jaw.

There are 32 teeth in the permanent dentition and 8 types of teeth: central incisors (4), lateral incisors (4), canines (cuspids) (4), first premolars (first bicuspid) (4), second premolar (second bicuspid) (4), first molars (4), second molars (4), and third molars (4) (Fig. 9.1).

The first primary tooth, which is usually the lower central incisor, erupts around 6 to 10 months of age, and all primary teeth have erupted by 30 months. Deciduous teeth start to shed at 6 years of age and usually all have shed by 11 or 12 years. Permanent tooth eruption starts at 6 to 7 years and is completed by 21 years with the third molars (wisdom teeth) (Idzik & Krauss, 2013).

Saliva

Saliva has antibacterial, antiviral, and antifungal properties that help balance the oral flora, prevent oral infections, and help maintain tooth enamel. Saliva facilitates speech, washes away food from around the teeth, neutralizes food and bacterial acids in the mouth, improves taste, and lubricates the mouth. It also makes food soft and easier to chew and swallow. Digestion of food starts in the mouth due to enzymes in saliva (Furness, Bryan, McMillan, Birchenough, & Worthington, 2013). Saliva is produced by three pairs of glands: the parotid, submandibular, and sublingual salivary glands (see Fig. 9.2). About

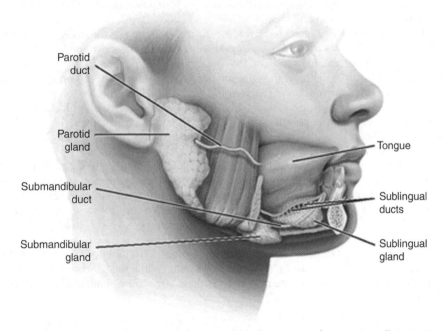

FIGURE 9.2 Salivary glands in the mouth. Reprinted with permission from McConnell, T. H., & Hull, K. L. (2011). *Human form, human function*. Philadelphia, PA: LWW.

10% of saliva is produced by minor salivary glands located in the labial, buccal, lingual, and palatal mucosa in the mouth. The saliva arch located in the brain controls the secretion of saliva. Chewing, smell, and taste of food stimulate the salivary center in the medulla, which then stimulates the nerves to the salivary glands for saliva production.

Oral Examination

The following equipment is needed:
- Good light source
- Gloves
- Tongue blade
- Gauze (2 × 2 or 4 × 4)
- Mouth mirror (optional)

The oral examination is performed to determine the health status of teeth and gums. The practitioner identifies any precancerous or cancerous oral lesions and, if needed, offers the patient anticipatory guidance (Clark et al., 2010). Systematic observation of symmetry of the face and lips begins the oral examination as well as the identification of any facial deformity, skin lesions or perioral lesions. To inspect the temporomandibular joint (TMJ), place the fingers gently over the TMJ and ask the patient to open and close the mouth a couple of times. Note any deviation or deflection, clicking or crepitus.

As in any physical examination, the face is examined for any abnormal lesions such as actinic keratosis (thick, scaly, and crusty patches of skin), lesions, and basal or squamous cell cancers. If the patient is a smoker or chews tobacco, the lips must be thoroughly examined, as they may show evidence of herpes, impetigo, or angular chelitis, which can also be caused by B_{12} deficiency, candidiasis, or poor fitting dentures. Nonhealing lesions could indicate skin cancer and should be referred.

The inside of the lips is checked by folding the upper lip up and the lower lip down in order to inspect the mucosa and the gums. Mucosa should be smooth, pink, and moist. Ulcerations or white patches are cause for concern. Note, if the gums are inflamed and/or if there is plaque or debris at the gumline or any gingival recession (gums shrinking away from teeth). This process is repeated for the inside of the cheeks, looking for the same evidence of smooth, pink, and moist mucosa and gums. Again, ulcerations are cause for concern, particularly in someone who uses any type of tobacco (including smokeless). This is the perfect time to discuss regular dental visits as well as brushing/flossing.

Periodontal disease (periodontitis) is deep inflammation of the gums, ligaments, and bony structures. Medications such as calcium channel blockers and anticonvulsants can cause gingival hyperplasia (swollen gums), making hygiene more difficult. Periodontitis is also associated with severe systemic complications such as heart disease, diabetes, and preterm labor, all of which are discussed later in this chapter.

Examine the anterior and posterior surfaces (if possible) of the teeth, noting discoloration, caries, plaque, trauma, and damaged or missing teeth. If a mouth mirror is not available, the patient is instructed to tilt the head backward. While the patient's head is tilted back, the hard and soft palates are inspected, as these areas can be high-risk area for oral cancers.

The tongue is an area that is common for the development of precancer or cancer and is often missed during an oral examination. The patient is asked to protrude the tongue in order to inspect the dorsum or anterior surface of the tongue. After asking the patient to protrude the tongue, the tip of the tongue is grasped with the gauze and moved to one side while retracting the cheek with a tongue blade, finger, or mouth mirror in order to visualize posterior lateral margins of the tongue (a cancer-prone area). This process is repeated in the opposite direction for the opposite margin of the tongue (see Fig. 9.3).

The posterior pharynx is examined for symmetry of size, and the supporting structures are also examined. A tongue blade will help with holding down the tongue to assist with visualization. Any areas of erythema, exudates, or ulceration are noted. The patient is asked to say "Ahhhh" to allow observation of movement of the uvula. The floor of the mouth is inspected and palpated by asking the patient to lift the tongue to the roof of the mouth.

The observation of any white lesion in the mouth should be referred to rule out cancer as oral cancer is the sixth most common cancer globally and the large majority of oral cancers are advanced at the time of detection (Brocklehurst, Kujan, O'Malley, Shepherd, & Glenny, 2013).

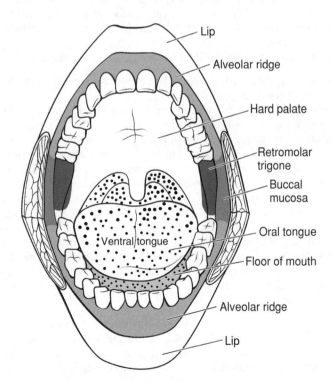

FIGURE 9.3 Common sites of oral cancer. (*Black dots* indicate areas where oral cancer can occur.) Reprinted with permission from Thorne, C. H., Bartlett, S. P., Beasley, R. W., Aston, S. J., Gurtner, G. C., & Spear, S. L. (2006). *Grabb and Smith's plastic surgery* (6th ed.). Philadelphia, PA: LWW.

Female Hormonal Changes throughout the Life span That Affect Oral Health

A woman's changing hormone levels influence her oral health throughout her life span. Health-care providers who understand these changes will be best equipped to address women's oral systemic health-care needs throughout puberty, menses, pregnancy, and menopause (Steinberg, Minsk, Gluch, & Giorgio, 2008).

Puberty

During puberty, surging levels of estrogen and progesterone will change the oral environment of every young woman, predisposing them to an increased risk of gingivitis and periodontal problems. Increased circulation and high concentrations of estrogen and progesterone allow for increased bacterial colonization (Thomas & Chitra, 2013). Changes in the oral microflora and resulting inflammatory response during puberty creates an altered gingival tissue that may lead to red, swollen, or bleeding gums. Mild cases of gingivitis respond to scaling and improved oral hygiene (Niessen et al., 2013).

Risk studies have shown that the best predictor for future caries is present caries, which is particularly important during puberty given the effect of hormones on the gingiva (Marinho, Worthington, Walsh, & Clarkson, 2013). Risk assessment of dental caries should be performed periodically and topical fluoride varnish applied to help prevent the formation of future caries.

The American Dental Association (Marinho et al., 2013) recommends:

- Fluoride varnish applied every 6 months will effectively prevent caries in the primary and permanent dentition of adolescents.
- High-risk populations (those with three or more caries in the past 3 years) will benefit from two or more applications of fluoride varnish.
- Other considerations surrounding the oral health of young women is that up to 50% of adolescent women have participated in oral sex (most without barrier protection), leading to further cause for oral health concerns. Several sexually transmitted infections can be transmitted orally, including syphilis, gonorrhea, herpes, HIV, chlamydia, and human papillomavirus (HPV), as oral sex is an efficient mode for transmission (Saini, Saini, & Sharma, 2010). The intact (healthy) mucosal membrane is a tough barrier and a protector from bacteria and viruses, but if the mucosal surface has been broken by a lesion, tear, gingivitis, or periodontal disease, a gateway is created to the bloodstream, leaving the mouth susceptible to over 150 species of bacteria. While the transmission of sexually transmitted infections through oral–genital contact is lower than through sexual intercourse, it is not without risk and should not be considered "risk-free behavior."

Health-care providers should perform an oral examination on all women during puberty, referring as necessary. The use of a barrier method during oral sex should be discussed with women who are participating in oral sex. Women should be advised to avoid oral sex with anyone who has a sexually transmitted infection, sores, or lesions on their genitals or sores or lesions on and in their mouths, as well as avoiding those with bleeding gums. In addition, all patients can be informed of the following:

- Wait to have oral sex at least 30 minutes after brushing or flossing teeth.
- Avoid oral sex after recent dental treatment or periodontal therapy (dental scaling and periodontal surgery).

- If body fluids are in the mouth, rinse with antibacterial mouthwash (Saini et al., 2010).
- Sexually active teens taking hormonal contraceptives may also have oral systemic health problems secondary to the use of oral contraceptives. Oral contraceptives (and the hormones they contain) create an increase in gingival irritation and a decrease in saliva, contributing to periodontitis.

Menses and Midlife Considerations

Elevated or decreased levels of sex hormones (estrogen and progesterone) can lead to oral health problems. Although menses can have no effect on a woman's oral health, some women may experience swollen gingival tissues, activation of herpes labialis, aphthous ulcers (canker sores), prolonged hemorrhage following oral surgery, and swollen salivary glands. Bleeding gums in days prior to menses will resolve once menses begins (Shourie et al., 2012).

Women taking hormonal contraceptives (oral, transdermal, or implanted) are particularly vulnerable to oral health concerns. A higher level of progesterone creates an exaggerated response by the body to the toxins from plaque. Hormonal contraceptive users experience changes in the composition of the saliva as well as a decrease in the amount of saliva, leading to oral health problems that can range from irritated gingiva to aggressive periodontitis (Thomas & Chitra, 2013). Low-dose contraceptives will lessen oral irritation, but any long-term use of low- or high-dose contraceptives may lead to an increased risk of periodontitis. Women should be advised to inform their dentist of hormonal contraceptive use, particularly if they need a tooth extracted. Hormonal contraceptive users are more likely to develop a painful condition post extraction known as dry socket. Extraction should take place on days that women take the "sugar pills," that is, on days 23 to 28 (Indian Dental Association, 2012).

Fertility

A recent study of more than 3,000 women (Hart, Doherty, Pennel, Newhnham, & Newnham, 2012) points to a correlation between poor oral systemic health and the amount of time that it takes a woman to become pregnant. Women without periodontal disease take approximately 5 months to conceive, while those with periodontal disease take 7 months or more. Non-Caucasian women were the most affected, because they appeared to have the highest level of inflammatory response when suffering from gum disease. A non-Caucasian woman with periodontal disease can take greater than 12 months to conceive. More study is needed to determine whether these results are statistically significant, but this correlation does raise the question about possible effects of poor oral health on fertility. A dentist consultation should be part of each woman's preconception counseling visit.

Pregnancy

Expectant mothers are often unaware of the implications of poor oral health for themselves, their pregnancy, and/or their unborn children (Council on Clinical Affairs, 2011). It is estimated that one in five women have never had dental care. Promotion of good oral systemic health during pregnancy not only affects the health of the pregnant woman but also has benefits for the fetus. Numerous studies show links between poor oral systemic health and premature birth, low birth weight, and preeclampsia, all life-threatening events. In addition, there is a correlation between periodontal disease and gestational diabetes (Council on Clinical Affairs, 2011).

At the beginning of pregnancy, it is not unusual for pregnant women to experience "morning" sickness (nausea and vomiting), which, in reality, occurs at any time of the day. Nausea and vomiting can contribute to erosion of tooth enamel. Rinsing the mouth after vomiting with one teaspoon of baking soda dissolved in a glass of water can help to avoid erosion. Teeth brushing during pregnancy can also bring on the same gagging or vomiting response. Again, rinsing with baking soda and water will limit the erosion of enamel (Clarke et al., 2010).

Hormonal changes during pregnancy contribute to the most common oral complaint during pregnancy, bleeding gums, or gingivitis. These symptoms generally surface at 2 months of gestational age and peak during the eighth month of pregnancy, affecting 25% to 75% of pregnant women (Clarke et al., 2010). It is well documented that vertical transmission from mother to child of mutans streptococci (MS), the bacteria that causes carries, is common. Unfortunately, MS can live in babies mouth, putting them at a disadvantage even before their teeth erupt (AAPD, 2011). All pregnant women should have a dental consultation to evaluate their own oral health and to reduce the risk of their children developing caries (AAPD, 2011). Dental treatment for tooth decay can be performed throughout pregnancy, but the ideal time is in the second trimester of pregnancy (13 to 26 weeks). During the second trimester, the gravid uterus is still small enough not to cause much pressure on the vena cava while reclining in a dentist chair. Pregnant women can be reassured that dental care during pregnancy is safe, including X-rays, local anesthesia, and pain medication. If the mother has not seen a dentist in the last 6 months, she should be referred. Delay in treatment could result in significant risk to the mother and the fetus.

Gestational diabetes mellitus (GDM) is a condition of carbohydrate intolerance that is detected during pregnancy (Nainggolan, 2013). Women with GDM are at risk for gestational hypertension, preeclampsia, and cesarean delivery and associated potential morbidities. In addition, the woman with GDM will have a sevenfold increased risk of developing diabetes later in life. The offspring of women with gestational diabetes are also at increased risk for macrosomia, neonatal hypoglycemia, hyperbilirubinemia, operative delivery, shoulder dystocia, and birth trauma (American College of Obstetrics and Gynecology, 2013).

Periodontitis and GDM have a bidirectional relationship. Pregnant women with periodontitis (approximately 15%) have the potential to affect blood glucose control and may contribute to the progression of the disease. Both diabetes mellitus and GDM add to the susceptibility of periodontitis and increased tooth loss as well as the above-named risks. Periodontitis has been shown to contribute to premature birth, thus increasing the risk for low birth weight and preeclampsia (a condition that exists only during pregnancy involving hypertension and proteinuria). Pregnant women with periodontitis have bacteria that may cause systemic inflammation leading to preterm labor. Studies have not yet shown that treatment of periodontal disease during pregnancy will improve outcomes; however, they do show that dental treatment of periodontal disease during pregnancy is safe. Safety is a common concern for pregnant women. Mothers should be seen by a dentist early in their pregnancy to prevent or correct any oral health conditions (Thomas & Chitra, 2013).

Pregnancy is a time of growth for many parts of the female body, and conditions that occur in the oral cavity are not exempt. Pyogenic granuloma (PG) or "pregnancy tumor" is a benign inflammatory lesion that is the most commonly found lesion in the oral cavity. Influenced by the hormones of pregnancy, PG can be found on the gingiva, the tongue, lips, or the buccal mucosa but most commonly appears on the labial aspect of the anterior maxillary region (Sun, Lei, Chen, Yu, & Zhou, 2013a). PG, if present, is usually noticed during the second month of pregnancy, reaching maximum growth at 8 months. Removal of a pregnancy tumor is recommended only when the tumor interferes with mastication or causes pain. PG usually resolves and disappears by 12 weeks postpartum. It is imperative that care providers are aware of this condition that can occur in 10% of pregnancies (Sun et al., 2013a) (Fig. 9.4). It is well established that many women during pregnancy have oral disease. While some oral conditions during pregnancy resolve after birth when the immune response returns to normal, bacteria can linger in the mother's mouth. The bacteria (Streptococcus mutans) can easily be transferred from mother to baby through saliva-sharing activities (sharing utensils, cleaning the pacifier with the mother's saliva). Mothers with high rates of caries will pass those oral bacteria to their babies, which can create caries where none existed (AAPD, 2011).

It is recommended that pregnant women should have an oral examination and be counseled to visit the dentist during the first prenatal visit. The oral examination and referral is documented on the chart, and the patient should be informed of the safety and preference of dental care during pregnancy for her health and that of the fetus. Encouraging good oral habits, including flossing, brushing twice daily, and limiting sweets, is part of pregnancy education (Clarke et al., 2010).

Postpartum

The postpartum visit is the perfect time for obstetricians/gynecologists, midwives, primary care providers, and postpartum nurses to encourage mothers to follow up with their own dental care (if it was delayed) and to educate them regarding how to take good care of the newborn's mouth. Such education, along with encouragement, will contribute to the prevention of childhood caries.

It is recommended that the newborn's mouth should be wiped out each day with a piece of damp cotton gauze or a clean soft cloth prior to the eruption of baby teeth (Clarke et al., 2010). This is best done before sleep when bacteria multiply. It is important to discourage the mother from putting the baby to sleep with the bottle (unless it has only water) or breast in his or her mouth. Fluoride products should be encouraged

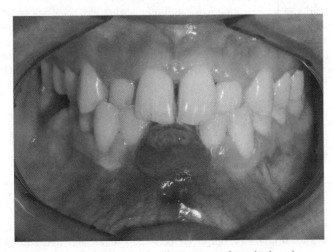

FIGURE 9.4 Pyogenic granuloma. Reprinted with permission from thinkstock.com.

as well as a diet low in sugar. Saliva-sharing activities (food, pacifier, bottles, etc.) should be strongly discouraged. Dental visits should begin early in life. "First visit by the first birthday" is the recommendation of the American Academy of Pediatric Dentists. Awareness of good oral habits has the potential to impact the future health of each child.

Menopause

Menopause (the cessation of menses for 12 months) results in a decrease in the amount of systemic estrogen and subsequent oral systemic changes, making women more susceptible to periodontal disease. If problems are diagnosed early, treatment can contribute to the avoidance of fracture and tooth loss. Oral pain and discomfort, burning sensation, mucosal atrophy, and osteoporosis resulting in a decrease of alveolar height and systemic bone loss (thus tooth loss) are not unusual (Burakoff, 2003). The decrease in estrogen can lead to loss of bone in the spine and hips, which can also result in tooth loss (Buencamino, Palomo, & Thacker, 2009). Many of the oral conditions that are attributed to menopause and medications are discussed in other areas of this chapter.

Menopausal women and postmenopausal women are at higher risk for osteoporosis and subsequent fragility fractures (Lo, Burnett-Bowie, & Finkelstein, 2011). Osteoporosis literally means "porous bones." It is a disease that weakens the bones and can lead to sudden and unexpected fractures, with women over the age of 50 being at greatest risk. Smoking and the use of alcohol increase the risk of fracture as does heredity and race (White and Asian women are most affected). Women taking hormone replacement therapy (HRT) may not experience oral problems as readily as their unmedicated counterparts, although HRT has mixed results depending on the oral–systemic health. Several studies have indicated that estrogen therapy protects against mandibular bone loss and diminishes the severity of periodontal disease in postmenopausal women (Haskin & Mobley, 2013; Mutneja, Dhawan, Raina, & Sharma, 2012).

The drying of vaginal tissue during menopause is widely known and attributed to the decrease in estrogen. The decrease in estrogen also contributes to the drying of the oral mucosa and can lead to menopausal gingivostomatitis, which is characterized by gingiva that bleeds readily, with an abnormally pale dry/shiny erythematous appearance (Mutneja et al., 2012). Unchecked gingivitis leads to periodontitis. Periodontitis leads to progressive and irreversible loss of bone and the periodontal ligament attachment as inflammation extends from the gingiva to the bone and ligament (Buencamino et al., 2009).

Oral Systemic Health Conditions

Burning Mouth Syndrome

Middle-aged and older women have the highest risk for burning mouth syndrome (BMS), the symptoms of which are typically described as a burning sensation of the oral mucosa without any apparent mucosal alteration (Sun et al., 2013b). The affected areas are usually the tip of the tongue and lateral edges, lips, and hard and soft palate. When there are no underlying dental or medical causes, and the pain or burning is unremitting and continuous for most of the day for 4 to 6 months, then the term BMS can be applied.

The pain is often relieved by eating or drinking and seldom interferes with sleep. Additional symptoms may be present such as xerostomia (dry mouth), bitter or metallic changes in taste, dry or sore mouth, and dysgeusia (dysfunction in the sense of taste). Reported prevalence rates in general populations vary from 0.7% to 15% and 12% to 18% for postmenopausal women. Many patients show evidence of anxiety, depression, and personality disorders (Karim, 2012; National Institute of Health [NIH], National Institute of Dental and Craniofacial Research [NIDCR], 2011). A thorough comprehensive assessment should include a detailed review of the woman's medical and dental history. Evaluation of symptoms includes the presence of parafunctional habits such as bruxism and tongue thrushing; and clenching, mechanical irritation, allergic reaction, infection, anemia, electrolyte and nutritional deficiencies as well as gastrointestinal, urogenital, psychiatric, neurologic, and metabolic disorders to determine either primary or secondary BMS. BMS is a diagnosis of exclusion and is made after physical examination inclusive of the extra- and intra-oral examination and laboratory workup to rule out other diseases such as diabetes and thyroid problems. Causes of BMS include damage to the nerves that control pain and taste, oral candidiasis, poorly fitting dentures or allergies to the denture materials, acid reflux disease, and hormonal changes.

Prevention/Treatment of Burning Mouth Syndrome

When local, systemic, or psychological factors are present, treatment or elimination of these factors usually results in a significant clinical improvement of oral burning and pain symptoms. If symptoms continue after the removal of potential causes, a therapeutic treatment plan should be designed around previous randomized controlled clinical trials outcomes. Drug therapy with topical capsaicin (pepper), the antioxidant food supplement α-lipoic acid, clonazepam, and anticonvulsants such as gabapentin may provide relief of oral burning or pain symptom. In addition, psychotherapy and behavioral feedback may help eliminate the BMS symptoms. The use of analgesia and hormones lacks sufficient evidence (Karim, 2012). Additional treatments include avoiding spicy or acidic foods such as tomatoes or oranges, brushing regularly with a soft brush and flossing daily, keeping the mouth moist, limiting alcohol and avoiding tobacco, using relaxation techniques, and adjusting or replacing irritating dentures (NIH, NIDCR, 2011). Ongoing psychological support, reassurance, and counseling should be offered as there is a considerable amount of stress related to BMS symptoms.

Oral HPV and Women

Oral HPV infection accounts for 40% to 80% of all oropharyngeal cancers (OPCs) (Fakhry & D'Souza, 2013). Poor oral health is an independent risk factor irrespective of tobacco smoking and oral sex practices. After analyzing data from the 2009 to 2010 National Health and Nutrition Examination Survey (NHANES), it was found that poor oral health was associated with a 56% higher prevalence of oral HPV infection in clients aged 30 to 69 years. Marijuana use is also linked to higher rates of infection, and research shows that the rates of HPV are 5% in nonusers, 8% in former uses, and 14% in current marijuana smokers (Bui, Markham, Ross, & Mullen, 2013).

In the United States, 40,000 people will be diagnosed with oral or pharyngeal cancer this year (Oral Cancer Foundation, 2013). Oral cancers are typically squamous cell carcinomas and, regardless of ethnicity, are more than twice as common in men as in women (American Cancer Society, 2013). Risk factors for women include tobacco use, heavy alcohol use, excessive sun exposure to the lips, and HPV. As with any cancer, early identification/screening and treatment is vital for survival. Over the past 20 years, HPV type 16 infection has been increasingly linked to OPC, and approximately 30% of people with OPC have HPV 16 E6 antibodies present (Kreimer, 2013). The most common sites for oral cavity and OPC are the tongue, tonsils, oropharynx, gums, floor of the mouth, and less commonly on the roof of the mouth.

Signs of Oral Cancer

- A sore, irritation, lump, or thick patch in the mouth, lip, or throat
- A white or red patch in the mouth
- A feeling that something is caught in the throat
- Difficulty chewing or swallowing
- Difficulty moving the jaw or tongue

Prognosis is significantly better when patients are diagnosed with HPV–positive oropharyngeal squamous cell carcinomas (HPV–OSCC) (82%) versus HPV–negative OSCC (57%) for 3-year overall survival. In the United States, currently more than half of the patients diagnosed with HPV–OSCC are alive 10 years after diagnosis (Fakhry & D'Souza, 2013).

Prevention/Treatment of Oral HPV in Women

Primary prevention of HPV–driven cancers via vaccination has been proven to be highly effective to prevent HPV 16/18 infection with randomized clinical trials providing strong evidence (Kreimer, 2013). Oropharyngeal HPV infection is usually acquired during sexual activity, and patient education should include HPV discussions. Currently, the Centers for Disease Control and Prevention (CDC) Advisory Committee on Immunization Practices (ACIP), recommends HPV vaccination for females between 11 and 12 years of age, as early as 9 years, and with a catchup vaccination scheme until 26 years of age. The vaccine is a series of three vaccines over a 6-month time frame. HPV–driven OPC is only a small percentage of the overall head and neck cancers detected, and counseling should be focused on tobacco and alcohol prevention strategies as they remain major risk factors for head and neck cancers globally. Written material regarding HPV–positive OSCC is available and may result in improved communication and understanding for the patients (Fakhry & D'Souza, 2013).

Additional primary prevention for oral cavity and OPC includes tobacco cessation and no excessive alcohol use, and limited exposure to ultraviolet (UV) radiation by using a sun protector factor (SPF) of at least 15 when outside with lip balm protection and a hat to avoid cancer of the lips. Good nutrition is important for maintenance of optimal oral health, and it is important that women who wear dentures have them properly fitted to prevent continuous oral irritation, which is a risk factor for oral cancer.

Secondary prevention of HPV–driven OPC includes the same as with all OPC—the oral cancer screening using visual/tactile assessment in routine screening annual examination. Oral HPV infection is more common in women between 30 to 34 years and 60 to 64 years. They have often been exposed to HPV for many years prior to having a diagnosis of malignancy (Fakhry & D'Souza, 2013). The NIDCR (2011) released a patient educational handout "Detecting Oral Cancer: A guide for health-care professionals." This oral cancer screening guide can be found on their website at http://www.nidcr.nih.gov/OralHealth/Topics/OralCancer/DetectingOralCancer.htm.

Special Considerations

Oral Health in Cancer Therapy

Utilizing a multidisciplinary team approach, the coordination of oral health care can improve a cancer patient's quality of life. Pretreatment oral health assessment is key as is offering oral health support during treatment and after treatment. Currently, the best evidence-based treatment guidelines for this specific population are available from the *Oral Health in Cancer Therapy: A Guide for Health Care Professionals*, third edition (Rankin, Jones, & Redding, 2012). This guide provides guidelines for oral health-care management across the life span for patients undergoing head and neck radiation, chemotherapy, and hematopoietic stem cell transplant treatments. Included are management guidelines for potential adverse side effects such as bisphosphonate-related osteonecrosis of the jaw (BRONJ) (discussed below), xerostomia, and oropharyngeal mucositis pain.

HIV–Infected Women

HIV–related morbidity and mortality rates have substantially reduced because of the active use of antiretroviral (ARV) medications, and HIV is now considered a chronic illness (Younai & Vincent-Jones, 2009). As a result, the number of women living with HIV has increased and the need for primary oral health-care services increased to retain or regain functional oral health in order to receive proper nutrition, prevent oral infections, and improve their quality of life. Health-care providers will need to diagnose and treat periodontal diseases in HIV–infected women. Women who are not receiving adequate medical care, are not responding to ARV therapy, or experiencing oral side effects of HIV–related disease may have urgent oral care needs. Oral soft-tissue lesions are associated with low CD4 counts and high viral loads, and may represent the first signs of HIV infection (Ryder, Nittayananta, Coogan, Greenspan, & Greenspan, 2012).

For women on ARV therapy, increase in HPV–related oral lesions and salivary gland disease has been reported (Younai & Vincent-Jones, 2009). Additionally, immune reconstitution inflammatory syndrome (IRIS) is experienced by 20% of women who start AVR, which has been reported to include oral candidiasis (the most common opportunistic infection) and parotid enlargement. Other commonly noted oral lesions are oral herpes, oral ulcers, and oral hairy leukoplakia in which Epstein–Barr virus is the etiological agent (Patton, 2014).

Prevention/Treatment of HIV in Women

HIV testing is available for anyone to self-test at home with oral fluid samples. All health-care providers should be offering universal HIV screening for all women either via rapid-point-of-care testing or venous blood. Treatment guidelines of HIV oral lesions and the more common opportunistic infections such as oral candidiasis and HSV are updated periodically and available from the CDC, National Institutes of Health, and HIV Medicine Association of the Infectious Disease Society of America (CDC, 2009).

Acute and Chronic Oral–Facial Pain

TMJ Disorders

A temporomandibular disorder relates to (a) orofacial pain at the jaw joint, muscles of mastication or other muscles of the head and neck region that control jaw function; (b) derangement of the joint due to a displaced disc, dislocated jaw, or direct injury; and (c) degenerative and/or inflamed joint disorder such as arthritis. It is more common in women than men and affects over 10 million Americans (de Souza, Lovato da Silva, Nasser, Fedorowicz, & Al-Muharraqi, 2012). The exact cause is unknown, but trauma to the jaw is sometimes implicated. Muscular pain is usually reproducible after palpation or resistance on examination. Pain with chewing is the most common symptom with other complaints of muscle stiffness in the jaw, locking or clicking of the jaw with decreased movement, grating, clicking when opening or closing the jaw, and a misfitting of how the upper and lower teeth close. Pain is often self-limited with topical and/or systemic pain treatment, but women can develop more long-term symptoms.

TMJ Osteoarthritis

Osteoarthritis (OA) of the TMJ is the most common arthritis in the TMJ and is associated with a bilateral or unilateral deep ache in the preauricular area with or without ear pain, coarse crepitus with or without clicking, and radiological evidence of bony changes and joint space narrowing (de Souza et al., 2012). Clinically, the patient may have joint tenderness on palpation and during function, limitation in opening, and crepitus.

Prevention/Treatment of TMJ Osteorthritis

Management is aimed at (a) decreasing joint pain, swelling, and reflex masticatory spasm and/or pain; (b) improving joint function; (c) stopping the progression of the disease; and/or (d) restoring the functions. First-line noninvasive treatment includes reassurance, education on how to rest the joint by reducing contributing factors such as excessive chewing by eating soft foods. Oral nonsteroidal anti-inflammatory agents as tolerated and muscle relaxants can be helpful. Topical ice and heat, massage, ultrasound, electrogalvanic simulation, and physical therapy modalities can all help to reduce inflammation and pain (de Souza et al., 2012). Minimally invasive modalities such as intra-articular injections of corticosteroids have limited benefit, and arthroscopy may be useful in the early diagnosis and management process. Less than 20% of patients require invasive treatments such as arthroplasty to reshape the articular surfaces. For severe TMJ OA, total joint replacement by graft or implants to salvage the joint is recommended (de Souza et al., 2012).

Intraoral Pain

Pain within the oral cavity is often directly caused by disease of the dentition, periodontium, soft and hard tissues of the mouth including the palate, floor of the mouth, buccal mucosa, and tongue. On examination, it is important to rule out pain associated with a particular area or structure in the mouth, which is done by percussion, palpation, or heat or cold testing. Sharp shooting pain may indicate dental caries, and swelling and/ or purulence in adjacent soft tissue may indicate a dental abscess. A referral to a dental professional is indicated (Kumar & Brennan, 2013).

Prevention/Treatment of Intraoral Pain

Conservative self-care practices are usually first line such as eating soft foods, applying topical ice, heat, avoiding excessive jaw movements like yawning, gum chewing, loud singing. Stress-reduction techniques and passive range of motion such as gentle jaw stretching and relaxation exercises may help to increase jaw movement. Nonsteroidal anti-inflammatory drugs (NSAIDs), such as ibuprofen, may provide temporary relief from jaw discomfort. Mouth guards may also help. Botox (botulinum toxin type A) in small doses has helped to alleviate pain due to nerve and the jaw muscle in clinical trials but is not FDA-approved for TMJ disorders (NIH, 2013).

Bisposphonate-Related Osteonecrosis of the Jaw

Bisphosphonates (BPs) are used to manage bone-related conditions such as osteoporosis, Paget disease, and skeletal-related events associated with malignancy from multiple myeloma, breast cancer, prostate cancer, thyroid cancer, lung cancer, and bladder cancer. In 2003, it was first reported that there was an association of BPs with osteonecrosis of the jaw (ONJ) in postmenopausal women (Khosla et al., 2012). Bisphosphonates are synthetic analogs that inhibit bone resorption with a consequent increase in bone mass largely due to refilling of the remodeling space and an increasing mineralization density. The mechanism by which bone resorption occurs is not fully understood. BPs are administered either orally or intravenously. BRONJ is now generally recognized as a very rare complication of long-term BPs at doses used to treat osteoporosis. Signs and symptoms of ONJ include swelling, pain, paresthesias, suppuration, soft-tissue ulceration, and intra-or extra sinus tracts. The highest incidence is for women who have been treated with intravenous BPs for underlying malignancy, dental extraction, oral bone-manipulation surgery, poor fitting dental appliances, intraoral trauma, glucocorticoid use, diabetes, and alcohol abuse. Prior to dental procedures, some researchers have suggested that women stop BPs for several months for improved dental outcomes such as implants. However, to date no data supports this. Treatment plans for ONJ include pain control and oral antimicrobial rinses to minimize the risk of oral infections (Khosla et al., 2012).

Periodontal Diseases

Periodontal disease is chronic inflammation of the supporting structures of the teeth, including the gingiva, periodontal ligament, root cementum, and alveolar bone (known as the periodontium). It is directly associated with poor oral hygiene maintenance, deregulated immune response, and advancing age (Romanos, Javed, Romanos, & Williams, 2012; Suvan, 2012). Prevalence ranges from 20% to 50% have been reported in the general population (Suvan, 2012). Patients with gingivitis (inflamed red gums) have a greater risk for chronic periodontitis and dental plaque is the primary factor for the exacerbation of dental caries formation and periodontal diseases (Sambunjak et al., 2012). Over the past decade, numerous research studies have investigated the potential association between periodontal disease and various chronic nonoral, systemic diseases and conditions. Periodontitis may be an independent risk factor for artherosclerosis, including stroke and coronary heart disease (CHD), metabolic syndrome, adverse pregnancy outcomes, and diabetes (Simpson, Needleman, Wild, Moles, & Mills, 2010). For some conditions, reviewed below, treatment of periodontitis leads to a reduction in the rates of some of these other diseases, lending further support that the association is reversible. An understanding of these correlations is important to allow health-care providers to counsel patients with periodontitis of their increased risks and for those with a chronic medical condition to be screened and treated for periodontal disease, as indicated.

Obesity

Periodontitis has been positively associated with obesity, and this association was more evident as obesity levels increased (Linden, Lyons, & Scannapieco, 2013). These findings indicate the need for early diagnosis and the inclusion of periodontal care in health-care programs for obese women (Pataro et al., 2012). Clinical evidence suggests that obese individuals have an increased oral-inflammatory response as well as an altered periodontal microflora. Fat tissue produces tumor necrosis factor alpha (TNF-α) and interleukin 6, which promote bone loss and inflammation. As host response to local bacterial challenge is a key factor in determining periodontitis susceptibility (Suvan, 2012), an increased inflammatory state as that found in obese individuals could predispose them to increased periodontal tissue destruction. Additionally, TNF predisposes the patient to diabetes as it causes insulin resistance (Suvan et al., 2012).

Diabetes

Diabetes and periodontal disease are two chronic diseases with a bidirectional relationship (Simpson et al., 2010). Clinically, patients suffer from gradual loss of tooth attachment in the alveolar bone, leading to periodontal pockets, receding gums, loose teeth, and eventually tooth exfoliation, which may result in changes in food preferences and choices, possibly affecting general health. Often, gums are red and swollen, bleed easily, and patients with periodontitis suffer from bad breath (Teeuw, Gerdes, & Loos, 2010). Periodontal disease may affect insulin release through proinflammatory mediators. The highly vascularized inflamed periodontium is a potential source of inflammatory mediators, such as TNF, which can affect glucose and fat metabolism (Telgi et al., 2013). TNF impairs insulin release by increasing the adipose tissue secretion of free fatty acids. Evidence suggests that this process weakens glycemic control in diabetic patients by raising insulin resistance (Telgi et al., 2013). Hence, chronic periodontitis, a predominantly gram-negative infection, may serve as a focal source for sustained entry of bacterially derived lipopolysaccharides and host-produced inflammatory mediators into the systemic circulation.

Periodontal therapy can effectively decrease hemoglobin A1c levels for diabetic patients (Telgi et al., 2013). Conversely, evidence supports that reducing blood glucose levels will also improve periodontal disease (Simpson et al., 2010). Patient education regarding diabetes self-care management should include information on gum disease prevention, promoting oral hygiene practices, and seeking professional treatment for periodontal disease detection and management. Education must emphasize that preventing and reducing inflammation caused by bacteria in the mouth can decrease blood glucose levels and have a positive impact on glycemic control. The glycated hemoglobin (HbA1c) level is a good indicator of glycemic control, and after treatment of periodontal disease, a 10% to 20% improvement in glycemic control can be seen (Mealey, 2006). After 3 or 4 months, scaling and root planing plus oral hygiene (with or without antibiotic therapy), compared with no treatment or usual treatment, a mean percent statistically significant difference in HbA1c of 0.40% was found (Simpson et al., 2010).

Coronary Heart Disease

Emerging evidence shows an association between periodontal disease and cardiovascular disease and, more specifically, CHD. Several studies indicated that participants with CHD have more periodontal disease independent of established common risk factors, such as diabetes and smoking, or other CHD risk factors, such as age, body mass index, lipid profile, hypertension, and demographic factors such as gender (Bokhari et al., 2012; Fisher, Borgnakke, & Taylor, 2010). Evidence supports the link between a reduction in C-reactive protein, fibrinogen, and white blood cell counts in patients with CHD (Bokhari et al., 2012).

Prevention/Treatment of Periodontal Disease

Despite many types of periodontal diseases, they all share the common characteristic of chronic inflammation, and therefore, professional and self-care treatment options are the same regardless of disease. Evidence supports that treatment of periodontal disease improves endothelial function and reduces atherosclerotic disease biomarker especially for patients with known diabetes and/or cardiovascular disease (Teeuw et al., 2013). Initially, therapy must start with the debridement of tooth calculus and the disruption of the oral biofilm by dental professionals, which reduces bleeding gums and deep pocket depths by shifting the amount of species during recolonization of periopathogens. Primary prevention with fluoride therapy and regular dental visits to control plaque formation are the most cost-effective treatment for prevention of caries and periodontal disease and avoidance of restorative treatment. This treatment promotes enamel remineralization. At home, patients should be taught to brush and floss as tooth brushing removes supragingival dental plaque, while flossing potentially could penetrate the interproximal dental area where periodontal disease is prevalent (Sambunjak et al., 2012).

Professional treatment includes root scaling and planing, systemic antibiotics, and mouth rinses such as 0.12% chlorhexidine. Scaling and root planing is a deep cleaning, nonsurgical procedure, which uses local anesthesia to remove plaque and tartar from above and below the gumline. Surgical treatment includes flap surgery to reduce pockets around the teeth. Bone grafts and surgery, soft-tissue grafts, and guided tissue regeneration are sometimes required when the tissue around the teeth is decayed and cannot be repaired with nonsurgical inventions. All health-care professionals can help their patients improve glycemic levels by controlling the inflammatory cytokines. Mental health assessment for depression is another vital component of the treatment plan as depression occurs frequently in patients with a chronic illness such as periodontal disease, diabetes, and CVD, and is associated with poorer health outcomes. Baumeister, Hutter, and Bengel (2010), in a Cochrane review of clinical trials on psychological treatment and antidepressant drugs in depressed patient with diabetes, found that antidepressant drugs have a positive effect on glucose levels.

Eating Disorders

A comprehensive oral health history and extraoral and intraoral clinical examination may reveal valuable client information about the presence or absence of eating disorders (EDs) during a routine general health visit, since patients with this disorder tend to avoid disclosure (Dynesen, Bardow, Petersson, Nielson, & Nauntofte, 2008). EDs are more common in adolescent females with a national prevalence rate of up to 5%. Anorexia nervosa (AN) and bulimia nervosa (BN) are the most common forms (Romanos et al., 2012), with AN having the highest mortality rate of any mental illness (National Association of Anorexia Nervosa and Associated Disorders [NAANAD], 2013). Females at low weight are not the only women to be screened for EDs. All episodes of precipitous weight loss, weight gain, or weight fluctuations in otherwise healthy females should be investigated for the possibility of an ED, including postbariatric surgery patients. A systematic review conducted by Suvan and colleagues (2012) found a positive association between overweight and obesity, and/or excessive body fat and prevalence of periodontitis.

AN and BN are both characterized by abnormal patterns of eating behavior, weight control, and altered perceptions about weight and body (NAANAD, 2013). Malnutrition and restriction of food is primarily associated with AN, whereas BN is characterized by binge eating followed by compensatory behaviors such as inappropriate laxative use, self-induced vomiting, and excessive exercise (Johansson, Norring, Unell, & Johansson, 2012). The orodental manifestations of EDs may include dental erosion, dental caries, negative alterations in salivary gland function and salivary secretion, periodontal disease, and disorders of the TMJ (Kim, Debate, & Daley, 2013; Romanos et al., 2012).

Compared with AN patients, BN patients reported worse oral health status, especially dental erosion, dry or cracked lips, and burning tongue syndrome. Dental erosion is the most distinct and consistent oral sign in patients with EDs, and the location of the erosion can help to distinguish between BN and AN. The chronic regurgitation of acidic gastric contents into the mouth causes demineralization and erosion of the enamel dentin, and hard tissue especially on the lingual/palatal and occlusal surfaces in BN (Romanos et al., 2012). On examination, the teeth have a smooth, glassy appearance with few stains or lines (Little, 2002) (Fig. 9.5).

Salivary glands and saliva flow rate are decompensated in patients with EDs, especially when treated with antidepressant medications, particularly the selective serotonin reuptake inhibitors (SSRIs), which cause xerostomia. On clinical examination, lips can be dry and cracked; parotid gland swelling "chipmunk cheeks" appearance may be present from swollen salivary glands (Dynesen et al., 2008).

Dental caries are more common due to a diet that consists of high sugar, which promotes cariogenic microbes in the mouth. Xerostomia from antidepressant side effects can additionally cause dental plaque to stagnate on teeth surfaces, facilitating cariogenic microbes to multiply in a mouth with poor oral hygiene and nutritional deficiencies such as vitamin C and vitamin D, leading to gingival bleeding and periodontal inflammation (Romanos et al., 2012).

Oral mucosa, oropharynx membranes, and soft palate may be traumatized from self-induced vomiting. Dry erythema and angular cheilitis (inflammation of the skin around the mouth and lips) may also be seen. In women with EDs, the TMJ and/or the muscles of mastication are usually involved. The evidence for TMJ disorders in women with EDs is limited, but Johansson and colleagues (2010) found dislocation and subluxation of the mandible condyle/s were occasionally present from excessive self-triggered vomiting.

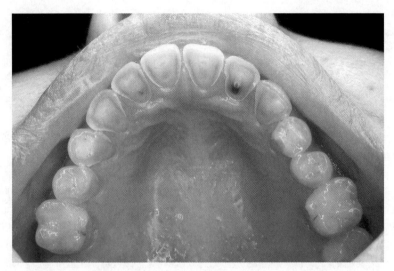

FIGURE 9.5 Location of dental erosion with eating disorders. Reprinted with permission from Scheid, R. C., & Weiss, G. (2011). *Woelfel's dental anatomy: Its relevance to dentistry* (8th ed.). Philadelphia, PA: LWW; and Courtesy of Carl M. Allen, DDS, MSD.

Sjögren Syndrome

Sjögren syndrome (SS) is an example of the many autoimmune diseases that primarily affect middle-aged women in the ratio of 9:1 female to male. It is a complex, chronic, inflammatory, systemic disease that affects the exocrine glands, especially the salivary and lacrimal glands, and is associated with dryness of the oral and ocular mucosae. Other exocrine glands found in the vagina, skin, respiratory, and gastrointestinal tract are also affected (Gonzalez, Sung, Sepulveda, Gonzalez, & Molina, 2013).

There are two types of SS: primary, in which xerostomia is the principal symptom, and secondary, in which the woman has another chronic inflammatory connective tissue disease such as rheumatoid arthritis, systemic lupus erythematous, or scleroderma (Gonzalez et al., 2013). Salivary gland dysfunction in SS causes a reduced saliva flow and quality, which may explain alterations in oral health such as difficulty with speaking, chewing, and swallowing. A higher level of caries-causing bacteria and candidiasis is present due to (a) the low saliva flow, (b) reduced mechanical flushing by saliva leading to food accumulation and dental plaque, (c) difficulty in maintaining adequate oral hygiene, and (d) increase in sugar from confectionary use or beverages that help with symptom relief (Pedersen & Nauntoofe, 2001). Depending on the progression of their disease, patients have varying amounts of saliva flow remaining. At night, some women may need to take sips of water, which can lead to sleep disturbances. Additional symptoms of chronic hyposalivation are glazed, sticky, and dry oral mucosal surfaces; the tongue appears fissured and/or lobulated, red, and dry with partial or complete atrophy of the filiform papillae. Some of the symptoms mimic oral candida infections and angular chelitis (papillary atrophy, dorsal tongue fissuring, and erythema of the oral mucosa with a burning oral sensation). In addition, specific tools to evaluate xerostomia are available such as the xerostomia questionnaire (XQ) and the xerostomia inventory (XI) (Furness et al., 2013). Other salivary and nonsalivary causes of xerostomia and hyposalivation are listed in Table 9.1.

TABLE 9.1	**Other Salivary and Nonsalivary Causes of Xerostomia and Hyposalivation**
Medications*	Diuretics, antidepressants, antipsychotics, antihistamines, anticonvulsants, incontinence
Systemic Diseases	SS, RA, sarcoidosis, poorly controlled DM, HIV infection and post-transplant recipients, HIV infection, hepatitis C virus
Irradiation	Radiotherapy treatment for head and neck and chemotherapy
Psychogenic Disorders	Depression, anxiety, social anxiety disorder
Local Factors	Salivary gland infection and obstruction, dehydration, mouth breathing, age-related changes to the tissues in the salivary glands
Autonomic Outflow Dysfunction	CVD, brain tumors, neurosurgical traumas affecting the peripheral nerves and CNS (e.g., trigeminal, facial, or glossopharyngeal nerves and nuclei salivatori)

*Over 500 medications have been reported to cause oral dryness through various proposed mechanisms (Femiano, 2008; Porter, 2004).
Adapted from Pedersen, A. M., & Nauntoofe, B. (2001). Primary Sjogren's syndrome: Oral aspects on pathogenesis, diagnostic criteria, clinical features and approaches for therapy. Pharmacotherapy, 2(9), 1415–1436.

Treatment of Xerostomia Symptoms

Salivary stimulation of the remaining functioning glands can be accomplished mechanically and is first-line treatment as it is least invasive. There is no effective therapy for primary SS, and all therapeutic treatment is aimed at alleviation of distressing symptoms of oral dryness. Second-line treatment can be chemotherapeutic agents. See Table 9.2 for treatment of xerostomia.

TABLE 9.2	**Treatment of Xerostomia**

Salivary stimulation by using sugarless gum or lozenges (use every 4 hours for 10 minutes at a time)
Assess for adequate hydration
Avoid cinnamon, strong mint, and heavy lemon
Children's fluoridated toothpaste if there is oral sensitivity to regular paste
Reduce or avoid liquids with alcohol or caffeine
Additional fluoride, such as 1.1% sodium fluoride paste once or twice a day
Oral hygiene regimen at a dental clinic every 3 months to control plaque, dietary education, and reduce caries
Topical antifungals if needed for uncomplicated and localized oral candidiasis
Acupuncture or mild transcutaneous electrical nerve stimulation (TENS)
Smoking cessation and alcohol reduction
Sucking ice chips or frequent sips of cold water may provide sufficient relief of mild symptoms
Systemic pharmacotherapies such as pilocarpine

Thyroid Disorder

In thyroid disorders, the oral manifestations seen on physical examination vary depending on the extent and length of time the thyroid disorder has been present. Women are four times more prone to thyroid disorders than men, and it becomes more common with increasing age. A lack of iodine in the diet is the most common cause of hypothyroidism as iodine is needed to produce an adequate amount of the thyroid hormone to perform daily cellular functions. The first laboratory change is an increase in thyroid-stimulating hormone and eventually a reduction in thyroxine levels. Prolonged and uncontrolled hypothyroidism causes many symptoms such as dull expression, puffy eyelids, course skin, dry nails, fatigue, depression, and anemia. In the oral cavity, an enlarged gingiva is associated with myxedema as a result of water retention and facial changes. Macroglossia, glossitis, salivary gland enlargement, and dysgeusia (distortion in the sense of taste) are all oral manifestations of prolonged hypothyroidism (Burkhart, 2013).

Hashimoto disease, which is 20 times more commonly diagnosed in women than in men, is an autoimmune disorder and is the most common form of hypothyroidism in the United States (Burkhart, 2013). Symptoms of an underactive thyroid include skin changes, depression, anxiety, fatigue, difficulty sleeping, and weight gain. When performing the extraoral examination, a goiter may be palpable. Lab tests will indicate positive antibodies against thyroglobulin and thyroperoxidase. Clinically, the patient may complain of fatigue, depression, anxiety, sleepiness, skin changes, and weight changes such as unintentional weight loss. Untreated hypothyroidism during pregnancy may lead to congential heart defects, and renal problems as well as a higher risk of cleft palate and learning disabilities in later life for the children.

Treatment

Both Hashimotos thyroiditis and Graves disease are treated with drug therapy, thyroid hormone replacement, and antithyroid medications, which inhibit the production of active thyroid hormone. Surgical removal of the thyroid or radioactive iodine therapy is often used, resulting in medication management of thyroid hormone postsurgery. An interprofessional team approach is recommended between endocrinologist, dentist, and primary care provider for early diagnosis, for avoidance of dental complications, and delivery of safe and optimal treatment.

Summary

Nearly every woman at some point in her life span, will experience tooth decay (caries) and periodontal disease (NIH, 2013). It is vital, that all health-care professionals, including nurses, critically integrate oral health into a patient's health history, physical assessment, and management plan. Lifestyle behaviors such as tobacco use, heavy alcohol use, and poor diet can adversely affect oral health, and every health-care provider can play a role in promoting healthier lifestyles for improved oral and general health (Steinberg, Hilton, Lida, & Samelson, 2013). An interprofessional approach and communication is required to provide holistic and comprehensive health care for all women.

References

American Academy of Pediatrics Children's Oral Health. (2011). Retrieved from http://www2.aap.org/oralhealth/index.html

American College of Obstetricians and Gynecologists (ACOG) (2013). *Gestational diabetes mellitus.* Practice Bulletin no. 137. Washington, DC: ACOG.

American Cancer Society. (2013). *Oral cavity and oropharyngeal cancer.* Atlanta, GA: Author.

Baumeister, H., Hutter, N., & Bengel, J. (2012). Psychological and pharmacological interventions for depression in patients with diabetes mellitus and depression. *Cochrane Database Systematic Reviews,* (12), CD008381. doi:10.1002/14651858.CD008381.pub2

Bokhari, S. A., Khan, A. A., Butt, A. K., Azhar, M., Hanif, M., Izhar, M., & Tatakis, D. N. (2012). Non-surgical periodontal therapy reduces coronary heart disease risk markers: A randomized controlled trial. *Journal of Clinical Periodontology, 39*(11), 1065–1074. doi:10.1111/j.1600-051X.2012.01942.x

Brocklehurst, P., Kujan, O., O'Malley, L. A., Shepherd, S., & Glenny, A. M. (2013). Screening pro-grammes for the early detection and prevention of oral cancer. *Cochrane Database Systematic Reviews,* (11), CD004150. doi:10.1002/14651858.CD004150.pub4

Buencamino, M. C., Palomo, L., & Thacker, H. L. (2009). How menopause affects oral health, and what we can do about it. *Cleveland Clinic Journal of Medicine, 76*(8), 468–475.

Bui, T. C., Markham, C. M., Ross, M. W., & Mullen, P. D. (2013). Examining the association between oral health and oral HPV infection. *Cancer Prevention Research, 6*(9), 917–924. doi:10.1158/1940-6207.capr-13-0081

Burakoff, R. (2003). Preventative dentistry: Current concepts in women's oral health. *Primary Care Update for Ob/GYNs, 10*(3), 141–146.

Burkhart, N. W. (2013). Hashimoto's thyroiditis. *Registered Dental Hygienist, 33*(3), 67–68.

Centers for Disease Control and Prevention. (2009). Guidelines for prevention and treatment of opportunistic infections in HIV-infected adults and adolescents. Recommendations from CDC, the National Institutes of Health and HIV Medicine Association of the Infectious Disease Society of America. *MMWR. Recommendations and Reports, 58*(RR-4), 1–206.

Chandna, S., & Bathla, M. (2011). Oral manifestations of thyroid disorders and its management. *Indian Journal of Endocrinology and Metabolism, 15,* S113–S116.

Clark, M. B., Douglass, A. B., Maier, R., Deutchman, M., Douglass, J. M., Gonsalves, W., . . . Quinonez, R. (2010). *Smiles for life: A national oral health curriculum* (3rd ed.). Society of Teachers of Family Medicine. Retrieved from www.smilesforlifeoralhealth.com

Council on Clinical Affairs. (2011). Guideline on perinatal oral health care. *American Academy of Pediatric Dentistry, 35*(6), 131–136.

de Souza, R. F., Lovato da Silva, C. H., Nasser, M., Fedorowicz, Z., & Al-Muharraqi, M. A. (2012). Inter-ventions for the management of temporomandibular joint osteoarthritis (Review). *Cochrane Library,* 1–20.

Dynesen, A. W., Bardow, A., Petersson, B., Nielsen, L. R., & Nauntofte, B. (2008). Salivary changes and dental erosion in bulimia nervosa. *Oral Surgery, Oral Medicine, Oral Pathology, Oral Radiology, and Endodontology, 106*(5), 696–707. doi.org/10.1016/j.tripleo.2008.07.003

Fakhry, C., & D'Souza, G. (2013). Discussing the diagnosis of HPV-OSCC: Common questions and answers. *Oral Oncology.* Retrieved from http://dx.doi.org/10.1016/j.oraloncology.2013.06.002

Fisher, M.A., Borgnakke, W.S., & Taylor (2010). Periodontal disease as a risk marker in coronary heart disease and chronic kidney disease. *Current Opinion in Nephrology and Hypertension, 19*(6), 519–526. doi: 10.1097/MNH.0b013e32833eda38

Fulmer, T., & Cabrera, P. (2012). The primary care visit: What else could be happening? *Nursing Research and Practice, 2012,* 720506. doi:10.1155/2012/720506

Furness, S., Bryan, G., McMillan, R., Birchenough, S., & Worthington, H. V. (2013). Interventions for the management of dry mouth: Non-pharmacological interventions (Review). *Cochrane Database of Systematic Reviews,* (9), CD009603. doi:10.1002/14651858.CD009603.pub3.

Gonzalez, S., Sung, H., Sepulveda, D., Gonzalez, M. J., & Molina, C. (2013). Oral manifestations and their treatment in Sjogren's syndrome. *Oral Diseases,* 1–9. doi:10111/odi.12105

Haber, J., Harnett, E., Hallas, D., Dorsen, C., Lange-Kessler, J., Lloyd, M., . . . Wholihan, D. (2014). Putting the mouth back in the head: HEENT to HEENOT. Unpublished manuscript.

Hart, R., Doherty, D. A., Pennell, C. E., Newnham, I. A., & Newnham, J. P. (2012). Periodontal disease: A potential modifiable risk factor limiting conception. *Human Reproduction, 25*(5), 1132–1342.

Haskin, C., & Mobley, C. (2013). The impact of women's oral health on systemic health. *Women and health* (2nd ed.). San Diego, CA: Elsevier.

Idzik, S., & Krauss, E. (2013). Evaluating and managing dental complaints in primary and urgent care. *Journal for Nurse Practitioners, 9*(6), 329–338. doi.org/10.1016/j.nurpra.2013.04.015

Indian Dental Association. (2012). Public community focus. Retrieved from http://www.ida.org.in/Public/CommunityFocus.aspx

Institute of Medicine. (2011a). *Advancing oral health in America.* Washington, DC: The National Academies Press.

Institute of Medicine. (2011b). *Building an oral health workforce.* Washington, DC: The National Academies Press.

Johansson, A.K., Johansson, A., Linell, L., Norring, C., & Carlsson, G.E. (2010). Eating disorders and signs and symptoms of temporomandibular disorders: A matched case-control study. *Swedish Dental Journal, 34*(3), 139–147.

Johansson, A.-K., Norring, C., Unell, L., & Johansson, A. (2012). Eating disorders and oral health: A matched case-control study. *European Journal of Oral Sciences, 120*, 61–68.

Karim, K. (2012). Diagnosis and management of burning mouth syndrome. *Dental Nursing, 8*(11), 717–721.

Khosla, S., Bilezikian, J. P., Dempster, D. W., Lewiecki, E. M., Miller, P. D., Neer, R. M., . . . Potts, J. T. (2012) Benefits and risks of bisphosponate therapy for osteoporosis. *Journal of Clinical Endocrinology Metabolism, 97*(7), 2272–2282.

Kim, J., Debate, R. D., & Daley, E. (2013). Dietary behaviors and oral-systemic health in women. *Dental Clinics of North America, 57*(2), 211–231. Retrieved from http://dx.doi.org/10.1016/j.cden.2013.01.004

Kreimer, A. R. (2013). Prospects for prevention of HPV-driven oropharynx cancer. *Oral Oncology.* Retrieved from http://dx.doi.org/10.1016/j.oraloncology.2013.06.007

Kumar, A., & Brennan, M. T. (2013). Orofacial pain differential diagnosis of orofacial pain and temporo-mandibular disorder. *Dental Clinics of North America, 57*(3), 419–428.

Linden, G. J., Lyons, A., & Scannapieco, F. A. (2013). Periodontal systemic associations: Review of the evidence. *Journal of Periodontology, 84*(4), S8–S19. doi:10.1902/jop.2013.1340010

Little, W. J. (2002). Eating disorders: Dental implications. *Oral Surgery, Oral Medicine, Oral Pathology, Oral Radiology, and Endodontology, 93*(2), 138–143. doi.org/10.1067/moe.2002.116598

Lo, J. C., Burnett-Bowie, S. A., & Finkelstein, J. S. (2011). Bone and the perimenopause. *Obstetrics and Gynecology Clinics of North America, 38*(3), 503–517.

Marinho, V. C., Worthington, H. V., Walsh, T., & Clarkson, J. E. (2013). Fluoride varnishes for pre-venting dental caries in children and adolescents. *Cochrane Database of Systematic Reviews*, (7), CD002279. doi:10.1002/14651858.CD002279.pub2

Mealey, B. L. (2006). Periodontal disease and diabetes: A two way street. *Journal of the American Dental Association, 137*(10 Suppl.), 26S–31S.

Mutneja, P., Dhawan, P., Raina, A., & Sharma, G. (2012). Menopause and the oral cavity. *Indian Journal of Endocrinology and Metabolism, 16*(4), 548–551.

Nainggolan, L. (2013). ACOG issues new practice bulletin on gestational diabetes. *Obstetrics and Gyne-cology, 122*, 406–416.

National Association of Anorexia Nervosa and Associated Disorders. (2013). Eating disorder statistics. Retrieved from http://www.anad.org/getinformation/about-eating-disorders/eating-disordersstatistics/?gclid=CMmi58meproCFRGi4AodOTgAJw

National Institute for Health. (2013). TMJ disorders (Publication No. 13-3487). Retrieved from http://www.nidcr.nih.gov/OralHealth/Topics/TMJ/TMJDisorders.htm

National Institute of Health, National Institute of Dental and Craniofacial Research. (2011, May). *Burn-ing mouth syndrome* (Publication No. 11-6288). Retrieved from http://www.nidcr.nih.gov

Newacheck, P. W., Hughes, D. C., Hung, Y. Y., Wong, S., & Stoddard, J. J. (2000). The unmet health needs of America's children. *Pediatrics, 105*(4), 989–997.

Niessen, L. C., Gibson, G., & Kinnunen, T. H. (2013). Women's oral health why sex and gender matter. *Dental Clinics of North America, 57*, 181–194.

Oral Cancer Foundation. (2013). Oral cancer facts. Retrieved from http://oralcancerfoundation.org/facts/index.htm

Oral Health Care During Pregnancy Expert Workgroup. (2012). *Oral health care during pregnancy: A national consensus statement.* Washington, DC: National Maternal and Child Oral Health Resource Center.

Pataro, A. L., Cosat, F. O., Cortelli, S. C., Cortelli, J. R., Abreu, M. H., & Costa, J. E. (2012). Association between severity of body mass index and periodontal condition in women. *Clinical Oral Investiga-tions, 16*, 727–734. doi:10.1007/s00784-011-0554-7

Patton, L. L. (2014). Progress in understanding oral health and HIV/AIDS. *Oral Diseases.* doi:10.1111/odi.12220

Pedersen, A. M., & Nauntoofe, B. (2001). Primary Sjogren's syndrome: Oral aspects on pathogenesis, diagnostic criteria, clinical features and approaches for therapy. *Pharmacotherapy, 2*(9), 1415–1436.

Rankin, K. V., Jones, D. L., & Redding, S. W. (Eds.). (2012). *Oral health in cancer therapy: A guide for health care professionals* (3rd ed.). Dental Oncology Education Program, Baylor Oral Health Foundation, Cancer Prevention and Research Institute of Texas.

Romanos, G. E., Javed, F., Romanos, E. B., & Williams, R. C. (2012). Oro-facial manifestations in patients with eating disorders. *Appetite, 59*, 499–504. doi.org/10.1016/j.appet.2012.06.016

Ryder, M. I., Nittayananta, W., Coogan, M., Greenspan, D., & Greenspan, J. S. (2012). Periodontal disease in HIV/AIDS. *Periodontology 2000, 60*, 78–97.

Saini, R., Saini, S., & Sharma, S. (2010). Oral sex, oral health and orogenital infections. *Journal of Global Infectious Diseases, 2*(1), 57–62.

Sambunjak, D., Nickerson, J., Poklepovic, T., Imai, P., Tugwell, P., & Worthington, H. V. (2012). Flossing for the management of periodontal diseases and dental caries in adults. *Cochrane Database of Systematic Reviews*, (12), CD008829. doi:10.1002/14651858.CD008829.pub2

Satcher, D. S. (2000). *Oral health in America: A report of the Surgeon General*. Rockville, MD: US Department of Health and Human Services, Public Health Service, National Institutes of Health, National Institute of Dental and Craniofacial Research. Retrieved from http://www.surgeongeneral.gov/library/oralheatlh/

Shourie, V., Dwarakanath, C. D., Prashanth, G. V., Alampalli, R. V., Padmanabhan, S., & Bali, S. (2012). The effect of menstrual cycle on periodontal health—A clinical and microbiological study. *Oral Health & Preventative Dentistry, 10*(2), 185–192.

Simpson, T. C., Needleman, I., Wild, S. H., Moles, D. R., & Mills, E. J. (2010). Treatment of periodontal disease for glycaemic control in people with diabetes (Review). *Cochrane Database of Systematic Reviews*, (5), CD004714. doi:10.1002/14651858.CD004714.pub2

Steinberg, B. J., Hilton, I. V., Lida, H., & Samelson, R. (2013). Oral health and dental care during pregnancy. *Dental Clinics of North America, 57*, 195–210.

Steinberg, B. J., Minsk, L., Gluch, J. I., & Giorgio, S. K. (2008). Women's oral health issues. In A. J. Clouse & K. Sherif (Eds.), *Women's health in clinical practice: A handbook for primary care* (pp. 273–293). Totowa, NJ: Humana Press.

Sun, W., Lei, L., Chen, L., Yu, Z., & Zhou, J. (2013a). Multiple gingival pregnancy tumors with rapid growth. *Journal of Dental Sciences*, http://dx.doi.org/10.1016/j.jds.2013.02.002 1–5.

Sun, A., Wu, K., Wang, Y., Lin, H., Chen, H., & Chiang, C. (2013b). Burning mouth syndrome: A review and update. *Journal of Oral Pathology & Medicine*, 1–7. doi:10.1111/jop.12101

Suvan, J., D'Aiuto, F., Moles, D.R., Petrie, A., & Donos, N. (2012). Association between overweight/obesity and periodontitis in adults. A systematic review. *Obesity Reviews, 12*, e381–e404.

Teeuw, W. J., Gerdes, V. E. A., & Loos, B. G. (2010). Effect of periodontal treatment on glycemic control of diabetic patients: A systematic review and meta-analysis. *Diabetes Care, 33*(2), 421–427.

Telgi, R. L., Tandon, V., Tangade, P. S., Tirth, A., Kumar, S., & Yadav, V. (2013). Efficacy of nonsurgical periodontal therapy on glycaemic control in type II diabetic patients: A randomized control clinical trial. *Journal of Periodontal Implant Science, 43*(4), 177–182. doi:10.5051/jpis.2013.43.4.177

Thomas, E. K., & Chitra, N. (2013). Periodontal changes pertaining to women from puberty to postmenopausal stage. *International Journal of Pharmacy and Biological Sciences, 4*(2), 766–771.

US Department of Health and Human Services. (2011). *Healthy People 2020: Understanding and improving health* (2nd ed., pp. 1–6). Washington, DC: US Government Printing Office.

Younai, F. S., & Vincent-Jones, C. (2009). Oral health and HIV infection: A chronic disease model. *Journal of California Dental Association, 37*(11), 811–819.

Zakrzewska, J. M., Forssell, H., & Glenny, A. M. (2005). Interventions for the treatment of burning mouth syndrome. *Cochrane Database of Systematic Reviews*, (1), CD002779. pub2. doi:10.1002/14651858.CD002779.pub2

Chapter 10

Resilience in Women

Anastasia Fisher, Diane C. Hatton,
and Ellen F. Olshansky

> *It is not the strongest of the species that survives,*
> *Nor the most intelligent that survives.*
> *It is the one that is the most adaptable to change.*
>
> —Charles Darwin (1859)

Introduction

Recent research has generated evidence for the concept of "resilience," which refers to the ability of a person to withstand stressors, maintain health and strength in the face of adversity, and maintain an optimistic attitude. Resilience is a recent concept that has been embraced in health and health care to reflect psychological well-being. As a newer clinical area, clearly more study is needed to understand how best to enhance resilience and how to understand the continuum of resilience among individuals. The purpose of this chapter is to present information on the concept of resilience, specifically in relation to optimal health for women. This chapter discusses the importance of resilience for health, how resilience is assessed, and how it can be achieved. The specific aims of this chapter are to

1. Discuss the concept of resilience with specific reference to women's health
2. Present ways to assess/measure/evaluate resilience
3. Present approaches to strengthening/increasing resilience in women

Importance of Understanding Resilience in Women

". . . prejudice, discrimination, war, violence, distorted interpretations of religious texts, physical and mental abuse, poverty, and disease fall disproportionately on women and girls" (Carter, 2014, p. 1). Former President Carter's poignant quote supports the relevance of an examination of resilience in women. Over the years, women have sought to achieve a sense of psychological strength as well as calmness and peacefulness as they (and all persons) are challenged with stresses of daily living. Sources of stress can be found everywhere, from internal fears, judgments, and anxieties to interpersonal issues, and to larger environmental/societal concerns. It is common to face multiple stressors on a daily basis. Being able to manage these stressors and to be resilient in the face of challenges is a key aspect of achieving optimal wellness. In fact, optimal wellness is unique for each woman as individual women experience particular challenges and stressors that are not necessarily the same for other women. In addition, and key to the concept of resilience, each individual woman responds to challenges and stressors in unique ways. For health-care providers to assist women in responding to their unique stressors, it is important to understand the individual woman's resilience as well as to assist in enhancing her resilience when appropriate.

Women have engaged in a myriad of health-seeking behaviors to mitigate stress, from classic psychoanalytic therapy to interpersonal or cognitive behavioral therapy, to other mind–body approaches. Different approaches work for different women. A key question is, why are some women better able to handle stress in their daily lives? And, if there is an answer to this question, then how might other women be helped to better manage their stress?

What is Resilience?

There are several definitions of resilience, but generally it refers to the interaction of psychological, social, environmental, and biological factors that allows a person to be mentally able to cope with adverse situations (Shanthakumari, Chandra, Riazantseva, & Stewart, 2013). Shanthakumari and colleagues stress that resilience is not a static concept, but is dynamic, involving ongoing interaction among many variables related to adversity, such as poverty, being in an abusive relationship, and personal attributes, social support, and larger contextual systems, such as schools and communities. Resilience, therefore, is not something one is born with and cannot be altered; rather, it is something that develops as one grows and develops, gains greater self-knowledge and more effective self-management skills (American Psychological Association [APA], 2014). Resilience emphasizes strengths rather than deficiencies. Others have described resilience as an individual's capacity to adapt to and recover from difficult circumstances (Carver, 1998; Tusaie & Dyer, 2004). The dynamic aspect of resilience is important, as Connor and Davidson (2003) emphasized that resilience is variable, changing due to multiple dimensions, such as context, time, age, gender, culture, and a person's varying life circumstances. Yu and colleagues (2014) examined resilience as it correlates with posttraumatic growth (PTG), a concept that describes a process wherein a person can grow as a result of having to cope with a difficult situation. These researchers have studied PTG as it interrelates with resilience, social support, and positive coping, recognizing that all of these factors contribute to PTG.

An important aspect of resilience is that it derives from a stance of health promotion, emphasizing one's strengths and abilities to overcome or to cope with difficulties, whether they are health situations or larger social contextual or individual situations. The APA (2014) identifies several factors contributing to resilience. The most salient factor is having caring supportive relationships within and outside of the family. Relationships that create and sustain love and trust, provide positive role models, and offer support and encouragement help to develop and strengthen resilient individuals. Jordan (1992, 2013) emphasized the importance of relationships in developing resilience in girls and women.

Detailed discussion of healthy relationships for both psychological and biological health is included in Chapter 16 of this book. Other factors associated with resilience include the capacity to make realistic plans and take steps to carry them out, a positive view of oneself and confidence in one's strengths and abilities, skills in communication and problem solving, and the capacity to manage strong feelings and impulses. These factors are very similar to those associated with promotion of mental health and general well-being (Ruddick, 2013). Wagnild and Young (1990, 1993) delineated five factors that are characteristic of resilience. These five factors are noted in the discussion of instruments to assess resilience, as these five interrelated factors are the foundation for the Resilience Scale (Wagnild, 2009).

Spirituality is an important aspect of resilience. Some people often reject a spiritual approach because they view spirituality as religion and they may not consider themselves to be "religious." However, another way to view spirituality is through the concept of "sacred space," as described by Burkhardt and Nagai-Jacobson (2013), who refer to "a home for the spirit, providing rest, stillness, nurture, and opportunities for opening to various connections" (p. 726). Spirituality is a way of creating a sacred space. Such a space may contribute to increased strength and resilience.

This relationship between well-being and resilience grounds the research of Siegel (2007). His work recognizes the similar ways in which well-being and resilience are promoted by secure attachment and mindful awareness and how these factors dovetail with the functions of the mid-region of the prefrontal cortex. He and other neuroscientists (Rutten et al., 2013) are engaged in identifying how patterned responses are wired in the brain (conditioning) and can derail resilience and how the brain rewires to develop new coping skills (neuroplasticity). "Resilience develops as the brain processes experience and translates that learning into neural circuitry" (Graham, 2013, p. 4). The prefrontal cortex is by far the single most integrative structure of the brain for supporting resilience; it is considered by some neuropsychologists to be an "evolutionary masterpiece" (Graham, 2010, p. 1). Because of this better understanding of brain science, we now know that we can "teach an old dog new tricks!" It is possible for us to improve our resilience through practice because our brain has the capacity for neuroplasticity, which allows new pathways to develop.

Three processes of brain change establish new patterns of coping. These processes include (1) new conditioning, (2) deconditioning, and (3) reconditioning (Graham, 2013). New conditioning involves intentional learning from our experiences, deconditioning requires taking a softened stance (self-compassion) toward deeply held beliefs and patterns in order to create mental space in our brain for new learning (Neff, 2013), and reconditioning helps rewire the neural circuitry for enhanced coping and resilience. Strategies to enhance these three processes are found in mindfulness practices. Graham (2013) suggests the following new conditioning exercise as a way to start rewiring our brains for enhanced resilience:

- Identify a habitual response to situations—impatience, anger, judgment—an old habit you want to change and something that you can use as a cue to rewiring your brain.
- Identify the new response you would like to substitute—such as pausing to reflect, approaching with curiosity, seeing the good, or calming down.
- Identify a way to cue yourself to change the usual response when it comes up. This can be a word, such as "slow down" or "breathe." Some people wear a bracelet or necklace with a favorite word or saying as a reminder; the aim here is to stop yourself from falling into the old patterned response and give yourself an opportunity for a new

response pattern to replace it. Saying the cue word to yourself while you are in a state of calmness or curiosity helps your brain to shift to this new state when it registers the cue.

- Practice the new pattern of response by saying your cue word while in the state you have chosen as the new experience (for example, calmness) as many times as needed. With practice, the new pattern will become the new habit.

The important conclusion from the research on the brain is the evidence that people can, in fact, learn new cognitive ways to approach stressors. Thus, individuals can learn and practice to develop greater resiliency.

Measuring/Assessing Resilience

Two instruments developed to measure/assess resilience are the Resilience Scale™ and the Connor–Davidson Resilience Scale (CD-RISC). The Resilience Scale™ has been used with male and female participants as well as a range of age groups and racial/ethnic groups. Developed from research with 810 community-dwelling older adults (Wagnild & Young, 1993), the original 25-item scale was based on a conceptual foundation consisting of five characteristics of resilience: perseverance, equanimity, meaningfulness, being self-reliant, and existential aloneness. An extensive description of these characteristics is beyond the scope of this chapter, but, briefly, Wagnild (2009) describes these characteristics as perseverance being persistence despite adversity, equanimity as a balanced perspective of life, meaningfulness as realizing life has purpose, self-reliant as believing in oneself, and existential aloneness as realizing each person is unique with some shared experiences and other experiences faced by oneself. Although Wagnild suggests further research will strengthen the scale, the research to date indicates this instrument has reliability and validity and has been used with a variety of populations.

The CD-RISC evolved from research and clinical work with men and women experiencing posttraumatic stress disorder (PTSD) and was conceptually based on resilience as a measure of stress coping ability. The intent of its authors was to develop a tool that could be useful in the treatment of anxiety, depression, and stress reactions. The original version consisted of 25 items. Two brief versions of 10 items (CD-RISC 10) and 2 items (CD-RISC 2) were later developed. The CD-RISC measures have demonstrated psychometric properties, and research using these instruments supports that resilience is modifiable and can improve with treatment. The CD-RISC has been used with a variety of populations and has been translated into other languages for international use (CD-RISC, 2013; Connor & Davidson, 2003).

Approaches to Increasing Resilience in Women

Strengthening or building resilience is a process. Each woman (and man, for that matter) will find some strategies more useful than others. This section includes some strategies that may be useful in building/strengthening resilience. This list of strategies was adapted from the APA (2014).

- **Increasing awareness.** For many women, mindfulness, which is the practice of awareness without judgment, is the foundational building block for resilience. Mindfulness practices have been taught for 2,500 years "as a reliable path that leads to release from suffering and to trust in our capacity to wisely and compassionately meet whatever comes our way" (Graham, 2013, p. 62). There are many mindfulness practices that lead to awareness and acceptance. Some of these include sitting and walking meditation, gardening, dancing, knitting, doing yoga, drumming, to name a few. Chapter 11 includes a more detailed discussion of self-healing approaches for women.

- **Making connections.** Good, kind relationships are key to becoming resilient. Healthy relationships are discussed in detail in Chapter 16. It is important for women to be able to accept help and support from those who care about her and who will listen to her with empathy. Helping others, too, can increase one's resilience. Making strong human connections is also part of engaging in meaningful activities. Becoming involved in activities that are meaningful will foster hope and help to put one's own situation into perspective. This engagement will also foster healthy relationships, leading to empathy and self-compassion, both important building blocks for resilience. Assisting others has mutual benefit.

- **Accepting change as a part of living.** Despite the occurrence of highly stressful events and suffering, individuals can be helped to learn to change how they view, interpret, and respond to events. Gaining a new perspective on one's self and situation can reduce stress.

- **Seeing events realistically.** Certain goals may not be attainable as a result of adversity or catastrophic circumstance. Acceptance of circumstances that cannot be changed can help give focus and energy to those things that can be altered.

- **Developing realistic goals and moving toward them.** Doing small things that make progress toward a goal can be meaningful and rewarding. It helps to set an intention each day to accomplish one thing that moves a person forward toward reaching a goal!

- **Taking actions.** In adverse situations, there may be areas in which a person can act constructively. Sometimes, some adverse situations cannot be changed, but there may be areas in which a person can act rather than detaching completely and hoping/wishing that things or events were different.

- **Looking for opportunities for self-discovery.** Out of adversity, people often learn a great deal about themselves, especially if they can reflect on their learnings. Sometimes, out of hardship come better relationships and new alliances, new meaning to experiences, more gratitude for small/simple things, more empathy for others, and increased appreciation for oneself and others. All of these elements are intrinsic to resilience.

- **Increasing self-compassion.** It is often the norm that women are their "own worst enemies," making harsh, demeaning statements to themselves about themselves. Developing self-compassion is not about being selfish or self-absorbed; it is about developing a soft, kind, open heart toward one's self and in doing so becoming more open and kind toward others.

- **Keeping things in perspective.** This is easy to say but not easy to do especially in the midst of what one perceives to be a crisis. It is important, if possible, to try to see events in the bigger context, being realistic rather than blowing events out of proportion. Taking time to take a breath and step back to see events from another perspective can help see things/events/situations/people in another way.

- **Maintaining a hopeful outlook.** An optimistic outlook enables a person to expect that good things will happen in life. It is common and, in fact, often second nature to worry about fears and concerns. Sometimes, through mindfulness meditation and cognitive therapy, women can learn to focus on the positive, what they want, the kinds of people with whom they want to spend their time, and their goals.

- **Taking good care of one's self.** Good self-care involves healthy eating, regular exercise, regular sleep patterns, a work-life in balance, and activities that provide meaning, relaxation, and fun. Paying attention to one's needs, feelings, and intuition provides the energy to deal with life more effectively, including those times when adversity occurs (APA, 2014; Fitzpatrick, 2013; Hawkins, Graham, Williams, & Zahn, 2009).

The strategies listed above are aimed at what a woman can do to build/strengthen her own resilience. Others have suggested the need to develop community-based, gender-sensitive interventions that support resilient communities and that ensure gender concerns are embedded in resilience-based actions (Ungar, 2013; United Nations Office for the Coordination of Humanitarian Affairs [OCHA], 2012).

Ungar (2013) defines resilience as the capacity of both individuals and their environments to interact in ways that optimize developmental processes (p. 256). Ungar's definition (2013) suggests that the capacity of individuals to navigate and negotiate for their needs is dependent on the capacity and willingness of their environment to meet those needs. More detail is presented on healing environments in Chapter 15. The macro- or community-level interventions suggested by this social–ecological definition of resilience involve building resilient households and communities through attention to disaster and violence-risk reduction, emergency preparedness, livelihood support, and social protection. Ungar (2013) supports an approach to resilience that builds on interventions that "first mitigate exposure to risk factors like violence, poverty, and social marginalization resulting from immigration, homophobia, and racism" (p. 263). He argues for research to identify how treatments vary when risk exposure is altered. Research reveals that disasters reinforce, perpetuate, and increase gender inequality, making bad situations worse for women and girls (OCHA, 2012, p. 1). To be effective and sustainable, the UN Office for the Coordination of Humanitarian Affairs (2012) recommends the following framework for building gender-sensitive resilience:

- **Analyze** gender differences in the affected community so that interventions are designed based on a gender analysis.
- **Design** humanitarian interventions that ensure women and girls can actually participate and benefit.
- **Ensure** access for women and girls, and monitor their participation so they have equal opportunity and access to needed services.
- **Ensure** that participation for women and girls is equal in vulnerability assessments and in prioritization and design of resilience-based projects that are built on their indigenous knowledge. Make sure that women are involved equally with men in choosing the assistance modality (food, vouchers) that best reflect their needs and reality.
- **Train** women and men equally.
- **Address** gender-based violence. During disasters, displacement from war, etc., sexual violence, exploitation, and abuse are all high-risk problems. All efforts must be made to identify and reduce these unintended effects.
- **Collect, analyze, and report sex-** and age-disaggregated data. These indicators provide more accurate data for targeted interventions.
- **Target** actions based on gender analysis. Set specific numbers/proportions of women participants in decision making-positions and in the projects as a whole. Ensure that women's capacity building allows for meaningful participation in decision-making.
- **Coordinate** actions with partners to ensure that gender issues are meaningfully incorporated into national policies that address risk reduction, climate change, and opportunity structures.

Conclusions

An essential part of wellness in women is enhancing resilience. As described in this chapter, resilience involves a focus on one's strengths, emphasizing ways to adapt to stressors and challenges, while learning to thrive to one's potential. The study of resilience is relatively new, but various techniques for increasing resilience were presented, while acknowledging that more research is needed to strengthen the evidence base.

References

American Psychological Association. (2014). *The road to resilience*. Retrieved from http://www.apa.org/helpcenter/road-resilience.aspx#

Burkhardt, M. A., & Nagai-Jacobson, M. G. (2013). Spirituality and health. In B. M. Dossey & L. Keegan (Eds.), *Holistic nursing: A handbook for practice*. Burlington, MA: Jones & Bartlett.

Carter, J. (2014). *A call to action: Women, religion, violence and power*. New York, NY: Simon & Schuster.

Carver, C. S. (1998). Resilience and thriving: Issues, models, and linkages. *Journal of Social Issues, 54*, 245–266.

CD-RISC. (2013). *Connor-Davidson Resilience Scale*. Retrieved from http://www.cd-risc.com/index.shtml

Connor, K. M., & Davidson, J. R. T. (2003). Development of a new resilience scale: The Conner-Davidson Resilience Scale (CD-RISC). *Depression and Anxiety, 18*, 76–82.

Darwin, C. (1859). *On the origins of species*. London, UK: John Murray.

Fitzpatrick, J. J. (2013). Resilience interventions. *Archives of Psychiatric Nursing, 27*, 111.

Graham, L. (2010, June). Neuroscience of resilience. *Wise Brain Bulletin*, Vol. 4,6 (6/10), 1–15. Retrieved from lindagraham-mft.net

Graham, L. (2013). *Bouncing back: Rewiring your brain for maximum resilience and well-being*. Novato, CA: New World Library.

Hawkins, S. R., Graham, P. W., Williams, J., & Zahn, M. A. (2009). *Resilient girls—factors that protect against delinquency. Girls Study Group: Understanding and responding to girls' delinquency*. Retrieved from http://www.ojp.usdoj.gov/ojjdp

Jordan, J. V. (1992). *Relational resistance*. Paper presented at the Stone Center Colloquium Series, Wellesley College, Wellesley, MA.

Jordan, J. V. (2013). Relational resistance in girls. In S. Goldstein & R. B. Brooks (Eds.), *Handbook of resilience in children*. New York, NY: Springer Science + Business Media.

Neff, K. (2011). *Self-compassion*. New York, NY: HarperCollins.

Ruddick, F. (2013). Promoting mental health and wellbeing. *Nursing Standard, 27*(24), 35–39.

Rutten, B. P. F., Hammels, C., Geschwind, N., Menne-Lothmann, C., Pishva, E., Schruers, K., . . . Wichers, M. (2013). Resilience in mental health: Linking psychological and neurobiological perspectives. *Acta Psychiatrica Scandinavia, 128*, 3–20.

Shanthakumari, R. S., Chandra, P. S., Riazantseva, E., & Stewart, D. E. (2013). "Difficulties come to humans and not trees and they need to be faced": A study on resilience among Indian women experiencing intimate partner violence. *International Journal of Social Psychology*. Advance online publication. doi: 10.1177/0020764013513440.

Siegel, D. J. (2007). *The mindful brain: Reflection and attunement in the cultivation of well-being*. New York, NY: W. W. Norton & Company.

Tusaie, K., & Dyer, J. (2004). Resilience: A historical review of the construct. *Holistic Nursing Practice, 18*, 3–8.

Ungar, M. (2013). Resilience, trauma, context, and culture. *Trauma, Violence & Abuse, 14*(3), 255–266.

United Nations Office for the Coordination of Humanitarian Affairs. (2012). *Gender and resilience*. Retrieved from http://www.unocha.org

Wagnild, G. M. (2009). A review of the resilience scale. *Journal of Nursing Measurement, 17*(2), 105–113.

Wagnild, G. M., & Young, H. M. (1990). Resilience among older women. *Image: The Journal of Nursing Scholarship, 22*, 252–255.

Wagnild, G. M., & Young, H. M. (1993). Development and psychometric validation of the Resilience Scale. *Journal of Nursing Measurement, 1*, 165–178.

Yu, Y., Peng, L., Chen, L., Long, L., He, W., Li, M., & Wang, T. (2013). Resilience and social support promote posttraumatic growth of women with infertility: The mediating role of positive coping. *Psychiatry Research, 215*, 401–405.

11

Self-care: Healing Energy and Other Complementary Therapies

Susan Thrane, Stephanie Deible, and Susan M. Cohen

Introduction

Attainment of optimal health is ideally accomplished by a partnership between the individual woman and her health-care provider(s). The partnership provides the foundation for both health care provided by the professionals and a woman's own self-care. Self-care is more than adherence to prescribed medications and lifestyle recommendations such as not smoking, wearing seat belts, or nutritional food choices. Self-care encompasses both preventative and health maintenance behaviors. Within the realm of self-care are healing energy modalities, including Reiki and meditation, which have shown promise in reducing stress, pain, and anxiety across women's life spans. In addition, there are several other self-care modalities such as guided imagery, prayer, acupuncture, and others. The evidence to support use by women for specific self-care modalities is generated from research. While meditation has been examined in research studies with both males and females, the studies presented in this chapter include only female participants or participant samples of at least 50% women. Areas particular to women's health such as menopausal hot flashes have been highlighted.

This chapter aims to

1. Present the history of Reiki and meditation, including a description of the Reiki method
2. Discuss the research to support Reiki, meditation, and other complementary self-care therapies as pertinent at various stages of women's lives
3. Present recommendations for teaching patients about self-care, specifically self-Reiki and meditation techniques

History of Reiki and Meditation

Both Reiki and meditation come from ancient traditions. Reiki is thought to have originated in the Himalayan region and brought to modern Japan in the early 20th century. Reiki was introduced to the Western world via Hawayo Takata in Hawaii

(Sierpina, 2001). Until recently, Reiki remained a secretive practice, taught only to initiates through apprenticeships. Reiki masters bring healing practices to clients that include intention-setting for health and wellness, light touching on the clothed body from the head to the feet, and a quiet environment. Reiki masters view themselves as conduits of energy meant to bring the client to a state of relaxation and receptiveness to healing states. The typical Reiki session lasts approximately 45 minutes to an hour with the client lying prone, clothed, and at ease. Individuals may be taught self-Reiki by a Reiki master, learning to perform this healing modality for themselves. Meditation also arises from ancient traditions. (See Box 11.1 for a description of how self-Reiki is performed.) Nearly every ancient civilization has some form of meditation practice, whether associated with religious practice or a component of the indigenous health system. Meditation is often either a guided imagery process led by a teacher or a recording or a relaxation-inducing practice that focuses on the breath as a means of reducing external stimuli. Mindfulness-based stress reduction (MBSR), as formulated by Kabat-Zinn (2013), has the individual bring awareness to the present without judging one's current situation or thoughts. Meditation is used to invoke a state that can be compared to Herbert Benson's relaxation response (Benson & Klipper, 1975). (See Box 11.2 for a description of how to begin meditating.) The mechanism of action for both Reiki and meditation has not been clearly elucidated at present. As with meditation, Reiki's mechanism of action may be an internal shift of cellular energy or may lie in the presence of a caring individual. Relaxation may also arise from ancient traditions that allow the individual to reduce stress and enhance the body's own healing mechanisms. Brain-imaging studies (fMRI) may bring clarity to the etiology of the effect of Reiki and meditation (Lazar et al., 2000; Short et al., 2010).

Box 11.1 Self-Reiki

Providing Reiki to yourself involves placing your hands on your body, breathing easily, and allowing energy to flow through you. It may enhance your self-Reiki to ask for your body to accept the ease and flow of energy. Set your intention. It is not necessary for your intention to be elaborate. Intentions include healing, rest, peace, relaxation, or whatever comes to mind. Reiki is a gift to yourself.

A process to guide energy flow includes placing your hands for 3 to 5 minutes at the following locations:

On top of your head; on your forehead; a hand over each eye; gently at your throat; one hand on your chest and the other on your solar plexus; and both hands just below your umbilicus.

After you finish the hand placement, silently thank yourself for bringing energy to and through yourself.

Box 11.2 Meditation

It is helpful to begin meditation with the help of resources. There are numerous books, recordings, and apps for meditation available. Jon Kabat-Zinn's book, *Full Catastrophe Living*, includes a full guide to learning MBSR. Beginners often find that using guided meditations such as the body scan or loving-kindness meditations is useful. This is particularly so if they are distracted by the constant flow of thoughts.

Women across the Life Span: Evidence for Use of Reiki and Meditation

Pregnancy, Birth, and Pediatrics

Giving birth has been thought of as a natural process until recently, when birth moved from the home to the hospital with the medicalization of childbirth becoming the norm. While this has certainly led to a significant decrease in maternal and perinatal mortality, it has also led to greater use of medication to assist with pain management. Complementary therapies offer a way for women to manage childbirth without invasive medical techniques, focusing on noninvasive interventions with the lowest possible risks. Effective support, particularly in managing pain during pregnancy, promotes health maintenance of both mothers and babies. Reiki and meditation are two examples of alternative therapies that increase options offered to women during pregnancy and childbirth.

Pregnancy and Birth

Anxiety is a major cause for discomfort in pregnant women, especially during labor and delivery. In a review of eight randomized controlled trials (N = 556), guided imagery, a form of meditation, has been found to be effective in decreasing anxiety in women during labor and delivery (Marc et al., 2011). Additionally, a study of pregnant women found that the same guided imagery course was effective in increasing knowledge about labor and delivery, decreasing pain levels in early and middle labor, increasing coping, decreasing postpartum depression, and increasing self-care (Marc et al., 2011). A longer length of labor can lead to exhaustion, stress, and possibly even need for assistance during delivery. A review of 12 studies (N = 1,397) found interventions combining yoga and meditation were effective in decreasing perceived stress and anxiety, shortening labor length, increasing birth weight, and decreasing the need for assisted births (Beddoe & Lee, 2008).

Another important factor surrounding pregnancy and labor is that of preterm labor and delivery. Relaxation therapy was examined in a review of 11 studies (N = 833), and was found to be effective for increased vaginal delivery instead of cesarean delivery, decreased stress and anxiety, and improved birth weight when combined with usual care (Khianman, Pattanittum, Thinkhamrop, & Lumbiganon, 2012). The review found no significant difference in preterm labor and delivery and no significant differences when relaxation therapy was used in lieu of standard care (Khianman et al., 2012).

Reiki is another technique that has been found helpful during childbirth. In a qualitative study exploring the utilization of complementary therapies in Israel, 13 midwives who practice in a hospital setting and routinely use complementary methods were asked about their use of several complementary methods. These midwives stated that using complementary therapies helps empower women to be in control of their bodies by preserving the "naturalness" of childbirth and reducing the dependency on technology, thus decreasing the medicalization of the birth process (Shuval & Gross, 2008).

Pediatrics

Children from birth onward can benefit from energy healing and other complementary therapies, particularly those involving touch, light touch, and distraction interventions such as stories, guided imagery, story or picture books, video games, cartoons, or music.

The specific complementary intervention chosen is guided by developmental stage. For example, for painful procedures such as heel sticks and vaccinations, infants respond well to touch, including kangaroo care, swaddling, and rocking; to sucking on pacifiers, either plain or dipped in sucrose; or to breast-feeding (Greenberg, 2002; Harrington et al., 2012; Johnston et al., 2003). Young children, as differentiated from infants, are able to remain calm when offered distractions and actually become more distressed when parents empathize and reassure them during painful procedures such as vaccinations (Schechter et al., 2007).

Energy therapy use with preterm infants is often a good adjunct treatment for various illnesses. Reiki therapy and therapeutic touch (TT) are especially useful and are often used in hospitals. Reiki therapy may be done with light touch or with the hands held above the infant in addition to TT, which is also a "hands off" type of therapy. Because preterm infants are often sensitive to external stimulation, including touch, using these treatments can be particularly helpful. In a study of TT use by nurses with preterm infants born at 23 to 37 weeks' gestation, researchers found that infants had a range of responses to TT. Infants who received treatments generally relaxed, slept better, experienced reduced heart and respiratory rates, and were better able to coordinate sucking, swallowing, and breathing during feedings (Hanley, 2008). Nurses felt that the babies' energy fields were more organized, and that their weight gain and well-being improved.

Many families who have children suffering from a chronic illness use complementary therapies. The most common therapies include prayer, natural products such as vitamins, herbs, and special diets (Cotton, Grossoehme, & McGrady, 2012; Paisley, Kang, Insogna, & Rheingold, 2011; Tomlinson, Hesser, Ethier, & Sung, 2011). In a survey of 213 families of children with cerebral palsy, 56% used some type of complementary therapy including prayer, massage, aqua therapy, acupuncture, and Reiki, with the majority using therapies once per week or more for symptom management, including muscle spasticity (Hurvitz, Leonard, Ayyangar, & Nelson, 2003). Seventy percent of families of children with sickle cell disease also used prayer, massage, and relaxation techniques for pain management (Yoon & Black, 2006). An integrative review of complementary therapy use with children who have cancer found that complementary therapies worked very well for pain management during painful procedures from blood draws to bone marrow biopsies as well as for pain and anxiety during general cancer treatments (Thrane, 2013).

Overall, Reiki, TT, and meditation have shown to be effective for a variety of situations affecting the young family. It is important for health-care providers to discuss and offer these treatments as adjunctive therapy for women and their families. Pregnant women may experience decreased stress and anxiety, improved coping, fewer medical interventions during labor, and a more "natural" labor and delivery process. Babies may show improved outcomes at birth, including increased birth weight and full-term delivery (Beddoe & Lee, 2008; Khianman et al., 2012). Children respond well to complementary therapies for painful procedures such as vaccinations and blood draws as well as for ongoing treatments for chronic illnesses. Families often prefer the addition of a complementary therapy rather than an additional medication because their children remain more active and better able to interact with family. Providers should be prepared to answer questions about the treatments they recommend, using up-to-date evidence and scientific data. Health-care providers must also offer information to their clients on the limits of these treatments while also emphasizing the complementary role of integrative medicine. Areas in which more research is needed on the role of complementary therapies include premenstrual syndrome (PMS) and dysmenorrhea.

Menopause

Women experiencing menopause may suffer from a variety of symptoms, including physical, cognitive, and emotional, ranging from mild to severe. Menopause, despite being a normal physiologic process that women undergo, has become medicalized through the common use of hormonal treatments for menopausal symptoms. However, evidence indicates conflicting results on safety and efficacy of both hormonal treatments as well as complementary approaches such as bioidentical hormones (Lewis, 2013). Thus, it is essential that further research be conducted and a variety of options explored for women suffering from symptoms often associated with menopause. There are a number of complementary therapies, some needing further research, that may help with some or all of these symptoms, including diet, exercise, dietary supplements, acupuncture, yoga, meditation, Reiki, and TT. In addition to promoting autonomy in this population, it is essential that providers encourage self-care to maintain quality of life while promoting overall wellness during this transition.

In a recent study of 110 women, it was noted that MBSR is effective for significantly reducing the number of bothersome hot flashes and night sweats while improving quality of life, sleep quality, anxiety, and perceived stress (Carmody et al., 2011). A systematic review of 18 clinical trials including 882 women showed that yoga and meditation programs were effective at improving menopausal symptoms including mood and sleep disorders, as well as musculoskeletal pain (Innes, Selfe, & Vishnu, 2010).

Canadian women found a variety of complementary therapies helpful for menopausal symptoms. In a survey of 423 Canadian women ranging in age from 39 to 63 (mean = 51.4) who were pre- to postmenopausal, 91% of the women used some type of complementary therapy (Lunny & Fraser, 2010). The therapies the women found moderately to significantly helpful were prayer (73%), relaxation techniques (71%), and TT/Reiki therapy (66%) (Lunny & Fraser, 2010). Older women with more education and more symptoms were more likely to use one or more complementary therapies.

In conclusion, meditation, TT, Reiki, and other complementary therapies have been shown to be effective at reducing or alleviating symptoms associated with menopause. Women with menopause often seek nonmedicinal treatments and self-care interventions that are easy to use and effective. Health-care providers can assist menopausal women to mitigate their symptoms by including complementary therapies as options for them.

Mood Disorders: Depression, Stress, and Anxiety

Depression

Mood disorders, particularly depression, often affect women. Women with mood disorders often suffer undiagnosed for a long time. By offering easy, cost-effective and self-care–oriented interventions, women both with and without a formal diagnosis have options for relief. For women with diagnosed depression who have been prescribed medication, complementary therapies may benefit them by offering side effect–free options that cannot be met with medications. Psychiatric medications are known to have side effects ranging from sleep impairment, driving impairment, decreased libido, and interference with daily activities. Sometimes, however, the benefits of medications outweigh the inconvenience of side effects, leaving patients with few options. Complementary therapies may, indeed, offer some options. This is particularly important for women with chronic mood disorders, where cost-effective, long-term strategies for treatment may be especially important. Even if women continue to require prescription medication, complementary therapies may help by enhancing the effects and possibly allowing a decrease in dosage (Tanay, Lotan & Bernstein, 2012).

The use of Reiki for mood disorders, specifically mild to major depression, has been studied with a variety of populations from college students to older, community-dwelling adults. In a study of depression in otherwise healthy young college students, 40 mostly female students were randomized into Reiki and control groups. Before the Reiki intervention, the students' depression was measured, and the students were categorized as having either high or low depression scores. At the 5-week follow-up after the Reiki intervention, the Reiki group had significant improvement in mood and a decrease in overall depression, anxiety, and stress in those students who had started with high depression scores (Bowden, Goddard, & Gruzelier, 2011). Using Reiki with older community-dwelling adults resulted in decreased depression, while, during the same time period, the control group experienced increased depression (Richeson, Spross, Lutz, & Peng, 2010).

Mindfulness-based techniques for reducing stress have been noted to improve mood and decrease depression. Some current findings on treating depression as a comorbidity of such conditions as cancer or fibromyalgia are addressed later in this chapter. A recent small study (N = 13) found that meditation improved coping with depression and anger in low-income older women (Szanton, Wenzel, Connolly, & Piferi, 2011). Another small study with men and women found that meditation was effective at decreasing negative thoughts, including experiential avoidance (avoiding experiences that trigger negative thoughts), while suffering from depression (Tanay et al., 2012).

Evidence indicates that mood and depressive symptoms show improvement with these complementary techniques. Women can be taught to engage in self-care by doing meditation and Reiki.

Anxiety, Stress, and Posttraumatic Stress Disorder

MBSR methods are effective for decreasing anxiety and stress in multiple settings and populations. These techniques have been found to be effective for reducing stress in young adult women nursing students (Kang, Choi, & Ryu, 2009). Additionally, "loving-kindness" meditation was effective at decreasing stress and stress-linked health disparities in African American women (Woods-Giscombe & Black, 2010).

Stress and anxiety seems to be a common reaction to modern life. Stress causes both emotional and physical responses. Physiological responses include increased cortisol, norepinephrine, and a disruption in serotonin levels. These hormones lead to changes in heart and respiratory rates, sleep disruption, decrease in immunity to illness, and alterations in appetite and mood. When Reiki was used in an oncology day clinic with patients receiving chemotherapy, participants experienced a significant decrease in anxiety after each Reiki session (Birocco et al., 2012). In a survey of 342 nurses, 99% had used a mind–body practice, such as prayer (94%), meditation (65%), or other mind–body practices (71%) such as healing touch or TT (39%), yoga or other mindful movement practice (34%), or guided imagery or hypnosis (25%), or Reiki or other energy healing (21%) (Kemper et al., 2011). In a study of 21 female health-care professionals experiencing burnout, participants experienced one Reiki session and one sham Reiki session. When comparing pretreatment to posttreatment measures of heart rate variability, body temperature, and cortisol, Reiki participants experienced an increase in heart rate variability, an increase in body temperature, but no change in cortisol levels (Diaz-Rodriguez et al., 2011). Two studies found that participants receiving Reiki experienced a significant increase in body temperature, a significant decrease in systolic blood pressure, and a subjective feeling of both physical and mental relaxation, all of which are indicative of a relaxation response (Wardell & Engebretson, 2001; Witte & Dundes, 2001). These changes in physiological symptoms indicate an effect on the parasympathetic response, which decreases the stress response (Harvard Health Publications, 2011). Overall, Reiki appears to decrease stress and increase relaxation.

Intimate partner violence and posttraumatic stress disorder (PTSD) are important women's health issues. Mindfulness experiences and training were shown to be effective in a small study (N = 10) to improve coping and stress in a minority, low-income population with PTSD and a history of intimate partner violence (Bermudez et al., 2013). It was mentioned in the study that standard psychotherapy should be used concurrently as meditation helps in coping with stress but does not specifically address underlying trauma. However, another small study (N = 20) in women suffering from PTSD as a result of intimate partner violence found that MBSR techniques were just as effective at decreasing sexual distress and were more effective at improving sexual arousal when compared with cognitive behavioral therapy (CBT) (Brotto, Seal, & Rellini, 2012).

For people who have suffered trauma resulting in depression or PTSD, complementary therapies can be an excellent adjunct to psychotherapy. In a study of 25 participants who had suffered trauma, including sexual abuse, and were undergoing psychotherapy, individuals received one of five different complementary healing techniques, one of which was Reiki therapy. After completing the complementary therapies, participants were asked about the helpfulness of the sessions and, overall, rated the complementary therapies as 8.6 on a scale of 0 to 10 for helpfulness (Collinge, Wentworth, & Sabo, 2005). There was a trend for higher perceived helpfulness for those with sexual or substance abuse histories. Participants were asked about their sense of interpersonal safety, bodily sensation, interpersonal boundary setting, and sense of bodily shame. Participants had an increased sense of safety, an increased level of bodily sensation (especially important for those who had suffered sexual abuse), an increased comfort level with boundary setting, and a decreased sense of bodily shame. These are very important findings for clients who have suffered trauma and abuse and for aiding select clients to make progress in their feelings of self-esteem and general mental health.

Alzheimer Disease

Crawford, Leaver, and Mahoney (2006) studied the use of Reiki therapy for adults with mild Alzheimer disease. After 4 weeks of twice-weekly treatments, those adults who received Reiki had higher scores on the Annotated Mini Mental State Examination (AMMSE), indicating improved memory, when compared with the control group who did not receive treatment. When comparing the Revised Memory and Behavior Problem Checklist scores before and after treatment, adults who received Reiki had significant improvement on tasks such as increased ability to remember recent events, improved concentration, decreased waking at night, decreased appearance of anxiety and sadness, and decreased feelings of failure (Crawford et al., 2006). The study authors suggest training caregivers in Reiki, so that caregivers may administer Reiki treatments frequently in order to improve family quality of life, decrease or delay outside nursing care, and delay the need for nursing homes. Caregivers can be taught to provide Reiki both for their family member and for themselves.

As shown in the above studies, complementary therapies are often helpful by themselves as a treatment for mood disorders, mild depression, stress, and even mild Alzheimer's.

However, with more serious conditions such as major depression and PTSD, complementary therapies should be used *in conjunction with* other conventional treatments such as psychotherapy. The therapies described help with stress and anxiety through increased relaxation that can be measured through parasympathetic response, including increased heart rate variability, increased body temperature, and decreased systolic blood pressure, which are all indicative of increased relaxation. These therapies are worth recommending to patients either alone or in conjunction with other therapies in order to decrease stress, anxiety, depression, PTSD, and mild Alzheimer disease.

Pain

Many people are wary of taking medication for pain owing to fears of addiction and untoward side effects. Complementary therapies are often helpful in many situations involving both acute and chronic pain.

Acute Pain

For acute and "short-term" pain (examples include stubbed toe, menstrual cramps, or surgery), complementary therapies include hot or cold packs, guided imagery, hypnosis, acupuncture, Reiki, and TT, which can be helpful in decreasing or relieving such discomfort. The use of complementary therapies for pain can help eliminate or decrease medication use depending on the situation and source of the pain, thus allowing better quality of life through less of the sedation associated with opioids.

Chronic Pain

Many older adults, a substantial number of whom are women, suffer from chronic pain with movement. In addition to the therapies noted for acute pain, other options such as meditation, yoga, tai chi, or qi gong are often helpful for more chronic pain such as arthritis. There is evidence for the use of Reiki and TT in chronic pain management. In a study of 20 community-dwelling adults with chronic pain, participants received a 45-minute Reiki session once per week for 8 weeks (Richeson et al., 2010). At the end of 8 weeks, the Reiki group had a statistically significant decrease in pain, while the wait-list control group had a statistically significant increase in pain (Thrane & Cohen, in press). Smith, Arnstein, Rosa, and Wells-Federman (2002) combined TT with CBT to examine whether the use of these two therapies combined would decrease pain in a group of 12 participants with chronic pain. While both the CBT alone and the CBT plus TT groups did have a decreased pain level, neither was statistically significant; however, the CBT plus TT group did have a larger decrease in pain than the CBT alone group (Smith et al., 2002).

Fibromyalgia

Pain from fibromyalgia remains a relatively unexplained condition in medicine. Women are frequently the sufferers of this chronic condition, which has limited effective treatments. One approach to this pain relief is MBSR. In a study of 43 women, aged 20 to 71, who suffered with fibromyalgia and were taught MBSR, while results showed non–statistically significant reductions in depression and anxiety, basal sympathetic nervous system activity was reduced, which may contribute to pain relief (Lush et al., 2009).

The study points to the need for increased clarification of the psychological and physiological responses in fibromyalgia. Another study (N = 31) followed women over 24 months and found long-term reduction in fibromyalgia symptoms through the use of transcendental meditation and yoga (Rasmussen et al., 2012). A randomized controlled trial of 177 women suffering from fibromyalgia, comparing MBSR to a wait-list control group, found significant improvement of depressive symptoms, anxiety, antidepressant use, and quality of life (Schmidt et al., 2011). These studies illustrate that MBSR may help some patients with fibromyalgia, but it is important to educate patients on the possible limits of effectiveness. When effective, MBSR techniques may offer an alternative to pain medications and the side effects associated with those medications.

Procedural Pain

Complementary therapies may be used to augment pain medications during procedures. Two studies examined the use of Reiki as an adjunct for pain management during screening colonoscopies (Bourque, Sullivan, & Winter, 2012; Hulse, Stuart-Shor, & Russo, 2010). Bourque and colleagues explored whether the use of Reiki therapy along with meperidine and midazolam would decrease meperidine use during colonoscopies: Although there was no statistical difference in medication use between the Reiki and sham Reiki groups, 4 out of 25 patients in the Reiki group did use less than 50 mg of meperidine, while the entire control group received more than 50 mg of the medication. Hulse and colleagues (2010) examined the use of Reiki therapy for anxiety prior to a colonoscopy. In this semirandomized study, the Reiki group had statistically higher levels of anxiety before the colonoscopy, and statistically lower levels of anxiety after the 15-minute Reiki treatment. Both studies recommend the use of Reiki for colonoscopies despite the lack of statistically significant differences because patients were very satisfied with the intervention and the staff noticed a difference in anxiety levels and medication use.

Postsurgical Pain

Both TT and Reiki therapy have been studied with postsurgical adults to examine pain relief. McCormack (2009) used TT with 90 participants randomly assigned to one of three groups: TT, a non–TT intervention (metronome use), and a control group. Within the TT group, participants experienced a significant decrease in pain, and when comparing the TT group with the other two groups, the TT group had significantly decreased pain scores, while both the non–TT group and the control group experienced increased pain scores (McCormack, 2009). Vitale and O'Connor (2006) used a Reiki intervention for pain and anxiety with women undergoing a hysterectomy. A 30-minute Reiki treatment was administered just prior to surgery and then again 24 hours postsurgery. When comparing the Reiki group with the usual care group, the Reiki group experienced significantly less pain 24 hours after surgery and used less pain medication (Thrane & Cohen, 2013).

Complementary therapies are often useful for both chronic and acute pain. Of course, not all types of pain will respond to complementary therapies any more than they will to conventional medications. Health-care practitioners understand that what works for one person and type of pain may not work for another. Complementary therapies such as meditation, Reiki, and TT have been shown to be effective in experimental conditions as described above. These therapies are all noninvasive with no known contraindications; thus, they may be acceptable options for many women.

Cancer Symptom Management

There are approximately 13.7 million cancer survivors in the United States, and over 1.6 million new diagnoses of cancer were expected to be made in 2014 (American Cancer Society, 2013). Cancer is now recognized as a chronic illness, and cancer survivors continue to experience mild to severe symptoms even years after treatment. Well over half of all cancer patients use some type of complementary therapy for symptom management (Brauer, El Sehamy, Metz, & Mao, 2010). Many of these therapies have not been well studied for safety, effectiveness, or indication for use with conventional cancer therapies. The legitimate problem with patient use of complementary therapies is that *providers rarely ask* about complementary therapy use and patients do not tell their providers about their use of complementary therapies, (Robinson & McGrail, 2004). Others, however, have been studied and may be recommended for symptom management in cancer survivors.

Complementary therapies are used by more than half of cancer patients. A survey of conventional cancer centers in the United Kingdom revealed that complementary healing practices such as Reiki and TT are either fully or partially accepted by 85% of responding centers, that 93% of providers in these centers view complementary therapies as very useful, and that the therapists feel that 79% of nonpractitioners see therapies as useful or very useful (Lorenc, Peace, Vaghela, & Robinson, 2010). Breast cancer patients are very likely to use some form of complementary therapy, with the most common being "activity-based" such as Reiki or meditation (71%), herbal or vitamin supplements (45%), or the use of topical preparations such as honey (26%) (Moran et al., 2013). The majority of complementary therapy users in this study felt that these therapies helped with symptoms such as stress (25%), or relief of symptoms related directly to cancer treatments (23%). For example, when comparing skin reactions (a side effect of radiation treatment) of those who used complementary therapies versus those who did not, complementary therapy users had significantly less severe skin reactions (Moran et al., 2013).

When formulating a plan for cancer care in women, it is essential that providers offer effective, feasible, and low-risk interventions to augment traditional treatment in order to support quality of life. MBSR techniques are easy to teach and implement, making it ideal for self-care. To maintain the holistic advantage in cancer care, providers should consider the use of MBSR for women with a diagnosis of cancer who are suffering from the side effects of cancer treatment. In women with all stages of breast cancer, improving quality of life should remain a high priority. MBSR and other forms of meditation have been shown to be effective in improving various aspects of quality of life for these women. In a recent study of 336 women, MBSR techniques were found to be effective in improving sleep quality in women with breast cancer (Andersen et al., 2013). In addition to sleep, MBSR was shown to be effective for improving sexual functioning and decreasing sexual distress (Brotto et al., 2012). A study of 229 women undergoing chemotherapy and radiation found MBSR was effective for decreasing mood disturbance, anger, anxiety, depression, fatigue, and confusion while improving emotional and functional well-being (Hoffman et al., 2012). Additionally, multiple studies have noted MBSR to be effective in improving quality of life, decreasing depression and anxiety, and improving well-being as well as enhancing spirituality in women suffering from breast cancer (Henderson et al., 2012; Nidich et al., 2009; Witek-Janusek et al., 2008).

Fatigue, even more than pain, is the most common treatment side effect reported by cancer patients (Morrow, Shelke, Roscoe, Hickok, & Mustian, 2005). Tsang, Carlson, and Olson (2007) investigated the use of Reiki with 16 cancer patients who had completed chemotherapy treatment. The Reiki intervention consisted of five once-daily sessions for 5 days followed by a 7-day washout period followed by two additional Reiki treatments during the next week. The control group consisted of resting for the same time period. The Reiki group had a statistically significant decrease in tiredness scores from pretreatment day 1 to posttreatment day 5 with a medium clinical effect size (Tsang et al., 2007). The Reiki group also had a significant decrease in pain with a medium effect size and a significant decrease in anxiety with a large effect size (Thrane & Cohen, 2013; Tsang et al., 2007).

Several studies have examined the use of Reiki therapy with cancer pain. In one study, Reiki was used for cancer patients receiving chemotherapy treatments in a day treatment center. For each session, participants experienced a statistically significant 50% decrease in pain after each session and a decrease in pain when comparing baseline pain scores with pain scores after the fourth session (Birocco et al., 2012). Marcus, Blazek-O'Neill, and Kopar (2013) asked cancer patients who had received Reiki treatments from volunteers about their experiences. Of the patients who received Reiki treatments in the infusion center, 94% had a positive experience, 89% said it was relaxing, 75% said they experienced decreased anxiety, and 45% said they had decreased pain levels (Marcus et al., 2013). Olson, Hanson, and Michaud (2003) examined Reiki therapy with cancer patients taking opioids for pain. Twenty-four participants were randomized either into the Reiki or the rest group. The Reiki group received two 90-minute treatments on days 1 and 4 of the week-long intervention. Reiki recipients experienced decreased pain, decreased diastolic blood pressure and heart rate on day 1, and decreased pain on day 4 (Olson et al., 2003). When comparing the Reiki group and the rest group, Reiki recipients had a medium clinical effect on day 1 for decreased pain ($d = 0.64$) and a large clinical effect for decreased pain on day 4 ($d = 0.93$) (Thrane & Cohen, 2013).

Despite the studies presented, there is still a dearth of research. Yet, several complementary therapies show promise for symptom management in cancer patients and cancer survivors. Both Reiki therapy and MBSR show potential, particularly for the reduction of pain and anxiety. Reiki and MBSR techniques may be taught to patients and family so that they may use them as self-care and for their loved ones. MBSR has shown promise for the improvement of sleep quality and for decreasing sexual distress in women undergoing cancer treatments.

". . . Reiki therapy may be considered a useful aid in the management of anxiety and pain during day hospital stay for cancer care; furthermore, offering Reiki therapy in hospitals could provide a global approach to cancer patients, which responds to their physical and emotional needs within a holistic vision of care" (Birocco et al., 2012, p. 294).

Complementary therapies including MBSR, Reiki, acupuncture, massage, yoga, and others help to empower women to take control of their symptoms in a way that suits their wishes and lifestyle.

Benefits to Health-care Providers

Self-care has been shown to be effective not only for patients, but also for health-care providers. Health-care providers frequently experience stress on the job, difficulty balancing work and other aspects of life, emotional challenges, and problematic situations. A recent report from the Centers for Disease Control and Prevention (CDC, 2008) labeled this phenomenon exposure to "occupational stress," and emphasized that such stress contributed to greater suicide and substance abuse rates in health-care providers over the general population. Complementary therapies may increase resiliency and coping in this population, which can be generalized to others in high-stress environments, including women at various life stages and situations (e.g., caregiving for older parents or for young children). A recent study of 82 health-care providers indicated that an 8-week program on integrative health-care training in Reiki, yoga, meditation, and sound healing was effective in decreasing stress and increasing confidence in ability to cope (Tarantino et al., 2013). Furthermore, this program emphasized self-care, allowing for personal growth and healing through a low-cost, low-risk treatment option.

Reiki level 1 was taught to health-care providers as a self-care method and to examine whether the providers would feel better able to care for their patients (Brathovde, 2006). This pilot study found that 70% of participants felt they had experienced a positive change in their perception of caring. Participants also felt more grounded, experienced an increase in self-care and caring behaviors, an increase in personal awareness, and the ability to be more mindful when working with patients (Brathovde, 2006). Cuneo and colleagues (2011) taught Reiki level 1 to nurses and encouraged them to practice self-Reiki for 3 weeks. Those nurses who practiced Reiki regularly during the 3-week period experienced a significant decrease in stress, while those nurses who occasionally practiced self-Reiki still experienced some decrease in stress. Finally, Vitale (2009) explored the experience of nurses who already practice Reiki for self-care. These nurses reported that Reiki makes them feel more connected to themselves and a higher power, that using self-Reiki during the day helps them become or remain calm even during stressful times, and decreases their stress in general. These studies demonstrate that using Reiki for self-care can be a very effective technique. Health-care providers know how important self-care is, but often do not make time for themselves. Complementary therapies such as Reiki, meditation, yoga, massage, and many other modalities are good ways to approach self-care. Reiki and meditation, in particular, can be done anywhere, and at any time, either during the workday or during non-working hours in order for providers to care for themselves, destress, recenter, and be better able to care for others.

Summary

This chapter has presented current research on various complementary healing modalities, many of which can be used by patients themselves. The importance of self-care in contributing to optimal healing was emphasized, with particular focus on Reiki and meditation, although several other complementary modalities were described. Examples of clinical situations were noted in which such modalities can be helpful in the healing process.

References

American Cancer Society. (2013, October 26). *Cancer facts & figures 2013.* Retrieved from http://www .cancer.org/acs/groups/content/@epidemiologysurveilance/documents/document/acspc-036845.pdf

Andersen, S. R., Wurtzen, H., Steding-Jessen, M., Christensen, J., Andersen, K. K., Flyger, H., ... Dalton, S. O. (2013). Effect of mindfulness-based stress reduction on sleep quality: Results of a randomized trial among Danish breast cancer patients. *Acta Oncologica, 52*(2), 336–344. doi:10.3109/02841 86X.2012.745948

Beddoe, A. E., & Lee, K. A. (2008). Mind-body interventions during pregnancy. *Journal of Obstetric, Gynecologic, and Neonatal Nursing, 37*(2), 165–175. doi:10.1111/j.1552-6909.2008.00218.x

Benson, H., Klipper, M.Z. (1975). *The relaxation response.* New York: Harper-Collins.

Bermudez, D., Benjamin, M. T., Porter, S. E., Saunders, P. A., Myers, N. A., & Dutton, M. A. (2013). A qualitative analysis of beginning mindfulness experiences for women with post-traumatic stress disorder and a history of intimate partner violence. *Complementary Therapies in Clinical Practice, 19*(2), 104–108. doi:10.1016/j.ctcp.2013.02.004

Birocco, N., Guillame, C., Storto, S., Ritorto, G., Catino, C., Gir, N., ... Ciuffreda, L (2012). The effects of Reiki therapy on pain and anxiety in patients attending a day oncology and infusion services unit. *American Journal of Hospice & Palliative Care, 29*(4), 290–294. doi:10.1177/1049909111420859

Bourque, A. L., Sullivan, M. E., & Winter, M. R. (2012). Reiki as a pain management adjunct in screening colonoscopy. *Gastroenterology Nursing, 35*(5), 308–312. doi:10.1097/SGA.0b013e3182603436

Bowden, D., Goddard, L., & Gruzelier, J. (2011). A randomised controlled single-blind trial of the efficacy of Reiki at benefitting mood and well-being. *Evidence-Based Complementary and Alternative Medicine, 2011*, 1–8. doi:10.1155/2011/381862

Brathovde, A. (2006). A pilot study: Reiki for self-care of nurses and healthcare providers. *Journal of Holistic Nursing, 20*(2), 95–101

Brauer, J. A., El Sehamy, A., Metz, J. M., & Mao, J. J. (2010). Complementary and alternative medicine and supportive care at leading cancer centers: A systematic analysis of websites [Research support, N.I.H., Extramural]. *Journal of Alternative and Complementary Medicine, 16*(2), 183–186. doi:10.1089/acm.2009.0354

Brotto, L. A., Erskine, Y., Carey, M., Ehlen, T., Finlayson, S., Heywood, M., ... Miller, D. (2012). A brief mindfulness-based cognitive behavioral intervention improves sexual functioning versus wait-list control in women treated for gynecologic cancer. *Gynecologic Oncology, 125*(2), 320–325. doi:10.1016/j.ygyno.2012.01.035

Brotto, L. A., Seal, B. N., & Rellini, A. (2012). Pilot study of a brief cognitive behavioral versus mindfulness-based intervention for women with sexual distress and a history of childhood sexual abuse. *Journal of Sex & Marital Therapy, 38*(1), 1–27. doi:10.1080/0092623X.2011.569636

Carmody, J. F., Crawford, S., Salmoirago-Blotcher, E., Leung, K., Churchill, L., & Olendzki, N. (2011). Mindfulness training for coping with hot flashes: Results of a randomized trial. *Menopause, 18*(6), 611–620. doi:10.1097/gme.0b013e318204a05c

Centers for Disease Control and Prevention [CDC] (2008). Exposure to stress occupational hazards in hospitals. www.cdc.gov retrieved 02-22-14.

Collinge, W., Wentworth, R., & Sabo, S. (2005). Integrating complementary therapies into community mental health practice: An exploration. *Journal of Alternative and Complementary Medicine, 11*(3), 569–574. doi:10.1089/acm.2005.11.569.

Cotton, S., Grossoehme, D., & McGrady, M. E. (2012). Religious coping and the use of prayer in children with sickle cell disease. *Pediatric Blood & Cancer, 58*(2), 244–249. doi:10.1002/pbc.23038

Crawford, S. E., Leaver, V. W., & Mahoney, S. D. (2006). Using Reiki to decrease memory and behavior problems in mild cognitive impairment and mild Alzheimer's disease. *Journal of Alternative and Complementary Medicine, 12*(9), 911–913. doi:10.1089/acm.2006.12.911

Cuneo, C.L., Curtis-Cooper, M.R., Drew, C.S., Naoum-Heffernan, C., Sherman, T., Walz, K., & Weinberg, J. (2011). The effect of Reiki on work-related stress of the registered nurse. *Journal of Holistic Nursing, 29*(10), 33–43.

Diaz-Rodriguez, L., Arroyo-Morales, M., Fernandez-de-Las-Penas, C., Garcia-Lafuente, F., Garcia-Royo, C., & Tomas-Rojas, I. (2011). Immediate effects of Reiki on heart rate variability, cortisol levels, and body temperature in health care professionals with burnout. *Biological Research for Nursing, 13*(4), 376–382. doi:10.1177/1099800410389166

Greenberg, C. S. (2002). A sugar-coated pacifier reduces procedural pain in newborns. *Pediatric Nursing, 28*(3), 271–277.

Hanley, M. A. (2008). Therapeutic touch with preterm infants: Composing a treatment. *Explore (New York, NY), 4*(4), 249–258. doi:10.1016/j.explore.2008.04.003

Harrington, J. W., Logan, S., Harwell, C., Gardner, J., Swingle, J., McGuire, E., & Santos, R. (2012). Effective analgesia using physical interventions for infant immunizations. *Pediatrics, 129*(5), 815–822. doi:10.1542/peds.2011-1607

Harvard Health Publications. (2011). *Understanding the stress response.* Retrieved from http://www.health.harvard.edu/newsletters/Harvard_Mental_Health_Letter/2011/March/understanding-the-stress-response

Henderson, V. P., Clemow, L., Massion, A. O., Hurley, T. G., Druker, S., & Hébert, J. R. (2012). The effects of mindfulness-based stress reduction on psychosocial outcomes and quality of life in early-stage breast cancer patients: A randomized trial. *Breast Cancer Research and Treatment, 131*(1), 99–109. doi:10.1007/s10549-011-1738-1

Hoffman, C. J., Ersser, S. J., Hopkinson, J. B., Nicholls, P. G., Harrington, J. E., & Thomas, P. W. (2012). Effectiveness of mindfulness-based stress reduction in mood, breast- and endocrine-related quality of life, and well-being in stage 0 to III breast cancer: A randomized, controlled trial. *Journal of Clinical Oncology, 30*(12), 1335–1342. doi:10.1200/JCO.2010.34.0331

Hulse, R. S., Stuart-Shor, E. M., & Russo, J. (2010). Endoscopic procedure with a modified Reiki intervention: A pilot study. *Gastroenterology Nursing, 33*(1), 20–26. doi:10.1097/SGA.0b013e3181ca03b9

Hurvitz, E. A., Leonard, C., Ayyangar, R., & Nelson, V. S. (2003). Complementary and alternative medicine use in families of children with cerebral palsy. *Developmental Medicine & Child Neurology, 45*(6), 364–370.

Innes, K. E., Selfe, T. K., & Vishnu, A. (2010). Mind-body therapies for menopausal symptoms: A systematic review. *Maturitas, 66*(2), 135–149. doi:10.1016/j.maturitas.2010.01.016

Johnston, C. C., Stevens, B., Pinelli, J., Gibbins, S., Filion, F., Jack, A., … Veilleux, A. (2003). Kangaroo care is effective in diminishing pain response in preterm neonates. *Archives of Pediatrics & Adolescent Medicine, 157*(11), 1084–1088. doi:10.1001/archpedi.157.11.1084

Kabat-Zinn, J. (2013). *Full catastrophe living: Using the wisdom of your body and mind to face stress, pain, and illness* (Rev. ed.). New York, NY: Random House.

Kang, Y. S., Choi, S. Y., & Ryu, E. (2009). The effectiveness of a stress coping program based on mindfulness meditation on the stress, anxiety, and depression experienced by nursing students in Korea [Randomized controlled trial]. *Nurse Education Today, 29*(5), 538–543. doi:10.1016/j.nedt.2008.12.003

Kemper, K., Bulla, S., Krueger, D., Ott, M. J., McCool, J. A., & Gardiner, P. (2011). Nurses' experiences, expectations, and preferences for mind-body practices to reduce stress. *BMC Complementary and Alternative Medicine, 11*(1), 26. doi:10.1186/1472-6882-11-26

Khianman, B., Pattanittum, P., Thinkhamrop, J., & Lumbiganon, P. (2012). Relaxation therapy for preventing and treating preterm labour. *The Cochrane Database of Systematic Reviews, 8*, CD007426. doi:10.1002/14651858.CD007426.pub2

Lazar, S. W., Bush, G., Gollub, R. L., Fricchione, G. L., Khalsa, G., & Benson, H. (2000). Functional brain mapping of the relaxation response and meditation. *Neuroreport, 11*(7), 1581–1585.

Lewis, R. (2013). ACOG revises guidelines on treating menopause symptoms. *Medscape Medical News.* Retrieved from http://www.medscape.com/viewarticle/818280

Lorenc, A., Peace, B., Vaghela, C., & Robinson, N. (2010). The integration of healing into conventional cancer care in the UK. *Complementary Therapies in Clinical Practice, 16*(4), 222–228. doi:10.1016/j.ctcp.2010.03.001

Lunny, C. A., & Fraser, S. N. (2010). The use of complementary and alternative medicines among a sample of Canadian menopausal-aged women [Research support, non-US Gov't]. *Journal of Midwifery & Women's Health, 55*(4), 335–343. doi:10.1016/j.jmwh.2009.10.015

Lush, E., Salmon, P., Floyd, A., Studts, J. L., Weissbecker, I., & Sephton, S. E. (2009). Mindfulness meditation for symptom reduction in fibromyalgia: Psychophysiological correlates. *Journal of Clinical Psychology in Medical Settings, 16*(2), 200–207. doi:10.1007/s10880-009-9153-z

Marc, I., Toureche, N., Ernst, E., Hodnett, E. D., Blanchet, C., Dodin, S., & Njoya, M. M. (2011). Mind-body interventions during pregnancy for preventing or treating women's anxiety [Review]. *The Cochrane Database of Systematic Reviews, 2011*(7), CD007559. doi:10.1002/14651858.CD007559.pub2

Marcus, D. A., Blazek-O'Neill, B., & Kopar, J. L. (2013). Symptomatic improvement reported after receiving Reiki at a cancer infusion center. *American Journal of Hospice and Palliative Care, 30*(2), 216–217 . doi:10.1177/1049909112469275

McCormack, G. L. (2009). Using non-contact therapeutic touch to manage post-surgical pain in the elderly. *Occupational Therapy International, 16*(1), 44–56. doi:10.1002/oti.264

Moran, M. S., Ma, S., Jagsi, R., Yang, T. J., Higgins, S. A., Weidhaas, J. B., … Rockwell, S. (2013). A prospective, multicenter study of complementary/alternative medicine (CAM) utilization during definitive radiation for breast cancer. *International Journal of Radiation Oncology, Biology, Physics, 85*(1), 40–46. doi:10.1016/j.ijrobp.2012.03.025

Morrow, G. R., Shelke, A. R., Roscoe, J. A., Hickok, J. T., & Mustian, K. (2005). Management of cancer-related fatigue. *Cancer Investigation, 23*(3), 229–239.

Nidich, S. I., Fields, J. Z., Rainforth, M. V., Pomerantz, R., Cella, D., Kristeller, J., … Schneider, R. H. (2009). A randomized controlled trial of the effects of transcendental meditation on quality of life in older breast cancer patients. *Integrative Cancer Therapies, 8*(3), 228–234. doi:10.1177/1534735409343000

Olson, K., Hanson, J., & Michaud, M. (2003). A phase II trial of Reiki for the management of pain in advanced cancer patients. *Journal of Pain and Symptom Management, 26*(5), 990–997. doi:10.1016/S0885-3924(03)00334-8

Paisley, M. A., Kang, T. I., Insogna, I. G., & Rheingold, S. R. (2011). Complementary and alternative therapy use in pediatric oncology patients with failure of frontline chemotherapy. *Pediatric Blood & Cancer, 56*(7), 1088–1091. doi:10.1002/pbc.22939

Rasmussen, L. B., Mikkelsen, K., Haugen, M., Pripp, A. H., Fields, J. Z., & Forre, O. T. (2012). Treatment of fibromyalgia at the Maharishi Ayurveda Health Centre in Norway II—A 24-month follow-up pilot study. *Clinical Rheumatology, 31*(5), 821–827. doi:10.1007/s10067-011-1907-y

Richeson, N. E., Spross, J. A., Lutz, K., & Peng, C. (2010). Effects of Reiki on anxiety, depression, pain, and physiological factors in community-dwelling older adults. *Research in Gerontological Nursing, 3*(3), 187–199. doi:*10.3928/19404921-20100601-01*

Robinson, A., & McGrail, M. R. (2004). Disclosure of CAM use to medical practitioners: A review of qualitative and quantitative studies [Review]. *Complementary Therapies in Medicine, 12*(2–3), 90–98. doi:10.1016/j.ctim.2004.09.006

Schechter, N. L., Zempsky, W. T., Cohen, L. L., McGrath, P. J., McMurtry, C. M., & Bright, N. S. (2007). Pain reduction during pediatric immunizations: Evidence-based review and recommendations. *Pediatrics, 119*(5), e1184–e1198. doi:10.1542/peds.2006-1107

Schmidt, S., Grossman, P.A., Schwarer, B., Jena, S., Naumann, J., & Walach, H. (2011). Treating fibromyalgia with mindfulness-based stress reduction: Results from a 3-armed randomized controlled trial. *Pain, 152*(2), 361–369.

Short, E. B., Kose, S., Qiwen, M., Borckardt, J., Newberg, A, George, M. S., & Kozel, F. A. (2010). Regional brain activation during meditation shows time and practice effects: An exploratory fMRI study. *Evidence-based Complementary and Alternative Medicine, 7*(1), 121–127.

Shuval, J. T., & Gross, S. E. (2008). Midwives practice CAM: Feminism in the delivery room. *Complementary Health Practice Review, 13*(1), 46–62. doi:10.1177/1533210107311471

Sierpina, V. (2001). *Integrative health care: Complementary and alternative therapies for the whole person.* Philadelphia: F.A. Davis.

Smith, D. W., Arnstein, P., Rosa, K. C., & Wells-Federman, C. (2002). Effects of integrating therapeutic touch into a cognitive behavioral pain treatment program. Report of a pilot clinical trial. *Journal of Holistic Nursing, 20*(4), 367–387.

Szanton, S. L., Wenzel, J., Connolly, A. B., & Piferi, R. L. (2011). Examining mindfulness-based stress reduction: Perceptions from minority older adults residing in a low-income housing facility. *BMC Complementary and Alternative Medicine, 11*, 44. doi:10.1186/1472-6882-11-44

Tanay, G., Lotan, G., & Bernstein, A. (2012). Salutary proximal processes and distal mood and anxiety vulnerability outcomes of mindfulness training: A pilot preventive intervention. *Behavior Therapy, 43*(3), 492–505. doi:10.1016/j.beth.2011.06.003

Tarantino, B., Earley, M., Audia, D., Adamo, C., & Berman, B. (2013). Qualitative and quantitative evaluation of a pilot integrative coping and resiliency program for healthcare professionals. *Explore, 9*(1), 44–47.

Thrane, S. (2013). Effectiveness of Integrative Modalities for Pain and Anxiety in Children and Adolescents with Cancer: A Systematic Review. *Journal of Pediatric Oncology Nursing, 30*(6), 320–332.

Thrane, S. & Cohen, S.M. (2013). Effect of Reiki therapy on pain and anxiety in adults: A in-depth literature review of randomized trials with effect size calculations. *Pain Management Nursing.* Published online doi:10.1016/j.pmn.2013.07.008

Tomlinson, D., Hesser, T., Ethier, M. C., & Sung, L. (2011). Complementary and alternative medicine use in pediatric cancer reported during palliative phase of disease [Research support, non-US Gov't]. *Supportive Care in Cancer, 19*(11), 1857–1863. doi:10.1007/s00520-010-1029-0

Tsang, K. L., Carlson, L. E., & Olson, K. (2007). Pilot crossover trial of Reiki versus rest for treating cancer-related fatigue. *Integrative Cancer Therapies, 6*(1), 25–35. doi:10.1177/1534735406298986

Vitale, A. T., & O'Connor, P. C. (2006). The effect of Reiki on pain and anxiety in women with abdominal hysterectomies: A quasi-experimental pilot study. *Holistic Nursing Practice, 20*(6), 263–272.

Vitale, A.T. (2009). Nurses' lived experience of Reiki for self care. *Holistic Nursing Practice, 23*(3), 129–145.

Wardell, D. W., & Engebretson, J. (2001). Biological correlates of Reiki Touch(sm) healing. *Journal of Advanced Nursing, 33*(4), 439–445.

Witek-Janusek, L., Albuquerque, K., Chroniak, K. R., Chroniak, C., Durazo-Arvizu, R., & Mathews, H. L. (2008). Effect of mindfulness based stress reduction on immune function, quality of life and coping in women newly diagnosed with early stage breast cancer. *Brain, Behavior, and Immunity, 22*(6), 969–981. doi:10.1016/j.bbi.2008.01.012

Witte, D., & Dundes, L. (2001, October). Harnessing life energy or wishful thinking? Reiki, placebo Reiki, meditation, and music. *Alternative & Complementary Therapies,* 304–309.

Woods-Giscombe, C. L., & Black, A. R. (2010). Mind-body interventions to reduce risk for health disparities related to stress and strength among African American women: The potential of mindfulness-based stress reduction, loving-kindness, and the NTU therapeutic framework. *Complementary Health Practice Review, 15*(3), 115–131. doi:10.1177/1533210110386776

Yoon, S. L., & Black, S. (2006). Comprehensive, integrative management of pain for patients with sickle-cell disease. *Journal of Alternative and Complementary Medicine, 12*(10), 995–1001. doi:10.1089/acm.2006.12.995

Chapter 12

Women and Herbal Medicine

Mahtab Jafari and Gabriel Orenstein

Introduction: Growth of Herbal Medicine Use

The therapeutic use of botanicals—commonly referred to as phytotherapy and herbal medicine—began thousands of years ago in medicinal practices around the world and has recently gained popularity in Western medicine. Herbal medicine is now considered an integral part of health care on a global scale. For many nations, herbal medicine is considered to be the first-line therapy; up to 50% of medicinals in China are traditional herbals, and for more than half of the children in African nations such as Nigeria and Ghana, the World Health Organization (WHO) reported that herbs are considered first-line therapy for malaria-related fevers. In the United States, a 2007 National Center for Complementary and Alternative Medicine (NCCAM) and the Centers for Disease Control and Prevention (CDC) joint survey indicated that 38% of adults use complementary and alternative medicine (CAM), with natural and herbal remedies being the most prominent modality (http://nccam.nih.gov/news/camstats/2007).

Over the past 50 years, there has been a steady growth of herbal medicine users in the United States (Kessler et al., 2011), predominated by middle-aged women (Tindle, Davis, Phillips, & Eisenberg, 2005). These women use herbs in a variety of conditions such as premenstrual syndrome (PMS), pregnancy-induced nausea and vomiting, insomnia, urinary tract infections (UTIs), menopausal symptoms (Posadzki et al., 2013), fertility enhancement (Rayner, Willis, & Burgess, 2011), and depression (Wu et al., 2007).

With high demand for herbal remedies, this multibillion dollar industry has grown steadily in the past decade, with many individual herbs grossing over $10 million annually (Lindstrom, Ooyen, Lynch, & Blumenthal, 2013). These products are no longer found only on the shelves of specialty natural products stores, but they appear in chain drug stores and supermarkets, with labels promoting the products as "natural," providing consumers with a relative sense of safety (Ernst, 1998). The increase in access to herbal remedies and their sales were mainly initiated with the Dietary Supplement Act of 1994, an amendment to the Federal Food, Drug, and Cosmetic Act, which does not require companies to obtain FDA approval for a dietary supplement before marketing it.

The ubiquity and general positive perception of herbal medicines—along with the growing trend of CAM and herbal medicine use in the United States—make it likely for health professionals to regularly care for patients who will be taking a variety of herbal remedies. Therefore, it is critical for health-care providers to be more informed about herbal medicines. There is a general assumption among herbal users that Western-trained clinicians are either opposed to or lack knowledge of phytotherapy (Blendon, DesRoches, Benson, Brodie, & Altman, 2001) and other forms of CAM (Robinson & McGrail, 2004), which leads to nondisclosure of herb use by as many as 67% of patients (Mehta, Gardiner, Phillips, & McCarthy, 2008) that can potentially result in herb–drug and herb–disease interactions. It is important that the clinician be aware of any herbal medicines the client is taking as they may interact with other medicines being prescribed by the clinician. Therefore, it is crucial for clinicians to inquire of their patients about any herbal use practices in order to avoid such interactions that could possibly compromise their patients' health.

Disclaimer: Many herbal users have reported using CAM therapies because of media influence (Wu et al., 2007), which is often not evidence-based. Even if a herb is deemed safe to treat a particular ailment—as reported in randomized clinical trials—it still runs the risk of interacting with pharmaceuticals adversely, containing contaminants such as heavy metals and pyrrolizidine alkaloids, or of being consumed incorrectly owing to obfuscated marketing (Bent, 2008). Clinicians should also pay attention to the quality of the studies and funding source. Another major issue with studies on herbal remedies is the lack of consistency among the products and lack of standardization of the herbs used in clinical trials.

The purpose of this chapter is to present a brief overview of seven selected herbal medicines that are either commonly used or are emerging in popularity in their use for common female ailments. Although the selected herbs may have some scientific evidence to support their use, their immediate substitution for pharmaceuticals may not be warranted. Even when a herbal remedy is deemed to be an appropriate therapy based on centuries of observed efficacy in traditional medical practices, the quality of the herbal supplements should be scrutinized in view of lack of regulation by the FDA (Ernst, 1998). Although the FDA does not regulate the manufacturing processes of the herbal supplements like pharmaceuticals, herbal supplements manufacturers can have their products and their manufacturing processes evaluated by the United States Pharmacopeial Convention (USP), which assesses the quality, strength, and even labeling of dietary supplements. The request for increased manufacturing transparency and potential verification by the USP does provide a greater level of credibility to herbal medicine because the USP standards are enforceable by the FDA and other government agencies (usp.org). Furthermore, certain herbs have conflicting evidence in regard to efficacy and safety, which may be partly because of the bioactive complexity inherent in the herbs, poor research methodology of published studies, or the use of nonstandardized materials. The herbs selected for presentation in this chapter are discussed in relation to the condition/ailment for which there is evidence to support their use. The seven herbs described are St. John's wort, kava, *Rhodiola rosea*, cranberry, chasteberry, black cohosh, and valerian.

In presenting each herb, the aims are to discuss

1. The ailment for which it is used
2. Scientific evidence for its use
3. Potential mechanisms of action
4. Side effects and drug interactions
5. Dosage

The data presented in this chapter is derived from an extensive literature review. A number of databases such as Webofknowledge, Natural Comprehensive Medicine, Natural Standard, American Botanical Council, and Cochrane were utilized in identifying the most researched herbs used in women's health. Owing to space constraints, remedies for ailments without female gender predominance—influenza, nausea, headaches, for example—were not considered. An initial search of the topic "herb" and containing "women" in the title furnished several hundred studies and reviews from Webofknowledge, 85 of which were relevant. Reviews and studies were compared with database meta-analyses and studies gathered from searching bibliographic references. The final groups of herbs were organized by ailment, with general use and application, potential mechanisms of action, side effects, and drug interactions as factors in determining safety and efficacy.

Ailments and Herbal Treatments

Depression and Anxiety: St. John's Wort, Kava, and Rhodiola rosea

Feelings of anxiety and depression can arise from stress and unfortunate events in life, but should not be present on a daily basis. When the feelings become chronic, such as for a period of 2 weeks or longer (Adaa.org/living-with-anxiety/women), it is considered a disorder. Depression and anxiety are more common in females (Piccinelli & Wilkinson, 2000), with depression being the most prevalent mental health disorder among women (World Health Organization, 2013). Gender disparity in regard to the propensity—as opposed to diagnosis—of depression and anxiety disorders has recently been challenged (Martin, Neighbors, & Griffith, 2013).

St. John's wort and kava are among the most researched herbs for depression and anxiety, respectively. *Rhodiola rosea* is an emerging herb for the treatment of anxiety and depression. While the number of trials is small relative to St. John's wort and kava, multiple studies reveal that *R. rosea* is a promising herbal remedy to manage anxiety and mild depression in women.

St. John's Wort (*Hypericum perforatum*)

Potential Mechanism of Action. St. John's wort is purported to have several potential pharmacological actions to account for its antidepressant function. The phloroglucinol derivative within the *H. perforatum* extract, hyperforin, has been shown to hinder synaptosomal uptake of γ-aminobutyric acid (GABA), noradrenaline, dopamine, l-glutamate, and serotonin (Chatterjee, Bhattacharya, Wonnemann, Singer, & Müller, 1998). This study was completed on rats and utilized methanolic (1.5% hyperforin), ethanolic (4.5% hyperforin), and CO_2 extracts (38.8% hyperforin). While the trial utilized an animal rather than a human model to parallel depression disorders, it demonstrated dose-dependent results that were comparable to imipramine (a tricyclic antidepressant [TCA]). The method by which *Hypericum* extract hinders syntaptosomal uptake of serotonin may be partly or fully explained by hyperforin's ability to elevate sodium [Na+], which is the driving force behind neurotransmitter transport, as demonstrated in *in vitro* experiments (Singer, Wonnemann, & Müller, 1999).

Inhibition of neurotransmitter degrading enzymes, monamine oxidase (MAO) and catechol-o-methyltransferase (COMT), has been demonstrated *in vitro* (Cott, 1997; Suzuki, Katsumata, Oya, Bladt, & Wagner, 1984; Thiede & Walper, 1994), and is purportedly caused by flavonoids, flavone glycosides, xanthone, and other lipid-soluble compounds of the *H. perforatum* extract (Thiede & Walper, 1994). A good example to compare this *in vitro* mechanism to the mechanism of pharmaceuticals is binding of GABA$_A$, as noted by Cott (1997). Benzodiazepines bind GABA$_A$ and can fix it into a conformation with higher affinity for GABA, bringing a further inhibitory effect of GABA and contributing to sedative and anxiolytic behavioral results. Extrapolating St John's wort inhibition of MAO and COMT in *in vitro* experiments to *in vivo* experiments should only serve as an example of potential translation from *in vitro* to *in vivo*. Recent *in vivo* studies found no significant change in MAO or COMT when *Hypericum* extract was used in animal models, so the mechanism is only applicable to *in vitro* studies currently (Sacher et al., 2011; Schroeder et al., 2004).

Other potential mechanisms include upregulation of serotonin receptors (Teufel-Mayer & Gleitz, 1997) and inhibition of substance P-inducing interleukin-6 synthesis (Fiebich, Höllig, & Lieb, 2001) and of dopamine β-hydroxylase (Kleber, Obry, Hippeli, Schneider, & Elstner, 1999). There is no single mechanistic explanation for the effects of *Hypericum*, but it is also possible that many of the above mechanisms work together on the nervous system.

Evidence. St. John's wort is considered a popular therapy for the management of depression, but the evidence is unclear and inconsistent. This is partly due to varying standardizations of *H. perforatum* extract and severity of dysfunction in subject populations. In the Hypericum Depression Trial Study Group (2002), a randomized placebo-controlled trial of 340 individuals with major depression, LI 160 formulation was used. This formulation is a common preparation with a standardized hypericin content of 0.12% to 0.28% (0.72 to 0.96 mg in 900 mg dose). A different preparation of St. John's wort—WS 5572—standardized to 5% hyperforin instead of standardized hypericin was used in another study (Kalb, Trautmann-Sponsel, & Kieser, 2001). In the study by Kalb and colleagues, individuals with mild to moderate depression instead of major depression were included. Another study utilized another formulation of *Hypericum* extract—WS 5570 (600 or 1,200 mg daily dose; 0.12% to 0.28% hypericin, 3% to 6% hyperforin)—for individuals with mild to moderate depression (Kasper, Anghelescu, Szegedi, Dienel, & Kieser, 2006). The study utilizing LI 160 recorded the *Hypericum* preparation as equally effective compared with placebo, while Kalb and colleagues and Kasper and colleagues found *Hypericum* extracts WS 5572 and WS 5570, respectively, to be significantly better than placebo in reducing depression, as measured by the Hamilton Depression Rating Scale (HAM-D) scores. There are many other dissimilar studies that are compared regularly in literature reviews. Meta-analyses reviewing and separating subject populations and medication standardizations are imperative to develop a better understanding of *Hypericum* efficacy.

Side Effects and Drug Interactions. Hyperforin has a high affinity for the pregnane X receptor, which regulates CYP3A4 (cytochrome P450 3A4), an enzyme that helps metabolize many different drugs (Moore et al., 2000). Binding to pregnane X leads to the induction of CYP3A4, which would increase the metabolism and decrease the bioavailability of drugs metabolized by this cytochrome P450 system. Since this drug–herb interaction can potentially result in a decrease in the efficacy of the drugs that use CYP3A4 for metabolism, lists of such pharmaceuticals should be reviewed prior to starting patients on St. John's wort (Henderson, Yue, Bergquist, Gerden, & Arlett, 2002; Ogu & Maxa, 2000). Owing to high variability among study methodologies, meta-analyses were used to identify common side effects. Although side effects are less common for St. John's wort when compared with conventional antidepressants, photosensitivity appears to be a common adverse effect with this herb, and patients should be advised to stay away from the sun or use sunscreen while taking St. John's wort. Gastrointestinal symptoms have also been reported with St. John's wort and should be monitored (Linde, Berner, & Kriston, 2008; Linde & Knuppel, 2005).

Dosage. St. John's wort's dosing range varies between 500 and 1,200 mg daily, with 900 mg/day being the most commonly used dosage. There are multiple standardizations, but the following formulations are considered the most common: LI 160 (900 mg daily dose; 0.72 to 0.96 mg hypericin/900 mg), WS 5572 (900 mg daily dose, 5% hyperforin content), WS 5570 (900 mg daily dose; 0.12% to 0.28% hypericin, 3% to 6% hyperforin).

Kava or Kava Kava (*Piper methysticum*)

Potential Mechanism of Action. The mechanism of action of kava as an anxiolytic is not completely known. The main active compounds in kava are kavalactones such as kavain, 5,6-dihydrokavain, methysticin, dihydromethysticin, yangonin, and desmethoxyyangonin. These putative active compounds have been reported to influence the central nervous system (CNS) by modulation of ion channels. High sodium influx and ion channel disequilibrium are linked to mood and several mental ailments (Imbrici, Camerino, & Tricarico, 2013). Kavain and methysticin inhibit Na+ channels (Gleitz, Gottner, Ameri, & Peters, 1996; Magura, Kopanitsa, Gleitz, Peters, & Krishtal, 1997) and noradrenaline reuptake (Seitz, Schüle, & Gleitz, 1997), and kavain and dihydromethysticin inhibit Ca+ channels and promote the action of ipsapirone, an endogenous serotonin agonist (Walden, von Wegerer, Winter, Berger, & Grunze, 1997). In addition to modulating ion channels, kava has also been shown to inhibit MAO-B (Uebelhack, Franke, & Schewe, 1998) and modulate GABA receptor binding (Jussofie, Schmiz, & Hiemke, 1994).

Evidence. Kava has been used for sedation in traditional medical practices. The plant appears promising in the management of symptoms associated with anxiety disorders, but the controversy surrounding kava-induced liver toxicity has resulted in a decrease in its use. Studies on the efficacy of Kava are generally small, but the methodology and evidence is consistent. A double-blind placebo-controlled study using WS 1490—a standardized product with 70 mg kavalactones/100 mg—showed that after only 1-week, patients who received this formulation had a significant improvement in their anxiety as measured on the Hamilton Anxiety Scale (HAMA) compared with patients who were on placebo (Lehmann, Kinzler, & Friedemann, 1996). The dosage of kava was three capsules daily—210-mg kavalactones daily—and continued for an additional 3 weeks, with HAMA scores continuing to improve. Another double-blind placebo-controlled study using WS 1490 in climacteric women showed the efficacy of kava in this patient population. This study (Warnecke, 1991) used the same kava dosage as Lehmann and colleagues' study. Again, after only 1 week, there was significant improvement in the HAMA score in the kava group compared with the placebo group. A more recent open study on perimenopausal women using kava also reported positive results with kava. After 1 month, there was a significant decrease in anxiety as measured by the State Trait Anxiety

Inventory (STAI) self-administered evaluation. The dosages of kava in the two groups that were included in this study were 100 and 200 mg daily with 55% kavaina.

In addition to placebo-controlled studies on the use of kava for anxiety, there are reports on the efficacy of kava in treating depression when compared with pharmaceuticals such as opipramol and buspirone (Boerner et al., 2003). In addition, d, l-kavain, a putative active compound in kava, has been reported to be as effective as oxazepam (Lindenberg & Pitule-Schödel, 1990). Kava has also been used to manage symptoms associated with benzodiazepine withdrawal (Malsch & Kieser, 2001).

Based on the current published studies, while there is substantial supportive evidence for the use of kava in the management of anxiety and depression, many of these studies lack the scientific rigor such as adequate duration of the study and/or adequate sample size. The variation in efficacy with kava could also be due to variabilities in gender, age, and GABA-transporter polymorphism (Sarris et al., 2013; Witte, Loew, & Gaus, 2005). These variables should be evaluated in future studies.

Adverse Effects and Drug Interactions. Hepatotoxicity is considered the main serious adverse effect with kava that warrants frequent monitoring with liver function tests. Hepatotoxicity has been reported in over 100 cases worldwide (Li & Ramzan, 2010) and has led to a ban on kava supplements in several countries. Allergic reactions, gastrointestinal complaints, and tachycardia have also been reported with kava.

Regarding hepatotoxicity, an animal study conducted over a long period with a high dosage found no signs of toxicity (Sorrentino, Capasso, & Schmidt, 2006). The exact mechanism for the liver damage is unknown, and it has been attributed to some of the active components of the plant and concurrent consumption of kava with alcohol (Li & Ramzan, 2010). Hepatotoxicity has also been attributed to the use of contaminated and moldy kava, as mycotoxin-producing *Aspergillus* bacteria species have been found in the extract (Teschke, Sarris, & Schweitzer, 2011).

Concomitant use of kava with any hepatotoxic or sedative drug should be avoided to prevent drug–herb interactions. Aside from alcohol, drugs posing a potential additive effect to the sedative properties of kava include pregnane steroids, pentobarbital, and benzodiazepines (Almeida & Grimsley, 1996).

Dosage. The recommended dose of kava is 300 mg daily with 70% or 55% kavalactones, pertaining to 210 and 165 mg kavalactones, respectively. Smaller doses such as 150 mg daily have been used as well.

Rhodiola rosea

Potential Mechanism of Action. It has been reported that *R. rosea* significantly inhibits MAO-A, which breaks down serotonin and norepinephrine (van Diermen et al., 2009). MAO inhibition is purportedly caused by some of the putative active compounds of *R. rosea* such as rosidirin, or a combination of rosidirin, cinnnamyl alcohol, triandrin, EGCG dimer, and rhodioloside (van Diermen et al., 2009). Although a number of active compounds have been suggested to contribute to CNS effects of this herbal extract, rhodioloside and tyrosol are suggested as the primary compounds contributing to the alleviation of symptoms associated with depression (Panossian et al., 2008).

Evidence. Preliminary studies on R. *rosea* in the management of anxiety and depression appear to be promising on the basis of a commonly used anxiety scale, HAMA (Bystritsky, Kerwin, & Feusner, 2008; Darbinyan et al., 2007). Although the sample size was very small in one of the studies (N = 10) and the study was not placebo-controlled, it addressed anxiety directly and the mean HAMA scores were significantly different compared with baseline. The formulation used in this study was Rhodax twice daily. Rhodax contains 170 mg R. *rosea* with 30 mg of each of the following: rosavin, rosarin, salidroside, rosin, rhodalgin, acetylrhodalgin, rosaridin, and rosaridol (Bystritsky et al., 2008). In another study, standard doses of Rhodiola *rosea* at 340 mg/day and 680 mg/day for 6 weeks were sufficient to significantly lower reports of somatization, emotional instability, and insomnia compared with placebo (Darbinyan et al., 2007). Rhodiola *rosea* appears promising as an adjunct therapy in combination with TCAs in treating psychopathological symptoms (Brichenko, Kupriyanova, & Skorokhodova, 1986). Animal studies with a standardized formulation of R. *rosea* (SHR-5, 3% rosavins and 0.8% salidroside) have also resulted in similar or potentially greater efficacy than conventional antidepressants such as fluoxetin (Panossian et al., 2008; Perfumi & Mattioli, 2007).

Side Effects and Drug Interactions. Reported side effects with R. *rosea* are generally mild and rare and include dry mouth and dizziness. At very high doses (>3 g/day), R. *rosea* may cause insomnia (Bystritsky et al., 2008). Multiple studies utilizing the standardized SHR-5 for applications similar to anxiety and depression reported no serious adverse events (Olsson, von Schéele, & Panossian, 2009; Spasov, Wikman, Mandrikov, Mironova, & Neumoin, 2000).

Dosage. The most commonly studied preparation of R. *rosea* extracts is SHR-5, which contains 3% rosavin and 0.8% salidroside (Spasov et al., 2000). There are also studies measuring additional putative compounds of R. *rosea* such as tyrosol and triandrin (Panossian, Hamm, Kadioglu, Wikman, & Efferth, 2013; Panossian, Wikman, Kaur, & Asea, 2012). The doses of SHR-5 in studies range from 100 mg daily to higher doses of 680 mg daily, with an average recommended dose of 360 mg/day (Darbinyan et al., 2007; Spasov et al., 2000).

Conclusion: St. John's Wort, Kava, and *Rhodiola rosea*

Although St. John's wort could be an attractive remedy in treating depression, more studies with uniform methodology are needed to prove its efficacy. In some studies, St. John's wort demonstrated superiority over placebo, while in others no improvement was reported compared with placebo. The metabolic pathway of *Hypericum* extract is CYP3A4, which is used by many other drugs. Caution should be practiced when St. John's wort is taken concomitantly with such drugs to avoid drug–herb interactions. Kava is widely used in treating anxiety disorders and has demonstrated efficacy and relative safety in multiple clinical trials. Since large and long-term studies are scarce, chronic and prolonged use is discouraged. Recent reports on kava-induced hepatotoxicity warrant close monitoring of liver function. Although R. *rosea* appears safe and promising in the management of anxiety and mild depression, additional long-term studies with larger sample sizes are needed to validate the use of this plant.

UTI: Cranberry (Vaccinium macrocarpon)

Introduction

UTI is a common medical problem, and it is estimated that 10.8% of women in the United States experience UTI annually, with an estimated one in three women visiting a primary care provider for UTI by age 26 (Foxman, Barlow, D'arcy, Gillespie, & Sobel, 2000). Recurrence can be common for those with a history of UTI, and risk of UTI can vary with age and sexual activity (Hooton et al., 1996). Although antibiotics are recommended to treat UTI, cranberry-based supplements were considered one of the top-selling herbs as adjunct preventive therapy in 2012 with sales over $60 million in the United States (Lindstrom et al., 2013).

Potential Mechanism of Action

Pathogenesis and virulence of UTI is determined by several factors, including bacterial adhesion, hemolysin, serum resistance, and type of capsular polysaccharide (Johnson, 1991). Early studies suggest urine acidification to have a bacteriostatic effect, but the change in pH appears insignificant or unnecessary in the management of UTI (Avorn et al., 1994; Liu, Black, Caron, & Camesano, 2006). The most popular mechanism of interest in UTI prevention is through inhibition of bacterial adhesion of *Escherichia coli* fimbriae. In a study using cranberry juice at 1:2 dilution, type 1 fimbriae, a mannose-sensitive adhesin, was inhibited by fructose, with an *in vitro* recording of almost no yeast aggregation (Zafriri, Ofek, Adar, Pocino, & Sharon, 1989). A more recent *in vitro* study has also determined that type A proanthocyanidins—included within the categories of flavonoids or polyphenols—decrease the mannose-resistant adhesin P-fimbriae in a dose-dependent manner (Gupta et al., 2007). This has been observed at a molecular level, with cranberry juice precipitating conformational change of P-fimbriae *in vitro* (Liu et al., 2006).

Evidence

While there is evidence promoting the use of cranberry for prevention of UTIs, inconsistent methodology leads to conflicting conclusions among studies. In one 2-month ex vivo study, cranberry juice (dried; polyphenolic content 3% m/m) at 1,200 mg/day yielded significantly less adherence by uropathogenic E. *coli* (Valentová et al., 2007). Stothers (2002) and Wing and colleagues (Wing, Rumney, Preslicka, & Chung, 2008) also reported favorable results for cranberry, with 250 and 240 mL of a standardized cranberry juice, in reducing UTI. Wing and colleagues estimated the standardized juice content to have 106 mg of proanthocyanidins. When compared with antibiotics trimethoprim (TMP; 100 mg) and trimethoprim–sulfamethoxole (TMP–SMX; 480 mg) for the management of UTI, cranberry appeared equivalent to TMP and inferior to TMP–SMX (Beerepoot et al. 2011; McMurdo, Argo, Phillips, Daly, & Davey, 2009). On the other hand, larger studies utilizing a 27% cranberry juice—an average of 112 mg proanthocyanidins/8 oz—concluded that the benefit of cranberry was insignificant compared with placebo (Barbosa-Cesnik et al., 2011; Stapleton et al., 2012). The use of different formulations and doses and lack of standardization in cranberry clinical studies pose challenges in interpreting the results of these studies. Proanthocyanidins are considered main active components in the cranberry when it comes to the prevention of UTI. Further studies considering proanthocyanidin content are needed in order to determine whether cranberry is an effective preventive measure for UTI.

Side Effects and Drug Interactions

Adverse events from continually taking cranberry supplements are few and minor, with many study durations being 6 months to 1 year. Adverse reports include gastrointestinal and vaginal irritation (Stapleton et al., 2012), nocturia (McMurdo et al., 2008; Valentová et al., 2007), sensitive nipples (McMurdo et al., 2008), and stomach acidity (Valentová et al., 2007). Multiple studies reported no serious adverse effects (Beerepoot et al., 2011; Kontiokari et al., 2001) or adverse reactions similar to those reported in the placebo group (Barbosa-Cesnik et al., 2011). Although cranberry studies lacked standardization because they recruited an expansive age range and employed different forms and dosages, cranberry appears to be safe. Two smaller studies administered high concentrations of the active constituents, phenolics (proanthocyanidins)—37% to children and 30% to adult women—and reported no serious adverse events (Afshar, Stothers, & MacNeily, 2012; Bailey, Dalton, Daugherty, & Tempesta, 2007). Cranberry juice can raise the risk for calcium oxalate and uric acid stones (Gettman et al., 2005). Persons with diabetes should also consume cranberry juice with caution because of its sugar content. Individuals taking warfarin should be cautious, as cranberry can potentially modulate the pharmacodynamics of warfarin and result in drug–herb interaction (Mohammed Abdul et al., 2008). CYP3A inhibitors have been identified in cranberry, which may account for the altered warfarin metabolism since warfarin uses CYP3A4 for metabolism (Kim et al., 2011).

Dosage

Different formulations of cranberry such as syrup, extract, and tablet have various bioavailability of proanthocyanidin, the primary active ingredient. In standardized formulations of cranberry, 36 to 72 mg/day is recommended as an effective dose to reduce bacterial adhesion (Howell et al., 2010). A pilot study indicated that a higher dosage of 100 mg/day of proanthocyanidin is also safe over a long period (Bailey et al., 2007).

Conclusion

According to the current literature, the efficacy of cranberry for prevention of UTI appears nonconclusive but safe. Larger studies using consistent methodologies and standardized formulation of cranberry need to be carried out to determine whether this plant is superior to placebo in UTI prevention. The high incidence of recurrent UTIs among women and the rise in antibiotic-resistant UTIs warrant additional well-designed studies with high enough concentrations of proanthocyanidins.

Premenstrual Syndrome: Chasteberry (Vitex agnus-castus)

Introduction

Pre Menstrual Syndrome (PMS) affects approximately 75% of menstruating women (http://www.mayoclinic.org/diseases-conditions/premenstrual-syndrome), and includes a wide array of symptoms, most of which are related to water retention (bloating, breast tenderness), negative affect (depression, anxiety), food (cravings), and pain (cramps and aches) (He et al., 2009). Up to 8% of women suffer from severe PMS, which may significantly affect their quality of life (Yonkers, O'Brien, & Eriksson, 2008). The broad array of symptoms and symptom severity, coupled with unknown etiologies for most of these symptoms, complicate the pharmacotherapy of PMS. This may draw more consumer attention to an over-the-counter "natural" PMS remedy such as chasteberry, which purportedly addresses multiple symptoms. Recent studies of chasteberry for the management of PMS symptoms positively support this multimodal remedy, even though the exact mechanisms of chasteberry in managing symptoms of PMS remain undetermined.

Potential Mechanism of Action

Etiology of PMS has been linked to several steroid hormones and neurotransmitters, and their relationship to each other in the hypothalamus–pituitary–ovarian axis, and the CNS (Yonkers et al., 2008). Chasteberry's ability to ameliorate symptoms of PMS is likely due to its action on the hypothalamic–pituitary–ovarian axis. It has been shown that dopaminergic diterpenes rotundifuran and $6\beta,7\beta$-diacetoxy-13-hydroxy-labda-8,14-dien in *V. agnus-castus* influence dopamine D_2 receptors *in vitro* (Meier, Berger, Hoberg, Sticher, & Schaffner, 2000). Since dopamine helps regulate prolactin levels (tuberoinfundibular pathway), the diterpenes could affect breast pain (mastalgia) associated with irregular prolactin levels. However, a clinical open study by Berger and colleagues (Berger, Schaffner, Schrader, Meier, & Brattström, 2000) recorded improvements in PMS symptoms without significant change in the women's physiologic prolactin levels. Dopamine manipulation could also contribute to decreasing the emotional irregularity (mood swings, depression, anxiety) via the mesocortical pathway. The extract has also been noted to bind estrogen receptors via flavonoids, including apigenin and penduletin (Jarry, Spengler, Wuttke, & Christoffel, 2006). *V. agnus-castus* also demonstrates an agonistic effect on the μ-opiate receptor (Webster, Lu, Chen, Farnsworth, & Wang, 2006), which is associated with analgesia and sedation. The evidence supporting chasteberry's influence on multiple receptors complicates the definition of an exact mechanism of action. However, this multireceptor influence lends support to the idea that the herb normalizes a multitude of PMS symptoms.

Evidence

The duration of placebo-controlled studies with chasteberry is generally over three menstrual cycles to assure evaluating the efficacy of chasteberry for various PMS symptoms. In one study of 162 women, chasteberry at 8-, 20-, and 30-mg Ze440 was compared with placebo. Efficacy was determined by scoring of the visual analogue scale (VAS), with attention to irritability, mood alteration, anger, headache, bloating, and breast fullness. With a symptom score reduction $\geq 50\%$ defining "responders," the 20-mg dose was the most effective, with 81% responders in the 20-mg group. The smaller dose of 8 mg (14% responders) was not significantly better than placebo (11% responders). The larger dose of 30 mg was not significantly better than the 20 mg dose, but it was still significantly better than placebo (Schellenberg, Zimmermann, Drewe, Hoexter, & Zahner, 2012). An older placebo-controlled trial utilizing 20-mg Ze440 was significantly superior to placebo in alleviating irritability, mood alterations, anger, headache, and breast tenderness (Schellenberg, 2001). In spite of these positive results, two other placebo-controlled studies reported that chasteberry lowered PMS symptoms, but the placebo response was too high to determine that the herb was effective (He et al., 2009; Ma, Lin, Chen, & Wang, 2010). The majority of non–placebo-controlled studies support the use of chasteberry as well. Although non–placebo-controlled studies may not provide us with definite answers, their data may be used to evaluate adverse effects profile of chasteberry (Berger et al., 2000; Loch, Selle, & Boblitz, 2000; Prilepskaya, Ledina, Tagiyeva, & Revazova, 2006). In these studies, different scales such as premenstrual tension syndrome (PMTS) scale, premenstrual syndrome diary (PMSD), VAS, and clinical global impression (CGI) were used to evaluate PMS symptoms. The evidence supporting chasteberry could be more conclusive if studies used the same scales. There are also studies comparing chasteberry to magnesium oxide (Di Pierro, Callegari, Speroni, & Attolico, 2009) and vitamin B_6 (Lauritzen, Reuter, Repges, Böhnert, & Schmidt, 1997). The latter study is sometimes referenced in support of the efficacy of chasteberry, but equivalence to vitamin B_6 is not meaningful as vitamin B_6 is not an established treatment for PMS symptoms.

Side Effects and Drug Interactions

Adverse effects are mild, with reports of nausea, acne and skin irritation/inflammation (Loch et al., 2000; Schellenberg, 2001), gastrointestinal problems (Loch et al., 2000), headaches (He et al., 2009; Schellenberg et al., 2012), erythematous rash, mild hypertension (Schellenberg et al., 2012), and menstrual disorders (Ma et al., 2010). No serious drug interactions have been reported. Since chasteberry can modulate various hormonal levels, women with diseases sensitive to hormone levels (e.g., breast and ovarian cancer) should be cautious. Oral contraceptive use does not appear to influence chasteberry efficacy (Berger et al., 2000), but women using such birth control methods should take caution for potential hormonal influences.

Dosage

A recent comparative dosage study of chasteberry (Ze440 formulation) concluded that an optimal dose (60% ethanol m/m, drug–extract ratio 6 to 12:1, standardized to casticin) was 20 mg daily, which corresponds to 180 mg of crude *V. agnus-castus* (Schellenberg et al., 2012). The dose of 20 mg was effective in an older study by the same authors as well (Schellenberg, 2001). Two other studies supporting chasteberry's use for PMS symptoms used different doses and extractions (BNO 1095), but the placebo responses were too high to determine whether this formulation was optimal (He et al., 2009; Ma et al., 2010).

Conclusion

There is growing evidence that chasteberry is effective in ameliorating multiple symptoms of PMS with few adverse events. Chasteberry appears to be a safe alternative treatment if PMS symptoms are mild or moderate and individuals are not responding to NSAIDs and SSRIs. In a study of women suffering from severe symptoms of PMS, although chasteberry appeared effective, placebo outcomes were also effective (He et al., 2009; Ma et al., 2010). The exact mechanism of action of the herb and the pathophysiology of the PMS symptoms are still unknown. The herb should be further researched in attempts to replicate positive clinical outcomes using consistent scales and standardized formulations.

Menopause: Black Cohosh (*Actaea racemosa* and *Cimicifuga racemosa*)

Introduction

Menopause is an inevitable hormonal transition for women, with characteristic hot flashes, insomnia, mood swings, night sweats, depression, breast pain, and many other symptoms. Until recently, hormone therapy (HT; estrogen, or estrogen + progesterone) was a standard approach to alleviating such symptoms in women. While HT is still used, the Women's Health Initiative (WHI) study created controversy about using HT, as long-term results were coupled with elevated risks of heart disease, stroke, and breast cancer (Rossouw et al., 2002). The findings of the WHI precipitated a decline in HT use (Hersh, Stefanick, & Stafford, 2004) and an increase in the use of popular herbal alternatives that contain isoflavones (phytoestrogens) such as soy-based products and red clover. Although these products are believed to be safe, the use of phytoestrogens could still be controversial in women with a history of hormone-sensitive cancers. Unlike phytoestrogenic products, black cohosh extract (BCE) does not influence systemic estrogenic activity. While some studies vary in methodology, they are mostly supportive of BCE use for treating menopausal symptoms.

Potential Mechanism of Actions

Black cohosh is thought to modulate menopausal symptoms through the activity of triterpene glycosides, but specific mechanisms are unknown. It is believed to act as a selective estrogenic receptor modifier (SERM), but does not influence breast or vaginal cytology. There are no systemic or breast cytology changes, as epithelial cells and estrogenic marker pS2 remained normal in extracellular components of nipple aspirate fluid (NAF) during a 12-week study (Ruhlen et al., 2007). Changes in endometrial thickness were not evident in Liske and colleague's (Liske et al., 2002) study. In another study, osteoblast activity was increased with black cohosh ethanolic extract, a bone-specific alkaline phophatase—a marker for bone formation (Wuttke, Seidlová-Wuttke, & Gorkow, 2003).

Aside from SERM activity, black cohosh may modify serotonin binding. A study on rats found that black cohosh isopropyl extract inhibits binding of [^{3}H]lysergic acid diethylamide to 5-HT$_7$, a 5-HT subtype concerned with thermoregulation (Burdette et al., 2003). The same study also demonstrated possible serotonin receptor agonistic effects, by elevating cAMP levels in 5-HT$_7$ transfected HEK293 cells (Burdette et al., 2003).

Evidence

An isopropanolic BCE demonstrates effective relief of menopausal symptoms in multiple randomized placebo-controlled 3-month studies. The Menopause Rating Scale (MRS) was used, which is a 10-point questionnaire, including somatic pains (muscle and joint pain), psychological symptoms (irritability, nervousness, depression, etc.), hot flashes, sleeping disorders, and urinary and sexual dysfunctions. In one study, the treatment group (40 mg isopropanolic BCE) experienced significant improvement compared with the placebo; all PMS subcategories significantly improved, except for the somatic symptoms (Osmers et al., 2005). A second study demonstrated significant improvement on the MRS as well, with hot flashes showing the greatest improvement (Ross, 2012). A smaller placebo-controlled study found the extract to be significantly better than placebo in respect to "atrophy" symptoms (vaginal dryness, sexual disorders, urinary complaints).

Other subcategories—psychological, somatic, and hot flashes—were "distinctly improved," but not significant compared with placebo (Wuttke et al., 2003).

While not placebo-controlled studies, two additional trials of isopropanolic black cohosh measured its efficacy with the Kupperman Index score (KI; similar scoring method as MRS) and demonstrated significant improvements in menopausal symptoms with black cohosh. In a study consisting of over 1,800 Hungarian women taking 40-mg BCE for 12 weeks, the women reported an average KI decrease of 17.64 points at the end of the study (Vermes, Bánhidy, & Ács, 2005). A smaller study with identical dosage and duration found a 48% average KI score improvement among women (Ruhlen et al., 2007).

A large placebo-controlled study contradicts BCE efficacy found thus far, with no significant difference in vasomotor frequency or intensity when compared with placebo (Newton et al., 2006). The dose of BCE was much higher in this study compared with that in any other studies. Further studies comparing different black cohosh doses are needed.

Side Effects and Drug Interactions

Black cohosh–induced hepatotoxicity has been reported in four cases. A review of these women and their health at initiation of the clinical tests noted that liver complications were evident prior to using black cohosh (Teschke & Schwarzenboeck, 2009). Additional studies monitoring liver enzymes during a 3-month period of BCE (40 mg) reported no hepatotoxicity with black cohosh (Osmers et al., 2005; Ross, 2012). There is also concern regarding women taking BCE who have a history of hormone-sensitive cancers and/or when HT is contraindicated. This concern is based on the fact that BCE may contain isoflavones such as formononetin. In clinical studies where vaginal cytology (endometrial thickness), breast cytology, and systemic estrogen levels were monitored, no abnormal changes were reported (Liske et al., 2002; Ruhlen et al., 2007; Wuttke et al., 2003). Nevertheless, women with compromised liver function or HT contraindication should be cautious, as the mechanism of action for BCE is still unknown. Adverse effects encompass gastrointestinal discomfort (Liske et al., 2002; Osmers et al., 2005; Ross, 2012; Ruhlen et al., 2007; Vermes et al., 2005), joint aches and musculoskeletal disorders (Liske et al., 2002; Osmers et al., 2005; Vermes et al., 2005), headaches, vaginal dryness, fatigue (Ruhlen et al., 2007), breast/nipple tenderness, fatigue, dysphagia (Ruhlen et al., 2007; Vermes et al., 2005), and allergic reactions (Vermes et al., 2005). Some of these symptoms may not be caused by BCE, as many appeared in placebo groups as well and could have been directly related to menopausal symptoms.

Dosage

Black cohosh should be standardized to triterpene glycoside content, usually 2.5%. Doses as high as 200 mg have been tested (Newton et al., 2006), but based on published studies, an effective and commonly tested dose appears to be an isopropanolic extract (Remifemin), 40 mg daily in liquid or tablet form. An aqueous ethanolic extract (58% vol/vol) of 40 mg daily has also been used successfully.

Conclusion

Black cohosh appears to be a promising safe alternative to HT to manage menopausal symptoms. Further studies to establish the effective dose and the exact mechanism of action of the herb should be performed.

Insomnia: Valerian (Valeriana officinalis)

Temporary sleep difficulty can result from factors such as elevated stress and anxiety, consumption of caffeine or alcohol, or changes in sleeping environment. When chronic, it is an insomnia disorder, and can stem from more serious neurological imbalances and medical disorders (Ohayon, 1997). The American Insomnia Survey (AIS) recorded insomnia in over 20% of the national population sample, with greater prevalence among women (Kessler et al., 2011). Those suffering from insomnia can experience a significant decrease in quality of life in addition to further dysfunction, including sequential comorbid depression (Katz & McHorney, 2002; Staner, 2010). Chapter 17 presents detailed information on promoting healthy sleep in women.

Potential Mechanism of Action

An exact mechanism of action of valerian for the management of insomnia is not established. This may be due in part to the variations in composition among valerian species, processing methodology, and environmental population factors (Houghton, 1999). *V. officinalis* is more commonly studied and contains the active constituents valepotriates (monoterpenes), valerinic acid, kessyl glycol, and other sesquiterpenes. These compounds influence GABA pathways, similar to mechanisms of the sedative and anesthetic, pentobarbital and diprivan (Propofol) (Nelson et al., 2002). Valerian elevates GABA levels—as demonstrated *in vitro*—by inhibition of GABA uptake and potentiation of K^+-stimulated GABA release (Ortiz, Nieves-Natal, & Chavez, 1999). Elevated GABA levels may also be due to significant levels of GABA within the herbal extract, but there is conflicting evidence (Ortiz et al., 1999). Lignans within valerian may also contribute to improved sleep, with one study reporting partial agonism of A_1 adenosine receptors (Schumacher et al., 2002).

Evidence

A relatively recent study that was almost double the size of any previous valerian study (N = 434) showed little difference between *Valeriana* (valerian forte 200 mg, 3 tablets before bed; equivalent to 3,600 mg *V. officinalis*) and placebo (Oxman et al., 2007). Sleep diaries were used throughout the study period, taking the tablets before sleeping for 14 days. Even though this study is larger than other published studies on valerian, owing to a number of methodological issues, researchers were not able to draw definitive conclusions. There are single ethanolic, valepotriate, or aqueous herbal extracts, as well as valerian–hops and valerian–lemon balm preparations (Taibi, Landis, Petry, & Vitiello, 2007). In addition, cohorts may be comprised of healthy individuals or those who experience primary, secondary, or comorbid insomnia (Taibi et al., 2007). Inclusion of the secondary and comorbid conditions may be confounding factors in interpreting the efficacy of valerian for the management of insomnia. The most studied *valerian* preparation is ethanolic extract LI 156 (Sedonium). This extract has been compared to benzodiazepines such as oxazepam (Dorn, 2000; Ziegler, Ploch, Miettinen-Baumann, & Collet, 2002), but quality placebo-controlled studies are limited, making it difficult to establish the efficacy of valerian (Bent, Padula, Moore, Patterson, & Mehling, 2006; Taibi et al., 2007).

Side Effects and Drug Interactions

Side effects are generally mild and may include dizziness, headache, diarrhea, gastrointestinal disturbances, and related symptoms (Taibi et al., 2007). The incidence of these side effects appears to be similar in the placebo group (Oxman et al., 2007). Consumers should be critical in selecting the herb manufacturer, as a recent consumer lab report indicated that a substantial percentage of valerian product labeling is inaccurate and possibly contaminated with lead (http://www.consumerlab.com).

Dosage

The most studied standardized preparation of valerian is LI 156 taken at 300 to 600 mg before sleeping (Taibi et al., 2007).

Conclusion

The efficacy of valerian is uncertain because of the highly variable research methodology across studies. While multiple trials both support and refute valerian for treating insomnia, there is a general consensus that the herb is safe. This may be a viable option for women who respond poorly to benzodiazepines and other sleep medications. Consumers should be cautious of the manufacturing company in view of recent reports of some products being contaminated with lead.

Summary

Herbal remedies have been used in traditional medical practices around the world for thousands of years. When prepared and recommended by indigenous and well-trained practitioners, they appear to be effective. When herbal remedies are used outside their traditional culture, their quality should be scrutinized due to lack of regulation by the FDA. Use of herbal medicine is prevalent in the United States, especially among women. The public perceives herbal remedies as a more natural, safe, and affordable treatment option. Scientifically unfounded statements through social media and advertising, peer community anecdotal evidence, and cultural practices may contribute to this view. As a result, many women embrace herbal therapies without consulting or communicating with their primary care provider. Such practices have the potential to be costly because of potential side effects, toxicity, and drug–herb and drug–disease interactions. Many well-researched herbs are not fully understood mechanistically and may contain heterogeneous and conflicting clinical results in regard to efficacy and safety. If health professionals initiate discussion of herbal medicine use and approach it from an objective and educated standpoint, patients may be more likely to share what herbal remedies they are utilizing. This practice advocates for a more open, safe, and comprehensive approach to care that can potentially lower incidences of acute illness and hospitalization due to herb–drug interactions.

References

Afshar, K., Stothers, L., & MacNeily, A. (2012). Cranberry juice for the prevention of pediatric urinary tact infection: A randomized controlled trial. *Journal of Urology, 188*, 1584–1587.

Almeida, J. C., & Grimsley, E. W. (1996). Coma from the health food store: Interaction between kava and alprazolam. *Annals of Internal Medicine, 25*(11), 940–941.

Avorn, J., Monane, M., Gurwitz, J. H., Glynn, R. J., Choodnovskiy, I., & Lipsitz, L. A. (1994). Reduction of bacteriuria and pyuria after ingestion of cranberry juice. *Journal of American Medical Association, 271*(10), 751–754.

Bailey, D. T., Dalton, C., Daugherty, F. J., & Tempesta, M. S. (2007). Can a concentrated cranberry extract prevent recurrent urinary tract infections in women? A pilot study. *Phytomedicine, 14*, 237–241.

Barbosa-Cesnik, C., Brown, M. B., Buxton, M., Zhang, L., DeBusscher, J., & Foxman, B. (2011). Cranberry juice fails to prevent recurrent urinary tract infection: Results from a randomized placebo-controlled trial. *Clinical Infectious Diseases, 52*(1), 23–30.

Beerepoot, M. A. J., ter Riet, G., Nys, S., van der Wal, W. M., de Borgie, C. A. J. M., de Reijke, T. M., ... Geerlings, S. E. (2011). Cranberries vs antibiotics to prevent urinary tract infections. *Archives of Internal Medicine, 171*(14), 1270–1278.

Bent, S. (2008). Herbal medicine in the United States: Review of efficacy, safety, and regulation. *Journal of General Internal Medicine, 23*(6), 854–859.

Bent, S., Padula, A., Moore, D., Patterson, M., & Mehling, W. (2006). Valerian for sleep: A systematic review and meta-analysis. *American Journal of Medicine, 119*, 1005–1012.

Berger, D., Schaffner, W., Schrader, E., Meier, B., & Brattström, A. (2000). Efficacy of *Vitex agnus castus* L. extract ze 440 in patients with pre-menstrual syndrome (PMS). *Archives of Gynecology Obstetrics, 264*, 150–153.

Blendon, R. J., DesRoches, C. M., Benson, J. M., Brodie, M., & Altman, D. E. (2001). Americans' views on the use and regulation of dietary supplements. *Archives of Internal Medicine, 161*, 805–810.

Boerner, R. J., Sommer, H., Berger, W., Kuhn, U., Schmidt, U., & Mannel, M. (2003). Kava-Kava extract Ll 150 is as effective as opipramol and buspirone in generalised anxiety disorder—An 8-week randomized, double-blind multi-centre clinical trial in 129 outpatients. *Phytomedicine, 10*(4), 38–49.

Brichenko, V. S., Kupriyanova, I. E., & Skorokhodova, T. F. (1986). The use of herbal adaptogens together with tricyclic antidepressants in patients with psychogenic depressions. *Modern Problems of Pharmacology and Search for New Medicine, 2*, 58–60.

Burdette, J. E., Liu, J., Chen, S., Fabricant, D. S., Piersen, C. E., Barker, E. L., ... Bolton, J. L. (2003). Black cohosh acts as a mixed competitive ligand and partial agonist of the serotonin receptor. *Journal of Agricultural and Food Chemistry, 51*, 5661–5670.

Bystritsky, A., Kerwin, L., & Feusner, J. (2008). A pilot study of *Rhodiola rosea* (Rhodax) for generalized anxiety disorder (GAD). *Journal of Alternative and Complementary Medicine, 14*(2), 175–180.

Chatterjee, S. S., Bhattacharya, S. K., Wonnemann, M., Singer, A., & Müller, W. E. (1998). Hyperforin as a possible antidepressant component of hypericum extracts. *Life Sciences, 63*(6), 499–510.

Cott, J. M. (1997). *In vitro* receptor binding and enzyme inhibition by *Hypericum perforatum* extract. *Pharmacopsychiatry, 30*, 108–112.

Darbinyan, V., Aslanyan, G., Amroyan, E., Gabrielyan, E., Malmström, C., & Panossian, A. (2007). Clinical trial of *Rhodiola rosea* L. extract SHR-5 in the treatment of mild to moderate depression. *Nordic Journal of Psychiatry, 61*(5), 343–348.

Di Pierro, F., Callegari, A., Speroni, M., & Attolico, M. (2009). Fast dissolving *agnus castus* fruit extract for the premenstrual syndrome: A controlled clinical trial. *NUTRA foods, 8*(1), 27–31.

Dorn, M. (2000). Efficacy and tolerability of baldrian versus oxazepam in non-organic and non-psychiatric insomniacs: A randomised, double-blind, clinical, comparative study. *Forsch Komplementarmed Klass Naturheilkd, 7*(2), 79–84.

Ernst, E. (1998). Harmless herbs? A review of the recent literature. *American Journal of Medicine, 104*, 170–178.

Fiebich, B. L., Höllig, A., & Lieb, K. (2001). Inhibition of substance P-induced cytokine synthesis by St. John's wort extracts. *Pharmacopsychiatry, 34*(Suppl. 1), S26–S28.

Foxman, B., Barlow, R., D'arcy, H., & Gillespie, B., & Sobel, J. D. (2000). Urinary tract infection: Self-reported incidence and associated costs. *Annals of Epidemiology, 10*(8), 509–515.

Gettman, M. T., Ogan, K., & Brinkley, L. J., Adams-Huet, B., Pak, C. Y. C., & Pearle, M. S. (2005). Effect of cranberry juice consumption on urinary stone risk factors. *Journal of Urology, 174*, 590–594.

Gleitz, J., Gottner, N., Ameri, A., & Peters, T. (1996). Kavain inhibits non-stereospecifically veratridine-activated Na+ channels. *Planta Medica, 62*(5), 580–581.

Gupta, K., Chou, M. Y., Howell, A., Wobbe, C., Grady, R., & Stapleton, A. E. (2007). Cranberry products inhibit adherence of P-fimbriated *Escherichia coli* to primary cultured bladder and vaginal epithelial cells. *Journal of Urology, 177*(6), 2357–2360.

He, Z., Chen, R., Zhou, Y., Geng, L., Zhang, Z., Chen, S., ... Lin, S. (2009). Treatment for premenstrual syndrome with *Vitex agnus castus*: A prospective, randomized, multi-center placebo controlled study in China. *Maturitas, 63*, 99–103.

Henderson, L., Yue, Q. Y., Bergquist, C., Gerden, B., & Arlett, P. (2002). St. John's wort (*Hypericum perforatum*): Drug interactions and clinical outcomes. *British Journal of Clinical Pharmacology, 54*, 349–356.

Hersh, A. L., Stefanick, M. L., & Stafford, R. S. (2004). National use of postmenopausal hormone therapy. *Journal of American Medical Association, 291*(1), 47–53.

Hooton, T. M., Scholes, D., Hughes, J. P., Winter, C., Roberts, P. L., Stapleton, A. E., ... Stamm, W. E. (1996). A prospective study of risk factors for symptomatic urinary tract infection in young women. *New England Journal of Medicine, 335*(7), 468–474.

Houghton, P. J. (1999). The scientific basis for the reputed activity of valerian. *Journal of Pharmacy and Pharmacology, 51*, 505–512.

Howell, A. B., Botto, H., Combescure, C., Blanc-Potard, A., Gausa, L., Matsumoto, T., ... Lavigne, J. (2010). Dosage effect on uropathogenic *Escherichia coli* anti-adhesion activity in urine following consumption of cranberry powder standardized for proanthocyanidin content: A multicentric randomized double blind study. *BMC Infectious Diseases, 10*, 1–11.

Hypericum Depression Trial Study Group. (2002). Effect of *Hypericum perforatum* (St. John's wort) in major depressive disorder: A randomized controlled trial. *Journal of American Medical Association, 287*(14), 1807–1814.

Imbrici, P., Camerino, D. C., & Tricarico, D. (2013). Major channels involved in neuropsychiatric disorders and therapeutic perspectives. *Frontiers in Genetics, 4*(76), 1–19.

Jarry, H., Spengler, B., Wuttke, W., & Christoffel, V. (2006). *In vitro* assays for bioactivity-guided isolation of endocrine active compounds in *Vitex agnus-castus*. *Maturitas, 55S*, S26–S36.

Johnson, J. (1991). Virulence factors in *Escherichia coli* urinary tract infections. *Clinical Microbiology Reviews, 4*, 80–128.

Jussofie, A., Schmiz, A., & Hiemke, C. (1994). Kavapyrone enriched extract from *Piper methysticum* as modulator of the GABA binding site in different regions of rat brain. *Psychopharmacology, 116*, 469–474.

Kalb, R., Trautmann-Sponsel, R. D., & Kieser, M. (2001). Efficacy and tolerability of hypericum extract WS 5572 versus placebo in mildly to moderately depressed patients. *Pharmacopsychiatry, 34*, 96–103.

Kasper, S., Anghelescu, I., Szegedi, A., Dienel, A., & Kieser, M. (2006). Superior efficacy of St. John's wort extract WS 5570 compared to placebo in patients with major depression: A randomized, double blind, placebo-controlled, multi-center trial. *BMC Medicine, 4*, 14.

Katz, D., & McHorney, C. (2002). The relationship between insomnia and health-related quality of life in patients with chronic illness. *Journal of Family Practice, 51*(3), 229–235.

Kessler, R. C., Berglund, P. A., Coulouvrat, C., Hajak, G., Roth, T., Shahly, V., ... Walsh, J. K. (2011). Insomnia and the performance of US workers: Results from the American insomnia survey. *Sleep, 34*(9), 1161–1171.

Kessler, R. C., Davis, R. B., Foster, D. F., van Rompay, M. I., Walters, E. E., Wilkey, S. A., ... Eisenberg, D. M. (2001). Long-term trends in the use of complementary and alternative medical therapies in the United States. *Annals of Internal Medicine, 135*, 262–268.

Kim, E., Sy-Cordero, A., Graf, T. N., Brantley, S. J., Paine, M. F., & Oberlies, N. H. (2011). Isolation and identification of intestinal CYP3A inhibitors from cranberry (*Vaccinium macrocarpon*) using human intestinal microsomes. *Planta Medica, 77*(3), 265–270.

Kleber, E., Obry, T., Hippeli, S., Schneider, W., & Elstner, E. F. (1999). Biochemical activities of extracts from *Hypericum perforatum* L. 1st communication: Inhibition of dopamine-beta-hydroxylase. *Arzneimittelforschung, 49*(2), 106–109.

Kontiokari, T., Sundqvist, K., Nuutinen, M., Pokka, T., Koskela, M., & Uhari, M. (2001). Randomised trial of cranberry-lingonberry juice and lactobacillus GG drink for the prevention of urinary tract infections in women. *British Medical Journal, 322*, 1–5.

Lauritzen, C. H., Reuter, H. D., Repges, R., Böhnert, K. J., & Schmidt, U. (1997). Treatment of premenstrual tension syndrome with *Vitex agnus castus*: Controlled, double-blind study versus pyridoxine. *Phytomedicine, 4*(3), 183–189.

Lehmann, E., Kinzler, E., & Friedemann, J. (1996). Efficacy of a special kava extract (*Piper methysticum*) in patients with states of anxiety, tension and excitedness of non-mental origin—A double-blind placebo-controlled study of four weeks treatment. *Phytomedicine, 3*(2), 113–119.

Li, X. Z., & Ramzan, I. (2010). Role of ethanol in kava hepatotoxicity. *Phytotherapy Research, 24*, 475–480.

Linde, K., Berner, M. M., & Kriston, L. (2008). St. John's wort for major depression. *Cochrane Library*, (4).

Linde, K., & Knuppel, L. (2005). Large-scale observational studies of hypericum extracts in patients with depressive disorders—A systematic review. *Phytomedicine, 12*, 148–157.

Lindenberg, D., & Pitule-Schödel, H. (1990). D, L-kavain in comparison with oxazepam in anxiety disorders: A double-blind study of clinical effectiveness. *Fortschritte der Medizin, 108*(2), 49–50.

Lindstrom, A., Ooyen, C., Lynch, M. E., & Blumenthal, M. (2013). Herb supplement sales increase 5.5% in 2012: Herbal supplement sales rise for 9th consecutive year; turmeric sales jump 40% in natural channel. *Journal of the American Botanical Council, 99*, 60–65.

Liske, E., Hänggi, W., Henneicke-von Zepelin, H. H., Boblitz, N., Wüstenberg, P., & Rahlfs, V. W. (2002). Physiological investigation of a unique extract of black cohosh (Cimicifugae racemosae rhizoma): A 6-month clinical study demonstrates no systemic estrogenic effect. *Journal of Women's Health & Gender-Based Medicine, 11*(2), 163–174.

Liu, Y., Black, M. A., Caron, L., & Camesano, T. A. (2006). Role of cranberry juice on molecular-scale surface characteristics and adhesion behavior of *Escherichia coli*. *Biotechnology and Bioengineering, 93*(2), 297–305.

Loch, E., Selle, H., & Boblitz, N. (2000). Treatment of premenstrual syndrome with a phytopharmaceutical formulation containing *Vitex agnus castus*. *Journal of Women's Health & Gender-Based Medicine, 9*(3), 315–320.

Ma, L., Lin, S., Chen, R., & Wang, X. (2010). Treatment of moderate to severe premenstrual syndrome with *Vitex agnus castus* (BNO 1095) in Chinese women. *Gynecological Endocrinology, 26*(8), 612–616.

Magura, E. I., Kopanitsa, M. V., Gleitz, J., Peters, T., & Krishtal, O. A. (1997). Kava extract ingredients, (+)-methysticin and (±)-kavain inhibit voltage-operated Na+-channels in rat CA1 hippocampal neurons. *Neuroscience, 81*(2), 345–351.

Malsch, U., & Kieser, M. (2001). Efficacy of kava-kava in the treatment of non-psychotic anxiety, following pretreatment with benzodiazepines. *Psychopharmacology, 157*(3), 277–283.

Martin, L. A., Neighbors, H. W., & Griffith, D. M. (2013). The experience of symptoms of depression in men vs women: Analysis of the national comorbidity survey replication. *JAMA Psychiatry, 70*(10), 1100–1106.

McMurdo, M. E. T., Argo, I., Phillips, G., Daly, F., & Davey, P. (2009). Cranberry or trimethoprim for the prevention of recurrent urinary tract infections? A randomized controlled trial in older women. *Journal of Antimicrobial Chemotherapy, 63*, 389–395.

Mehta, D. H., Gardiner, P. M., Phillips, R. S., & McCarthy, E. P. (2008). Herbal and dietary supplement disclosure to health care providers by individuals with chronic conditions. *Journal of Alternative Complementary Medicine, 14*(10), 1263–1269.

Meier, B., Berger, D., Hoberg, E., Sticher, O., & Schaffner, W. (2000). Pharmacological activities of *Vitex agnus-castus* extracts in vitro. *Phytomedicine, 7*(5), 373–381.

Mohammed Abdul, M. I., Jiang, X., Williams, K. M., Day, R. O., Roufogalis, B. D., Liauw, W. S., … McLachlan, A. J. (2008). Pharmacodynamic interaction of warfarin with cranberry but not with garlic in healthy subjects. *British Journal of Pharmacology, 154*, 1691–1700.

Moore, L. B., Goodwin, B., Jones, S. A., Wisely, G. B., Serabjit-Singh, C. J., Willson, T. M., … Kliewer, S. A. (2000). St. John's wort induces hepatic drug metabolism through activation of the pregnane X receptor. *Proceedings of the National Academy of Sciences of the United States of America, 97*(13), 7500–7502.

Nelson, L. E., Guo, T. Z., Lu, J., Saper, C. B., Franks, N. P., & Maze, M. (2002). The sedative component of anesthesia is mediated by GABAA receptors in an endogenous sleep pathway. *Nature Neuroscience, 5*(10), 979–984.

Newton, K. M., Reed, S. D., LaCroix, A. Z., Grothaus, L. C., Ehrlich, K., & Guiltinan, J. (2006). Treatment of vasomotor symptoms of menopause with black cohosh, multibotanicals, soy, hormone therapy, or placebo. *Annals of Internal Medicine, 145*, 869–879.

Ogu, C. C., & Maxa, J. L. (2000). Drug interactions due to cytochrome P450. *Proceedings (Baylor University Medical Center), 13*(4), 421–423.

Ohayon, M. M. (1997). Prevalence of DSM-IV diagnostic criteria of insomnia: Distinguishing insomnia related to mental disorders from sleep disorders. *Journal of Psychiatric Research, 31*(3), 333–346.

Olsson, E. M., von Schéele, B., & Panossian, A. G. (2009). A randomized double-blind placebo controlled parallel group study of SHR-5 extract of *Rhodiola rosea* roots as treatment for patients with stress related fatigue. *Planta Medica, 75*(2), 105–112.

Ortiz, J. G., Nieves-Natal, J., & Chavez, P. (1999). Effects of *Valeriana officinalis* extracts on [^{3}H]Flunitrazepam binding, synaptosomal [^{3}H]GABA uptake, and hippocampal [^{3}H]GABA release. *Neurochemical Research, 24*(11), 1373–1378.

Osmers, R., Friede, M., Liske, E., Schnitker, J., Freudenstein, J., & Henneicke-von Zepelin, H. H. (2005). Efficacy and safety of isopropanolic black cohosh extract for climacteric symptoms. *Obstetrics and Gynecology, 105*(5), 1074–1083.

Oxman, A. D., Flottorp, S., Håvelsrud, K., Fretheim, A., Odgaard-Jensen, J., ... Bjorvatn, B. (2007). A televised, web-based randomized trial of an herbal remedy (valerian) for insomnia. *PLoS One, 2*(10), e1040.

Panossian, A., Hamm, R., Kadioglu, O., Wikman, G., & Efferth, T. (2013). Synergy and antagonism of active constituents of ADAPT-232 on transcriptional level of metabolite regulation of isolated neuroglial cells. *Frontiers in Neuroscience, 7*(16), 1–17.

Panossian, A., Nikoyan, N., Ohanyan, N., Hovhannisyan, A., Abrahamyan, H., Garielyan, E., & Wikman, G. (2008). Comparative study of Rhodiola preparations on behavioral despair of rats. *Phytomedicine, 15*, 84–91.

Panossian, A., Wikman, G., Kaur, P., & Asea, A. (2012). Adaptogens stimulate neuropeptide Y and Hsp72 expression and release in neuroglia cells. *Frontiers in Neuroscience, 6*(1), 1–12.

Perfumi, M., & Mattioli, L. (2007). Adaptogenic and central nervous system effects of single doses of 3% rosavin and 1% salidroside *Rhodiola rosea* L. extract in mice. *Phytotherapy Research, 21*, 37–43.

Piccinelli, M., & Wilkinson, G. (2000). Gender differences in depression: Critical review. *British Journal of Psychiatry, 177*, 486–492.

Posadzki, P., Lee, M. S., Moon, T. W., Choi, T. Y., Park, T. Y., & Ernst, E. (2013). Prevalence of complementary and alternative medicine (CAM) use by menopausal women: A systematic review of surveys. *Maturitas, 75*, 34–43.

Prilepskaya, V. N., Ledina, A. V., Tagiyeva, A. V., & Revazova, F. S. (2006). *Vitex agnus castus*: Successful treatment of moderate to severe premenstrual syndrome. *Maturitas, 55S*, S55–S63.

Rayner, J., Willis, K., & Burgess, R. (2011). Women's use of complementary and alternative medicine for fertility enhancement: A review of the literature. *Journal of Complementary Medicine, 17*(8), 685–690.

Robinson, A., & McGrail, M. R. (2004). Disclosure of CAM use to medical practitioners: A review of qualitative and quantitative studies. *Complementary Therapies in Medicine, 12*, 90–98.

Ross, S. M. (2012). A standardized isopropanolic black cohosh extract (remifemin) is found to be safe and effective for menopausal symptoms. *Holistic Nursing Practice, 26*(1), 58–61.

Rossouw, J. E., Anderson, G. L., Prentice, R. L., LaCroix, A. Z., Kooperberg, C., Stefanick, M. L., ... Ockene, J. (2002). Risks and benefits of estrogen plus progestin in healthy postmenopausal women. *Journal of American Medical Association, 288*(3), 321–333.

Ruhlen, R. L., Haubner, J., Tracy, J. K., Zhu, W., Ehya, H., Lamberson, W. R., ... Sauter, E. R. (2007). Black cohosh does not exert an estrogenic effect on the breast. *Nutrition and Cancer, 59*(2), 269–277.

Sacher, J., Houle, S., Parkes, J., Rusjan, P., Sagrati, S., Wilson, A. A., & Meyer, J. H. (2011). Monoamine oxidase A inhibitor occupancy during treatment of major depressive episodes with moclobemide or St. John's wort: An [11c]-harmine PET study. *Journal of Psychiatry Neuroscience, 36*(6), 375–382.

Sarris, J., Stough, C., Bousman, C. A., Wahid, Z. T., Murray, G., Teschke, R., ... Schweitzer, I. (2013). Kava in the treatment of generalized anxiety disorder: A double-blind, randomized, placebo-controlled study. *Journal of Clinical Psychopharmacology, 33*, 643–648.

Schellenberg, R. (2001). Treatment for the premenstrual syndrome with agnus castus fruit extract: Prospective, randomized, placebo controlled study. *British Medical Journal, 322*, 134–137.

Schellenberg, R., Zimmermann, C., Drewe, J., Hoexter, G., & Zahner, C. (2012). Dose-dependent efficacy of the *Vitex agnus castus* extract ze 440 in patients suffering from premenstrual syndrome. *Phytomedicine, 19*, 1325–1331.

Schroeder, C., Tank, J., Goldstein, D. S., Stoeter, M., Haertter, S., Luft, F. C., & Jordan, J. (2004). Influence of St. John's wort on catecholamine turnover and cardiovascular regulation in humans. *Clinical Pharmacology & Therapeutics, 76*(5), 480–489.

Schumacher, B., Scholle, S., Hölzl, J., Khudeir, N., Hess, S., & Müller, C. E. (2002). Lignans isolated from valerian: Identification and characterization of a new olivil derivative with partial agonistic activity at A1 adenosine receptors. *Journal of Natural Products, 65*, 1479–1485.

Seitz, U., Schüle A., & Gleitz, J. (1997). [^{3}H]-Monoamine uptake inhibition properties of kava pyrones. *Planta Medica, 63*(6), 548–549.

Singer, A., Wonnemann, M., & Müller, W. E. (1999). Hyperforin, a major antidepressant constituent of St. John's wort, inhibits serotonin uptake by elevating free intracellular Na$^+$. *Journal of Pharmacology and Experimental Therapeutics, 290*(3), 1363–1368.

Sorrentino, L., Capasso, A., & Schmidt, M. (2006). Safety of ethanolic kava extract: Results of a study of chronic toxicity in rats. *Phytomedicine, 13*(8), 542–549.

Spasov, A. A., Wikman, G. K., Mandrikov, V. B., Mironova, I. A., & Neumoin, V. V. (2000). A double-blind, placebo-controlled pilot study of the stimulating and adaptogenic effect of *Rhodiola rosea* SHR-5 extract on the fatigue of students caused by stress during an examination period with a repeated low-dose regimen. *Phytomedicine, 7*(2), 85–89.

Staner, L. (2010). Comorbidity of insomnia and depression. *Sleep Medicine Reviews, 14*, 35–46.

Stapleton, A. E., Dziura, J., Hooton, T. M., Cox, M. E., Yarova-Yarovaya, Y., Chen, S., & Gupta, K. (2012). Recurrent urinary tract infection and urinary *Escherichia coli* in women ingesting cranberry juice daily: A randomized controlled trial. *Mayo Clinic Proceedings, 87*(2), 143–150.

Stothers, L. (2002). A randomized trial to evaluate effectiveness and cost effectiveness of naturopathic cranberry products as prophylaxis against urinary tract infection in women. *Canadian Journal of Urology, 9*(3), 1558–1562.

Suzuki, O., Katsumata, Y., Oya, M., Bladt, S., & Wagner, H. (1984). Inhibition of monoamine oxidase by hypericin. *Planta Medica, 50*(3), 272–274.

Taibi, D. M., Landis, C. A., Petry, H., & Vitiello, M. V. (2007). A systematic review of valerian as a sleep aid: Safe but not effective. *Sleep Medicine Reviews, 11*, 209–230.

Teschke, R., Sarris, J., & Schweitzer, I. (2011). Kava hepatotoxicity in traditional and modern use: The presumed pacific kava paradox hypothesis revisited. *British Journal of Clinical Pharmacology, 73*(2), 170–174.

Teschke, R., & Schwarzenboeck, S. (2009). Suspected hepatotoxicity by Cimicifugae racemosae rhizoma (black cohosh, root): Critical analysis and structured causality assessment. *Phytomedicine, 16*, 72–84.

Teufel-Mayer, R., & Gleitz, J. (1997). Effects of long-term administration of hypericum extracts on the affinity and density of the central serotonergic 5-HT1 A and 5-HT2 A receptors. *Pharmacopsychiatry, 30*(Suppl. 2), 113–116.

Thiede, H. M., & Walper, A. (1994). Inhibition of MAO and COMT by hypericum extracts and hypericin. *Journal of Geriatric Psychiatry and Neurology, 7*, S54–S56.

Tindle, H. A., Davis, R. B., Phillips, R. S., & Eisenberg, D. M. (2005). Trends in use of complementary and alternative medicine by US adults: 1997–2002. *Alternative Therapies in Health and Medicine, 11*(1), 42–49.

Uebelhack, R., Franke, L., & Schewe, H. J. (1998). Inhibition of platelet MAO-B by kava pyrone-enriched extract from *Piper methysticum* Forster (kava-kava). *Pharmacopsychiatry, 31*(5) 187–192.

Valentová, K., Stejskal, D., Bednář, P., Vostálová, J., Číhalík, Č., Večeřová, R., … Šimánek V. (2007). Biosafety, antioxidant status, and metabolites in urine after consumption of dried cranberry juice in healthy women: A pilot double-blind placebo-controlled trial. *Journal of Agricultural and Food Chemistry, 55*(8), 3217–3224.

van Diermen, D., Marston, A., Bravo, J., Reist, M., Carrupt, P., & Hostettmann, K. (2009). Monoamine oxidase inhibition by *Rhodiola rosea* L. roots. *Journal of Ethnopharmacology, 122*, 397–401.

Vermes, G., Bánhidy, F., & Ács, N. (2005). The effects of remifemin on subjective symptoms of menopause. *Advances in Therapy, 22*(2), 148–154.

Walden, J., von Wegerer, J., Winter, U., Berger, M., & Grunze, H. (1997). Effects of kawain and dihydromethysticin on field potential changes in the hippocampus. *Progress in Neuro-Psychopharmacology & Biological Psychiatry, 21*, 697–706.

Warnecke, G. (1991). Psychosomatic dysfunction in the female climacteric. Clinical effectiveness and tolerance of kava extract ws 1490. *Fortschritte der Medizin, 109*(4), 119–122.

Webster, D. E., Lu, J., Chen, S. N., Farnsworth, N. R., & Wang, Z. J. (2006). Activation of the μ-opiate receptor by *Vitex agnus-castus* methanol extracts: Implication for its use in PMS. *Journal of Ethnopharmacology, 106*, 216–221.

Wing, D. A., Rumney, P. J., Preslicka, C., & Chung, J. H. (2008). Daily cranberry juice for the prevention of asymptomatic bacteriuria in pregnancy: A randomized, controlled pilot study. *Journal of Urology, 180*(4) 1367–1372.

Witte, S., Loew, D., & Gaus, W. (2005). Meta-Analysis of the efficacy of the acetonic kava-kava extract ws 1490 in patients with non-psychotic anxiety disorders. *Phytotherapy Research, 19*, 183–188.

World Health Organization. (2013, May). *Fact Sheet No. 134*. Retrieved from http://who.int/ mental_health/resources/gender/en

Wu, P., Fuller, C., Liu, X., Lee, H., Fan, B., Hoven, C., Mandell, D., … Kronenberg, F. (2007). Use of complementary and alternative medicine among women with depression: Results of a national survey. *Psychiatric Services, 58*(3), 349–356.

Wuttke, W., Seidlová-Wuttke, D., & Gorkow, C. (2003). The Cimifuga preparation BNO 1055 vs. conjugated estrogens in a double-blind placebo-controlled study: Effects on menopause symptoms and bone markers. *Maturitas, 44*(Suppl. 1), S67–S77.

Yonkers, K. A., O'Brien, P. M. S., & Eriksson, E. (2008). Premenstrual syndrome. *Lancet, 371*, 1200–1210.

Zafriri, D., Ofek, I., Adar, R., Pocino, M., & Sharon, N. (1989). Inhibitory activity of cranberry juice on adherence of type 1 and type P fimbriated *Escherichia coli* to eukaryotic cells. *Antimicrobial Agents and Chemotherapy, 33*(1), 92–98.

Ziegler, G., Ploch, M., Miettinen-Baumann, A., & Collet, W. (2002). Efficacy and tolerability of valerian extract LI 156 compared with oxazepam in the treatment of non-organic insomnia—A randomized, double-blind, comparative clinical study. *European Journal of Medical Research, 7*(11), 480–486.

Chapter 13

Pharmacologic Approaches to Wellness and Disease Prevention in Women over the Life Span

Diana N. Krause

To promote wellness in women, there is often the need to supplement healthy lifestyle choices with medications, both prescription and nonprescription. This chapter focuses on prescription medications. Drugs may be given to relieve *acute* conditions (e.g., headache, allergy, infection), improve well-being for those with underlying *chronic* conditions (e.g., depression, arthritis, hypothyroidism), or *prevent* the development of disease (e.g., stroke, osteoporosis, diabetes). Contraceptive drugs enhance a woman's welfare by enabling her to plan pregnancy, which benefits mother and baby as well as the family.

Women's use of prescription drugs involves a number of special considerations that have been historically underappreciated. Recent developments like the US National Institute of Health's (NIH) Women's Health Initiative (http://www.nhlbi.nih.gov/whi) are helping to bring these considerations to light and incorporate them into perspectives on therapy for women. Important variables include male–female differences in drug effects, changing requirements over a woman's life span, and unique health needs of women.

This chapter presents

1. Male–female differences in drug response
2. Implications of life span changes in women on drug use
3. Unique health needs of women in relation to drug use
4. Common drug classes used by women over the life span

Male–Female Differences in Drug Response

There is a growing awareness that women and men can differ in their susceptibility to disease and their response to therapeutic drugs (Baggio, Corsini, Floreani, Giannini, & Zagonel, 2013). Unfortunately for women, much of what is known about current drugs comes from studies in males. Up until 1993, women were routinely excluded from US clinical drug trials (Merkatz et al., 1993). This was based on the misguided assumption that women would show similar responses, coupled with safety concerns for women of childbearing age. As discussed below, male–female differences have been found in both the *pharmacokinetic* and *pharmacodynamic* aspects of drugs. However, in spite of these known differences, research in males continues to dominate both preclinical animal studies and clinical trials. Women and their care providers need to be aware of the male bias in the knowledge base and stay alert for new findings relevant to optimizing therapy in females.

Pharmacokinetics describes what happens to a drug in the body, that is, how it is absorbed, distributed, metabolized, and excreted. Pharmacokinetic variables impact how well a drug works and its potential for side effects; thus, fine-tuning these variables for use of a drug in women is crucial for achieving successful outcomes. For many drugs, the pharmacokinetic profile differs between men and women. Pharmacokinetic factors can increase the risk of adverse effects in women by increasing the level of drug exposure for a given dose. In general, women tend to be smaller, so the "standard" dose determined from trials in men may, in fact, be an overdose in women. Sexual dimorphism in body composition also causes differences in drug distribution, such as increased storage of fat-soluble drugs in women. Women are generally slower at processing drugs in the GI tract (absorption) and the kidney (excretion) (Spoletini, Vitale, Malorni, & Rosano, 2012).

Drug levels in men and women also can differ because rates of drug metabolism may not be the same. For example, females metabolize diazepam, prednisolone, caffeine, and acetaminophen somewhat faster than men. However, propranolol, chlordiazepoxide, and lidocaine are metabolized slower by women. Female sex hormones have been shown to alter the expression of key P450 metabolizing enzymes in the liver; they decrease CYP1A2, CYP2E1, and CYP2D6 but increase CYP3A4 (Spoletini et al., 2012). The latter enzyme is responsible for the metabolism of almost half of the medications currently in use, including many antidepressants, anxiolytics, analgesics, anticholesterols, antihypertensives, anticoagulants, antibiotics, and sex steroids. Thus, these medications are generally cleared faster in women, which could result in lower levels and shorter duration of action.

Pharmacodynamics refers to the actions of the drug on the body. Women may respond differently than men to a drug with respect to either desired beneficial effects and/or non-desired side effects. The underlying bases for sex differences in biological responses are not entirely clear, but may result from the influence of sex hormones, sex chromosomes and their regulation of gene expression, or from sex-related changes that occur during development. An example of pharmacodynamic differences is seen in the response to some pain medications. Women have better pain relief with morphine as compared with men (Niesters et al., 2010). Another illustration of sex differences comes from recent trials investigating the use of low-dose aspirin in primary stroke prevention. This therapy was shown to be effective in women but not in men (Berger et al., 2006).

Drug-related cardiac arrhythmia is an example of a serious adverse reaction that is more common in women (Anthony, 2005). This problem is caused by drugs that prolong the QT interval in the EKG, such as certain antihistamines, antibiotics, antipsychotics, and antiarrhythmics. Women have a higher baseline QT interval and are more likely to inherit mutations in potassium channel genes that increase their risk of drug-induced long QT syndrome and torsades de pointes, a potentially fatal arrhythmia. Female sex hormones also affect potassium channel function, resulting in longer QT intervals during the menses and ovulation phases of the menstrual cycle (Yang & Clancy, 2012).

In general, women are more likely to have adverse reactions to drugs as compared with men (Reidl & Casillas, 2003). Contributing factors may be that women tend to use more medications and are more likely to report side effects. As discussed above, drugs tested primarily in males may not be optimized for use in women. Whatever the cause, it is always prudent to monitor women for potential adverse drug events.

Individual Variability: Pharmacogenomics

Customizing drug use for women is part of an emerging focus on developing *individualized* medicine optimized for each patient. This concept is fueled by advances in understanding genetic variations in proteins important for drug action. *Pharmacogenomics* addresses how a person's genetic makeup impacts his or her response to medication.

So far, most studies have focused on genetic variations in enzymes that metabolize drugs, in particular the liver cytochrome P450 enzymes (Ingelman-Sundberg, Sim, Gomez, & Rodriguez-Antona, 2007; Sim, Kacevska, & Ingerman-Sundberg, 2013). These differences are an important cause of individual variability in the response to a given drug treatment. For example, polymorphisms in the P450 enzyme CYP2C9 alter responses to the widely used drugs glipizide (antidiabetic), warfarin (anticoagulant), and phenytoin (anticonvulsant). If an individual has a "slow" form of the enzyme, the drug may not be broken down as fast as expected and result in higher blood levels and adverse effects. On the other hand, a fast metabolizer may clear the drug too quickly to achieve full benefit. P450 polymorphisms also contribute to racial and ethnic variability in drug responses. For example, poor metabolizing forms of CYP2D6 are more prevalent in African Americans and Asians as compared with other populations. Thus, patients in these groups may require dose adjustment or discontinuation of drugs that are inactivated by CYP2D6. Common examples are β-blockers (antihypertensive) and selective serotonin reuptake inhibitors (SSRIs; antidepressant).

Some drugs require metabolic processing to become active, for example, conversion of codeine to morphine by the enzyme CYP2D6. If someone expresses the gene for the "slow" form of this enzyme, they may not achieve the desired benefit of pain relief. Conversely, a person with the "ultrarapid" form of CYP2D6 may produce too much active metabolite. In one extreme case, a woman who was an undiagnosed rapid metabolizer was taking codeine for postpartum pain. The elevated levels of morphine she produced were passed in her breast milk to her infant who died of opiate poisoning (Koren, Cairns, Chitayat, Gaedigk, & Leder, 2006).

Thus, better understanding of the polymorphisms in P450 genes that affect drug metabolism can provide a more rational basis for selecting the appropriate drug and drug dosage for an individual who has been genotyped. Research is continuing to identify other genetic polymorphisms that affect pharmacokinetic and/or pharmacodynamic parameters. The promise of pharmacogenomics is safer and more effective drug treatment for each individual.

Drug Use Over a Woman's Life Span

The number and the type of drugs used by women vary over the life span. Recent data from the US National Center for Health Statistics (2013) provide a snapshot of the most common drugs taken by women. Their report shows that use of prescription drugs by women increases over the life span. About 65% of older women (65 years and older) reported using three or more medications over a 30-day period, in contrast to less than 15% of young adult women (18 to 44 years old) who took three or more drugs.

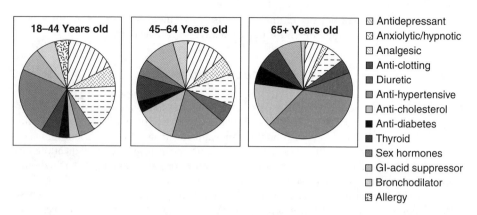

FIGURE 13.1 The usage of commonly prescribed drug classes by women in different age groups: 18 to 44 years, 45 to 64 years, and 65 years and older. Pie charts were constructed using data from the 2013 report of the US National Center for Health Statistics (2013) on women who took at least one prescription drug during a 30-day period, 2007 to 2010. For each age group, the relative usage of each drug class is shown.

The percentage of middle-aged women (45 to 64 years old) who used three or more drugs was about 40%.

The type of drugs that are most frequently used by women also varies depending on their age, as shown in Figure 13.1 (US National Center for Health Statistics, 2013). Younger women are more likely to be taking sex hormone–related medications and drugs to suppress depression, anxiety, and pain. Middle-aged women reported taking fewer hormones, but took more drugs to combat cardiovascular disease, specifically agents to lower cholesterol and blood pressure. Women in this age group also took a substantial amount of drugs for depression, anxiety, and pain. In older women, however, cardiovascular drugs made up the largest proportion of drugs taken. Clearly, the health needs of women change as they age. Moreover in older women, age-associated decline in renal clearance and drug metabolism can increase the risk of drug toxicity; usually lower doses are warranted. The increased use of multiple drugs (polypharmacy) with age also increases the likelihood of potentially harmful drug–drug interactions.

A major impact on a woman's well-being over her life span comes from the varying influence of sex hormones and changes in reproductive status. Premenopausal women are concerned about menstrual changes, contraception, infertility, and pregnancy. Postmenopausal women must deal with the consequences of losing ovarian hormone production. Each of these conditions poses special considerations for drug therapy. Fluctuations in sex hormones can precipitate the need for drugs, such as with menstrual migraine, cramps, and mood changes, or postmenopausal osteoporosis. Moreover, the effectiveness, pharmacokinetics, and side-effect profile of ongoing drug therapy may be altered when hormone levels fluctuate over the course of menstrual cycles or pregnancy (Isoherranen & Thummel, 2013). Administration of exogenous sex hormones for contraception or hormone replacement therapy can have similar effects on drug therapy. Female sex hormones alter processes involved in drug absorption, metabolism, and excretion as well as targeted drug action at receptors, ion channels, enzymes, and molecular signaling pathways. Dosing may need to be adjusted to achieve optimal therapeutic effects and/or avoid adverse actions, particularly with drugs that have a narrow therapeutic index.

TABLE 13.1	FDA Drug Categories of Teratogenic Risk during Pregnancy
Category	**Description**
A	No risk to the fetus as determined in controlled studies of drug in pregnant women
B	No evidence of risk in humans: Animal studies show no risk; however, there are no controlled human studies OR animal studies show risk but human studies do not
C	Risk cannot be ruled out: Animal studies show risk, but no adequate human studies. For drugs in this category, potential benefits may outweigh potential risks; caution is advised
D	Positive evidence of risk to human fetus. Benefits may outweigh potential risks in serious conditions
X	Contraindicated in pregnancy: Fetal risks outweigh potential benefits

Use of prescription drugs during pregnancy and lactation is a situation unique to women that requires careful balancing of the potential benefit to the mother with potential adverse and/or teratogenic actions on the baby. The US Food and Drug Administration (FDA) categorizes drugs according to their potential to cause birth defects during pregnancy (Table 13.1). However, in many cases, this potential is not really known or is extrapolated from preclinical tests in cells or animals. Risks to the fetus may differ over the course of pregnancy depending on critical periods of development; the first trimester is often the most vulnerable to drug effects. Following birth, drugs that can pass into the mother's milk are of particular concern for breast-fed infants.

The health status of the mother also may change during pregnancy. Some conditions may remit during pregnancy (migraine); while others may emerge that require treatment, such as preeclampsia, gestational diabetes, and postpartum depression. Thus, management of medications during this time can be complex and may require that a drug be stopped or substituted with a safer alternative in specific trimesters or throughout the course of pregnancy, delivery, and/or the postpartum period.

Drugs for Conditions of Particular Concern for Women

Obviously, women have unique pharmacologic needs for managing reproductive health and changes in reproductive status. Many of the drugs used are related to female sex hormones. In addition, women are particularly prone to certain types of medical conditions. Depression, anxiety, and pain are observed more frequently in women than in men. Women have increased risk for autoimmune diseases such as rheumatoid arthritis, thyroid disorders, lupus, and multiple sclerosis. Osteoporosis, irritable bowel syndrome, and urinary tract problems are other conditions that are more likely to occur in women. Thus, drug classes that treat these disorders are among those most commonly prescribed for women (see Fig. 13.1).

Common Drug Classes Used in Women Across Their Life Span

The intent of the remainder of this chapter is to briefly review drug classes that are used frequently by women across their life span to enhance health and well-being (Fig. 13.1). The focus is on commonly prescribed drugs and/or drugs for particular concerns of women. Although it is impossible to cover all aspects of prescription drugs in one chapter, more in-depth information can be obtained in the many pharmacology texts available, including two recent books focused on women (King & Brucker, 2011; Mitchell, 2012). There are also excellent Web-based sites that specifically address drug research and therapy in women, such as the NIH Office of Research on Women's Health (http://orwh.od.nih.gov/index.asp) and the FDA Office of Women's Health (http://www.fda.gov/AboutFDA/CentersOffices/OC/OfficeofWomensHealth/default.htm). To supplement the following text, key aspects of common drug classes are summarized in table form.

Drugs Related to Sex Hormones and Reproductive Health

Women have unique needs for drugs related to female sex hormones and female reproductive health. As shown in Figure 13.1, a significant portion of the drugs taken by younger women are forms of the ovarian hormones, estrogen and progesterone, that are used primarily for birth control. Older women also are prescribed sex hormones as replacement therapy to alleviate postmenopausal symptoms.

Drugs to Prevent Pregnancy

Birth control pills are the most common form of reversible contraception used by women. Most pills are a combination of a synthetic estrogen and a synthetic progestin, but some formulations contain only progestin (Table 13.2). In currently available contraceptives, hormone levels are relatively low, as compared with the first generation of birth control pills, in order to minimize side effects. In addition to oral formulations, which are taken daily, more long-term delivery methods are available for hormonal contraception: transdermal patches, vaginal rings, injections (every 12 weeks), or implants under the skin (every 3 years). Metabolism and side effects of the different synthetic hormones and formulations can vary among women, so individuals may have a specific preference.

Common side effects of contraceptive drugs are breast tenderness, nausea and gastrointestinal discomfort, headaches, changes in vaginal discharge, and irregular vaginal bleeding. Most of these effects disappear within the first months of treatment. Formulations that only contain progestin are more likely to cause unpredictable bleeding or amenorrhea, as well as possible weight gain from fluid retention, decreased peristalsis, constipation, or bloating. With combination contraceptives, adverse effects may also occur from the estrogen component. Most serious is an increased risk for forming blood clots, which can lead to venous thromboembolism, myocardial infarction, and ischemic stroke. Thrombosis is primarily a concern in women who smoke or have existing cardiovascular risk factors. Hormonal contraceptives are not recommended in women who are over 35 and smoke, have cardiovascular risk factors, coagulopathies or history of embolism, breast cancer, or liver disease. Interestingly, hormonal contraceptives can also lower levels of endogenous free testosterone. A potential negative consequence is decreased libido, but a positive benefit is reduction in acne.

TABLE 13.2 Endocrine Drugs

Desired Effect	Drug Class	Examples	Side Effects
Sex Hormones			
Prevent pregnancy (contraceptives)	Synthetic estrogen and progestins		
	Oral	Ethinyl estradiol (EE) + progestin (norethindrone)	Nausea, breast tenderness, thrombosis
		Progestin only	Irregular bleeding
	Patch	EE + norelgestromin	
	Injection/implant	Medroxyprogesterone/ etonogestrel	
	"Morning after"	levonorgestrel	
Induce abortion	Progesterone receptor blocker	Mifepristone	
	17β-Estradiol		Blood clots, stroke, breast cancer, gallbladder disease, high blood pressure
Reduce menopausal symptoms; hormone replacement	Synthetic oral estrogens	Conjugated equine estrogens	
	Progestins	Medroxyprogesterone	
	SERMS	Raloxifene, ospemifene	
Thyroid			
Replace thyroid	Levothyroxine	Synthroid	Hyperthyroidism, atrial fibrillation, bone loss
Decrease thyroid	Thionamides	Methimazole	Hypothyroidism
Diabetes			
Replace insulin	Insulins	Insulin, insulin lispro, insulin glargine	Hypoglycemia
Lower blood glucose	Oral antidiabetics		
	Biguanides	Metformin	GI upset
	Sulfonylureas Meglitinides	Glipizide Repaglinide	Weight gain, hypoglycemia
	DPP-4 inhibitors	Sitagliptin	Pancreatitis (rare)
	α-Glucosidase inhibitors	Acarbose	GI upset
	Thiazolidinediones	Pioglitazone	Edema, weight gain, CV and hepatic risk

GI, gastrointestinal; CV, cardiovascular; SERM, selective estrogen receptor modulator; DPP, dipeptidylpeptidase.

"Emergency" contraception or "morning after" pills are hormonal contraceptives that are used to prevent pregnancy following unprotected sex, contraceptive failure, incorrect use of contraceptives, or in cases of sexual assault. For this purpose, a short course of oral steroid hormones is taken within 72 hours of sexual intercourse. Progestin drugs that are formulated specifically for this purpose, such as Plan B, are most effective and have fewer side effects than combination pills containing both estrogen and progestin.

If a pregnancy does occur that must be terminated, there is an "abortion pill" that can be used. Mifepristone is a sex steroid analog that blocks progesterone receptors and causes shedding of the uterine lining. It has been approved by the FDA for terminating intrauterine pregnancies of up to 49 days' gestation. It is used in conjunction with the synthetic prostaglandin misoprostol that causes softening of the cervix and uterine contractions.

Hormone Replacement After Menopause

Following the loss of ovarian hormones at menopause, some women need medication to cope with the problems of hot flashes, night sweats, and vaginal dryness and irritation. Risk of osteoporosis also increases with loss of estrogen. *Hormone replacement therapy* can be used to alleviate these symptoms. However, because of concern for possible serious and/or long-term risks, the current recommendation is for hormones to be used at the lowest dose for the shortest time necessary. Evidence suggests that the most appropriate time of therapy is in the early stages of menopause.

The use of hormone replacement in postmenopausal women has generated considerable controversy, particularly following the landmark NIH Women's Health Initiative Trial of conjugated equine estrogens (CEEs) plus medroxyprogesterone acetate in healthy postmenopausal women (Rossouw et al., 2002). This trial concluded that the overall risks (increased risk of breast cancer, thromboembolism, and cardiovascular disease) exceeded the benefits for primary disease prevention (lower risk of fractures and colorectal cancer). Subsequent studies have tried to determine whether certain factors can be addressed to lower the risks of hormone therapy, for example, type of hormone analog, formulation, and dose; age at initiation; or patient selection based on individual traits, history, and preexisting conditions (Chen, 2011; Howard & Rossouw, 2013). Ongoing research may eventually lead to more optimal hormone replacement regimens.

Current choices for hormone replacement (Table 13.2) include oral estrogenic compounds such as CEEs. Other formulations are available that deliver either CEEs or the primary form of endogenous estrogen, 17β-estradiol, via a transdermal patch or cream, vaginal insert or cream, or by injection. In addition, there are combination pills that also contain a progestin, primarily to counteract the ability of estrogen to stimulate endometrial cancer in women with an intact uterus.

Common, but mild, side effects of hormone replacement include painful or tender breasts, vaginal spotting, nausea and vomiting, stomach cramps and bloating, fluid retention, headaches, hair loss, and vaginal yeast infection. For some women, hormone medications may increase their risk of blood clots, stroke, gallbladder disease, liver problems, and breast cancer. Thus, hormone therapy is not recommended for women who are at risk for breast cancer or have cardiovascular, clotting, or liver disorders. Endometrial cancer is a risk for women who have an intact uterus and are only taking estrogen without a progestin.

In addition to hormone replacement, drugs called "selective estrogen receptor modulators" (SERMs) are available to treat specific menopausal symptoms (Table 13.2). These drugs are estrogen analogs that can have either agonist or antagonist effects, depending on the specific tissue affected. Raloxifene is a prototypic SERM that has estrogen-like effects on bone and is used to prevent osteoporosis in menopausal women. Conversely, it has antiestrogenic effects in breast and endometrial tissue and can actually lower the risk of breast cancer (Cummings et al., 1999). Raloxifene does not relieve hot flashes, but it does act like estrogen to increase clotting risk.

Another SERM, ospemifene, was approved by the FDA in 2013 for relief of moderate to severe dyspareunia (painful intercourse), a symptom of vulvar and vaginal atrophy due to menopause. The availability of this drug may put more focus on a problem that has not received adequate attention in menopausal women. Adverse effects of ospemifene include estrogen-like risks of deep-vein thrombosis, stroke, and endometrial cancer (in the absence of progestin).

To avoid the risks associated with hormone therapy, other types of medications can be used for certain menopausal symptoms. In particular, drugs that specifically prevent bone loss are used in postmenopausal women at risk for osteoporosis. *Bisphosphonates* (alendronate, risedronate, ibandronate, and zoledronate) are considered first-line therapy and are given long term to increase bone density and prevent fractures (Miller & Derman, 2010). In 2013, the FDA approved the first nonhormonal alternative for treating moderate to severe hot flashes associated with menopause. A low-dose formulation of paroxetine, an SSRI, is used for this indication, in contrast to the higher doses given to treat depression. Evidence suggests paroxetine may not be as effective as estrogen replacement, but it offers a viable alternative for women in which hormones are contraindicated.

Drugs for Thyroid Dysfunction

As shown in Figure 13.1, thyroid medications represent a significant proportion of the drugs taken by women in all age groups. Thyroid dysfunction is one of the most common endocrine disorders seen in primary care, and it occurs more frequently in women than in men. This disparity likely reflects the fact that autoimmunity and ovarian hormones are common contributors to thyroid dysfunction.

*Hypo*thyroidism is the most prevalent thyroid problem, and replacement of thyroid hormones is critical for a woman with this condition (Almandoz & Gharib, 2012). Symptoms include fatigue, memory problems, depression, weight gain, hoarseness, hyperlipidemia, and bradycardia. Hypothyroidism can also cause ovulatory dysfunction, the leading cause of impaired female fertility, and stabilizing thyroid levels reduces menstrual irregularities and risk of polycystic ovary syndrome. Levothyroxine (T_4), a synthetic thyroid hormone, is most commonly used as replacement therapy (Table 13.2). Usually, women with hypothyroidism must take thyroid therapy on a chronic basis throughout their life span. Adverse effects primarily occur if too much thyroid is given, resulting in risk of atrial fibrillation, accelerated bone loss, heat intolerance, weight loss, or tremors. Conversely, some women exhibit the latter symptoms because they have thyroid conditions that cause overproduction of endogenous thyroid hormone. *Hyper*thyroidism is treated with thionamides (methimazole or propylthiouracil), drugs that inhibit thyroid synthesis.

Drugs for Diabetes Mellitus

Diabetes is a common endocrine disorder of carbohydrate metabolism that causes sustained high blood glucose levels. If untreated, it can lead to serious, potentially fatal complications, including cardiovascular disease, kidney failure, nerve damage, and blindness. The incidence of type 2 diabetes in women is on the rise, coincident with increases in obesity, sedentary lifestyle, and metabolic syndrome (Beckles & Thompson-Reid, 2001). Diabetes is treated with lifestyle changes along with insulin analogs and oral diabetic drugs (Table 13.2).

Patients with *type 1 diabetes* are usually diagnosed in childhood or adolescence; and because they lack insulin, they require hormone replacement for life. Human insulin and various analogs are either short-acting (insulin, insulin lispro) to treat postmeal spikes in glucose or longer-acting (insulin glargine) to lower basal glucose levels. Insulins must be injected subcutaneously once or multiple times each day; currently available injector pens or continuous infusion pumps offer the most convenient options. Hypoglycemia is the most common and serious side effect of taking insulin.

A unique condition that affects women is *gestational diabetes mellitus,* in which carbohydrate intolerance/insulin resistance occurs for the first time during pregnancy. Pregnancy can also increase the risk of diabetic complications in women who are already diabetic. To protect both mother and baby, it is vitally important to control blood glucose levels during pregnancy, whether the patient has type 1, type 2, or gestational diabetes. Insulin preparations are the traditional treatment during pregnancy. Oral antidiabetic drugs (described below) also are used; metformin, acarbose, and sitagliptin are in FDA Pregnancy Category B, and all others are in Category C. Of the oral agents, metformin and glyburide are most frequently used, although they both cross the placenta and should be used with caution (Paglia & Coustan, 2009).

Type 2, the most common form of diabetes, is typically diagnosed during middle age ("adult-onset diabetes"), but its prevalence is increasing in younger age groups as well. A progressive resistance to insulin occurs in the tissues, and insulin secretion is not inadequate to control blood glucose. Type 2 diabetes is managed with lifestyle modifications, oral antidiabetic agents, and/or insulin. Monotherapy with one drug may be sufficient, but as the disease progresses, use of multiple drugs may be needed to control glucose levels.

Oral antidiabetic drugs can be divided into five classes that act in different ways to lower blood glucose (Table 13.2). *Biguanides*, such as metformin, suppress glucose production and are often used as initial therapy. Unlike many other oral antidiabetics, they do not cause weight gain, which can be a benefit for obese patients. Biguanides also do not cause hypoglycemia. However, gastrointestinal upset is a common side effect that may be managed by adjusting the dosing. Caution is advised for older adults with impaired renal function as metformin can cause lactic acidosis.

Sulfonylureas, such as glipizide, and short-acting *meglitinides*, like repaglinide, are two drug classes that promote insulin release from the pancreas. They are effective in lowering blood glucose, but they may cause weight gain or hypoglycemia. A newer approach for stimulating insulin release is the use of *dipeptidylpeptidase 4 (DPP-4) inhibitors* such as sitagliptin. These drugs enhance the action of incretins, which are peptide hormones released from the GI tract in response to food to stimulate pancreatic insulin secretion. DPP-4 inhibitors help lower blood glucose without causing hypoglycemia and do not cause weight gain.

α-*Glucosidase inhibitors*, such as acarbose, are drugs that delay carbohydrate absorption and are taken with meals. They do not affect weight, but may cause some GI distress. The final drug class of oral antidiabetics is the *thiazolidinediones*, which includes pioglitazone. These drugs are effective in reducing insulin resistance by increasing glucose utilization and reducing glucose production. However, because of side effects such as edema, weight gain, liver problems, and increased risk of congestive heart failure, thiazolidinediones are generally used as adjunct or second-line drug options. Women of childbearing years should be cautioned that thiazolidinediones may increase the chance of pregnancy, since these drugs can induce ovulation as well as reduce the efficacy of contraceptives. Thiazolidinediones also increase the risk of bone fractures in women.

Weight-Loss Drugs

Weight-loss strategies are a frequent concern for women and often involve a combination of diet control and exercise. However, with the alarming rise of obesity and associated disease risks, there is new emphasis on the development of pharmacotherapies for overweight patients. Drug options have been limited, but recently the US FDA approved several new medications for treatment of obesity. Most of the available drugs act to suppress appetite, namely lorcaserin, phendimetrazin, phentermine, and the combination of phentermine/topiramate. These drugs are not recommended for patients with a history of heart attack, stroke, irregular heartbeat, or overactive thyroid. Another option, orlistat, works by blocking fat absorption in the gut. In most studies, women lost about 5% to 10% of their initial body weight over a year on prescription weight-loss drugs, taken in conjunction with a diet and exercise program. Even a 5% to 10% reduction in weight decreases cardiometabolic risk and obesity-related morbidity and mortality (Sweeting, Tabet, Caterson, & Markovic, 2014).

Drugs Affecting Mental Health

Women are twice as likely as men to suffer from depression and anxiety, the two most common mood disorders (King, Johnson, & Gamblian, 2011; Seedat et al., 2009). Women of childbearing age may experience premenstrual mood disorders and/or perinatal depression, which affects about 10% of women in the first postpartum year. Risk of depression also increases at midlife, around the time of menopause. These conditions negatively impact a woman's ability to cope with ordinary events and/or experience pleasure; fortunately, they can be effectively managed using antidepressant and/or anxiolytic drugs. As shown in Figure 13.1, these medications comprise a significant portion of the drugs taken by women aged 18 to 64 years old.

Antidepressants

The most commonly prescribed antidepressants are called "selective serotonin reuptake inhibitors" and include citalopram, escitalopram, fluvoxamine, fluoxetine, paroxetine, and sertraline (Table 13.3). For many women, these medications improve mood with relatively few side effects. Several weeks are usually needed to achieve a positive result, and effectiveness can be enhanced if the drug is combined with counseling or psychotherapy. Each SSRI has a slightly different side-effect profile and elimination half-life. Most of the common adverse effects, such as nausea, headache, jitteriness, dizziness, anhedonia, sweating, or vivid dreams, tend to subside after a few weeks of treatment. Some women experience changes in weight or sexual dysfunction, such as decreases in libido or organisms. If adverse effects persist, a lower dose or an alternative SSRI may be better

TABLE 13.3	CNS Drugs/Pain Medications		
Desired Effect	**Drug Class**	**Examples**	**Side Effects**
Antidepressant	SSRIs	Fluoxetine, sertraline	GI upset
	SNRIs	Venlafaxine, duloxetine	GI, CV effects
	Tricyclics	Imipramine	Sedation, weight gain, CV effects
	MAO inhibitors	Tranylcypromine	Sedation, weight gain, orthostatic hypotension
	Atypical	Bupropion	GI upset
Antianxiety	Benzodiazepines	Alprazolam, lorazepam	Sedation, withdrawal
Induce sleep	Benzodiazepines	Temazepam, triazolam	Habituation, withdrawal
	Nonbenzodiazepines	Zolpidem, eszopiclone	Anterograde amnesia
	Antihistamines	Diphenhydramine	Dry mouth, next-day drowsiness, tolerance
	Melatonin	Ramelteon	
Relieve Pain			
Mild/moderate pain relief	NSAIDs	Aspirin	GI, ulcer, bleeding
		Acetaminophen	
		Ibuprofen	GI distress, ulcer
	COX-2	Celecoxib	CV risk
Moderate/severe pain relief	Opioid narcotics	Codeine	Constipation, nausea, sedation, addiction, dependence
		Morphine	
		Hydrocodone	
Chronic Pain Relief			
Antimigraine	Triptans	Sumatriptan	CV risk
	Antiseizure	Topiramate	Drowsiness, ataxia, paresthesias, weight loss
Relief of neuralgia	Antiseizure	Gabapentin, pregabalin	Drowsiness, blurred vision, edema
	Antidepressant	SNRIs, tricyclics	

GI, gastrointestinal; CV, cardiovascular; SSRI, selective serotonin reuptake inhibitor; SNRI, serotonin–norepinephrine reuptake inhibitor; MAO, monoamine oxidase; NSAID, nonsteroidal anti-inflammatory drug; COX, cyclooxygenase.

tolerated. Discontinuation of these drugs should be done gradually to avoid withdrawal symptoms. All SSRIs are in FDA Pregnancy Category C, except for sertraline (Cat. B) and paroxetine (Cat. D). SSRIs must be used with caution in children, adolescents, and young adults under 25 years, as these drugs may cause a paradoxical increase in suicidal ideation in some younger patients.

Several newer antidepressants affect other monoamine neurotransmitters in addition to serotonin (Table 13.3). Serotonin–norepinephrine reuptake inhibitors (*SNRIs*) include venlafaxine, duloxetine, and desvenlafaxine. These drugs share many similarities with SSRIs. They are more effective for some patients but may also cause additional sides effects, such as dry mouth or elevated blood pressure. SNRIs are classified in FDA Pregnancy Category C, and there is concern that babies delivered to mothers who take SNRIs in the last half of pregnancy may exhibit withdrawal symptoms of difficulty breathing, feeding problems, and tremors. Another drug option is bupropion, known as an *atypical* antidepressant. It has additional effects on dopamine uptake that does not occur with SSRIs and SNRIs. Some women prefer this drug, as it does not cause weight gain or affect sexual desire and may improve attention and alertness. However, bupropion can cause dry mouth, nausea, constipation, insomnia, headache, tremor and, of most concern, seizures. Older types of antidepressants, namely *tricyclic antidepressants and monoamine oxidase inhibitors*, are also used; but they are usually reserved as second-line options for treating depression. The older drugs can be very effective; however, they also have more side effects than SSRIs or SNRIs.

Antianxiety Drugs

Benzodiazepines are the primary class of drugs used for relief of anxiety symptoms, such as those associated with traumatic stress, panic attacks, or depression. Drugs of this class, such as alprazolam, lorazepam, and diazepam all have a similar effect, but they differ in how quickly they work, their duration of action, and other pharmacokinetic properties. The main side effect is drowsiness, and they potentiate the effects of other CNS depressants such as alcohol or barbiturates. Because of the potential for tolerance and withdrawal symptoms, it is recommended that benzodiazepines only be taken on a short-term basis (up to 1 month).

Drugs for Insomnia

Women frequently seek medication for sleeping problems; and in fact, insomnia occurs more often in women than in men. Hormonal changes appear to be a factor, as insomnia is associated with the menstrual cycle, pregnancy, postpartum period, and most commonly, during menopause. Several classes of "sleeping pills" are available (Table 13.3).

Benzodiazepines are commonly prescribed for insomnia, usually at higher doses than those used to treat anxiety. More recently, *nonbenzodiazepines* such as zolpidem, eszopiclone, and zaleplon have been developed to promote sleep. Their mechanism of action is similar to that of benzodiazepines, but they have fewer adverse effects and more desirable pharmacokinetic properties such as quick onset and/or short duration of action to avoid next-day sleepiness. With all of these drugs, tolerance and rebound insomnia can occur with chronic dosing; thus, short-term use is recommended. The shorter-acting drugs, in particular, can also cause anterograde amnesia, a condition in which the person does not remember things that happened after taking the drug. This effect is the basis for abuse of some potent benzodiazepines as "date rape" drugs. Another concern is the increased vulnerability of older women to side effects of sleeping pills such as daytime sedation and confusion. Ataxia and unsteadiness also are more likely and increase the risk of falls and bone fractures. Lower doses of benzodiazepines and nonbenzodiazepines are recommended for older patients.

Antihistamines that cause drowsiness are available as nonprescription sleeping pills. These drugs, however, have a number of adverse effects, and tolerance develops to limit effectiveness. Another treatment option is the use of melatonin, a hormone that is normally produced at night to regulate circadian rhythms. *Melatonin*, or the melatonin-like drug ramelteon, is used to help patients who have difficulty falling asleep or experience insomnia due to jet lag or shifted work schedules.

Drugs to Alleviate Pain

Pain is a common symptom of many conditions, and pain medications are frequently used by women of all ages (Fig. 13.1). Both over-the-counter and prescription drugs are used to relieve acute and chronic types of pain.

Nonsteroidal Anti-inflammatory Drugs for Mild to Moderate Pain

Aspirin and other nonsteroidal anti-inflammatory drugs (NSAIDs), such as ibuprofen, naproxen, and acetaminophen, are widely used for relief from mild to moderate pain. They effectively produce analgesia without causing sedation, loss of consciousness, or dependence. NSAIDs are used for headache, muscle aches, toothache, menstrual cramps, postoperative pain, painful injury, and inflammatory conditions like rheumatoid arthritis or osteoarthritis. They also reduce fever. Doses are lower in over-the-counter preparations as compared with prescription uses, and often NSAIDs are formulated in combination with other types of medications. NSAIDs inhibit the cyclooxygenase enzymes (COX), and most of them act nonselectively on both COX-1 and COX-2 isoforms. Drugs within this class differ somewhat in dosing regimens and side-effect profiles, and responsiveness to a particular drug can vary among individuals. NSAIDs generally have minimal side effects with short-term use. The most common adverse effects are gastrointestinal, such as heartburn, nausea, and gastric distress. Of most concern is the risk of gastric ulceration and bleeding with chronic use.

Several unique properties of individual NSAID drugs should be noted. Aspirin has additional antiplatelet actions that increase the risk of bleeding and may exacerbate a bleeding ulcer or increase menstrual bleeding if taken for dysmenorrhea. Chronic use of high doses of aspirin may cause renal impairment. Acetaminophen is unique in that it primarily acts via the CNS and has no effects on gastric irritation, platelets, or inflammation. However, it may increase hypertension in women and cause liver damage if used chronically at high doses and/or in combination with chronic alcohol consumption. Acetaminophen is considered safe for short-term use during pregnancy and breast-feeding. Other NSAIDs are generally not recommended during pregnancy, and, in particular, are contraindicated during the third trimester.

COX-2 Selective NSAID

Celecoxib is a selective inhibitor of COX-2 that is used to treat mild to moderate pain and inflammation. It was developed to avoid effects on COX-1 located in the gastrointestinal tract and platelets, as inhibition of COX-1 leads to the ulceration and bleeding seen with nonselective NSAIDs. Celecoxib is particularly useful for alleviating pain caused by arthritis (osteoarthritis, rheumatoid arthritis, or juvenile rheumatoid arthritis). It is also used to treat painful menstrual periods and to relieve other types of short-term pain. The most common side effects are diarrhea, bloating, sore throat, and cold-like symptoms. The most serious concern with celecoxib is that it may increase the risk of heart attacks and other adverse cardiovascular events.

Opioid Analgesics for Moderate to Severe Pain

Opioid analgesics, also known as narcotics, are very effective at relieving moderate to severe pain (Table 13.3). Commonly used drugs of this class are morphine, codeine, hydrocodone, oxycodone, propoxyphene, and meperidine. One of the primary indications for opioids is relief from severe *acute* pain following surgery or serious injury. Opioids are also used during childbirth as they suppress pain but do not interfere with a woman's ability to push during labor. Other indications include a variety of *chronic* pain syndromes, such as osteoarthritis and chronic low back pain.

Opioid drugs can be administered by a variety of routes: oral, rectal, parenteral, transdermal, buccal, intranasal, or epidural. There is considerable variation among individuals in both analgesic response and manifestation of side effects. Some of the contributing factors, as discussed above, are genetic differences in drug metabolism and pain sensitivity and sex differences in opioid receptor responses. Available drugs vary in their actions on μ- and κ-opioid receptor subtypes. Morphine, which is selective for μ-receptors, has greater efficacy in women as compared with men (Niesters et al., 2010).

One of the most prevalent and bothersome adverse effects of opioids is constipation. Other common side effects include sedation, nausea, and vomiting. Opioids may interfere with menstruation by limiting the production of luteinizing hormone. When given during labor, opiates cross the placenta and can produce side effects in the baby, such as CNS depression, respiratory depression, impaired early breast-feeding, altered neurological behavior, and decreased ability to regulate body temperature.

With chronic opiate use, tolerance develops to the analgesic effects; and abrupt discontinuation of the drug causes withdrawal symptoms such as diarrhea, nausea, vomiting, muscle pain, anxiety, and irritability. Opioid narcotics also produce a strong sense of euphoria that can lead to addiction. A major concern with opioids is the risk of physical and psychological dependence with prolonged use. Many women treated for chronic pain disorders later become addicted to opiates like hydrocodone and oxycodone. Sometimes, heightened concerns regarding dependence and addiction result in a patient not being prescribed adequate drug for pain management. On the other hand, there is a growing concern about narcotic overdose in women. Women between the ages of 25 and 54 are most likely to be admitted to the emergency room because of narcotic misuse or abuse. Women aged 45 to 54 have the highest risk of dying from an overdose of prescription painkillers (US Centers for Disease Control and Prevention, 2013). The occurrence of overdose in women is increasing at a faster rate than in men (US Centers for Disease Control and Prevention, 2013). A number of factors likely contribute: women are more likely to have chronic pain, be prescribed narcotic analgesics, be given higher doses, and use them for longer periods as compared with men. Women typically have less body mass than men, making it easier to overdose. Thus, it is important to prescribe only the quantity needed for pain relief and monitor the patient for substance abuse and mental health problems.

Drugs for Chronic Pain Syndromes

Certain chronic pain syndromes, such as migraine and fibromyalgia, can be managed with drugs other than opioid narcotics.

Antimigraine Drugs

Migraine headache is a chronic pain syndrome that disproportionately afflicts women (Office on Women's Health, US Department of Health and Human Services, 2012). Women are more frequently affected and tend to have more painful, longer lasting headaches, and more symptoms like nausea and vomiting as compared with men. Ovarian hormones also are a factor; migraine attacks often occur around the time of the menses (menstrual migraine), and they tend to abate after menopause and in the later stages of pregnancy. Migraine is most common in women aged 20 to 45.

There are two types of drug treatment for migraine: acute abortive treatment to treat symptoms when they occur, and preventive treatment to decrease the frequency and severity of attacks (Table 13.3). Milder headaches may be managed with NSAIDs, sometimes combined with caffeine. However, overuse of these drugs can actually cause rebound headaches. The primary prescription remedy for migraine symptoms is a class of drugs known as *triptans*, such as sumatriptan and zolmitriptan. They are not recommended for patients with cardiovascular disease.

A variety of medications may be given on a chronic basis to try to reduce the frequency of migraine attacks; however, none of them affect acute symptoms. Certain antiseizure drugs, such as topiramate, gabapentin, and valproate, are helpful in some patients. Other types of drugs used to prevent migraine are cardiovascular drugs like β-blockers, antidepressants like amitriptyline or venlafaxine, and injections of botulinum toxin (Botox). Hormone therapy may help prevent attacks in some women with menstrual migraine.

Drugs for Chronic Neuropathic Pain

Severe, chronic pain can result from neuropathic conditions caused by diabetes, shingles, fibromyalgia, or a spinal cord injury. These neuralgias can be treated with drugs originally developed for epilepsy or depression. Gabapentin and pregabalin are antiseizure drugs with a unique mode of action that also suppresses nerve pain. Side effects include drowsiness, dizziness, nausea, and difficulty concentrating. Antidepressants, particularly SNRIs and tricyclics, are also useful for reducing neuropathic pain.

Cardiovascular Drugs

To maintain good health, women need to manage their cardiovascular risk factors. Risks of heart disease and stroke are low for young women, but they increase after menopause. In particular, chronic high blood pressure and elevated cholesterol can lead to heart attack, stroke, and other cardiovascular disorders. Both of these risk factors are typically controlled using prescription medications, which increase in use as women age (Fig. 13.1).

Drugs to Lower Blood Pressure

Blood pressure is regulated by controlling blood volume, vascular tone, and cardiac output via neural and hormonal reflexes. Antihypertensive drugs target these various mechanisms, and often drugs of several classes are combined in order to increase effectiveness (Table 13.4). For most patients, antihypertensive drugs must be taken chronically to keep blood pressure in the normal range. However, because patients do not feel symptoms of high blood pressure (the "silent killer") and may also experience drug side effects, adherence to taking their medicine can wane over time, leading to unnecessary disease progression and complications. Feedback from regular blood pressure checks can help motivate the patient.

Diuretics lower blood pressure by decreasing blood volume. These drugs act on the kidney to induce excretion of salt and water. *Thiazides*, such as hydrochlorothiazide, are the

TABLE 13.4	**Cardiovascular Drugs**		
Desired Effect	**Drug Class**	**Examples**	**Side Effects**
Lower blood pressure	Diuretics	Hydrochlorothiazide Furosemide	Hypokalemia, alkalosis
		Spironolactone	Hyperkalemia, acidosis
	ACE inhibitors	Captopril	Cough, hyperkalemia
	ARBs	Losartan	Hyperkalemia
	β-Blockers	Atenolol, metoprolol	Lightheadness, dizziness bradycardia, fatigue
	Calcium channel blockers	Nifedipine	Tachycardia, flushing
		Diltiazem, verapamil	Bradycardia
Lower cholesterol	Statins	Atorvastatin	Muscle pain
Suppress clot formation	Anticoagulants	Warfarin	Bleeding
		Dabigatran	Bleeding, GI distress
	Antiplatelets	Low-dose aspirin	Bleeding, ulcer
		Clopidogrel	Bleeding

ACE, angiotensin-converting enzyme; ARB, angiotensin receptor blocker; GI, gastrointestinal.

initial drug choice for many hypertensive patients. These drugs are cost-effective, well tolerated, and are particularly efficacious in elderly and African American patients. Hydrochlorothiazide is a Pregnancy Category B drug. *Loop diuretics* such as furosemide are more potent diuretics and are usually reserved for patients with more severe hypertension. Both thiazides and loop diuretics can cause hypokalemia and metabolic alkalosis. Sometimes, a *potassium-sparing diuretic*, such as spironolactone, is added to a thiazide drug to prevent hypokalemia.

Drugs that target the *angiotensin* system are effective at lowering blood pressure and generally well tolerated by patients. ACE inhibitors, such as captopril, prevent the formation of angiotensin II, a potent vasoconstrictor, by inhibiting angiotensin-converting enzyme (ACE). Angiotensin receptor blockers (ARBs), such as lorsartan, prevent the action of angiotensin II at its AT_1 receptor. A common side effect of ACE inhibitors is a dry, persistent cough, which can be alleviated by switching to an ARB. Hypotension and dizziness, especially on initial dosing, and hyperkalemia are side effects of ACE inhibitors and ARBs. Both drug classes are contraindicated in pregnancy.

Blood pressure also can be lowered using drugs that inhibit sympathetic nerve action. Antagonists at β-adrenergic receptors, or β *blockers*, are the most common drugs of this type. They decrease heart rate, cardiac output, and renin release via β_1-receptors in the heart and kidney. Drugs specific for the β_1-receptor subtype, such as atenolol and metoprolol, are preferred because they lower blood pressure without affecting β_2-receptors in lungs. Nonselective β_1/β_2 blockers can trigger bronchoconstriction and are contraindicated in asthmatic patients. Side effects of β-blockers include bradycardia, lightheadedness, dizziness, and fatigue. They can also increase blood glucose in diabetics. Certain β-blockers are considered safe during pregnancy, but others such as atenolol are in FDA Pregnancy Category D and should not be used.

Calcium channel blockers are another drug class used to treat hypertension. Often, they are given as a second-line or adjunct medication; however, in African Americans, calcium channel blockers may be more effective than β-blockers, ACE inhibitors, or ARBs (Ferdinand & Armani, 2007). Dihydropyridines, such as nifedipine, are calcium channel blockers that act preferentially to relax blood vessels. Side effects include reflex tachycardia, flushing, and dizziness. Verapamil and diltiazem are two calcium channel blockers of unique structure that have significant effects on the heart and may cause bradycardia.

Drugs to Lower Cholesterol

Elevated blood cholesterol increases the risk of developing heart disease and stroke. In particular, levels of low density lipoprotein (LDL) cholesterol are of most concern. LDL transports cholesterol to the tissues, such as blood vessels where it contributes to atherosclerosis. In contrast, high density lipoprotein (HDL) is protective because it transports cholesterol to the liver to be metabolized. Estrogen increases HDL, which helps lower cholesterol during childbearing years. Women over 55 tend to have higher cholesterol levels and are most likely to receive anticholesterol drugs to lower their risk of cardiovascular disease (Fig. 13.1).

HMG-CoA reductase inhibitors, known as *statins*, are the first-line treatment for lowering levels of LDL (Table 13.4). Examples include atorvastatin, lovastatin, pravastatin, rosuvastatin, and simvastatin. Drug therapy is best combined with a low-fat diet, weight loss, and exercise to achieve normal cholesterol levels. The drugs differ in potency, and individuals show variable responses, in part due to genomic polymorphisms in metabolic enzymes. Common side effects of statins are muscle aches, cramps, soreness, or weakness (myalgia), and GI distress. Females tend to be more at risk for statin side effects. All statins carry a Pregnancy Category X and are contraindicated for women who are pregnant or breast-feeding. There are other drug options for lowering cholesterol. Ezetimibe, a cholesterol absorption inhibitor, and bile acid sequestrants such as cholestryramine decrease cholesterol from the diet. Fibrates and niacin (nicotinic acid) are other drug options used to lower LDL, and they also raise HDL.

Drugs to Prevent Blood Clots

Pathological blood clots, called thrombi, cause life-threatening conditions such as heart attack, stroke, and pulmonary embolism. Women have unique risks for thrombosis during pregnancy and when taking birth control pills or postmenopausal hormone therapy. Women with atrial fibrillation and/or cardiovascular disease have increased risk for ischemic stroke. Anticoagulants and antiplatelet drugs are used to prevent and treat harmful blood clots (Table 13.4). For all of these drugs, the primary adverse effect is increased risk of bruising and bleeding.

Anticoagulants ("blood thinners") include injectable heparins and oral medications like warfarin and the recently approved drugs dabigatran, rivaroxaban, and apixaban. Anticoagulants are used to suppress blood clotting in deep veins of the legs and pelvic area (deep-vein thrombosis). This condition can occur in pregnancy or after prolonged immobilization or surgery and lead to pulmonary embolism. Anticoagulants also inhibit clot formation due to prosthetic heart valves or atrial fibrillation, which is more common in older women. Warfarin is the most commonly used drug of this class. It is taken orally, but has a narrow safety margin and multiple drug interactions that require patients to be monitored on an ongoing basis. Warfarin has teratogenic effects and is contraindicated in pregnancy (Cat. X). Direct thrombin inhibitors, like dabigatran, are a new class of oral anticoagulants. They may cause GI distress (stomach pain, heartburn, and nausea) and increase risk of bleeding; however, they do not require lab monitoring. Dabigatran is classified in Pregnancy Category C. Injectable heparin formulations are another option that can be used safely in pregnancy since these drugs do not cross the placenta.

Antiplatelet drugs such as aspirin and clopidogrel, are used to prevent formation of arterial clots that cause stroke and heart attack (Table 13.4). Aspirin is used in low doses, which are effective for this indication and minimize GI adverse effects. For primary prophylaxis in women at risk, aspirin was found effective for prevention of stroke but not heart attack (Berger et al., 2006). The reverse was true for men. In women over 55, the potential benefit of aspirin to decrease stroke risk is considered to outweigh the risk of GI bleeding (US Preventive Services Task Force, 2009). For secondary prevention, low-dose aspirin is effective following either stroke or heart attack. Clopidogrel is another commonly used antiplatelet drug with less GI side effects than aspirin. Both agents increase risk of bleeding.

GI Disorders/Antiacid Drugs

When gastrointestinal symptoms such as heartburn and abdominal pain are frequent and/or severe, the underlying cause is often dyspepsia, gastroesophageal reflux disease (GERD), or peptic ulcer that requires drug treatment. Women are more at risk for nonulcerative dyspepsia than men, and hormonal fluctuations of the menstrual cycle can make symptoms worse. More than half of all pregnant women experience heartburn. Thus, it is not surprising that drugs to treat acid reflux and peptic ulcer are commonly taken by women of all ages (Fig. 13.1). Over-the-counter antacids are often used to relieve symptoms along with drugs that decrease secretion of gastric acid and help heal an inflamed esophagus or stomach ulcer, *histamine H2 receptor blockers* and *proton pump inhibitors*. These drugs are available over-the-counter in low doses and by prescription for higher doses (Table 13.5). All are considered safe to take during pregnancy, even during the first trimester.

H_2 blockers, such as cimetidine, famotidine, nizatidine, and ranitidine, do not act as quickly as antacids, but they give longer relief from heartburn and are particularly effective when taken prior to a meal. These drugs are well tolerated, and side effects are rare. Proton pump inhibitors, such as omeprazole, lansoprazole, esomeprazole, pantoprazole, and rabeprazole, block acid production for a longer period of time. They work well for heartburn symptoms but also protect damaged esophageal tissue from acid, allowing it to heal. Side effects include headache, diarrhea, abdominal pain, bloating, constipation,

TABLE 13.5	**Gastrointestinal/Allergy/Asthma Drugs**		
Desired Effect	**Drug Class**	**Examples**	**Side Effects**
GI			
Reduce acid	H_2 antagonists	Ranitidine, famotidine	
	Proton pump inhibitors	Omeprazole	Diarrhea, nausea, headache
Antiasthma			
Quick relief to improve breathing	β_2-Agonsts, short-acting	Albuterol (inhaled)	Nervousness, tremor
	Muscarinic antagonists	Ipratropium	Dry mouth, cough
Prevent attacks	Inhaled corticosteroids	Fluticasone, beclomethasone	Thrush, hoarseness
	Long-acting β-agonists	Salmeterol	Nervousness
	Leukotriene inhibitors	Zileuton, montelukast	Headache, heartburn
Antiallergy			
Relieve symptoms	Antihistamines	Fexodfenadine, loratadine, cetirizine	
Emergency treatment	Epinephrine injection	EpiPen	

GI, gastrointestinal.

nausea, and gas. Many ulcers are induced by *H. pylori* infection, and in these cases, a combination of antibiotics and acid-reducing medicines is the most effective treatment.

Drugs for Asthma

Asthma is a chronic condition that affects a significant number of both men and women, but symptoms are often more severe in women, especially during childbearing years. In particular, asthma may worsen during the menstrual period, suggesting an influence of ovarian hormones. Drugs to control asthma are frequently prescribed to women of all ages (Fig. 13.1). These drugs are considered safe to use during pregnancy, and, in fact, it is important for the mother to control asthma attacks to ensure normal breathing and adequate blood oxygenation for her and her baby.

There are two main types of antiasthma drugs (Table 13.5). The first category consists of bronchodilators that are used acutely during an asthma attack to open the airways and improve breathing. These drugs are often referred to as reliever or rescue drugs, and they are given using an inhaler to quickly deliver the drug to the lungs. *Short-acting β2-adrenergic agonists*, such as albuterol and metaproterenol, are the first-line treatment. Drug delivery via inhalation minimizes the risk of systemic side effects, but sometimes, nervousness, tremor, tachycardia, headache, nausea, or dizziness is reported. The other main type of rescue inhalation drug is a *muscarinic antagonist* like ipratropium or tiotropium. These drugs may not be as effective as β_2-agonists for asthma, but they are frequently used to restore breathing in chronic obstructive pulmonary disease (COPD), another respiratory disease that is more likely seen in older patients. Common side effects of the muscarinic antagonists are dry mouth, cough, headache, nausea, and dizziness.

Asthmatics are usually given a second type of drug to take on a chronic basis to prevent recurrent attacks. These prophylaxic drugs are also given for seasonal allergic rhinitis and to prevent exercise-induced bronchospasm. They do not relieve symptoms but chronically suppress inflammation in the lungs and reduce airway sensitivity. *Inhaled corticosteroids*, such as fluticasone, beclomethasone, and budesonide, are commonly prescribed for this purpose. Side effects include oropharyngeal candidiasis (thrush), hoarseness, and throat irritation, but systemic effects of corticosteroids are minimized by using the inhalation route of delivery. A long-acting β-agonist such as salmeterol and formoterol is often given in combination with the inhaled corticosteroid to potentiate the latter drug's effects. Another option for asthma prevention is to use a drug that affects *leukotrienes*, important endogenous mediators of lung inflammation. Zileuton inhibits leukotriene synthesis, while drugs like montelukast and zafirlukast block the leukotriene $CysLT_1$ receptor.

Antiallergy

Antiallergy medication is the final class of drugs that is indicated in Figure 13.1 as commonly prescribed for women. These drugs are available in both over-the-counter and prescription forms. Histamine is the cause of the majority of symptoms associated with an allergic reaction, such as nasal congestion, irritated eyes, skin rash and itching, bronchoconstriction, and stomach cramps. *Histamine H1 receptor antagonists* are used to block histamine's actions. Second-generation antihistamines such as fexodfenadine, loratadine, and cetirizine are preferred because they have highly selective actions and are nonsedating. Side effects of the second-generation antihistamines include photosensitivity, tachycardia, and prolongation of the QT interval. Loratadine and cetirizine are classified in FDA Pregnancy Category B; fexofenidine is in Category C.

An extremely severe allergic reaction is called anaphylaxis. Although rare, if not treated quickly, anaphylaxis can cause very serious health concerns and even death. *Epinephrine* injections are used to counter these symptoms. Patients at risk should have this drug available for emergency use. Autoinjectors such as the EpiPen are convenient for this purpose.

Conclusion

Prescription medications have a significant role in helping women maintain good health and well-being over their life span. This chapter briefly covers examples of the drugs that are most commonly used by women. Drug treatment of women presents unique concerns and complexities, depending on factors such as age, hormonal and reproductive status, and genetics. As discussed here, there is a growing appreciation of differences and issues that must be considered in optimizing the use of medications in women. As this trend continues in the future, all women will benefit from greater understanding and attention to women's needs with respect to drug therapy.

References

Almandoz, J. P., & Gharib, H. (2012). Hypothyroidism: Etiology, diagnosis, and management. *Endocrinology and Metabolism Clinics of North America, 96*, 203–221.

Anthony, M. (2005). Male/female differences in pharmacology: Safety issues with QT-prolonging drugs. *Journal of Women's Health, 14*, 47–52.

Baggio, G., Corsini, A., Floreani, A., Giannini. S., & Zagonel, V. (2013). Gender medicine: A task for the third millennium. *Clinical Chemistry and Laboratory Medicine, 51*, 713–727.

Beckles, G. L. A., & Thompson-Reid, P. E. (Eds.). (2001). *Diabetes and women's health across the life stages: A public health perspective.* Atlanta, GA: US Department of Health and Human Services, Centers for Disease Control and Prevention, National Center for Chronic Disease Prevention and Health Promotion, Division of Diabetes Translation.

Berger, J. S., Roncaglioni, M. C., Avanzini, F., Pangrazzi, I., Tognoni, G., & Brown, D. L. (2006). Aspirin for the primary prevention of cardiovascular events in women and men: A sex-specific meta-analysis of randomized controlled trials. *Journal of the American Medical Association, 295*, 306–313.

Chen, W. Y. (2011). Postmenopausal hormone therapy and breast cancer risk: Current status and unanswered questions. *Endocrinology and Metabolism Clinics of North America, 40*, 509–518.

Cummings, S. R., Eckert, S., Krueger, K. A., Grady, D., Powles, T. J., Jane A., … Jordan, V. C. (1999). The effect of raloxifene on risk of breast cancer in postmenopausal women. Results from the MORE randomized trial. *Journal of the American Medical Association, 281*, 2189–2197.

Ferdinand, K. C., & Armani, A. M. (2007). The management of hypertension in African Americans. *Critical Pathways in Cardiology, 6*, 67–71.

Howard, B. V., & Rossouw, J. E. (2013). Estrogens and cardiovascular disease risk revisited: The Women's Health Initiative. *Current Opinion Lipidology, 24*, 493–499.

Ingelman-Sundberg, M., Sim, S. C., Gomez, A., & Rodriguez-Antona, C. (2007). Influence of cytochrome P450 polymorphisms on drug therapies: Pharmacogenetic, pharmacoepigenetic and clinical aspects. *Pharmacology & Therapeutics, 116*, 496–526.

Isoherranen, N., & Thummel, K. E. (2013). Drug metabolism and transport during pregnancy: How does drug disposition change during pregnancy and what are the mechanisms that cause such changes? *Drug Metabolism and Deposition, 41*, 256–262.

King, T. L., & Brucker, M. C. (Eds.). (2011). *Pharmacology for women's health.* Sudbury, MA: Jones & Bartlett.

King, T. L., Johnson, R., & Gamblian, V. (2011). Mental health. In T. L. King & M. C. Brucker (Eds.), *Pharmacology for women's health* (pp. 750–791). Sudbury, MA: Jones & Bartlett.

Koren, G., Cairns, J., Chitayat, D., Gaedigk, A., & Leder, S. I. (2006). Pharmacogenetics of morphine poisoning in a breast-fed neonate of a codeine-prescribed mother. *Lancet, 368*, 704.

Merkatz, R. B., Temple, R., Sobel, S., Feiden, K., Kessler, D., & the Working Group on Women in Clinical Trials. (1993). Women in clinical trials of new drugs: A change in Food and Drug Administration policy. *New England Journal of Medicine, 329*, 292–296.

Mitchell, D. (2012). *The women's pill book: Your complete guide to prescription and over-the-counter medications.* New York, NY: St. Martin's Press.

Miller, P. D., & Derman, R. J. (2010). What is the best balance of benefit and risks among anti-resorptive therapies for postmenopausal osteoporosis? *Osteoporosis International, 21*, 1793–1802.

Niesters, M., Dahan, A., Kest, B., Zacny J., Stijnen, T., Aarts, L, & Sarton, E. (2010). Do sex differences exist in opioid analgesia? A systemic review and meta-analysis of human experimental and clinical studies. *Pain, 151*, 61–68.

Office on Women's Health, US Department of Health and Human Services. (2012). Migraine fact sheet. Retrieved from http://www.womenshealth.gov/publications/our-publications/fact-sheet/migraine.html

Paglia, M. J., & Coustan, D. R. (2009). The use of oral antidiabetic medications in gestational diabetes mellitus. *Current Diabetes Reports, 9*, 287–290.

Reidl, M. A., & Casillas, A. M. (2003). Adverse drug reactions: Types and treatment options. *American Family Physician, 68*, 1781–1790.

Rossouw, J. E., Anderson, G. L., Prentice, R. L., LaCroix, A. Z., Kooperberg, C., Stefanick, M. L., … Writing Group for the Women's Health Initiative Investigators. (2002). Risks and benefits of estrogen plus progestin in healthy postmenopausal women: Principal results from the Women's Health Initiative randomized controlled trial. *Journal of the American Medical Association, 288*, 321–333.

Seedat, S., Scott, K. M., Angermeyer, M. C., Berglund, P., Bromet, E. J., Brugha, T. S., … Kessler, R. C. (2009). Cross-national associations between gender and mental disorders in the World Health Organization World Mental Health Surveys. *Archives of General Psychiatry, 66*, 785–795.

Sim, S. C., Kacevska, M., & Ingelman-Sundberg, M. (2013). Pharmacogenomics of drug-metabolizing enzymes: A recent update on clinical implications and endogenous effects. *Pharmacogenomics Journal, 13*, 1–11.

Spoletini, I., Vitale, C., Malorni, W., & Rosano, G. M. C. (2012). Sex differences in drug effects: Interaction with sex hormones in adult life. In V. Regitz-Zagrosek (Ed.), *Sex and gender differences in pharmacology, handbook of experimental pharmacology* (Vol. 214, pp. 91–105). Berlin, Germany: Springer-Verlag.

Sweeting, A. N., Tabet, E., Caterson, I. D., & Markovic, T. P. (2014). Management of obesity and cardiometabolic risk—Role of phentermine/extended release topiramate. *Diabetes Metabolic Syndrome and Obesity, 12*, 35–44.

US Centers for Disease Control and Prevention. (2013, July 2). Prescription painkiller overdoses: A growing epidemic, especially among women. Retrieved from http://www.cdc.gov/vitalsigns/PrescriptionPainkillerOverdoses/index.html

US National Center for Health Statistics. (2013). *Health, United States, 2012: With special feature on emergency care.* Hyattsville, MD: Author.

US Preventive Services Task Force. (2009). Aspirin for the prevention of cardiovascular disease. US Preventive Services Task Force recommendation statement. *Annals of Internal Medicine 150*, 396–404.

Yang, P. C., & Clancy, C. E. (2012). In silico prediction of sex-based differences in human susceptibility to cardiac ventricular tachyarrhythmias. *Frontiers in Physiology, 3*, 360.

14

Healing Arts: Movement in the Form of Pilates

Diane Diefenderfer

Introduction

The human body and its capacity for movement is a key aspect of health and wellness. From the time we are children, we bend and stretch, stoop and twist, jump and run, all without much thought or concern about body mechanics or kinesthetic awareness. We may be fortunate to enjoy this uninhibited freedom of movement throughout our lifetime, appreciating our physical being for the divine mechanism it truly is. Others may experience various health issues and life circumstances making even the simplest everyday tasks painful or debilitating. From one end of the spectrum to the other, whether fit as a fiddle or feeling creaky upon arising from bed each morning, women can learn to appreciate their bodies at any age, shape, or physical limitations. One particular way to do so is by learning to discover the body from the inside out. The "healing arts" refers to dance therapy, music therapy, and art therapy. Within these broader categories are many specific therapies. This chapter presents one example of a "healing art," in this case the Pilates Method of body contrology, including the history of Pilates and the experience of the author, as both a student and a teacher of Pilates in embracing it as a healing art. The importance of understanding and practicing correct breathing techniques, finding a strong abdominal center, and achieving healthy alignment and posture will be emphasized. Finally, as the body, mind, and spirit are interconnected, the joy of movement may be discovered, ultimately becoming a healing art.

Background/Literature on Pilates

As a long-time practitioner of Pilates as well as a teacher of the Method, I have witnessed and experienced the benefits of Pilates as one specific exercise/modality. The scientific literature confirms these benefits; however, one must be cautious with the findings because such literature is scant, supporting the need for further rigorous research in this area. Bernardo (2007) conducted a critical review of the scientific literature, finding 277 articles, 39 of which were published in refereed journals, with 3 of those being quasi-experimental designs. Findings, while providing support for Pilates as an effective way to improve flexibility, abdominal and lumbo-pelvic stability, and muscular activity, also indicate the need for additional research that incorporates an experimental design and that clearly defines the Pilates Method. Caldwell, Harrison, Adams, and Triplett (2009) found that college-age students who completed a semester of regular Pilates training experienced improved self-efficacy and mood state, with a trend toward improved sleep quality as well. An observational, prospective study of 47 adults, 45 of whom were women, indicated that Pilates is correlated with increased flexibility (Segal, Hein, & Basford, 2004). These authors found that it was challenging to establish findings of improved body composition, health status, and posture, but they suggest that further focused study with larger samples and appropriate control groups is needed. A group of adults with chronic low back pain who participated in a program of Pilates focused on core stability, experienced decreased back pain after 6 weeks of the program (Gladwell, Head, Haggar, & Beneke, 2006). Jago, Jonker, Missaghian, and Baranowski (2006) conducted a small clinical trial of 11-year-old girls, with those in the Pilates group experiencing improved body composition as measured by a decrease in BMI after 4 weeks, indicating that there may be evidence that Pilates is effective in contributing to managing obesity. A more recent experimental design study (Kloubec, 2010) revealed that Pilates led to improvement in abdominal endurance, hamstring flexibility, and upper body muscular endurance.

How do I look? How do I feel? How often do women ask themselves these questions on a daily basis throughout their lifetimes? What are women most concerned with? Do women imagine what others see when they look at them? To what extent does this affect how they feel about themselves? And do women's feelings about appearance relate to how they feel physically? Does a woman's actual physical condition influence (or even create) her body image? Ask a female teenager how important looking good/feeling good is to her, and it is likely that appearance is foremost in important factors. When presenting the same question to a woman who has struggled with illness, injury, or physical disabilities, her primary concern is undoubtedly the desire to be pain-free, healthy, and alive. Thus, women's own sense of wellness is relative to how they feel physically as well as the value they place on their appearance but more importantly their ability to embrace all that their bodies offer.

Through the Pilates Method of exercise, body conditioning, and mindful movement, women have become knowledgeable about the complexities of the human body, finding joy and fascination in functional, and at times, even beautiful movement. Popular media often emphasizes the importance of achieving a beautifully toned and conditioned body as a link to confidence and self-esteem. This desire to look good, even great, drives many women to the gym, studio, and track in an effort to improve their outward physical appearance. Beyond physical appearance, the benefits of exercise are significant, including stress reduction, weight maintenance, and boosting immunity even when the initial motivation is directed toward other goals. The alleviation of stress and anxiety may be achieved through some kinds of exercise, particularly cardiovascular activity, as stated by Michael Otto, PhD, coauthor of *Exercise for Mood and Anxiety* (cited in Girdwain, 2013, p. 47), "A proven way to ease anxiety naturally is with a bout of cardio." Exercise may also improve one's moods to actually increase happiness. Researcher Sonja Lyubomirsky, and author of *The How of Happiness: A Scientific Approach to Getting the Life You Want*, states that "Exercise may well be the most effective instant happiness booster of all activities" (cited in Monroe, 2012, p. 47). There are many reports on the positive physical and emotional aspects of health. Art Weltman, PhD, and director of exercise physiology, University of Virginia, states, "Fast-paced walking, when combined with healthy eating, is hugely effective for weight loss" (cited in Everett, 2013, p. 37). Additionally, exercise is a great builder for our immune system according to David Katz, MD, founding director of the Yale University Prevention Research Center, who said, "When it comes to preventing health problems, exercise is one of the best medicines we have" (cited in Girdwain, 2013, p. 47).

Women are finding that many forms of healing arts lead to elevation in mood and improved physical well-being. Yoga, Tai Chi, Gyrokinesis, and Zumba dance are but a few examples of these forms of exercise. From a women's wellness perspective, however, it is important to understand how to encourage women to engage in these various healing arts. A key question is to understand why some women find it difficult to do so. Stress, age, bad habits, old injuries, lack of motivation, low self-esteem, to name some examples, all can contribute to poor physical health and, paradoxically, often make it difficult for women to begin a program of healing arts. Women with chronic back pain find it difficult to perform even the simplest day-to-day tasks such as standing, doing daily chores, or everyday activities. Others have hip, knee, or shoulder pain from years of sports activities, long since abandoned. Some are still valiantly attempting to participate in a physical activity that they typically enjoy, yet their pain, lack of mobility, and even fear of injury hold them back. The once pleasurable becomes the impossible. Many women have undergone joint replacement and simply want to return to normal daily function. Then there are those who have suffered with the challenges of various cancers or other health conditions. These women represent many other women who would benefit from practicing Pilates. The next section is presented from a very personal perspective of the author, who discovered Pilates after being engaged in dance, finding Pilates to be uniquely helpful, which led her to bring Pilates to others as a healing art.

"The benefits (of Pilates) span a decade and a half and have helped me overcome fourteen months of surgeries and chemotherapy to treat my ovarian cancer. They also help me cope with the aches and pains of an aging body. My body is healthy now. I am cancer-free, strong and flexible. And at the age of 65, I am still able to lead an active and productive life" (Donna T).

The Pilates Method

I first discovered the Pilates Method in 1978 while dancing with the Los Angeles Ballet. Or rather, it found me! Two teachers from The Ron Fletcher Studio for Body Contrology, Diane Severino and Michael Podwal, came to the ballet company to assist with rehearsals of a new modern dance piece, something a bit foreign for us classically trained ballet dancers. Their mission was to teach us efficient use of our abdominals, contractions and release, spinal articulation, and fundamentals of core control. This all seemed very odd to me as did dancing barefoot rather than in pointe shoes! After a few rehearsals, Diane and Michael invited me to come to their studio, free of charge, to experience the Pilates Method. Being somewhat curious and eager to attempt anything that might improve my dance technique, I bravely set out to give this Pilates "thing" a try.

I'll never forget the first time I walked into that studio. There were the most unusual-looking contraptions spaced about the room: horizontal sliding apparatus with ropes, springs and bars, a taller four-poster type "bed" resembling some kind of medieval torture rack, and a metal device that not only looked like a guillotine but, as I later learned, was named so as well! In one corner was the "Electric Chair!" There were other pieces of unique equipment, including small and large barrels, rings, and even simple mats on the floor. I wondered exactly how any of this would relate to my work as a dancer and what on earth had I gotten myself into? There were about four or five clients and two instructors, and no one looked like they were suffering. Instead, I noticed the quiet intensity and focus of the students and the calm, encouraging directions given by the teachers. No music accompanied this program. In its place was the steady cadence of deep breathing, sometimes brisk and percussive, other times so slow and rich that I wondered at the possibility of how far the lungs could stretch.

History of the Pilates Method: Joseph Pilates

Joseph Hubertus Pilates was born near Düsseldorf, Germany, in 1880. As a sickly, frail youth, he was determined to overcome his weaknesses by engaging in bodybuilding, gymnastics, diving, and skiing. He was so successful that he became a model for anatomy charts. Moving to England in 1912, Pilates found work as a boxer and circus performer as well as an instructor in self-defense. While interned with other German nationals at the outbreak of World War I, he began teaching his fellow inmates about health and fitness as well as bodybuilding. He later claimed that because of his regimen, none of the internees succumbed to the influenza epidemic that killed thousands in 1918 (Friedman & Eisen, 1980, p. 9). After emigrating to the United States in 1926, Joseph Pilates, along with his wife Clara, opened a studio in New York City and began teaching his method of body contrology. He wrote in *Return to Life,*

> Contrology is complete coordination of body, mind and spirit. Through Contrology you first purposefully acquire complete control of your own body and then through proper repetition of its exercises you gradually and progressively acquire that natural rhythm and coordination associated with all your subconscious activities. (Pilates & Miller, 1945, p. 5)

Pilates was truly ahead of his time in his belief in mind–body fitness, a term so frequently used today. He sought to teach his students to become kinesthetically aware with the mind and body functioning as a unified entity. He went on to state, "Contrology develops the body uniformly, corrects wrong postures, restores physical vitality, invigorates the mind and elevates the spirit" (Pilates & Miller, 1945, p. 5).

Sounds great! Is this possible, and if so, how is this achieved? Can anyone learn this method? Is it simple or complicated, attainable for the average individual, a miracle? Many people went to the original Pilates studio for help. Movie stars such as Katherine Hepburn, Lauren Bacall and Jill Clayburgh, opera star Roberta Peters, and socialites such as Gloria Vanderbilt and Peggy Guggenheim regularly came to Joe's studio. George Balanchine, director of the New York City Ballet, and Martha Graham, modern dance pioneer, sent their dancers to Pilates. Legendary dancer Jacques D'Amboise became a devotee, claiming,

> The Pilates Method makes me feel exhilarated and absolutely wonderful. The exercises are excellent for strengthening and stretching the entire body, especially the lower abdomen and back. If all people did the Pilates Method there would be a good deal less back trouble. (Friedman & Eisen, 1980, p. 2)

Ordinary folks were regulars as well; Joe and his wife Clara would work with anyone who walked through the door. Two of his early students, Ron Fletcher (1921–2011) and Romana Kryzanowska (1923–2013), who would later become my teachers, were among a very few who would carry on Joe's work after his death in 1967.

Fundamentals of the Pilates Method

Joseph Pilates designed his method based on six fundamental principles, each an integral part of the complete program, interrelated and essential to the successful practice of the work. These six principles are (1) concentration, (2) control, (3) centering, (4) precision, (5) fluid movement, and (6) breath.

Complete mental *concentration* is imperative while practicing the Pilates Method to ensure every attention to detail is realized, as the entire body is fully involved. From the beginning focus of an exercise, through the preparatory position, to the full execution of the movement, *control* is vital. Without proper control, injury and poor habits can occur. Pilates believed in complete control of the mind over the body. He often referred to a quote from Friedrich von Schiller, German poet and philosopher, "It is the mind (Geist) [in German] itself which builds the body" (Friedman & Eisen, 1980, p. 7). *Centering* in the Pilates Method refers to control emanating from the abdominal area, perhaps one of the most important of the fundamentals to ensure proper support for the entire body. Ron Fletcher referred to this area as the "girdle of strength," necessary for the body to move with energy, balance, and power. *Precision* is critical as every movement in the Pilates Method is to be performed with a detailed specificity, refined and beautiful in its execution, rather than haphazard or meaningless. *Fluid movement* requires strength and control coming from a firm center, with even pacing and clear articulation. *Breath* is an integral component of the Pilates Method, vital to life yet often not given the full focus it deserves. As Joe Pilates so simply stated, "Breathing is the first act of life and the last" (Pilates & Miller, 1945, p. 9). Something to think about! He continued, "To breathe correctly you must completely exhale and inhale, always trying very hard to 'squeeze' every atom of impure air from your lungs in much the same manner that you would wring every drop of water from a wet cloth" (Pilates & Miller, 1945, p. 9). And as Joe would implore his students and later my teachers, Ron Fletcher and Romana Kryzanowska, "You must OUT the air to IN the air!"

New Beginning

In my first hour of Pilates instruction, I learned about the importance of breath, correct use of the abdominals, spinal articulation, and alignment. Beginning with breath, not only had it never been discussed in ballet school, I had never given it any real thought except during those awkward times on stage when I found myself out of it! I thought I had strong abdominals because my belly was flat (I was fortunately rather skinny), and I didn't think engaging my center had that much to do with dancing. I knew I had nice posture from ballet training, but what did spinal articulation really mean anyway? As for working toward optimal alignment, why was it so crucial to work in parallel when, after all, I was a ballerina who only needed to be "turned-out"?

Though I was a dutiful student and respectful of my teachers, I only halfheartedly appreciated the Pilates work in the beginning. While I certainly was humbled by my obvious lack of abdominal control and naiveté concerning alignment, I didn't really begin to appreciate the method until after my first knee surgery. Owing to the rigors of classical ballet, combined with the natural bow I had in my legs, not yet corrected by Pilates, I found myself with a torn meniscus. Only surgery could repair the problem, and the arthroscopic procedure was not particularly invasive. Weeks of conventional physical therapy were certainly beneficial, yet I became rather panicked that while the post-op treatment was good for the knee, the rest of my body was falling apart. How would I return to dance? Could I get back what I had lost in those 6 to 8 weeks? Had I taken my body for granted? In my opinion, injury and illness surely can be a great motivator to work toward rehabilitation and wellness, and I found myself eager to learn all I could and practice the Pilates Method.

First I had to learn how to breathe. Beyond the obvious fact that **breath** is vital to life, I had never given much thought to the benefits of focused, rich breathing. With each full inhalation, oxygen is sent into the bloodstream to fuel the body and nourish the cells. Taking deep breaths may help reduce stress and tension as well as calm the nerves (in my case, prior to going on stage). The breath in the Pilates Method sets the tempo for the exercises, much like a metronome keeps the pace for a musician—it becomes the music for the movement. When utilizing a percussive breath pattern, along with conscious control of one's center, the abdominals become involved, movement is coordinated, and the body naturally warms up. Ron Fletcher would implore his students not to be stingy breathers....I surely didn't want to be one of those! Instead, what I began to experience was the wonderful sensation of stretching my lungs, like muscles, filling them with fresh air, and expanding my thoracic muscles, followed by the thorough emptying of the lungs with a continuous and complete exhalation. At first, I became light-headed, much like the experience of blowing out too many candles on a birthday cake, but was really the natural result of all that pure oxygen coursing through my bloodstream and entering my brain. Bit by bit, I found it unnatural *not* to keep a steady breath pattern during my Pilates practice. I was able to relax and experience a natural flow of movement throughout even the most challenging exercise sequences.

Abdominal awareness? My center? I had no idea how much there was to learn and improve upon. When asked to pull my navel to my spine and elongate my back in a supine position on the mat or Pilates apparatus, I found it nearly impossible to do so. My back swayed, my ribs flared upward and outward, and I had little to no pelvic stability. Sure, I could kick my legs up high and leap about the ballet studio, but maybe this weakness had something to do with inadequate balance, stability, and control? My teachers patiently explained to me how movements that emanate from a strong center could be more graceful and fluid, at the same time being less likely to cause imbalances and injury. They guided me through the simplest of exercises to help me discover how my abdominals supported my back and stabilized my pelvis. I was taught how to use my breath, fully inhaling and exhaling to initiate movement, maintain fluidity, and aid in recruiting my deepest abdominals. In time, the exercises intensified, I became stronger, and my flat stomach was now not only firm but also provided a wonderful connection to my low back. This newfound sense of power and strength resulted in a freedom of movement I had never before realized.

Articulation of the spine was yet another new concept for me, and while I had flexed, extended, twisted, and rotated my spine as a human as well as a dancer, I had little appreciation of how important a healthy, well-functioning spine really could be. When first asked to sit on a mat on the floor and slowly roll through my spine, one vertebra at a time until I lay flat, I found myself lowering in large segments, not very smoothly and not even arriving in a straight line. To reverse the process was even more difficult, a result of weak abdominals and lack of musculoskeletal connectivity. It seemed I couldn't successfully articulate my spine until I achieved abdominal awareness and strength. Again, time, patience, and encouragement from my teachers made all the difference. I loved hearing Ron say (when rolling down through the spine), "think of your spine like a strand of pearls and slowly and deliberately lay one beautiful pearl down, then the next one, then the next...." I couldn't not use my abdominals! I also learned how to correct slight postural faults, lengthening my entire spine, avoiding both an excessive lordotic curve as well as a "tucked" pelvis. Using my abdominals, standing straighter and taller, lifting my ribs away from my hips, helped create space between the vertebral discs, which reduced pressure on the spine. Not only did my spine feel fantastic, my flexibility improved, I felt a wonderful sense of complete centering and control, *and* to this day, my back has remained injury free.

> The art of Contrology proves that the only real guide to your true age lies not in years or how you think you feel but as you actually are as infallibly indicated by the degree of natural and normal flexibility enjoyed by your spine throughout life. If your spine is inflexibly stiff at 30, you are old; if it is completely flexible at 60, you are young. (Pilates & Miller, 1945, p. 12)

As I faced the mirror in the studio, standing with my feet and legs hip width apart, I noticed how bowed my legs really were. My **alignment** needed some work! Without engaging the correct muscles, my knees failed to "track" or align correctly over my toes when bending my knees. This misalignment, compounded by the balletic demands of external rotation or "turn-out" plus years of jumping and landing, twisting and turning, had taken its toll. It was no wonder I had knee problems. With painstaking practice and attention to detail, my teachers and I worked diligently to retrain the muscles necessary to maintain proper alignment of my legs throughout full range of motion. Primarily utilizing the Universal Reformer apparatus, in a supine position and using spring resistance, I performed multiple sequences of bending and extending my legs, simulating the plie movement essential to dance. At first, I worked only in a parallel position, using both legs and then one leg at a time to notice irregularities. There were several. It seemed I had been favoring my stronger side, only to place more demands on that leg to the detriment of both. I learned to properly engage external rotators and adductors to bring my legs into a more truly parallel stance. Much work was needed to strengthen my vastus medialis obliques (VMO) to protect the entire knee joint. Also important was the correct firing of the gluteus muscles, not to the point of gripping and tucking the pelvis but while maintaining a neutral pelvis connected to a strong abdominal center. This method of regaining strength and proper alignment, while working around my knee injury, was significant to me as a dancer. Dr. James G. Garrick, Orthopedic Surgeon, St. Francis Hospital, San Francisco, stated, "The exercises allow you to strengthen movements that you're going to use in life, whether that life is being on a ballet stage or carrying groceries to your car" (as cited in Gavenas, 1992, p. 104).

The beautiful thing about the entire process was that I learned I had control over my body and the infinite manner in which I could use it as a means of artistic expression. I successfully resumed my dancing career with a newfound joy and confidence. Upon retiring many years later, I chose to share the benefits of the Pilates Method and healthy movement practices with other women, enabling them to feel strong and confident in body, mind, and spirit.

Inspiration

"What I love about my Pilates experience is that, even after 4 years as a student, I am still learning. A tiny adjustment in my form can mean the difference between just doing an exercise and controlling an exercise. My instructor knows the body thoroughly and has guided me to a stronger core, a straighter posture, and an awareness of my muscles that

I never had. I finish each workout feeling strengthened and toned, yet with a sense of relaxation and well-being. Pilates will be with me for life" (Beth H).

I am challenged, delighted, and *inspired* each and every day by the women I teach who are mindful movers, thoughtful and intelligent, and far more interested in how they feel and move than in their outward physical appearance. These women, no matter their age, shape, or physical limitations, seek their own optimal fitness: of the body, mind, and spirit. They want to stand tall with beautiful posture and carriage, conveying the grace and elegance that comes with inner strength and confidence. Rather than a workout of mindless repetitions or forcing the body into unnatural positions, the emphasis is to make the conditioning and Pilates practice an artful movement experience. As my mentor Ron Fletcher so eloquently stated,

> Every body is beautiful. Every body is divinely inspired, superbly designed, awesome in the complex way it's put together and wonderful in the simple, economical way it works. Every body can be vital, strong and flexible, moving through life with grace and assurance, totally healthy—not just some of the time but most of the time. Every body can be improved, inside and outside, because the body potential is hardly ever realized. (Fletcher, 1978, p. 17)

Over a period of many years of study and continued practice, I learned from Ron Fletcher hundreds of Pilates exercises, on the floor and on various apparatus, original work he learned from Joe and Clara, as well as multiple variations and modifications. More importantly, he emphasized quality, refinement, and detail, never just going through the motions of an exercise. He was relentless, in the best possible way, in his quest to find meaning and joy in each and every movement. It is his legacy, originated from his work with Joseph Pilates, that I strive to share with others. Let us go forward to experience the same....

Experiencing Movement Fundamentals

Let's Breathe!!!

There are various ways to bring air in and out of the lungs, including inhaling and exhaling through the nose, mouth, or variations on both, and while other activities and disciplines may call for different techniques, in the Pilates Method, we consistently focus on inhaling through the nose and exhaling through the mouth. It's difficult to fill the lungs while in a slumped or slouched position, so now is the time to bring good posture into the picture (and more on that in a bit). Stand up tall, feet and legs parallel, hip width apart, arms relaxed down at your sides (if necessary for support, you may sit at the forward edge of a firm chair, knees bent and feet comfortably on the floor, hands relaxed on your lap). Begin simply by taking a full breath in through your nose, feeling the sensation of the lungs expanding in three directions: forward, out to the sides, and into your back, then exhaling with slightly pursed lips, slowly and thoroughly emptying the lungs of carbon dioxide. A helpful image is to picture your lungs functioning like a bellows used to fuel a fire with oxygen; the flexible sides of the chamber, your lungs, expand to draw air in, then compress to force the air out. Continue with your breathing, imagining how full and then how empty you can make those two sacs. To better understand the function of the rib cage and thoracic muscles during this breathing process, place your hands on your ribcage with fingertips just beneath your sternum. As you take a deep breath, notice how your fingers and hands open and separate much like the ribs expanding, making room for the lungs to fill. As you exhale, the fingers close together as the ribcage narrows once again around the now empty lungs. Continue breathing deeply and perhaps more slowly, completely filling your lungs and then thoroughly emptying them each time. As quoted earlier, "out the air to in the air," Joseph Pilates taught that the lungs must be completely empty before fresh, new air can be brought in. At this point, the student (you) may feel a bit light-headed, like you have just blown up a very large balloon. Good for you! You are feeling the wonderful results of forcing all that oxygen into your body, nourishing the cells, creating energy and vitality.

The breath in the Pilates Method is directly related to the flow and tempo of the movements; sometimes deep, luxurious breathing will accompany an exercise performed slowly and with the utmost control. Other times, movement patterns may be swift with breathing to match, inhaling and exhaling quickly and more forcefully. Percussive breathing is a related technique incorporating beat, sound, and a good dose of mental concentration. We'll practice bringing air into the lungs in two parts or halves to make a full dose, and then exhale in two parts until empty...in, in, out, out. The inhalation sound will be similar to a quiet sniff, sniff, and the exhale a shush, shush. Continuing with a steady percussive beat as though keeping time with a metronome or tick tock of a clock, breathing in, in, out, out, in, in, out, out...inhale/inhale (your lungs are full) exhale/exhale (your lungs are empty)...sniff, sniff, shush, shush, sniff, sniff, shush, shush...continue for 10 full sets. You may now certainly feel a bit light-headed, and perhaps a little silly making all this noise and *thinking* so much about breathing. I know I did in the beginning, yet I was also aware of fully oxygenating my entire being for the first time. I think the fantastic thing is that while focusing on my breath, timing, coordination, and expansion and contraction of my lungs and ribs and thoracic muscles, I had little time to think or worry about anything else. Hopefully, you too will experience how breath in itself can be a full mind–body experience, helping with focus on the here and now.

If you wish to challenge your mind/body/breath to focus a bit deeper, you may try a longer breath pattern. Instead of taking one full inhalation in two parts, you can try three, then four, and even five. Let's try the four-part breath...in, in, in, in....out, out, out, out...10 times. You may wish to picture your lungs filling in fourths—one quarter of air in, then another to make a half, three quarters, finally four quarters, and your lungs are full. Now empty in fourths, exhaling in the same pattern as you inhaled. It takes practice, control, and concentration to not gulp all the air in at one time, rather filling those two chambers, sacs, balloons, however you like to picture your lungs, in increments of four. Inhale two, three, four, exhale two, three, four...keep going and enjoy the command of controlled, focused rich breathing. Remember to keep the steady beat!

I walk a lot and often practice timing my steps with my breath, keeping a steady cadence and rhythm, often challenging myself to see how deeply I can breathe in and then how long it takes to fully exhale. I may inhale for 4 counts as I take 4 steps and exhale for 8, or even inhale for 5 and exhale for 10 with a corresponding stride. Before I know it, I've walked quite a long way and found the experience relaxing and invigorating at the same time. However you chose to experience this Pilates style breathing, I hope you will appreciate the idea of exercising your lungs, the sensation and awareness of oxygenating your entire system, and the mind, body, breath connection.

Finding Your Center/Abdominal Connectivity

With all of that conscious breathing, you may have already become aware of your abdominal area. Great! We most definitely want to make the connection. In the Pilates Method, the center is described as the area of the body that forms a continuous band, front and back, from the bottom of the rib cage to the line across the hipbones (Friedman & Eisen, 1980, p. 15). Rather than going into anatomical detail (rectus abdominus, internal and external obliques, and transverse abdominus), we can think of our center as the commonly named "abs," belly, or tummy.

Standing tall as earlier, place your hands on your lower belly, below the navel and just above the pubic bone. As you relax the area beneath your fingers, you may notice that the low abdominals are distended or a bit lax. Now, try engaging those lower tummy muscles, thinking of pulling your navel back toward your spine; the area beneath your hands a firming girdle. I like to think of those low, deep, transverse muscles as the "seat belt" which aids in connecting and supporting the abdominals to the low back and creating pelvic stability. As well as the traditional Pilates cue to "pull **navel to spine**," I also suggest the image of bringing the pubic bone toward the sacrum.

Let us now practice incorporating deep breathing with abdominal awareness. This may be challenging if you have practiced other forms of breathing techniques, but give it a try. Our goal is a flattering, flat stomach but, more importantly, strong abdominals to support a healthy back. Taking a full inhalation and exhalation, you may find that your belly distends and you've lost the navel to spine connection. Remember that in the Pilates Method we are breathing deeply into the lungs. "Lots of people get into the habit of breathing low in the belly, which can lead to distended stomach muscles. Good breathing begins in the chest area, not in the belly" (Fletcher, 1978, p. 31). While the abdominal cavity may enlarge as the diaphragm moves downward allowing the lungs to fill during inhalation, we don't want to let the low belly completely relax and "hang out." Keeping your hands over your low abdominal area, begin to inhale, trying to maintain firmness and control, navel to spine, pubic bone to sacrum. As you exhale completely, continue to focus on this area, making an even deeper connection. You may imagine your seat belt becoming tighter, your belly button even closer to your spine and your tummy firmer and flatter. You will probably find it much easier to keep your belly flat during exhalation rather than inhalation, but keep at it. Not only are you practicing the art of conscious, deep breathing, you are also performing a rather simple yet effective abdominal exercise, finding your center from within.

Spinal Awareness and Articulation

Moving onto the floor allows us to experience our abdominal–spinal connection, with breath of course, in a supine position. Ideally, using a firm, yet comfortable mat is best; if not, a nicely padded carpet will do. First, lie down on your mat, on your back, legs and arms stretched out, hands (palms up) and feet completely relaxed. Keep your neck long, chin neither tucked nor arched, jaw relaxed, and head straight. You may close your eyes and for a few moments, just breathe. Feel which parts of your body are pressed into your mat. Are there spaces here and there? Are some areas flatter than others? Is your back arched? It's all fine; you are gathering information about your body. Try to get rid of undue tension, both in mind and body, and simply be present in the moment. Most women will notice an arch or space in the mid-back, as this is the natural lordotic curve in the waist area. Under the neck is a similar curve, normal and desirable. Keep breathing and feeling your body. Now, slowly bend your knees, bringing the soles of your feet to a parallel position on your mat, 6 to 8 inches apart and 10 to 12 inches from your buttocks. Place your arms comfortably at your sides, palms facing down. You should now feel a change in your spinal alignment, with more of your lower back touching the mat. In this lengthened position, we can begin to experience the technique of **imprinting** the spine, feeling each vertebra in its place along the mat. Imagining your body from top to bottom, keep the neck long with focus directly to the ceiling, continuing to make sure you don't tuck the chin into the throat or overly extend the neck up and back. (Some women may find it comfortable to place a small pillow or rolled up towel under the back of the skull, *not* under the neck, as this can exaggerate an already overly extended cervical spine.) We still want to maintain a slight lordotic curve in the neck area. Shoulders should be flat and down, with a lovely openness across the chest and sternum. Think of your heart pointing to the ceiling. The ribcage will continue to open and close as you breathe, without flaring the ribs to the ceiling. We remember the lungs open in all directions, so now is a perfect time to think of inhaling into your back, or in this case, into your mat. Go ahead and feel the width of your beautiful back as it fans open to allow air in. Then exhale and sense the narrowing of the entire cage. Remember to keep those shoulders down…they don't need to rise or tense to take a breath. We now come to the area that may be the most problematic of all, the mid to low back. Without unduly forcing the spine down, I encourage you to take another deep breath, and as you exhale, pull your belly button down and into your back, allowing gravity to assist you in diminishing the space or tunnel under your waist. *Do not* tuck the pelvis; rather keep it neutral, pubic bone to sacrum, sacrum to mat. It is of utmost importance to maintain a stable and neutral pelvic alignment for a healthy back. I like to think of the pelvis as a flat, horizontal plane with hip bones even, as though I could balance a ruler from bone to bone in a level, straight line. Continue to breathe in and out, slowly and completely, feeling your abdominals pull in and down toward your spine, each vertebra, all the way down to your tailbone connecting to the mat. You have successfully imprinted your spine! If you would like to think of lying in wet sand while experiencing this sensation, you would arise to find you had left a wonderful imprint of your beautiful back.

Beginning in the imprinted position, you may now wish to experience a subtle articulating movement combining abdominal activization with lumbar spinal flexion and engagement of the gluteal muscles and pelvic floor. Take a deep inhalation while the sacrum is anchored to your mat, then as you slowly exhale, engage the low band of abdominals across your hip line and tip the lower back and sacrum up and slightly off the mat, thinking of pointing your pubic bone toward the ceiling (this is a posterior pelvic tilt). At the same time, engage or tighten your buttocks muscles and think of drawing your "sitz bones" or ischial tuberosities together. As you draw these bones toward one another, the pelvic floor can become activated and strengthened. In this flexed spine position, it is possible to feel a concave scoop of the lower abdominals, deeply contracting the transverse abdominals. There is no need to lift the sacrum more than a few inches off the mat to experience this exercise. Repeat several times, breathing slowly and making sure to return to a neutral pelvis with each new breath. To activate the inner thigh muscles (adductors), simply place a medium-sized ball—a soccer-size ball is good—between your knees, and gently squeeze it while performing the exercise.

Taking this movement a bit further, you may experience a full **pelvic press**. (This may seem a bit like the yoga pose known as the bridge, but they differ.) Begin with the same breath in neutral pelvis, and then slowly exhale as you initiate the movement from the deep transverse abdominals, lifting the sacrum off the mat. Continue to peel one vertebra at a time, sequentially from the mat until you are firmly supported on your upper shoulder area, arms still long at your sides, head and neck in straight, neutral alignment. At the peak of travel, there should be a long diagonal line from your knees, to your hip and pelvic area, to your shoulders. It is important to keep the knees and feet in equal parallel alignment throughout the exercise, and if it's helpful to hold the ball, you may do so. When you have reached the top, take another deep breath, and then as you slowly exhale, reverse the process by rolling back down onto your mat one vertebra at a time, remembering the pearl imagery mentioned earlier.

Rolling through the spine one vertebra at a time is a significant cue in much of the Pilates work. It aids in spinal articulation, alignment correctives, and finding balance in the body. So often we tend to favor a "strong" side, causing the weaker side to become less involved and therefore even weaker. Our abdominals play a huge role in this spinal movement as you may experience in this next exercise. The classic **roll-up** begins in a supine position (and that may be attempted later.) Let us first find how to roll down through the spine. Begin by sitting up on your mat with your knees bent and parallel in line with your feet. You may wish to support yourself with your hands behind your thighs, or rest them at your sides. Sitting as tall as you can, lengthening your spine, and reaching your crown to the ceiling, take a deep breath. With an exhale, begin by contracting in the abdominals, and slowly roll down to your mat, one vertebra at a time until you are lying flat, as earlier during the "imprinting" of the spine. If you found that you descended in larger segments of your back, your feet popped off the mat, and your shoulders became tense, you are not alone! This is a difficult movement to execute smoothly and requires the utmost control, abdominal strength, and fluidity. Practice will help. To enjoy more of a challenge, try the roll-up, in which you reverse the movement, rolling back up, vertebra, by vertebra, by vertebra. Now you have experienced full spinal articulation! Remember, this is *not* a sit-up but a rolling movement. Finally, the classic Pilates roll-up is performed from a completely outstretched position, legs straight with inner thighs connected, feet pointed, arms extended over the head, back long, and navel pulled toward the spine. Bring arms to a perpendicular line (inhale), lift head toward the frame of your arms, continuing to roll off the mat one vertebra at a time until your armpits are over your hips, arms reaching past your toes (exhale), flex your feet (inhale), roll back down *one vertebra at a time* (exhale) until your body is once again long and streamlined on your mat. This movement requires the utmost consistent abdominal control, and, as always, remember to breathe.

Alignment

Returning to a standing position will allow us to consider our alignment, and it may be especially helpful to use a mirror in the beginning. I would like to emphasize that I find it best to ultimately achieve healthy alignment and posture without a mirror image, utilizing your own kinesthetic and proprioceptive awareness. However, checking in a mirror or with an experienced instructor is fine at first.

Stand tall with your feet in parallel about hip width apart and your arms relaxed at your sides. Beginning with the feet, we want to have equal weight on our foot centers, that is, a tripod of support comprising three points of contact with the floor: (1) the ball of the foot under the big toe, (2) the ball of the foot under the little toe, and (3) the heel. Many women have the tendency to supinate or roll toward the outside of the foot, or pronate, rolling inward toward the instep. Perhaps only one foot does this. Look down at your feet, and check and double check that your 10 toes are pointing forward in the same direction, and feel your weight on both feet evenly, on those tripods. I still remember my mentor Ron saying, "people just don't pay enough attention to their feet! No wonder so many people have foot problems, with women in high heels suffering the most." Now, lift all 10 toes up off the floor. Press the toes back down into the floor as though you are grabbing the floor like a cat, trying to feel all the toes working equally. Repeating several times may help strengthen and articulate feet and toes that are weary and ignored!

Working up the legs, we want to pay particular attention to the alignment of the entire leg, from the hip to the knee to the foot. Try feeling the sensation of "pulling up" the leg muscles, a cue we use in dance to engage the quadriceps correctly without gripping the knee joint. Properly engaged thigh muscles may help the knee to track correctly in line with the hip and foot. (Many women will find that their legs are not perfectly aligned in a straight line but may have knock-knees or bowed legs, like me. These deviations may be corrected to a certain extent under the guidance of an expert teacher using a variety of exercises done on Pilates equipment.) Now, carefully bend your knees slightly, and see if your knees are pointing forward in the same direction as your toes. Hold for just a moment, then straighten the legs to the starting position, maintaining alignment throughout. Try repeating this simple movement, a plie in dance, continuing to be mindful of the knees tracking exactly over the feet, all in parallel.

The alignment of the pelvis and hipbones was discussed earlier when lying on the mat and imprinting the spine. Now that you are standing, you will want to check that your hipbones are in an even line, parallel with the floor. Referring to the experience on the mat, we want to keep the pelvis in a "neutral" position with the tailbone pointing down to the floor, neither tucking the pelvis allowing the pubic bone to swing forward nor swaying the low back into an excessive lordotic curve. Many women may be unaware of uneven pelvic alignment, thinking one leg is shorter/longer than the other when, in fact, the hips and pelvis may not be evenly lined up. It is essential that the abdominal muscles be activated to stand up straight and support the entire lumbopelvic structure. The abdominal activation and pelvic awareness exercises you experienced earlier while lying on your mat are useful to remember while standing.

Next, take a look at your rib cage, sternum, and shoulder area. As you take a deep breath, do your shoulders lift? Go ahead and lift them, and upon exhaling, try feeling as though your hands are holding light weights and your arms are growing longer and longer at your sides, pressing your shoulders down evenly (one may be higher or lower from holding a bag or a child on the same side every day!) I often use a cue that seems to work well for most women—imagine you are wearing the most beautiful diamond necklace—lifting your sternum or breastbone and opening beautifully across your chest while keeping your shoulders down. A nice exercise is to shrug your shoulders while inhaling, then press the shoulders down while exhaling, feeling the scapula/shoulder blades depressed into the back.

Finally, take a look at your head and neck alignment. Often, there is unevenness in this area from holding a phone, child, purse, etc., on one side. Sometimes, there is a tendency to tuck the chin down or inward. Try maintaining an even and healthy alignment in this area by using the well-known imagery of holding a book on the top of your head.

Ten Tips—From Head to Toe

Now that you are aware of your posture and alignment, abdominal muscles supporting the back and pelvis and the sensation of full breath, you may feel a greater sense of power and control emanating from your center. The following 10 simple exercises, included in Box 14.1, may be practiced daily, enabling you to experience the healing art of mindful movement and awareness of your own body.

Box 14.1 Ten Tips—From Head to Toe

From the tall, standing posture described earlier and always breathing:

1. Bring your chin gently forward over your chest, stretching the back of your neck; carefully lift the chin slightly up toward the ceiling, opening the throat; return to center; turn the head to the right, center, left, center, finding the profile position evenly to both sides. Repeat as desired.

2. Shrug your shoulders, lifting them high up toward your ears; press them down, arms long at the sides of the body; roll the shoulders forward, up, back, center; reverse the circle. Repeat 5 times.

3. With palms turned upward and shoulders down, sweep arms out to the side and up to the ceiling; at the top, turn palms downward and press arms back to your sides. Repeat 10 times. Clasp hands together behind your derriere with arms straight and feel the shoulders down and the sternum lifted; hold for a few counts.

4. Extend straight arms out to the side, making a horizontal line from the fingertips of one hand, across the chest, to the fingertips of the other hand. You will be in a "T" shape. Begin with palms facing floor, then turn palms to ceiling. Continue palms up, down, up, down rapidly changing from one to the other. Try 25 sets.

5. Simply standing tall, squeeze your buttocks muscles and engage the pelvic floor, holding for a few counts. Repeat 10 times.

6. With a straight back and legs in good parallel alignment, bend your knees, keeping your heels on the floor; hold the position for a few counts; return to straight knees. Repeat 10 times.

7. Feeling your feet (no shoes) firmly pressed to the floor and on your foot centers, lift all 10 toes up; return toes; lift heels, finding balance evenly on the balls of your feet; return. Repeat 10 times.

8. Transfer your weight to your left side and lift your right leg off the floor; extend the right leg forward, inches from the floor with the foot nicely pointed; while balanced, flex your foot, pulling the toes back toward your shin bone; point the foot and toes. Repeat about 5 times, then change legs. You will need to practice keeping your strong center throughout to maintain balance.

9. From your tall standing position, you may experience the roll down. Begin rolling head forward, then allow shoulders to roll forward (arms are relaxed and long at your sides), continue rolling vertebra by vertebra until you are all the way forward, hands toward the floor. You may wish to bend your knees slightly at any time throughout the movement. Return to the starting posture, moving slowly through the spine until you are once again standing tall. Repeat 5 times.

10. Close your eyes. Feel yourself in space, rooted to the floor, lengthened and streamlined from head to toes (and heels). Your legs are stretched, your buttocks muscles are engaged, your navel is toward your spine, and pubic bone toward sacrum. Your arms are relaxed at your sides with shoulders pressed down and chest elegantly lifted, head held high. Open your eyes, awake, aware, and alive in your body.

While many of the exercises in this chapter come directly from the classical Pilates repertoire, many others are movement sequences designed to aid the reader in experiencing her own body awareness and joy of movement. Sometimes, the simplest exercises done with thoughtfulness and precision are the most valuable in achieving mind–body equanimity and a sense of peacefulness: the ultimate hoped for result.

Conclusion

Six months ago, I underwent total knee-replacement surgery (the arthroscopic surgery 30 years earlier was to the other knee). One might ask, "Why, after so many years of dedicated Pilates practice, did I need to have a new knee?" A combination of the aging process and osteoarthritis, brought on in large part by many years of dance, had resulted in a knee joint that was bone-on-bone and quite unstable. My MRI showed very little left in the way of ligaments, and I found walking more than a few blocks painful. After months of thinking that I could "power through," I took advice from a trusted physical therapist and wise counsel from my orthopedic surgeon, and decided the surgery was inevitable. It is noteworthy to mention that due to the many years of Pilates conditioning, my doctor believed I was in great shape going into the surgery and to expect a terrific outcome. Of course, I was terrified!

The surgery was successful. After a tough first-week postsurgery and wondering if I had made the right decision, things started to turn around. Fortunately, I was very motivated to faithfully perform my rehabilitation exercises, guided by a wonderful home care therapist. Then, when I began sessions at a clinic featuring Pilates as part of their therapy practice, I was tickled. Exactly 3 weeks after the surgery, I made a note in my diary— "Movement feels good!" I was once again relishing the joy of movement—stretching, reaching, twisting, even extending and bending my knee quite well. I was delighted to find my body as a whole once again, enjoying the physicality I so desired. Within 6 weeks, I had made significant progress and was honored to be somewhat of a "star" in my orthopedic surgeon's eyes. Most important was how I felt about myself, grateful to have the knowledge and ability to take care of my physical well-being and to appreciate my body for the uniquely wonderful mechanism it is. My hope is for other women to discover the same.

References

Bernardo, L. M. (2007). The effectiveness of Pilates training in healthy adults: An appraisal of the research literature. *Journal of Body Work and Movement Therapies, 11*(2), 106–110.

Caldwell, K., Harrison, M., Adams, M., & Triplett, N. T. (2009). Effect of Pilates and taiji quan training on self-efficacy, sleep quality, mood, and physical performance of college students. *Journal of Body Work and Movement Therapies, 13*(2), 155–163.

Everett, J. (2013, April). Ready, set, walk it off! *Health*, 37–38.

Fletcher, R. (1978). *Every body is beautiful* (pp. 17–75). Philadelphia, PA: J. B. Lippincott.

Friedman, P., & Eisen, G. (1980). *The Pilates Method of physical and mental conditioning* (pp. 2–26). Garden City, NY: Doubleday.

Gavenas, M. L. (1992, June). The dancer's workout. *Fitness*, 104.

Girdwain, J. (2013, May). Fix it with fitness. *Health*, 47–50.

Gladwell, V., Head, S., Haggar, M., & Beneke, R. (2006). Does a program of Pilates improve chronic non-specific low back pain? *Journal of Sports Rehabilitation, 15*, 338–350.

Jago, R., Jonker, M. L., Missaghian, M., & Baranowski, T. (2006). Effect of 4 weeks of Pilates on the body composition of young girls. *Preventive Medicine, 42*(3), 177–180.

Kloubec, J. A. (2010). Pilates for improvement of muscular endurance, flexibility, balance, and posture. *Journal of Strength and Conditioning Research, 24*(3), 661–667.

Monroe, M. (2012, September). The happiness factor: Part two. *IDEA Fitness Journal,* 47–55.

Pilates, J. H., & Miller, W. J. (1945). *Return to life: Through contrology* (pp. 3–18). New York, NY: J. J. Augustin.

Segal, N. A., Hein, J., & Basford, J. R. (2004). The effects of Pilates training on flexibility and body composition: An observational study. *Archives of Physical Medicine and Rehabilitation, 85*(12), 1977–1981.

15

Healing Environments

Nancy Lieberman Neudorf

Introduction: Mutuality between Women's Health and the Environment

To benefit and detriment alike, women's health and the environment are inextricably linked. The contributions to the health of the "exposome" (the environmental exposures over one's lifetime) are gaining attention among health-care providers and researchers. In ways both obvious and subtle, our health is influenced by our physical surroundings and the social context within which we function. Healing environments are those milieus that foster the physical, mental, and spiritual health of individuals and communities. At minimum, they provide the requirements for biological life: clean air, water, soil, and food. At best, they offer a wide range of resources and choices, liberating the organism to pursue its unique and optimal state of wellness. When discussing environment, it is useful to delineate and distinguish among three major components: the natural, built, and social environments, as conceptualized in Figure 15.1.

The **natural environment**—the air, water, food, and soil that is assimilated into our biological processes—affects our health in ways that are fairly obvious and well understood. The physical realities of the **built environment**—freeways, power plants, sidewalks, buildings, and parks, for example—may be observed, but the effects on health may occur via linkages that require explication. Features of the **social environment**—gender roles, opportunity, income, family, the media, lifestyle—have been found to influence health, yet the specific pathways are elusive, and potential prescriptions to improve health are still controversial. Table 15.1 summarizes the key aspects of the natural, built, and social environments. Currently available research does reveal much evidence of the healing power of the natural, built, and social environments. Sadly, many studies also demonstrate their potential harm.

Each of the environments depicted in Figure 15.1 and Table 15.1 has the potential to promote the health of women. For example, there are abundant therapeutic resources available in the **natural environment**: just a view of nature from a hospital window has been shown to speed recovery from illness (Raanaas, Patil, & Hartig, 2012); watching animals can improve mood (Townsend, Maller, Leger, & Brown, 2003); and the sound of

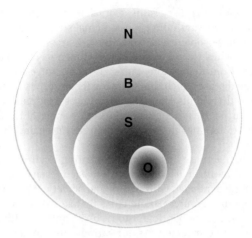

The relationship of the organism to its environment(s)

N   natural environment

B   built environment

S   social environment

O   the organism (individual woman or community)

FIGURE 15.1 Relationship of the organism to its environment.

flowing water may reduce pain (Kline, 2009). The **built environment**, when thoughtfully designed, can result in walkable neighborhoods where residents manage their weight better than those in a car-dependent community (Arkin, Braverman, Egerter, Williams, & Robert Wood Johnson Foundation, 2013; Dannenberg, Frumkin, & Jackson, 2011) and are thus at lower risk for heart disease, diabetes, and some cancers (Frumkin & McMichael, 2008; Wilkinson, Marmot, & World Health Organization, 1998). Friends and family, important attributes of the **social environment**, can help one to sustain improved health habits (Vrazel, Saunders, & Wilcox, 2008). These are but a few examples of the environment's capacity to nurture women's health.

The environment has the potential to threaten women's health as well. Environmental hazards are thought to contribute to more than 80% of illnesses reported by the World

TABLE 15.1	Three Components of the Environment: Natural, Built, Social
Component	**Examples**
Natural	Air, water, food, land, climate, chemicals, microbes
Built	Urban development, community design, transportation, energy, waste, life indoors
Social	Economic, educational opportunities, social support cohesion, societal attitudes, addictions, media

Health Organization (WHO; Prüss-Üstün, Corvalán, & WHO, 2006). The health of women is suffering in many ways from environmental stress. Heart disease, cancers, and stroke, all believed to have some causative factors in stress, comprise 50% of deaths in women in the United States (http://www.cdc.gov/women/lcod/index.htm). Women suffer disproportionately from depression, eating disorders, digestive problems, domestic violence, autoimmune diseases, including type I diabetes, lupus erythematosis, arthritis, multiple sclerosis, and thyroid disorders (Schiller, Lucas, National Health Interview Survey, & National Center for Health Statistics, 2012). In most of these disease processes, there are particularly strong links to environmental causation and/or exacerbation (Dannenberg et al., 2011).

Furthermore, human activity has a hand in creating environmental harm. In addition to making unhealthy lifestyle choices, we engage in behaviors that do not always acknowledge our interdependence with nature and society. We depend on fuel sources that pollute our life-giving resources, build cities that isolate us in cars and present barriers to walking and socialization, attempt to resolve conflicts with aggression, and are unfair to the vulnerable in our society. As our various environments grow unhealthy, so do we.

Nevertheless, women and their environments can be mutually beneficial. Recognizing their reciprocal relationship, women can live in and care for their surroundings in a symbiotic fashion. Improving the health of their environment, even in small ways, improves their own health and that of their communities. Truly preventive health care encompasses the environment as a major influence on women's physical and mental health. To achieve optimal wellness, it is critical that we harness the healing power of the environment and learn to live more harmoniously with it.

Healers have long recognized the contribution of the environment to individual and community health. Florence Nightingale spoke of making the environment conducive to health when she described how to make hospitals more welcoming and healing to patients (Nightingale, 1859; Nightingale & McDonald, 2001). In 1992, both the WHO and the International Council of Nurses (ICN) issued statements advising health-care practitioners to consider environmental protection essential to human health. The American Nurses Association (ANA) recognized the interconnectedness of human and environmental health in their 2007 policy statement and called for nursing leadership to address environmental injustice (ANA & Congress on Nursing Practice and Economics, 2007). Most recently, the American Congress of Obstetricians and Gynecologists (ACOG) and the American Society for Reproductive Medicine (ASRM) have called for action to identify and reduce toxic environmental agents (ACOG, 2013).

Recognizing the importance of the environment in disease prevention and health promotion, clinicians need to address environmental factors with women and communities to reduce health risks and encourage ecologically sound health habits.

This chapter focuses on environmental aspects of health promotion for women with the goal of understanding the important role of the environment in healing, and our role in shaping it to achieve its maximum benefits. Specifically, this chapter addresses

1. Influences on women's health of the natural, built, and social environments
2. The relationship of the environment to women's health across the life span
3. Actions to foster environmental and individual health in women and communities
4. The role of the health-care provider in facilitating environmental health

Influence of the Natural, Built, and Social Environments on Women's Health

The Natural Environment

The natural world contains everything required for biological life: clean air and water, nourishing food, and fertile land. We are what we eat, drink, breathe, and absorb. Therefore, contamination of any of these components is likely to endanger women's health. Sadly, the quality of these life-giving resources is deteriorating, at least in part due to human activities. As we increase our understanding of what is harmful, we have an obligation to improve our practices.

Air

A very widespread stressor to public health is the pollution of urban air by particulate matter and ozone, which results primarily (80% in the United States) from the combustion of fossil fuels in industrial processes, energy generation, and vehicles. In the United States, nearly half of the population lives in cities where pollution readings often exceed the national air quality standards. Air pollution levels are highest within 200 feet of busy roadways; exposure drops off to background levels by approximately 1,000 feet (McConnell et al., 2006; Zhu, Hinds, Kim, & Sioutas, 2002).

Other common contributors to fouled air may include cigarette smoke, carbon monoxide (also from fossil fuel combustion), mold (where conditions are warm and humid), volatile organic compounds (VOCs) from chemicals used in household products, and airborne diseases (influenza, tuberculosis, SARS). The health effects from these airborne substances may range from mucosal irritation, dizziness, nausea, to sudden death (US Department of Health and Human Services, Office on Women's Health, 2009).

Polluted air has been classified as a carcinogen by the WHO's cancer agency (Wild & Stewart, 2014). Studies have also demonstrated associations between air pollution and respiratory ailments (particularly asthma), cardiovascular disease, and infections (Dannenberg et al., 2011; US Environmental Protection Agency [EPA], 2013).

Water

Even in the developed world, traces of cleaning chemicals, pesticides, pharmaceuticals, parasites, bacteria, minerals, heavy metals, and VOCs may be found in the water. Urban and agricultural runoff, inadequate treatment, weather patterns, and improper disposal of toxic and pharmaceutical waste are among the causes. Depending on dose and duration of exposure, the effects from impure water can range from mild gastrointestinal distress to cancer or developmental, neurological, cardiac, immune, and reproductive disorders.

As there is no substitute for many of its uses, attention must be paid not only to water quality, but future supply as well. Large amounts of water are expended on energy and industrial processes, and on food production. In light of fouled supplies, increased demand, population growth, energy generation, industrial process, efforts to privatize the resource, loss due to warming temperatures, and the fact that there is no substitute, "peak freshwater" is even more critical to human health than "peak oil."

Food

A varied, colorful, plant-based diet, as described at www.choosemyplate.org, is generally recommended for optimal health. However, our present industrial food system arouses concerns about food quality as well as the environmental footprint of its production. It emphasizes volume rather than biodiversity, is very resource intensive, and is heavily reliant on the use of pesticides, chemicals, fossil fuels (for production and long-range transportation), water, grain, and pharmaceuticals (for livestock). Setting aside the perils of resource depletion and the advisability of a meat-based diet, the resultant food may be contaminated with hormones, heavy metals, dioxins, herbicides, and diesel particulates. Local or traditional farming is actually able to feed more people a wider variety of food than is our current industrial food system (Pimentel, Hepperly, Hanson, Douds, & Seidel, 2005).

Even locally grown and organic food (grown without hormones, pesticides, or antibiotics) is subject to damage from air, water, or soil contamination. Proper food handling, which includes washing surfaces and hands thoroughly, separating raw meats from other foods, cooking foods to the proper temperature, and refrigerating them promptly (www .fda.gov), can help mitigate this concern.

Caution with seafood consumption is also warranted owing to possible contamination as well as concerns about overfishing. Larger fish contain dangerous levels of mercury, which is known to be a neurotoxin. Raw fish eaten as sushi may include endangered fish.

Land

Multiple health and economic benefits can be derived from green and blue open spaces. Open spaces provide habitats for a rich world of biodiversity, retain and filter water, save billions in storm water management costs, and help mitigate air pollution. Trees beautify landscapes, cool temperatures, and absorb carbon dioxide from the atmosphere. Lakes and oceans deliver economic, recreational, and environmental benefits. Studies show that parks help reduce blood pressure, increase fitness, reduce crime, increase property value, trigger stress reduction, and promote community cohesion (Changelab Solutions, 2013). Water views and sounds can prompt an increased sense of well-being and improved concentration (Huynh, Craig, Janssen, & Pickett, 2013).

But adverse agricultural practices, urban sprawl, airborne contaminants, microbial pathogens, and drought can clear growth, ruin habitats, and degrade the water and soil, rendering it less fit for food cultivation and habitation. Habitat fragmentation and destruction can lead to pressure on species and eventual extinction. The interdependency among various life forms makes the acceleration of species loss a real concern for human destiny.

Climate

Climate determines where and how humans live. We depend on its cycles and derive energy from the tides, sun, and wind. It regulates our entire ecosystem and biological rhythms.

Twelve of the hottest years on record occurred in the last 15 years. Scientists have ascertained that the planet's climate is becoming hotter and more humid, most likely due to emissions from greenhouse gases such as carbon (CO_2) and methane (CH_4). The former comes mainly from fossil fuel combustion, the latter primarily a result of livestock production (Frumkin & McMichael, 2008).

Climate change is already causing more extremes in weather events, demonstrated by an increase in fires, storms, floods, and drought. There is evidence of new and increased numbers of infectious pathogens and vectors of disease, as well as changing habitats and growth cycles. The effects of climate change are expected to continue to cascade, eventually causing the polar icecaps to melt, the sea level to rise significantly, violence and competition for resources to increase, and millions of climate refugees to flee their homes.

This current and looming public health crisis has been well described by Frumkin and McMicheal (2008), and Bill McKibben of 350.org, "a global grassroots movement to solve the climate crisis" (www.350.org), and many others. Clearly, climate change poses major challenges to women's health.

Chemicals and Microbes

We are surrounded and occupied by innumerable chemicals and microbes. While much is yet to be learned about the difference between those that are beneficial and those that are harmful, and at what doses, some of them are well known to pose a threat to women's health. According to the WHO, toxicity may be increased for women, who have a higher percentage of body fat to store lipophilic chemicals than men. Nearly 300 chemicals, many known to be harmful to humans, have been identified in body fat and breast milk (WHO, 2010).

These chemicals and microbes pose considerable concern in the perinatal community. In September 2013, a joint statement was issued by ACOG and ASRM, calling for action by health-care providers, scientists, manufacturers, and lawmakers to identify and prevent toxic substances from being introduced into the environment (ACOG, 2013).

There are many examples of chemical substances that impact health. In particular, radiation, which is present in sunlight, harnessed for nuclear energy, and emitted from electronics, can have adverse effects on humans. Hormone disrupters such as bisphenol A (BPA) and phthalates are found in vinyl and plastic products. Parabens are found in some hygiene products such as toothpaste and shampoo. Pressed wood cabinets and furniture may contain formaldehyde. These chemicals can cause health problems ranging from mucosal irritation to respiratory problems, reproductive damage, and cancer (US Department of Health and Human Services, Office on Women's Health, 2009).

Microbial agents are increasingly resistant to drugs. According to the Centers for Disease Control and Prevention (CDC, 2013), drug-resistant infections, caused by antibiotic use in animals and overuse of antibiotics, cost $26 billion and kill more than 23,000 people annually.

The Built Environment

Driven by the wish to have the required services of civilization efficiently delivered to us, we modern humans tend to congregate near one another, in cities and towns. The built environment is how we have designed our common space and arranged to live together.

The infrastructure for water, electricity, plumbing, and fuel is created and maintained by the municipal government. The city policy-makers are also charged with regulating land use: determining where there will be homes, where commerce can occur, and what land will remain open for public use. Local governments adopt detailed standards for building codes, energy generation, sidewalks, water management, transportation networks, and public safety.

The world population is anticipated to increase from its current 7 billion residents to 10 billion by the turn of the next century (Frumkin & McMichael, 2008). The world will become increasingly urbanized, making it imperative that our cities and buildings are designed not only with an eye to promoting human health, but to easing, if not reversing, human pressures on the health of our environment.

Urban Development and Community Design

Women's health is greatly influenced by the design of a community. Are the neighborhoods safe, clean, and affordable? Is it possible to find adjacent employment, education, elder and childcare? Is there a range of transportation alternatives to suit all ages? Are there nearby opportunities for physical recreation and time in nature? Is healthy food easily accessible? Are there gathering places? Is the community engaged and involved in decision making? Unfortunately, in many US cities, the answers to most of these questions is "no."

In previous decades, urban design separated housing from sanitation and industry to protect the public health. The advent of the private automobile made the suburban lifestyle possible. However, there is a dawning awareness that urban "sprawl" is inefficient and very costly in terms of fossil fuel use, time wasted in traffic, motor vehicle accidents, and social disconnection.

Increasingly, young people and retirees are seeking a walkable urban lifestyle with cultural amenities, convenient employment access, and transit. Cities are building mixed-use neighborhoods, offering employment, commercial, and educational centers alongside living spaces. Streets are "complete"—built for pedestrians, bicyclists, wheelchairs, transit, and cars. Housing is denser in the mixed-use model to support public transit; neighborhood parks substitute for private yards and offer chances for social bonds to form among residents.

Transportation

In our society, mobility is key to a good life. Getting to work, to school, to entertainment, to recreation, to visit with friends and family—freedom of movement is a must. Where a private automobile is the only mobility choice, the social and activity options for children, older adults, and women without a car are severely limited. Women feel fewer social ties to neighbors (Wilkinson et al., 1998). Dependency on cars leads to a higher rate of motor vehicle accidents, diminished air quality, and increased obesity (Frumkin, Frank, & Jackson, 2004).

For health, as well as significant economic benefit, active transportation is preferred. Walking and bicycling, with public transit bridging the gaps, result in improved physical and mental health outcomes, fewer injuries, and reduced carbon emissions (Frumkin et al., 2004, Frumkin & McMichael, 2008; Wilkinson et al., 1998).

Designing for walkability includes several components. It is important to include neighborhoods with a mix of incomes and uses; "complete" streets to accommodate all users; schools, workplaces, interesting destinations, and town centers located within 2 miles; a comprehensive network of safe, off-street bike lanes; and houses and buildings situated closer to the street with parking in the back.

Bike- and car-sharing programs consist of fleets of bicycles or cars for short-term rental strategically located in an urban area. These programs have been shown to reduce traffic congestion, improve air quality, support transit systems, save money, and boost tourism.

Energy

As has been noted, the burning and production of fossil fuels (coal, petroleum, and natural gas) for society's energy requirements contaminates the air we breathe, the water we drink, and the soil in which we grow our food. Fossil fuels are a major contributor to geopolitical conflicts and to global climate change. As our population increases and our energy needs intensify, it is foolhardy and dangerous to continue to explore for and rely on them.

Fortunately, nature provides alternatives. Solar photovoltaic electricity generation, solar thermal passive water heating, wind turbines, geothermal power, and hydroelectric power can all be harnessed safely, securely, and without detriment to human health. In addition, a green and renewable energy economy has the potential to create full employment by retrofitting our carbon nation while saving billions of dollars. As an example, the renewable retrofit of the Empire State Building in New York City paid for itself in 3 years and continues to save $4.4 million annually (http://www.esbtour.com/d/).

Waste

The worldwide production of municipal waste will double in the next 10 to 15 years. The average American recycles about one-third of the waste he or she produces. There is enough energy discarded in the average bag of kitchen trash to light a 100-watt bulb for 24 hours (Flanigan, 2013).

Food waste makes up 14% of the landfills where it becomes a source of methane, a greenhouse gas even more detrimental than carbon dioxide. Plastic wastes also pack landfills, or end up in the ocean, harming wildlife. Only 20% to 29% of plastic bottles are recycled (EPA, 2010), and these un-recycled bottles take 450 years to decompose (EPA, 2014).

Plastic water bottles are a noteworthy menace to health, requiring 3 L of water to produce just 1 L of bottled water. The polyethylene (PET) plastic bottles contain toxic chemicals, notably BPA, which can seep into the water, particularly when the bottle is subjected to heat. Each bottle uses the equivalent of one-fourth a bottle of fossil fuel in production and transportation (Pacific Institute, 2007). In light of these facts and the mounting concerns about privatization of water, a basic human right, carrying a thermos instead of buying bottled water seems like a reasonable thing to do.

Proper disposal of hazardous waste allows for conservation of energy and resources, recycling of valuable materials, and diversion of toxic pollutants. Electronics, batteries, pharmaceuticals, used oil, and light bulbs are among the items that require proper disposal. Local waste management or the EPA (www.epa.gov) can provide further details.

Life Indoors

Americans, on average, spend 23 hours a day inside. Depending on ventilation, which is worse in older buildings, indoor air pollutants can reach levels two to five times higher than outdoors. A sampling of common indoor air pollutants include carbon monoxide from heating systems, formaldehyde and VOCs in building materials and furnishings, and secondhand smoke (to which girls may be more vulnerable than boys) (Holmen et al., 2002).

One can also be exposed to additional health threats within buildings. Toxic contaminants such as pesticides and infectious microbes may be tracked indoors on footwear. Artificial lighting, particularly at night, has been shown to alter circadian rhythms and sleep, contributing to obesity (Wyse, Selman, Page, Coogan, & Hazlerigg, 2011) and some breast cancers (Bauer, Wagner, Burch, Bayakly, & Vena, 2013).

On the other hand, buildings can provide a shelter and safe haven. Attention to the indoor surroundings can have an enormous influence on women's health and well-being. Natural light can produce positive effects on mood and cognition (Kent et al., 2009). Greenery, the sounds of running water, and the presence of pets and fish, have been shown to be healing (Huynh et al., 2013). Stimulating the senses with pleasant colors, aromas, views of nature, meaningful pictures, art, and music can all create positive conditions for health.

The Social Environment

The social environment might be described as personal circumstances, societal conditions, and social norms. Personal circumstances include elements such as one's available resources and opportunities, gender, and ethnic group. Societal conditions address several factors, such as the bonds that exist between neighbors, the transparency of the local government and its responsiveness to women's concerns and input, and the local crime rate. Social norms refer to the written or unwritten rules of behavior prevalent in a community. The social environment is where we humans interact with one other and negotiate our social contract. By understanding the social circumstances that bring about health, we can work to change the social norms that will contribute to a healthier society.

Economic and Educational Opportunity

The National Women's Law Center (www.nwlc.org) highlights the critical nature of poverty as a women's issue, indicating that of all poor adults, almost 60% are women, and that 50% of children in poverty are part of women-headed households. This is striking because poverty rates are particularly high for single mothers, women of color, and older women who live by themselves. Women working full time in the United States earn 81¢ for every dollar earned by a man (US Department of Labor, Bureau of Labor Statistics, 2012).

Multiple studies show that poverty leads to inferior health outcomes. It drives the choice of neighborhood, which in turn determines safety, housing quality, food access, and exposure to nature and recreational opportunities. Low socioeconomic status is linked to increased smoking, poor diet, increased alcohol intake, increased stress, and increased exposure to injury and violence (Arkin et al., 2013; Chehimi, Cohen, & Valdovinos, 2011; Wilkinson et al., 1998).

Similarly, lack of education leads to decreased control over one's circumstances, fewer choices, and material deprivation. Lack of knowledge and resources make a woman less healthy by initiating a cascade of poor outcomes, causing her to endure a high baseline level of stress. Chronic stress leads to inflammation, which is a causal factor in autoimmune disease, heart disease, cancer, lung disease, and obesity (Schweitzer, Gilpin, & Frampton, 2004; Wilkinson et al., 1998).

Social Support and Cohesion

This factor is an enormously powerful force for good health, especially in women. Women of all ages tend to thrive where relationships are strong and encouraged. Social support and a network of caring and trusting relationships have been shown to improve coping, stress management, mental health, health behaviors, and adherence to medical regimens. Evidence also indicates that if a woman feels supported, she is less susceptible to acute illnesses and less likely to develop chronic illness (Uchino, 2009). On a population level, social support and cohesion are key to social justice, equitable access to opportunity, civic involvement, volunteerism, caring about one's neighbors, and a safe and healthy community.

Societal Attitudes, Addictions, and the Media

Women face gender discrimination in almost every society. They hold fewer positions in government, earn less money, and are physically victimized more often than men. This power differential results in stress and risks to mental and physical health. Societal addictions present a threat to women's health. Alcohol and substance abuse can lead to violent behavior and female victimization as well as driving under the influence. Addiction to "screens," as described below, can be the cause of accidents when driving while distracted, or other antisocial behavior.

The pervasiveness of computers, televisions, tablets, and smartphones is reducing social interaction and increasing isolation. The ubiquity of this compelling "entertainment" is causing a reliance on external stimulation, reducing the time spent being still and self-reflective. Studies show mixed results for health. One study (Bessière, Pressman, Kiesler, & Kraut, 2010) documented increased depression when computer use was for health purposes, but reduced depression when computers were used to connect with family and friends. On the basis of findings associating excessive media use with obesity, attention problems, and entrée to inappropriate content, the American Academy of Pediatrics has advised the limiting of screen time to 1 to 2 hours of quality programming for children older than 2, as well as the establishment of "screen-free zones" in the home, so that other activities may be encouraged.

As the mouthpiece of society, the media reflects the zeitgeist—the thoughts and norms that influence and exemplify the current culture—all the while attempting to attract advertising revenue. Societal attitudes, biases, and attention-grabbing entertainment all have a profound, if difficult to quantify, effect on the health of women.

The media's representation of women presents a huge barrier to female safety, equity, health, and empowerment. Sexual images of women prevail in marketing campaigns, movies, and video games. Drug use and smoking is alluring. Story lines rarely feature powerful women, career women, or female leaders. Portrayals of unrealistic body shapes are pervasive (Smith, Choueti, Prescott, & Pieper, n.d.). These media messages lead to eating disorders, poor self-esteem, violence against women, and gender norms that limit the opportunities available to women. Society suffers when half of the population is not fully heard.

Women's Health across the Life Span in Relationship to the Environment

A female's vulnerability and susceptibility to risk factors in her physical and social milieus can vary greatly according to her age and developmental stage. While a woman's genetics, beliefs, values, and choices are important variables, it is possible to make some general statements about the impact on health that a woman's surroundings may exert at various points in her life. Women's motivation to make constructive changes also varies across the life span. This section addresses environmental vulnerabilities and susceptibilities of women at various life stages as well as motivation by women to improve their environmental health. More in-depth discussion related to the health-care provider's role in encouraging constructive behavioral changes is included in a later section, but behavioral changes are briefly discussed at each significant point in a woman's life span.

Infancy and Early Childhood

Susceptibility and Vulnerability to Risk Factors

Owing to their rapidly developing bodies, increased metabolic requirements, proximity to the ground, primitive hygiene habits, and propensity for placing things into their mouths, all infants and young children, including female, are extremely vulnerable to pollutants in the natural environment. Early childhood exposure to lead, for example, can cause damage to the renal, circulatory, and nervous system, in severe cases leading to permanent brain damage (US Department of Human and Health Services, Office on Women's Health, 2009). Infants and toddlers are very sensitive to noise ("New WHO Guidelines for Community Noise," 2000) in the built environment. As they are entirely dependent on others for their survival, their social environment is that of their caretakers. The bond between caretaker and infant is essential to proper social and physical development. A weak emotional relationship or limited stimulation may yield potentially lifelong repercussions of ill health (Wilkinson et al., 1998).

Motivation and Ability to Practice Environmental Care

The behaviors of infants and toddlers are mainly instinctual, and they have very little agency to act on anything beyond getting their basic needs met. Yet, the seeds can be planted at this stage for a lifelong motivation to respect the natural world, and to treat others fairly and with kindness.

School Age

Susceptibility and Vulnerability to Risk Factors

Children are more vulnerable to environmental risks than are adults. Worldwide, one in four diseases is thought to be caused by the environment, but in children that ratio increases to one in three. The primary causes of death in this age group are related to injuries and accidents, and mental health issues are the predominant cause of ill health (Prüss-Üstün et al., 2006).

Repeated or chronic contacts with toxins at this age can result in diseases later in life. For example, significant exposure to UV rays during childhood may increase the risk of developing melanoma or cataracts at an older age (US Department of Health and Human Services, Office on Women's Health, 2009). The built environment impacts this age group, insofar as it allows for active and independent mobility, contact with nature, and a healthy school setting. The social environment becomes particularly important at this stage of life, as children begin to interact with the world on their own. The "Adverse Childhood Experience" (ACE) study (www.cdc.gov/ace), initiated in 1995, was among the first to demonstrate that various types of abuse, neglect, and stressors in childhood led to many physical and mental health problems such as substance use, depression heart disease, and unintended pregnancies. Females in the study were far more likely to suffer sexual and emotional abuse, as well as to have experienced four or more ACEs, which increased the risk and severity of negative health consequences.

Poverty in childhood can affect children's short- and long-term health outcomes by constraining options for living conditions and education. In addition, poverty has been shown to have a strong influence on the development of a child's brain (Luby et al., 2013).

Adolescence can be a stressful time for a girl to navigate. Her emerging sexuality, combined with society's messages regarding gender roles, beauty, and popularity, may contribute to the increased incidence of depression, self-harm, eating disorders, risk-taking, sexually transmitted diseases, violent victimization, and unintended pregnancies found in this age group (Johnson, Roberts, & Worell, 1999).

Motivation and Ability to Practice Environmental Care

Children are lovers of nature, open to the concept of interconnectedness and care for the earth. Teens are imagining their future, beginning to take responsibility for their actions, and establishing their adult health practices. Given supportive family and community environments, sufficient opportunities, and accurate information, girls in this age group are both motivated and able to engage in ecologically sound habits, and to break free of the social constraints on their potential.

The Reproductive Years

Susceptibility and Vulnerability to Risk Factors

Pregnant women and their developing fetuses are highly vulnerable to nearly all of the health hazards in each of the environments described earlier in this chapter. Owing to the sensitivity of the brain and other developing organs during this critical period of life, unfavorable physical or social circumstances can lead to untoward consequences over the lifetime of the unborn child. As an example of threats during pregnancy inherent in the physical environment, evidence demonstrates an increased incidence of behavior problems (Perera et al., 2013), low birth weight (Pedersen et al., 2013), prematurity (Kloog, Melly, Schwartz, Ridgway, & Coull, 2012), and autism (Roberts et al., 2013) in children born to women exposed to blighted air. Adverse social conditions, such as poverty and social exclusion, are also linked to poor fetal development via intermediary associations with smoking, poor nutrition, and lack of prenatal care (Wilkinson et al., 1998).

Motivation and Ability to Practice Environmental Care

During pregnancy and young motherhood, a woman is often anxious to protect the environments surrounding her developing fetus and young child, and may be receptive to fine-tuning her health habits. A clinician is likely to find her very motivated to practice environmental care, and capable of adopting recommended new routines.

Older Women

Susceptibility and Vulnerability to Risk Factors

By virtue of the limited regenerative abilities, preexisting diseases, weakened immune systems, and cumulative lifetime exposures that are associated with the aging process, the health of older women may be significantly impacted by environmental factors.

In the natural environment, poor air quality is associated with an increased risk for stroke, heart attack, aggravation of respiratory difficulties, and cognitive decline in seniors. Dementia and cancers have been linked to long-term exposure to pesticides (US Department of Health and Human Services, Office on Women's Health, 2009). The extreme weather events and excessive heat, and infectious organisms related to climate change present greater challenges to the health of older women (Luber & McGeehin, 2008).

The built environment presents challenges to the health of older women as well. Cracked or absent sidewalks, noise, poor lighting, and inaccessible buildings all diminish independence and well-being.

As women tend to live longer than men, older women are often alone. Social activity may be restricted, transportation options limited, and finances inadequate. Older women are at risk for injury, isolation, victimization, and depression in an unfavorable social environment.

Motivation and Ability to Practice Environmental Care

Older women may be at a particularly receptive stage, and open to activism. Finding themselves unburdened by the demands of a full household, they may be experiencing what human potential scholar Jean Houston (Houston, 2013) calls "postmenopausal zest." Pondering their legacy and their grandchildren's future, they may turn their energies and wisdom toward community engagement and search for reliable advice regarding community health promotion. Provided they have the physical health and the required resources, older women may be powerful advocates for environmental protection and social change.

Actions that Foster Individual, Community, and Environmental Health

What exists in the environment that can harm us? What is our individual or communal contribution to the threat? By investigating the potential hazards in their client's unique environment, a health-care provider may more effectively counsel a woman or community in risk prevention.

Conversely, by what means is it possible for the environment to nurture human and community health? Clinicians can also prescribe ways for women to take advantage of this powerful support to create true "healing environments."

Personal Planetary Approaches

Clearly, an individual has little control over environmental threats such as the outdoor air that they breathe or the transportation alternatives available in their community. However, they can make modifications in their personal habits, homes, and businesses that will mitigate potential environmental harm to them and their families. Often, these actions are restorative to the earth as well as beneficial to individuals. They can then set positive examples for others and influence their community (city, school, workplace, place of worship). Table 15.2 lists a sample of individual choices that have been shown to benefit human and/or environmental health.

TABLE 15.2	Personal Planetary Habits for Health
Breathe cleaner air	If possible, live and work close to greenery and at least 1,000 feet from busy roadways Allow no smoking in your car, home, or close vicinity Ventilate all fuel-burning devices in your home (e.g., over cooktop); keep filters clean and appliances in good repair Open the windows for ventilation whenever possible Choose only low VOC carpets and paints Cultivate multiple houseplants
Value and conserve water	Use water sparingly; turn it on and off as needed (as opposed to running continuously) when brushing teeth, shaving, or washing dishes Repair leaking toilets and faucets Plant water-saving and native landscapes (no lawns); install smart water irrigation systems Carry a thermos; limit your purchase of water in plastic bottles
Nourishing food and farming	Eat lower on the food chain: less meat, more produce. The production processes are less energy intensive and better for your health Eat a wide variety of foods, local and organic if possible Grow food and/or participate in community-supported agriculture (CSA) Do not microwave foods in or under plastic Avoid seafood known to contain high levels of mercury: shark, swordfish, king mackerel, tilefish. Canned light tuna has less mercury than albacore Avoid products containing palm oil—palm plantations are one of the major causes of rainforest destruction Eat only meats that are grass-fed or chicken that was free-range Trim fat off meats, which may store pesticides Wash and scrub produce under running water, peel skin, or trim outer leaves Food facts for women http://www.fda.gov/Food/ResourcesForYou/Consumers/ucm2006969.htm
Love the land	Plant a variety of trees and plants in your yard or neighborhood. Create an appealing habitat for birds and insects Spend more time in nature—studies show it improves women's moods Appreciate the outdoors and our interconnectedness

(continued)

TABLE 15.2	Personal Planetary Habits for Health *(continued)*
Climate comfort	Use a programmable thermostat Keep indoor humidity at <60% in the summer and between 25% and 40% in the winter Support environmental protection organizations Consider the purchase of carbon offsets to compensate for the climate change costs of the high emission activities you choose (www.nativeenergy.com)
Reduce toxic and infectious exposures indoors and out	Handwashing! Keep immunizations up to date Follow procedures for safe food preparation and handling Clean anything that goes in the mouth; prevent children from eating dirt or paint chips Take shoes off at the door Clean regularly to reduce dust, dander, and other allergens; use nontoxic cleaning and personal products Install and maintain carbon monoxide and smoke detectors Practice nontoxic pest control; prevent infestations by barriers or traps, removing food and water sources Stop using pesticides and fertilizers Use a nontoxic dry cleaner Use an extender with cell phone; do not carry on your body; minimize use when pregnant or near children Wear sunscreen, hats, and sunglasses for UV protection; limit time outdoors between 10 a.m. and 4 p.m. when UV radiation levels are highest. *Never* use tanning beds Practice safe sex; strive to limit intimacy to those with whom you are willing to share pathogens See ACOG's "Environmental Chemicals—Stay Safe During Pregnancy" (www.acog.org)
Be safe and in charge	Plan your pregnancies—do your part to reduce overpopulation. www.plannedparenthood.org Learn basic self-defense Be alert and aware of your surroundings, minimize distractions such as talking on a cell phone Carry a cell phone set to an emergency number Keep car doors locked at all times Do not open a door to anyone unknown to you Stay in well-lit, populated areas Walk or jog with a partner Carry some kind of personal defense such as pepper spray, a whistle, or alarm Be prepared. Follow recommendations re: emergency preparedness at Red Cross. www.redcross.org/prepare Participate in your community's emergency response team (CERT) training
Make your transportation more active, less stressful, and more fun	Walk, bike, take transit, or commute. Reduce your vehicle miles travelled (VMT), and enjoy the benefits to your body, mind, spirit, and bank account. Interact more with your community while contributing a little less noise and traffic congestion Take the stairs until you are 90 or beyond, if possible Consider driving an electric or hybrid car

TABLE 15.2	Personal Planetary Habits for Health *(continued)*
Intelligent energy	Turn off appliances when they are not in use; use power strips to streamline the process Use energy star appliances and LEDs; keep appliances in good working order; insulate your home. www.consumerenergycenter.org Install solar panels Install solar thermal or tankless water heaters
Manage your waste	Reduce, reuse, and recycle. Only then consider discarding Bring unwanted prescription medicines, old batteries, electronics, used LEDs, and all hazardous materials to hazardous waste collection sites Whenever possible, use reusable bags, cups, and food storage Compost your organic waste; leave grass clippings and leaves on the lawn Participate in the sharing economy via Zipcar, Tradesy, or Lyft, etc; make use of underutilized resources as an entrepreneurial opportunity; focus on the usefulness of a commodity, rather than ownership
Healing home	Employ natural light wherever possible Reduce light trespass to reinforce circadian rhythm and improve sleep, immunity, and energy—use room-darkening shades, remove lights from computers, phones, and clocks from bedroom Bring nature inside with plants, moving water, pets Stimulate your senses and emotions in ways that are pleasant. Pay attention to aromas, colors, high ceilings, art, photos, meaningful objects, pets, ergonomics, and music or nature sounds Avoid injury. Ensure clear pathways, safe wiring and cords. Utilize contrasting colors, soft flooring, clear passage, and grab bars to promote safety for older adults
Economics and education	Pursue educational opportunities and develop useful skills Educate yourself, friends, and family about environmental health and choices. www.greenpeace.org, www.grist.org and many others Support pay equity for women
Build community	Extend your time and caring to people around you—kindness usually begets more kindness Stay connected to people who respect and value you. Live near them if possible Join an environmental group Advocate for environmental health; contact and educate decision makers in your community
Beware what you buy (into)	Place a daily limit on screen time; consider a media-free weekend day Buy soaps and detergents without formaldehyde or parabens Buy clothing from nontoxic companies. (www.greenpeace.org/detox) Support local green businesses Financially support and enjoy the merchandise from companies that remove toxins from their products and processes. www.Betterworldshopper.com, a work in progress, grades companies on their social and environmental practices Buy products from companies that promote positive images of women in their advertising Evaluate the environmental and social impacts of companies in which you invest your resources

Community Approaches

Cities, schools, hospitals, and businesses are all making the link between the environment and impacts to health, productivity, and the economy. They can avail themselves of many of the same approaches outlined in "personal planetary habits" above. They may choose to make purchases with an eye toward sustainability and reduced waste. They may pursue an organization-wide nutrition policy that focuses on organic foods that are locally sourced. They can consider a ban on styrofoam, bottled water, and plastic bags.

Local governments make public policy determinations, possess land use authority, and allocate public funds on behalf of the community. Schools, hospitals, and businesses have control over the policies of their organizations, the design of their spaces, and the range of human services they will provide. Thus, the consequences of their decisions are far-reaching. Unfortunately, these decisions are not always informed by data regarding health impacts and opportunities. At worst, this can lead to a decline in community health; at minimum, to not getting the full benefit of the resources spent.

Just as each woman has different values, beliefs, and goals for herself, so too does each community define its own best health. Table 15.3 presents general recommendations for cities and organizations to consider.

TABLE 15.3	Community Actions for Health
Health-promoting policies www.changelabsolutions .org www.policylink.org www.lgc.org	Ensure widespread community outreach and engagement. The stakeholders know what they need and what they are motivated to do about it
	Work across sectors to achieve the best possible results for resources expended
	Review all major development and resource expenditures for potential health impacts via checklists, health professional review, or health impact assessments (see www.humanimpact.org)
	Whenever possible, make the healthy thing the easy thing to do—people are most likely to go with the default option
	Consider adopting Leadership in Energy and Environmental Design (LEED) standards for buildings and/or for neighborhood design (LEED-ND)
	Adopt smoke-free ordinances
	Purchase alternative energy vehicles for fleets
	Prohibit idling of buses on site
	Consider styrene and plastic bag bans
	Reduce, reuse, recycle, and, where possible, recover as energy via various "waste to energy" designs
	Adopt green policies for cleaning and landscaping
	Adopt wellness policies for nutrition and physical activity
	Consider restrictions on inappropriate marketing
	Adopt living and equal-wage ordinances
	Enforce laws against driving while intoxicated and/or distracted
Barrier-free design www.smartgrowthamerica .org www.designinghealthy communities.org	Design for walkability and bikability—think people, not cars
	Design for safety via Crime Prevention Through Environmental Design principles (www.cptedtraining.net)
	Ensure that roadways are designed to welcome all users—see "Complete Streets" guidelines (www.smartgrowthamerica.org/ complete-streets)

TABLE 15.3	**Community Actions for Health** *(continued)*
	Protect wetlands and streams, watersheds, and natural open space
	Plant native tree and plants; use recycled water for irrigation
	Subscribe to superior storm water management standards such as reduced impervious surfaces and water-retention ponds
	Build parks and pleasing outdoor spaces, even small ones, wherever possible
	Plan for and build connected networks of well-lit off-street bike and pedestrian trails across the entire community; bridges across busy roadways
	Incentivize the development of mixed-use neighborhoods
	Supply and support affordable public transit
	Explore bike- and car-share opportunities
	Use caution when approving sensitive land uses such as housing, schools, or hospitals near sources of air pollution like busy roadways or industrial sites
	Ensure an adequate supply of adaptable, affordable housing in a variety of types near jobs
	Install solar panels, energy-efficient lighting, and central air filtration on public buildings
	Take advantage of energy cogeneration opportunities where possible
	Investigate the WELL standard for health-promoting buildings by Delos Living—company states economic premiums of 10%–30% achieved with increased costs of only 3%–5%
Health education and services www.preventioninstitute .org www.rwjf.org	Support school-based and community health centers
	Install community gardens
	Ensure convenient availability of healthy food
	Educate and raise awareness to promote a new water ethic
	Offer on-site health education classes, wellness programs, fitness facilities, screenings, and/or immunization and blood drives
	Ensure availability of affordable child care
	Provide convenient recycling, organic waste, and hazardous waste disposal
	Develop partnerships with the academic community to generate research and apply evidence-based practice

Role of Nurses and other Health-Care Professionals

Prevention

As providers of health care, our job is not only to mend injured bodies and spirits, but to practice prevention by making assessments and recommending therapies far upstream of the medical office. We need to take environmental histories from our patients and help them understand the link between the health of the environment and their own health. It is possible for our health advice to include actions they can take to heal their surroundings.

Society needs health experts to weigh in on policy development and the allocation of public resources, advocating for the decisions that maximize opportunities and minimize impediments to community health.

Raising Individual and Community Awareness

There is no doubt that the planet is ailing, and causing harm to human health. Conversely, individuals and communities must protect the planet. Nature will do its best to heal itself, but our current practices are overwhelming it. As individuals, we need to protect our health and practice environmental care. As a society, we must stop relying on and pouring resources into environmentally disastrous systems and products. We should consider our health as well as that of the environment when we commit our time and money to a decision. We ought to act fairly and be kind and open to one another. We have got to be willing to be flexible.

Health-care providers, more than most, are in a position to help inspire environmental healing by leading constructive changes. Women seek health advice. Clinicians, particularly nurses, are a trusted source. Health-care providers understand the value of prevention and are likely to first observe the consequences of a toxic environment. Our prescriptions can include appropriate evidence-based interventions.

As previously noted, women have a reciprocal relationship with the environment. They must learn not only to avoid incurring harm from, but also to avoid causing harm to, their various environments. However, as health-care providers well know, it can be challenging to effect actual change in clients' behaviors. Fogg (2011) posited that three things must be present simultaneously for behavior change to occur. There must be a **trigger** to act plus the **motivation** and **ability** to do so.

Just as a woman's vulnerability to environmental threats can vary across the life span, so too can this behavior change triad. The passage of certain development milestones may **trigger** her awareness and/or increase her receptivity to information. Particular stages in a woman's life may find her more or less **motivated** and/or **able** to "go green." Cognizant of this, a clinician might more effectively raise her clients' awareness and prescribe steps to help her meet her own environmental and personal health goals.

As health advisors, nurses and other health professionals have privileged access to a good part of our clients' internal environment—their beliefs, values, and choices. It is important to respect women's values, determine their knowledge and awareness level, and assess their resources in order to advise them of the most effective health-promoting behaviors.

Many women experience anxiety about the earth and our environmental future. It is important to acknowledge their fears about the future, to let them know that they are not alone, and that there are actions they can take toward healing. It is essential that women understand that their choices matter—the more positive activity, the more healing. Empowering women with actions they can take will boost their spirit and strength.

Prevention starts in the community. That is where projects are planned, land use decisions are made, and significant resources are spent. Unfortunately, cities and corporations do not commonly seek health advice, although they are increasingly aware of the health hazards of urban life and society, and hungry for data and best practices.

While behavior change at the community level is challenging because developers and governing bodies are not always open to making changes to their usual routines, it is crucial to find ways to be part of early planning discussions so that health effects may be taken into account. It is important to influence and craft polices to expend resources efficiently and wisely, thereby promoting health.

Increasingly, health professionals are entering the policy-making arena. They are consultants, government staffers, business owners, members of school or other governing boards and commissions, and elected officials. Their health expertise and focus can lead to the adoption of public policies that support health-promoting natural, built, and social environments.

Education and Recommendations

It is crucial to address environmental health with clients. ACOG (2013) specifically recommends that environmental health be included in the health history. Education must be integrated into a health-care visit in order to assist clients to make the link between the health of the environment and the health of their family and communities, and to guide them to discover where they may be acting against their own self-interests. Clients can be taught to take advantage of the healing power of nature and to show it the most possible respect.

Health-care providers must educate themselves, their clients, their students, and their colleagues about the human health effects of the natural, built, and social environments. Further, it is important that health-care providers develop partnerships with public health departments, businesses, schools, and local governments to bring screening and education into the community.

In addition to drugs, therapies, and surgeries, health professionals can confidently prescribe evidence-based actions that lead to environmental healing, resulting in benefit both to women and to their communities. While it is common for health providers to write a prescription for an expensive medicine with unpleasant side effects, ironically it is much less common to write a prescription for daily walks in nature, meatless Mondays, and unwired weekends.

Evidence-Based Prescriptions for Environmental Health

There are many health-promoting, cost-effective, and evidence-based environmental actions to recommend with confidence. Tables 15.2 and 15.3 summarize planetary habits and community habits, respectively, that will enhance the health of the individual and the environment.

Advocacy and Research

Health professionals can advocate for harmony-inducing policies, a green economy, cleaner fuels, and transportation choices via public testimony and media appearances. They are able to promote research to study community problems, and identify areas where research is needed to make evidence-based recommendations.

Health professionals should push for good information about safe levels of chemicals and microbes. They can publicly support shifting the burden of proof to the manufacturers before approvals, as well as the costs of remediation and disposal if damage is done.

Changing Social Norms

Social norms change slowly, one person at a time, one community at a time, across multiple sectors. By empowering women and local communities to act, we unleash their potential to create a world where living well with nature and each other is the norm.

Call to Action

Facing the hard truth about environmental degradation and its devastating effects on human health can be overwhelming. No one person is able to solve the massive problems created by our unhealthy environments, but we can each take action within our realm of influence. This is an exciting opportunity for nurses and other clinicians to actively engage in prevention. It is possible for clinicians to spread strength and resilience and healing to themselves, their patients, and their communities. Environmental health counseling must be included in the promotion of health and wellness across a woman's life span.

References

American College of Obstetricians and Gynecologists Committee on Health Care for Underserved Women, American Society for Reproductive Medicine Practice Committee, & The University of California, San Francisco Program on Reproductive Health and the Environment (2013, January 1). Exposure to toxic environmental agents. ACOG Committee Opinion No. 575. *Fertility and Sterility, 100*(4), 931–934.

American Nurses Association & Congress on Nursing Practice and Economics. (2007). *ANA's principles of environmental health for nursing practice with implementation strategies.* Silver Spring, MD: American Nurses Association.

Arkin, E., Braverman, P., Egerter, S., Williams, D., & Robert Wood Johnson Foundation. (2013). *Time to act: Investing in the health of our children and communities: Recommendations from the Robert Wood Johnson Foundation Commission to Build a Healthier America.* Washington, DC: Robert Wood Johnson Commission to Build a Healthier America.

Bauer, S. E., Wagner, S. E., Burch, J., Bayakly, R., & Vena, J. E. (2013). A case-referent study: Light at night and breast cancer risk in Georgia. *International Journal of Health Geographics, 12*, 23.

Bessière, K., Pressman, S., Kiesler, S., & Kraut, R. (2010, January 1). Effects of internet use on health and depression: A longitudinal study. *Journal of Medical Internet Research, 12*, 1.

Center for Disease Control and Prevention. (2013). *Threat report 2013: Antimicrobial resistance.* Atlanta, GA: Author.

Changelab Solutions. (2013). *This land is our land: A primer on public land ownership and opportunities for recreational access.* Retrieved from http://changelabsolutions.org/sites/default/files/This_Land_is_Our_Land_FINAL_20130722.pdf

Chehimi, S., Cohen, L., & Valdovinos, E. (2011, January 1). In the first place: Community prevention's promise to advance health and equity. *Environment and Urbanization, 23*, 1, 71–89.

Dannenberg, A. L., Frumkin, H., & Jackson, R. (2011). *Making healthy places: Designing and building for health, well-being, and sustainability.* Washington, DC: Island Press.

Flanigan, T. (2013, June 28). Trash: The big picture. *Ecomotion EcoNet News, 15*, 10.

Fogg, B.J. (2011). *What causes behavior change?* http:www.behaviormodel.org,

Frumkin, H., Frank, L. D., & Jackson, R. (2004). *Urban sprawl and public health: Designing, planning, and building for healthy communities.* Washington, DC: Island Press.

Frumkin, H., & McMichael, A. J. (2008, January 1). Climate change and public health: Thinking, communicating, acting. *American Journal of Preventive Medicine, 35*(5), 403–410.

Holmen, T. L., Barrett-Connor, E., Clausen, J., Langhammer, A., Holmen, J., & Bjermer, L. (2002). Gender differences in the impact of adolescent smoking on lung function and respiratory symptoms. The Nord-Trondelag Health Study, Norway, 1995–1997. *Respiratory Medicine, 96*(10), 796–804.

Houston, J. (2013, November). Women's creativity and the emerging new story. Women's Empowerment Initiative, Lecture conducted at University of California, Irvine.

Huynh, Q., Craig, W., Janssen, I., & Pickett, W. (2013). Exposure to public natural space as a protective factor for emotional well-being among young people in Canada. *BMC Public Health, 13*, 407.

Johnson, N. G., Roberts, M. C., & Worell, J. (1999). *Beyond appearance: A new look at adolescent girls.* Washington, DC: American Psychological Association.

Kent, S. T., McClure, L. A., Crosson, W. L., Arnett, D. K., Wadley, V. G., & Sathiakumar, N. (2009). Effect of sunlight exposure on cognitive function among depressed and non-depressed participants: A REGARDS cross-sectional study. *Environmental Health, 8*, 34.

Kline, G. A. (2009, January 1). Does a view of nature promote relief from acute pain? *Journal of Holistic Nursing: Official Journal of the American Holistic Nurses' Association, 27*(3), 159–166.

Kloog, I., Melly, S. J., Schwartz, J., Ridgway, W. L., & Coull, B. A. (2012, August 6). Using new satellite based exposure methods to study the association between pregnancy PM2.5 exposure, premature birth and birth weight in Massachusetts. *Environmental Health: A Global Access Science Source, 11*, 1.

Luber, G., & McGeehin, M. (2008, January 1). Climate change and extreme heat events. *American Journal of Preventive Medicine*, *35*(5), 429–435.

Luby, J., Belden, A., Botteron, K., Marrus, N., Harms, M. P., Babb, C., Nishino, T., ... Barch, D. (2013, December 1). The effects of poverty on childhood brain development. *JAMA Pediatrics*, *167*(12), 1135.

McConnell, R., Berhane, K., Yao, L., Jerrett, M., Lurmann, F., Gilliland, F., ... Peters, J. (2006, January 1). Traffic, susceptibility, and childhood asthma. *Environmental Health Perspectives*, *114*(5), 766–772.

New WHO guidelines for community noise. (2000, January 1). *Noise & Vibration Worldwide*, *31*, 24–29.

Nightingale, F. (1859). *Notes on nursing: What it is and what it is not*. London, England: Dover.

Nightingale, F., & McDonald, L. (2001). *Florence Nightingale on public health care*. Waterloo, Ontario, Canada: Wilfrid Laurier University Press.

Pacific Institute. (2007). *Bottled water and energy: Getting to 17 million barrels*. Retrieved from http://pacinst.org//wp-content/uploads/sites/21/2013/04/bottled_water_factsheet.pdf

Pedersen, M., Giorgis-Allemand, L., Bernard, C., Aguilera, I., Andersen, A.-M. N., Ballester, F., . Slama, R. (2013, January 1). Ambient air pollution and low birthweight: A European cohort study (ESCAPE). *The Lancet Respiratory Medicine*, *1*, 9.

Perera, F. P., Wang, S., Rauh, V., Zhou, H., Stigter, L., Camann, D., ... Majewska, R. (2013, January 1). Prenatal exposure to air pollution, maternal psychological distress, and child behavior. *Pediatrics*, *132*(5), 1284–1294.

Pimentel, D., Hepperly, P., Hanson, J., Douds, D., & Seidel, R. (2005, July 1). Environmental, energetic, and economic comparisons of organic and conventional farming systems. *Bioscience*, *55*(7), 573–582.

Prüss-Üstün, A., Corvalán, C., & World Health Organization. (2006). *Preventing disease through healthy environments: Towards an estimate of the environmental burden of disease*. Geneva, Switzerland: World Health Organization.

Raanaas, R. K., Patil, G. G., & Hartig, T. (2012, January 1). Health benefits of a view of nature through the window: A quasi-experimental study of patients in a residential rehabilitation center. *Clinical Rehabilitation*, *26*(1), 21–32.

Roberts, A. L., Lyall, K., Hart, J. E., Laden, F., Just, A. C., Bobb, J. F., ... Weisskopf, M. G. (2013, January 1). Perinatal air pollutant exposures and autism spectrum disorder in the children of nurses' health study II participants. *Environmental Health Perspectives*, *121*(8), 978–984.

Schiller, J. S., Lucas, J. W., National Health Interview Survey, & National Center for Health Statistics. (2012). *Summary health statistics for US adults: National Health Interview Survey, 2011: Data from the National Health Interview Survey*. Hyattsville, MD: US Dept. of Health and Human Services, Centers for Disease Control and Prevention, National Center for Health Statistics.

Schweitzer, M., Gilpin, L., & Frampton, S. (2004, January 1). Healing spaces: Elements of environmental design that make an impact on health. *Journal of Alternative & Complementary Medicine*, *10*(1), S71–S83.

Smith, S. L., Choueti, M., Prescott, A., & Pieper, K. (n.d.). *Gender roles & occupations: A look at character attributes and job-related aspirations in film and television* [executive report]. Retrieved from Geena Davis Institute on Gender in Media website: http://www.seejane.org/downloads/full-study-gender-roles-and-occupations-v2.pdf

Townsend, M., Maller, C., Leger, L., & Brown, P. (2003). Using environmental interventions to create sustainable solutions to problems of health and wellbeing. *Environmental Health*, *3*(1), 58–69.

Uchino, B. (2009, January 1). Understanding the links between social support and physical health: A life-span perspective with emphasis on the separability of perceived and received support. *Perspectives on Psychological Science*, *4*(3), 236–255.

US Department of Health and Human Services, Office on Women's Health. (2009). *The environment and women's health: Frequently asked questions*. Retrieved from http://www.womenshealth.gov/publications/our-publications/fact-sheet/environment-womens-health.html

US Department of Labor, Bureau of Labor Statistics. (2012). *The editor's desk: Women's earnings as a percent of men's in 2010*. Retrieved from http://www.bls.gov/opub/ted/2012/ted_20120110.htm

US Environmental Protection Agency. (2010). *Municipal solid waste generation, recycling, and disposal in the United States: Facts and figures for 2010*. Retrieved from http://www.epa.gov/wastes/nonhaz/municipal/pubs/msw_2010_rev_factsheet.pdf

US Environmental Protection Agency. (2013). *Our built and natural environments: A technical review of the interactions between land use, transportation, and environmental quality*. Washington, DC: US Environmental Protection Agency, Development, Community, and Environment Division.

US Environmental Protection Agency. (2014). *Marine debris timeline*. Retrieved from http://www.epa.gov/gmpo/edresources/debris_t.html

Vrazel, J., Saunders, R. P., & Wilcox, S. (2008, January 1). An overview and proposed framework of social-environmental influences on the physical-activity behavior of women. *American Journal of Health Promotion, 23*(1), 2–12.

Wild, C. P., & Stewart, B. (2014). *World cancer report 2014.* Geneva, Switzerland: World Health Organization.

Wilkinson, R. G., Marmot, M. G., & World Health Organization. (1998). *The solid facts: Social determinants of health.* Copenhagen, Denmark: Centre for Urban Health, World Health Organization.

World Health Organization. (2010). *Protecting children's health in a changing environment: Report of the fifth ministerial conference on environment and health.* Geneva, Switzerland: Author.

Wyse, C. A., Selman, C., Page, M. M., Coogan, A. N., & Hazlerigg, D. G. (2011, January 1). Circadian desynchrony and metabolic dysfunction; did light pollution make us fat? *Medical Hypotheses, 77*(6), 1139–1144.

Zhu, Y., Hinds, W. C., Kim, S., & Sioutas, C. (2002, January 1). Concentration and size distribution of ultrafine particles near a major highway. *Journal of the Air & Waste Management Association, 52*(9), 1032–1042.

Chapter 16

Healing Relationships

Robynn Zender and Ellen F. Olshansky

Introduction

Relationships have received increasing attention in both popular and academic literature, especially with the recent explosion in knowledge of the neurobiological processes of human interactions. It has become clear that women's relationships, including spousal, parental, work, and friendships, interact with their own personality, cognitive and psychological makeup; genetic predispositions; relational history; and physiology to impact health and well-being. The deepening understanding of the social nature of the human species has informed research in the fields of psychology, sociology, neuroendocrinology, immunology, epidemiology, and medicine/health, prompting cross-disciplinary investigation and, in some cases, creating new disciplines. Women, in particular, possess a different biological organization than men, which yields distinct motivations, capacities, behaviors, and health-related outcomes relative to relational and social states. This chapter presents the latest research on the effects of relational connection and disconnection on women's health and the constituents and facilitators of healthy and unhealthy relational behavior. The chapter aims to

- Describe what is meant by relationships
- Explain why human beings are "social animals"
- Discuss how relationships contribute to the health status of women
- Present specific aspects of the importance of relationships at various stages of a woman's life
- Discuss how health-care providers can facilitate relational health in women

What Is Meant by "Relationships"

A relationship is defined as "a connection, association, or involvement" (Dictionary.com Unabridged, 2013). Depending on the level through which they are viewed, relationships have atomic, microscopic, and molecular aspects, moving onto whole beings interacting with others, and up to the largest relationships between individuals and the environmental, political, social, and spiritual contexts in which they are situated. In this discussion of human relationships, the unit of reference is the individual as a whole, in interaction with internal and external environments, most often viewed within dyadic exchange.

Healthy relationships enable growth and survival. Traditional psychological frameworks, however, identify healthy psychological development as composed of separation and autonomy. These traditional constructs of individualism are, in fact, so ingrained in society that they are the unquestioned and often unconscious reference for determining reality in Western civilization (Jordan, 1997). What has become increasingly understood, however, is that we grow through and toward relationships throughout our lives. Healthy development is contingent upon individuals engaging in healthy interpersonal relationships, and ultimately, we grow not toward separation, but toward greater connection with others (Jordan, Kaplan, Miller, Stiver, & Surrey, 1991; Miller, 1986). Indeed, in a 75-year prospective cohort study of 268 male Harvard students from the classes of 1938 to 1940, where a multitude of physical, economic, personality, and social factors were evaluated at regular intervals, the state of one's relationships rated as the top predictor of health and happiness (Vaillant, 2012). Healthy relationships consist of empathy, authenticity, and mutuality, all of which lead to growth-fostering human connections.

Growth-enhancing connection is characterized first by mutual empathy: an emotional–cognitive (feeling–thinking) movement where each person sees, knows, and feels the responsiveness of the other person (Jordan, 2000). Mutual empathy leads to a flow in exchange of more thoughts and feelings, altering each person's cognitive–emotional understanding and, as the interaction progresses, the relationship grows and evolves. This is an expansive experience that leads to a sense of mutual empowerment where all participants experience themselves as effective human beings (Miller & Stiver, 1997). The results of relational connection are the present-moment experiences of what Jean Baker Miller (1986) referred to as "the five good things": (1) increased "zest" (vitality); (2) increased ability to take action (empowerment); (3) a clearer picture of one's self, the other, and the relationship (clarity); (4) increased sense of worth; and (5) a desire for more connection—for more relationships beyond that particular relationship (Jordan & Hartling, 2002; Miller & Stiver, 1997). The concept of "mutuality" is a key component of effective relational exchange, and differs from the term "reciprocity," which implies an equally balanced "tit for tat." Mutuality involves affecting the other and being affected by the other, where one extends oneself out to the other and is also receptive to the impact of the other. It is characterized by an openness to influence, emotional availability, and a constantly changing pattern of responding to and affecting the other's state. There is both receptivity and active initiative toward the other (Jordan, 1986). Mutuality does not mean sameness or equality, but rather is a way of relating; a shared activity in which each (or all) involved is participating as fully as possible (Miller & Stiver, 1997, p. 43). "Movement toward mutuality" in relationships entails a dynamic process in which the individuals are increasingly able to be authentic, and authentically responsive to each other's thoughts and feelings (Miller & Stiver, 1997, p. 54). "In order for one person to grow in a relationship, both people must grow" (Jordan & Walker, 2006, p. 3). From many such growth-enhancing connections, one can build the resilience to sustain psychological development, and it is from the lack of these experiences that the reverse occurs (Miller & Stiver, 1997, pp. 30–31), where a draining of one's resources through disconnection can lead to depression (Jack, 1991; Kaplan, 1986; Miller & Stiver, 1997), confusion (Miller, 2008), and physical disease (Adler, 2002, 2007; Levenson & Gottman, 1983; Riess & Marci, 2007; Suchman & Matthews, 1988; Wilce, 2003).

One must have a well-differentiated sense of self, as well as an ability to appreciate and be sensitive to the differentness as well as the sameness of another person, in order to engage empathically (Jordan, Surrey, & Kaplan, 1991, p. 29). Differentiation, in relational terms, departs from the ideas of Freudian thought that autonomy is a process of growing toward independence in separation. Autonomy, defined relationally, incorporates a person's ability to be responsible to others and take into account relational consequences of one's own actions (Fishbane, 2001). Relational autonomy includes both clarity about one's own needs and desires, and a willingness to be moved by another (Fishbane, 2001). Thus, relational capacity is a sort of catch-22: one gains clarity about one's self (that is, differentiates) through connection with others, yet one must have some degree of clarity of self in order to enter into connection. The term "relational paradox" has been used to describe impediments to establishing empathic connection, where we keep large parts of ourselves out of connection, even though we yearn deeply to connect (Miller & Stiver, 1997). Because of previously experienced harm or violations that occur within the desires and attempts to connect (which happens to all of us to some degree throughout our lifetimes), we develop strategies of disconnection. While these strategies are preferable to physical isolation, they cost an individual greatly in terms of disconnection from one's self, a lack of clarity about one's feelings, and creating a sense of inauthenticity; in short, disconnection hinders the potential for empathy and thus, reduces our potential to develop fully (Jordan, 1997, cited by Fedele, 2004, p. 217).

Connection with others is the primary motivating force in people's lives, and isolation (not defined as "being alone," but as feeling locked out of the possibility of human connection [Hawkley & Cacioppo, 2010; Miller, 2008]) is a primary source of human suffering (Jordan & Walker, 2006). Indeed, solitary confinement is the ultimate threat and punishment within the prison setting (Shalev, 2008; Smith, 2006). Effected through movement in relational connection, individuals develop and grow toward more differentiated states, with relational development superseding self-development; that is, the development of autonomy and the self occurs through relationships with others, rather than the contrary, and the deepening capacity for relationship and relational competence is the principal goal of an individual's development (Surrey, 1991). These types of present moment strengthening interchanges correlate with positive biological and emotional health-related outcomes (Zender & Olshansky, 2012). Such exchanges represent a vital, though as yet under-recognized, source of healing.

Humans Are Social Animals

Modern biology reveals humans to be fundamentally emotional and social creatures, with the original purpose of our brains being to manage our physiology, optimize our survival, and allow us to interact and flourish (Immordine-Yang & Damasio, 2007). As social animals, we form groups that extend beyond the individual. Group social structures evolved along with biological and cognitive mechanisms to improve chances of individual and species survival (Cacioppo, Hawkley, Norman, & Berntson, 2011).

Survival in contemporary society relies less on physical strength and stamina, and more on psychological and relational fitness. In fact, relational fitness as much as competition, has contributed to adaptation and survival. Even Darwin noted the evolutionary advantages of socially cooperative behavior (Axelrod & Hamilton, 1981; Costa, 2013). For the most part, we are no longer fighting for our lives from cold, starvation, injury, and infection, but rather from poverty, stress, and social isolation (De Vogli, Chandola, & Marmot, 2007; Marmot & Wilkinson, 2009; Sapolsky, 2004). It is these latter constructs through which relational capacity acts to directly and indirectly impact health.

The fundamentally social nature of humans is evident also in the immune system. Similar to the brain, human immune systems evolve and function in social contexts (Wilce, 2003). The immune system communicates via molecular signals with the brain and body, where the body is integrated within larger systems of society (Tauber, 2000). The effects of stress and relational resonance on changes in immunity markers have shown up in most aspects of the immune system, including the lethality of killer T cells, the levels of various interleukins (IL) in the bloodstream, numbers of lymphocytes in circulation, and glucocorticoid concentrations and sympathetic nervous system action when the release of IL-1 from monocytes activates the hypothalamic–pituitary–adrenocortical (HPA) axis. Prolonged stress inhibits protein synthesis, the building blocks of immune cells, and suppresses the body's ability to fight infection and disease (Cozolino, 2006). Prolonged stressful conditions also shrink the thymus gland, which slows the maturation of T cells.

Men and women succeed socially through different mechanisms, with biological substrates motivating distinct social behaviors. Oxytocin is one hormone implicated in behavior motivation in both sexes. Oxytocin in women is produced in response to socially connective experiences (breast-feeding, touch, sexual activity), and in times of social distress (social conflict, threats, and inadequate social support), to support social activity in both situations through providing positive emotions, as well as activating attempts to secure social connections, respectively (Taylor, 2011). Administered oxytocin has been shown to increase one's capacity and motivation for social engagement through increasing heart rate variability (HRV), an important function in responding relationally (Kemp et al., 2012). Interestingly, neither the change in motivation nor HRV was accompanied by any detectable changes in mood states, indicating that it may increase the *capacity* for engagement without necessarily provoking behavior in that direction. Similarly, vasopressin, a neuropeptide involved in vasoconstriction and resorption of water by the kidneys, has more recently been identified as an active facilitator of social behaviors and processes that initiate and maintain social relationships (Kemp et al., 2012). Endogenous plasma levels of vasopressin are associated with having a larger social network, fewer negative marital interactions, less attachment avoidance, more attachment security, and greater spousal social support (Gouin et al., 2012). Similar to the action of oxytocin, vasopressin's association with social behaviors may be mediated by individual and contextual factors in terms of gender differences and situations of distress (Bartz, Zaki, Bolger, & Ochsner, 2011; Taylor, Saphire-Bernstein, & Seeman, 2010).

Both oxytocin and vasopressin have demonstrated an association with faster wound healing, where men and women with the highest oxytocin had faster wound healing, as did women with greater vasopressin levels (Gouin et al., 2010). Oxytocin and vasopressin appear to dampen responses to some threats, allowing for greater behavioral acts of generosity, caregiving, and approach-oriented emotions in response to threatening faces (Baumgartner, Heinrichs, Vonlanthen, Fischbacher, & Fehr, 2008; Thompson, George, Walton, Orr, & Benson, 2006). It has been posited, too, that oxytocin and vasopressin may be biological factors in the caregiving behavioral system that suppresses avoidance tendencies in response to the potential cost or loss that may be incurred from helping others (Poulin, Holman, & Buffone, 2012).

The right hemisphere of the brain is more strongly activated in women during appraisals of social interactions, which correlates with greater empathic capacity in women versus men (Rueckert & Naybar, 2008). Women demonstrate more dramatic physiological responses to relational interactions of any valence, be they positive, negative, neutral, or ambivalent. Self-silencing within relationships, defined as "the inability to manifest and affirm in relationships aspects of self that are central to one's identity" (Jack, 1999, p. 225), although perhaps occurring equally in men and women (depending on one's perception of self-silencing [Smolak, 2010]), demonstrate greater detrimental effects in women. Self-silencing is associated with decreased self-esteem, decreased possibility for intimacy, feelings of a loss of self, and a greater risk for depression and disordered eating (Jack & Dill, 1992; Locker, Heesacker, & Baker, 2012). Women show greater distress when functioning within incongruent role expectations, such as networking or social brokering. Role expectations for women in brokering positions are often inconsistent with women's values, given many women's decreased emphasis on control and improving one's relative position within a social network (Carboni & Gilman, 2012). Likewise, social support in times of stress reduces the physiological stress response, as well as detrimental effects of stress (Wohlgemuth & Betz, 1991). As much as humans require the satisfaction of satiating their hunger, thirst, and sexual drive, they have the need to maintain rewarding social relationships (Taylor, 2011).

Relationships and Health

Relationships affect health through complex and interwoven mechanisms, including behavioral, psychosocial, and physiological/biological. Behavioral mechanisms refer to health-related actions (such as medication adherence, seeking out medical help, smoking, alcohol, nutrition) that are often mediators that explain the relationship between stress and physical health outcomes (Cohen & Lemay, 2007; Karelina & DeVries, 2011). Social control theory purports that support networks encourage healthy behaviors and discourage unhealthy behaviors (Cacioppo et al., 2011), and offer exchanges in social resources (Cohen, 2004).

Similarly, the psychological context of relationships in humans and primates can modulate the linkage between physical stressors and subsequent stress response (Sapolsky, 2007). In fact, the stress response can be initiated by certain psychological contexts, in the absence of any physical stressor (Sapolsky, 2007). Psychological stress is at the core of understanding why chronic stress is pathologic, thus leading to both acute and chronic illness. Psychological stress can result from the anticipation of stressful events (i.e., dreading a meeting with an adversary), the perception of hardship (i.e., worrying, hypochondriasis), and the actual stress of a social, psychological, or physical nature (i.e., relational discord, loss, injury, illness). The two psychosocial stressors imparting the strongest effects on health, both physical and psychological, from a population perspective are social isolation and poverty.

A greater degree of high-quality social interactions extends one's life span, reduces morbidity of several diseases and disorders (including cerebrovascular and cardiovascular disease [CVD], depression, recovery from cancer, wound healing, autoimmune diseases, and inflammation-sensitive diseases [e.g., kidney disease, arthritis]), improves quality of life, and provides greater meaningfulness for women (Cohen et al., 2007; Fagundes, Lindgren, & Kiecolt-Glaser, 2013; Myers, 1999; Seeman, 2000; Strating, Suurmeijer, & Van Schuur, 2006; Uchino, 2006). In addition to impacting health behaviors, social relationships improve health through immunological, neural, and hormonal activity that alters physiological, emotional, and cognitive experiences and behavioral choices (Karelina & DeVries, 2011; Lakey & Orehek, 2011; Zender & Olshansky, 2012). It is in this way, too, that toxic relationships provoke inflammatory, sympathetic, and hormonal stress responses that diminish our ability to cope and heal.

Mortality

The impact of social relationships on life expectancy appears to be at least as large as that of smoking, obesity, sedentary lifestyle, and high blood pressure (Holt-Lunstad, Smith, & Layton, 2010; House, Landis, & Umberson, 1988; Sapolsky, 2004). A 50% higher risk for mortality correlates with having low social support, as high social support predicts lower CVD risk, the leading cause of death in the United States (Uchino et al., 2013). Russ and colleagues (2012) found a dose–response relationship between psychological stress (including depressive and anxiety symptoms, social dysfunction, and low self-confidence) and mortality that increased from 20% risk with the lowest reports of stress, to a twofold increase among those with very high stress. Conversely, a 50% increased likelihood of survival exists for individuals with stronger social relationships (Holt-Lunstad et al., 2010). Using multiple dimensions to assess social integration, an even stronger association was found: a 91% increase in the odds of survival. This finding rivals that of well-established risk factors (diet, smoking, etc.). Interestingly, the *belief* that stress is harmful, in combination with an individual's report of the amount of stress he or she is under, may increase the risk of premature death by 43% (Keller et al., 2012). If this association is causal, 20,000 excess deaths per year occurred during the study period from stressed people believing that stress is harmful. Conversely, the amount of stress reported in this study did not increase one's risk of mortality independent of the appraisal, and neither did experiencing high levels of stress while believing that stress has little effect on health (Keller et al., 2012). Changing one's appraisal of stress from that of "harm" to "helpful," where the stress response is accepted as the body's way of meeting a challenge, and that such a response is helpful and good, reduces vascular resistance to the stress and increases cardiac efficiency, which proves to be an adaptive response that attenuates pathological effects of stress on the cardiovascular system (Jamieson, Nock, & Mendes, 2012).

Mortality risk from stress may also be attenuated through enacting helping behaviors (Poulin, Brown, Dillard, & Smith, 2013). Helping behaviors, such as transportation, errands, shopping, housework, and child care, directed toward friends, neighbors, or relatives who did not live with them, buffered the effects of stressful events such that stress was not a predictor of mortality for those who engaged in helping behavior. Conversely, each additional stressful event in the Poulin et al. study (2013) predicted a 30% relative increase in mortality risk among those who did not engage in helping behaviors. The authors concluded that the health benefits of helping behaviors derive specifically from stress-buffering processes as a result of such actions (Poulin et al., 2013).

Morbidity

There is ample evidence linking social support to aspects of the cardiovascular, neuroendocrine, and immune systems, which is consistent with the beneficial role of social support across different diseases (Kamiya, Timonen, Romero-Ortuno, & Kenny, 2013; Uchino, 2006). Positive outcomes associated with supportive relationships include better recovery from cancer treatment, reduced stress, reduced physiological reactivity to stressful events, and a longer life span (Fagundes et al., 2013; Jaremka, Lindgren, & Kiecolt-Glaser, 2013) faster wound healing (Gouin & Kiecolt-Glaser, 2011), better dental and oral health (Tsakos et al., 2013), lower cancer mortality (Holt-Lunstad et al., 2010) reduced risk of respiratory infections (Cohen, Doyle, Skoner, Rabin, & Gwaltney, 1997), and lower risk of cognitive decline (Bennett, Schneider, Tang, Arnold, & Wilson, 2006).

Cardiovascular Disease

Systemic inflammation is consistently associated with CVD, its antecedents, and its outcomes (Steptoe & Kivimaki, 2012). Short-term psychosocial stress (such as an episode of intense anger, or acute sadness or bereavement) can trigger acute myocardial infarction, and chronic stress experienced at work and within one's family and social life is associated with a 40% to 50% increase in the occurrence of coronary heart disease (Kivimäki et al., 2006; Orth-Gomér et al., 2000; Steptoe & Kivimaki, 2012). Social support (emotional support, rather than instrumental support) tends to lower blood pressure reactivity (a risk for the development of CVD), and decrease atherosclerosis in women at high risk for developing heart disease (Uchino, 2006). The renin–angiotensin–aldosterone system (RAAS) has been neglected in social relationships research as a mechanism through which depression and social isolation may promote CVD (Häfner et al., 2012). The RAAS is a hormonal system that regulates blood pressure and fluid balance systemically via vasopressin production. The RAAS has a well-documented influence on the development and progression of CVD. Stress activates the RAAS, stimulating a range of processes that exacerbate cardiovascular injury, including oxidative stress (Leopold et al., 2007; Stehr et al., 2010), inflammation (Gekle & Grossmann, 2009), and insulin resistance (Lastra, Dhuper, Johnson, & Sowers, 2010). Häfner and colleagues (2012) discovered that living alone nor depressive symptomatology individually were associated with activation of the RAAS, but the combination of living alone and depressive symptomatology yielded a highly significant increase in aldosterone and renin levels (Häfner et al., 2012). This study demonstrated that, under the condition of chronic stress, depressed individuals may have a hyperactive RAAS response to stress, which could explain the known increased risk of CVD in this group.

Mental Health

Many studies correlate psychological stress and disorders, in the forms of depression, anxiety, isolation, self-silencing, absence of social support, examination stress, caregiver stress, major life events (loss of job, death of a spouse, etc.), and negative relationships, with an increased risk for certain disease outcomes such as CVD, Alzheimer disease, diabetes, cancer, osteoporosis, reduced resistance to viral infections, poorer wound healing, poorer response to vaccinations, dental periodontitis, and autoimmune disease (Kiecolt-Glaser, McGuire, Robles, & Glaser, 2002; Littrell, 2008). Furthermore, the relationship between depression and inflammation is bidirectional in that depression enhances inflammation and inflammation promotes depression (Jaremka, Lindgren, et al., 2013). Both situations also activate social disengagement behaviors (Dickerson, Kemeny, Aziz, Kim, & Fahey, 2004).

Resources such as close personal relationships that diminish negative emotions may enhance health in part through their positive impact on immune and endocrine regulation (Kiecolt-Glaser et al., 2005). For example, older women who report having trusting and satisfying relationships demonstrate lower levels of inflammatory markers (IL-6) than those with less satisfying relationships, as do ovarian cancer survivors reporting greater perceptions of closeness and intimacy in personal relationships (Kiecolt-Glaser, Gouin, & Hasoo, 2010). Conversely, mood states affect physiologic biomarkers, such that depression, anxiety, and anger and hostility enhance the production of IL-6, contribute to immune dysregulation through proinflammatory cytokine overproduction, and activate both the sympathetic–pituitary–adrenal medullary axis and the HPA axis (Kiecolt-Glaser et al., 2005).

Depression can also arise as a product of social rejection (mediated through biological mechanisms). Because social exclusion and rejection disrupt social bonds, and humans possess a basic drive to maintain a positive social status, rejection threatens self-preservation, and initiates a cascade of physiological, emotional, and cognitive responses. Social rejection implies a devaluation of a person by others, which can trigger self-diminishing thoughts (i.e., "I'm bad, unlovable, and of no value."). Such responses can be short-lived, but for those vulnerable to depression, the cyclical nature of negative thoughts and emotions can continue, moving toward greater disengagement and withdrawal (Kemeny, 2009; Slavich, O'Donovan, Epel, & Kemeny, 2010).

Relationships Throughout a Woman's Life Span

Prenatal

The period of prenatal development is a crucial time when biophysical processes are programmed for lifelong trait responses and behaviors, and is impacted heavily by the uterine environment's response to maternal physiology, behavior, and environment. In fact, fetal and maternal responses to stress appear to be coprogrammed, that is, programmed in parallel, which has implications for long-term child development and mother–child interactions (Sandman, Davis, Buss, & Glynn, 2012). Maternal cortisol in response to psychosocial stress impacts neonatal stress regulation, and decreases maternal affective responses to stress, alters memory, and increases the risk for postpartum depression (Davis, Glynn, Waffarn, & Sandman, 2011), suggesting a bidirectional exchange between maternal and placental physiology. Interestingly, a fetus's placenta acts as a "compressed hypothalamic–pituitary system," producing its own hormones, neuropeptides, growth factors, and cytokines (Entringer, Buss, & Wadhwa, 2010, p. 509). The degree to which stress hormones are experienced by the fetus, and maternal perceptions of stress, both vitally impact fetal nervous system organization and maternal adaptation during pregnancy. Pregnancy is also a critical period in a woman's life in which neural architecture is remodeled for the remainder of her life span. Such maternal programming includes changes in affective responses (dampened psychological and physiological responses to adverse events), biologically-mediated cognitive function (estradiol and cortisol trajectories predict memory recall and working memory), and depression, with the most sensitive gestational period for programming postnatal maternal mood being 25 weeks (Entringer et al., 2010).

Key periods of exposure exist during the prenatal time frame, with stressful events early in pregnancy perceived as more unpleasant by the mother, and may more greatly impact fetal development than with stress occurring late in the pregnancy (Sandman et al., 2012). On the other hand, although the maternal biological stress response progressively attenuates as a pregnancy progresses, late-stage prenatal stress is associated with offspring psychopathology and low birth weight (Rice et al., 2010). Great variation exists in newborn developmental "plasticity," that is, in the baby's differential biological sensitivity to their immediate environmental context (Pluess & Belsky, 2011). More sensitive babies are considered more "plastic," more malleable, to both positive *and* negative environments, whereas less "plastic" neonates respond less strongly to both positive and negative conditions. This malleability is seen in both physiological stress reactivity, as well as in infants' display of temperament, which then impacts parenting behavior quality and socioemotional functioning. It is posited that a baby's plasticity is programmed in utero, in response to maternal adversities (or ease) and cortisol activity. Interactions between stressful prenatal environments and genetic makeup can also promote or dampen the postnatal plasticity of a fetus (Pluess & Belsky, 2011). This prenatal stress programming, and subsequent postnatal physiological and behavioral reactivity, may contribute to creating a difficult and less cohesive childhood relationship within one's family. Pregnant women's recalled childhood stress has thus been associated with perceived stress during pregnancy, and with perceived social support in both childhood and as an adult (Kingston, Sword, Krueger, Hanna, & Markle-Reid, 2012).

Other evidence of neonates' development in relation to maternal factors include maternal depression predicting degree of right brain amygdala and neural fiber coherence and organization, and axonal integrity (Rifkin-Graboi et al., 2013); maternal positive affect in pregnancy extending the length of gestation (Voellmin, Entringer, Moog, Wadhwa, & Buss, 2013); maternal psychosocial stress predicting earlier delivery; placental corticotrophin-releasing hormone (CRH) in response to prenatal stress (psychosocial stress and other stress, such as nutritional, or environmental) predicting the rate of fetal growth and size at birth, and neonatal, childhood, and adult adiposity; reorganization of central neural pathways that program energy balance set points (leptin, ghrelin, peptide YY function) (Entringer et al., 2012); increased glucocorticoid exposure reducing pancreatic β-cell mass, lowering insulin content, and increasing the risk for metabolic diseases later in life (Entringer et al., 2010); maternal psychosocial stress, programming fetal cytokine and other immune responses (Entringer et al., 2008), HPA–axis activity (Entringer et al., 2009; Wüst, Entringer, Federenko, Schlotz, & Hellhammer, 2005), and newborn leukocyte telomere length, a biomarker that may predict age-related diseases and mortality (Entringer et al., 2013). Maternal stress in these studies was measured by number and types of adverse events: relationship conflicts, death of someone close, severe illness of a loved one, severe financial problems, having had a car accident, job loss, worry over birthing a disabled infant, globally-perceived stress, response to the Trier Social Stress Test (where a panel of judges negatively evaluate an individual performing an unprepared public speaking activity), and reports of depression, and state and trait anxiety (Robinson et al., 2011).

Early Childhood

The topic of social influences on brain development in early childhood forms the foundation of scientific inquiry into the psychophysiology of relationships. Other people are humans' primary environment. We survive initially based on the ability of our caregivers to detect our needs and intentions. If we are successful in relationships, we will have food, shelter, protection, and, for some, children of our own (recognizing that not all persons choose to have children or may experience infertility) (Cozolino, 2006). Stable attachment patterns (either health-promoting or health-defeating) are apparent by the end of the first year of life, established through experience-dependent right hemisphere linkage with a caregiver, and mediated through visual contact, vocalizations, and touch (Cozolino, 2006; Schore, 2001). Reactivity of cortisol secretion is highly dependent on attachment security (McEwen, 2003).

Familial relationships form the basis of our relational capacities, and are the primary pathways for transgenerational propagation of behavior, be they adaptive or otherwise. Babies acquire the most basic and enduring relational knowledge within the first year of life, where the infrastructure for the development of empathic capacity, attachment style, social competence, and emotional and physiological regulation is formed. It is well documented that caregiver–infant social interaction directly impacts central and peripheral nervous system development. Specifically, mutually responsive eye gaze, caregiver responsiveness to infant behavior, and physical touch facilitate right hemisphere and vagal nerve development, hippocampal size and structure, and formation of socioemotional regulation physiology (Porges, 1996; Schore, 2001). Parental care in an infant's early life contributes to the development of an internal perception by the infant as being worthy of love and caring, directs hippocampal volume, and patterns of the cortisol stress response that endure throughout life (Engert et al., 2010). Warm family environments, defined by expression of affection; parental involvement, monitoring, and directing of child behavior; and modeling of appropriate regulatory and social behavior in caregivers' relationships produces secure childhood attachments that lead to development of adaptive regulatory systems and behaviors, healthier social relationships and competencies, and better physical and mental health in adulthood.

Growing up in a risky family or harsh familial climate characterized by overt conflict, cold, unsupportive or neglectful relationships, inadequate parenting, household chaos, or deficient nurturing increases one's risk for chronic disease, especially CVD, autoimmune disorders, and premature death in adulthood (Miller & Chen, 2010; Repetti, Taylor, & Seeman, 2002). The effects of these harmful environments create deficits in children's control and expression of emotions, and deficits in social competence through physiologic dysregulation that accumulates over time and leads to adverse physical and mental health (Repetti et al., 2002).

Early life influences on lifelong patterns of emotionality and stress responsiveness is well established, and occurs through physiological formation of brain structures. These initial structural configurations set an individual up for later health or illness, and ultimately alter the rate of brain and body aging (McEwen, 2007; Repetti et al., 2002). Chronic illnesses may have their developmental roots in experiences from long ago, where deeply reinforced experiences have created (often unconscious) patterns of thinking, behaving, and interacting that are physiologically motivated, and may be quite resistant to change. That relational connection can alter this physiology for the better, and that disconnection through dismissiveness and objectification can reinforce it, is miraculous, and of fundamental importance.

Long-lasting consequences of childhood experiences are thought to persist into adulthood through physiological/neuroendocrine functioning in response to stress, leading to patterns in emotional processing that affect social competence and behavioral self-regulation (Repetti et al., 2002). Early disruptions continue to impact future developmental stages. Chronic sympathetic–adrenomedullary activation may lead to wear and tear on the cardiovascular system, leading eventually to chronic heart disease (Repetti et al., 2002). Because HPA activity modulates such a wide array of somatic functions, persistent activation of this system promotes immune deficiency, growth inhibition, delayed sexual maturity, hippocampal damage, cognitive impairment, and psychological problems (Repetti et al., 2002; Sapolsky, 2004). Dysregulation in the serotonergic system has been tied to depression, suicidality, aggression, and substance abuse. Genetic predisposition and family environment interact together in affecting these neurochemical systems (McEwen, 2010; Repetti et al., 2002). Over time, small perturbations in the body's regulatory system may accumulate, leading to multiple vulnerabilities. Body images, developed from infancy on, gain predispositions that set up later health or disease, ranging from mental illness to cancer to broken legs to querulous immaterial complaints. The problem arises when we ignore the fact that these predispositions are programmable (Comfort, 1979).

Adolescence

Adolescence is a distinct developmental stage socially and biologically, marked by puberty at the beginning, and being less defined as to its end. The discrepancy between physical maturity and social role maturity has widened since the 1800s. During these earlier centuries, attainment of physical maturity coincided for the most part with the completion of education, and gaining employment, marriage, and children. Today, however, the age at menarche occurs at roughly 12 to 13 years of age, while engagement in education can be lifelong and marriage and children may occur anytime through the 40s and possibly beyond. Such patterns make a clear demarcation of the end of adolescence difficult (Sawyer et al., 2012).

People aged 10 to 24 years comprise one-quarter of the world's population, the largest percentage in history, and coincides with a reduction in infectious disease, malnutrition, and early life mortality, even though the health of this group has improved significantly less than that of young children. Although chronic disease marks the health focus in developed nations, some of the most pressing problems among adolescents concern sexually transmitted infections; suicide; homicide; mental illness; substance misuse; and more socially-determined predictors such as intrafamilial difficulties, school, and sexual orientation violence; poverty; and racial and ethnic inequality (Blum, Bastos, Kabiru, & Le, 2012).

Adolescent periods are observable in other species in addition to humans in terms of behavioral observations of sensation- and novelty-seeking, risk-taking, fighting with parents, increases in peer-directed social interactions, and increased per-occasion alcohol intake (Spear, 2013). A major challenge of adolescence is reconciling the asynchronous maturation of socioemotional and cognitive systems. Cognitive, top-down impulse control is underdeveloped compared to the socioemotional neural systems, which are triggered by the onset of puberty and provide greater reward experiences through dopamine and oxytocin activation with social and emotional stimuli, promotion of sensation-seeking, preferences for peer companionship, sexual interest, and a desire for separation from the family unit (Casey, Getz, & Galvan, 2008). Thus, it is not that adolescents believe themselves invulnerable to risks (Millstein & Halpern-Felsher, 2002), or that they are incapable of sound judgment (Reyna & Farley, 2006), but that social and emotional triggers that are appraised unconsciously and intuitively, rather than deliberately, often override intellectual inhibition and result in the greater risk-taking behaviors so typical in this age group (Shulman & Cauffman, 2014). Indeed, full maturation of the human brain is not complete until about the age of 25 years.

The parent–child relationship shapes the context, style, and meaning of a teen's relationship with individuals outside the family. Teens with greater parental support delay their first sexual encounter, are more likely to use condoms, and expect sex to occur only within relationships, rather than casually. Parenting that builds sexual autonomy (volition and control in sexual decision making) through parental communication, monitoring, and transmission of sexual values through day-to-day interactions and role modeling may promote healthier and more satisfying sexual experiences for adolescents (Parkes, Henderson, Wight, & Nixon, 2011). However, precocious engagement in romantic and sexual relationships in adolescence is thought to undermine healthy adolescent development, and high-quality maternal parenting and supportive peer relationships can reduce the number of serious relationships and sexual encounters of adolescents (Roisman, Booth-LaForce, Cauffman, & Spieker, 2009). Sexual and reproductive health is important to address with adolescents and their parents. The degree of "connectedness" an adolescent experiences directly impacts teen pregnancy and sexually transmitted infection rates. Domains of connectedness significantly protective of sexual and reproductive health include family connectedness, general and sexuality-specific parent–adolescent communication, parental monitoring, and peer, partner, and school connectedness. Overly controlling parenting behaviors tend to impart greater sexual risk behaviors in adolescents (Markham et al., 2010).

Friendships can be adaptive. The fact that many mammalian species develop friendships that last years, including horses, elephants, hyenas, dolphins, and chimpanzees (Seyfarth & Cheney, 2012), indicates an evolutionary origin of friendship that enables survival and health. Adolescents' social capital is defined by quantity (breadth) and quality (depth) of their relationships. The extensiveness of a friendship network and the degree of high-quality relationships across contexts contribute interpersonal assets and opportunities to a teen as he or she adjusts to the transition to young adulthood (Pettit et al., 2011). For females and males alike, friendships enhance skills: males often gain greater competitive ability, and women experience less stress, greater survival of their infants, and longer life spans than would exist without such friendships (Seyfarth & Cheney, 2012). But peers can also promote risk-taking, unsafe, and unhealthy behaviors. There is robust and consistent support for the role of peers in alcohol use, smoking, aggressive and illegal behaviors, nonsuicidal self-harm, depressive symptoms, eating problems, body image concerns, and values and beliefs around academic motivation and achievement and prejudiced attitudes (Brechwald & Prinstein, 2011). Interestingly, even sleep behaviors are known to be influenced by adolescent peers and, in the situation of shortened sleep patterns of 6 to 7 hours per night, may instigate drug use through mediating factors of conduct, cognitive, and emotional problems (Mednick, Christakis, & Fowler, 2010). The social environment in which lesbian, gay, and bisexual teens live, measured by the proportion of same-sex couples, proportion of registered voters supportive of gays, presence of gay–straight alliances in schools, and nondiscrimination and antibullying school policies, significantly contributes to suicide attempts in this population (Hatzenbuehler, 2011).

Role models for adolescents also impact their health behaviors, with teacher, family member, and athlete role models promoting more positive health behaviors, and peer and entertainer role models associated with riskier health behaviors (Yancey, Grant, Kurosky, Kravitz-Wirtz, & Mistry, 2011). Likewise, experiencing less chronic interpersonal stress in the late teen years results in lower expression of inflammatory signal markers, and a less pronounced IL-6 response to a microbial challenge. These biological markers relative to social stress may demonstrate a mechanism through which inflammation-sensitive diseases such as depression and heart disease are diminished or enhanced (Miller, Rohleder, & Cole, 2009). Finally, the use of social network sites through electronic media have both positive and negative impacts on adolescent development and health. Because this age is marked by shifts toward independence and establishing a unique identity, social media can offer a venue to "try on" different identities while remaining anonymous. Learning to refine the capacity for self-control, nuanced interactions involved with being tolerant and respectful of others' viewpoints, gaining peer acceptance and feedback, and using online social networks to strengthen off-line relationships with peers are other positive effects of social media use among teens. Negative aspects of social media include exposure to cyberbullying and sexual predators, and engaging in more violent, sexual, and substance use behaviors (Pujazon-Zazik & Park, 2010).

Goals for a healthy adolescence include being academically engaged, emotionally, socially, and physically safe and healthy, and possessing a positive sense of self,

self-efficacy, and life and decision-making skills (Blum et al., 2012). It is a time period in which many patterns of adult health and behavior are established, and should be placed center stage if we are to impact population health across diverse conditions.

Midlife

Midlife comprises a long and rather nebulous period in life in which much growth, change, and maturation occurs. With the life expectancy of women increasing from 40 years of age in 1900 to 80.2 in 2006, interests, motivations, roles, and resources in social relationships undergo great changes that impact women's health. Women invest in their relationships across the life span in different ways than do men, with many and distinct shifts in their most significant relationships, which may have a direct relationship to changes in a woman's reproductive stage. For instance, women invest more heavily in creating and maintaining pair bonds than do men during reproductively-active periods in their lives (Palchykov, Kaski, Kertész, Barabási, & Dunbar, 2012). As women age, however, attention tends to shift away from one's spouse and toward a group of contacts that change dynamically in importance based on the transition in reproductive stages from choosing a mate, to child rearing, to investing as a grandparent. Men, on the other hand, demonstrate little variance in their most significant relational contacts across the life span (Palchykov et al., 2012).

Midlife women transition through that many life phases that may include marriage and parenthood, work and career activities, caregiving roles across multiple generations, and hormonal cycles and shifts that occur through monthly menses cycles, pregnancy, lactation, and menopause. In general, midlife may be defined generally as life between the ages of 40 and 60 years; however, it may be better defined by the primary changes, conflicts, and characteristics of this phase of life, and as a period in one's life when old values are questioned and new directions are sought (Boston, 2006).

A variety of health implications relative to social relationships in this life period include many factors. Many women derive a greater sense of well-being from and preference for friends more than relatives (Waite & Harrison, 1992). Childless women, single mothers, or full-time homemakers are more likely to report poorer health than women who hold multiple roles (McMunn, Bartley, Hardy, & Kuh, 2006). Psychosocial health status is affected by biological changes of weight gain, decreasing eyesight, diminishing energy, a stressful familial environment, and fear of aging and loneliness (Singh & Singh, 2006). Women in a stable relationship (co-habitation or marriage) tend to enjoy better sleep quality (Troxel et al., 2010).

Despite appearances to the contrary, menopause and midlife crises may be largely socially constructed rather than biologically determined (Ward, Scheid, & Tuffrey, 2010). Experiencing more intense menopausal symptoms occurs more readily in cultures where lower social class and greater male domination reduce a woman's social and financial autonomy. Menopausal symptoms such as vasomotor activity, joint pain, and some psychosomatic disorders are evinced through feeling more socially degraded and of less aesthetic and social value, whereas women of higher social class with greater autonomy report few physical symptoms of menopause and little change in their social value (Delanoe et al., 2012). It has been posited that biology and culture interact to create "local biologies," where menopausal symptoms vary according to local perceptions of the inherent value of a woman, rather than merely her reproductive capacity (Lock, 1993, 2002, 2007).

Marital strain joins social isolation as a psychosocial risk factor for negative health outcomes that is similar in magnitude to more traditional risk factors, such as physical activity and smoking (Jaremka, Glaser, Malarkey, & Kiecolt-Glaser, 2013). Marital discord has been identified as a risk factor for morbidity in the form of major depressive illness, worsened prognoses among women with coronary heart disease, and overall increased mortality (Kiecolt-Glaser et al., 2005). Familial discord increases the odds of relapsing from a mood or psychiatric disorder, heightens susceptibility to respiratory infections, delayed wound healing, accelerated emergence of metabolic syndrome, and CVD morbidity and mortality (Miller et al., 2009). Prolonged social stress can foster exacerbations of immune conditions such as multiple sclerosis and rheumatoid arthritis (Marin, Martin, Blackwell, Stetler, & Miller, 2007). A review by Wanic and Kulik (2011) found that negative and hostile behaviors during marital conflict promoted elevations in cardiovascular activity, altered hormones related to stress, and dysregulated immune function in women, and may be attributed to women being more relationally dependent on and subordinate to men.

Menopause/Older Women

Aging, though often fraught with physical and cognitive decline, can also be a period of great satisfaction and meaning, attributed strongly to an individual's social and relational environment. While women's need for social relationships continue as they age and the consequences of being isolated also continue, women's social and emotional lives do change. Emotions become more predictable and stable as women's life experiences facilitate their resilience (Charles & Carstensen, 2010). The natural decrease in biological, physical, and cognitive abilities intermingle with resources of a lifetime of successful adaptation to demarcate old age as a unique time period rich with challenge and meaning.

Aging women naturally and actively prune their social network from a greater number of casual contacts to a smaller cohort of more intimate, familiar, emotionally close, and meaningful contacts, with the number of emotionally close companions remaining mostly stable throughout life (Fung, Stoeber, Yeung, & Lang, 2008). Older people derive greater satisfaction from interaction with family than do younger adults (Carstensen, Mikels, & Mather, 2006; Charles & Piazza, 2007). Network size and constitution change over the life span, with the exception of the family network, which tends to remain fairly stable. Some networks are important only through specific age ranges, such as work and friend networks as social transitions take place. Furthermore, personal and friend networks decrease in size over the last 35 years of life (Wrzus, Hänel, Wagner, & Neyer, 2013), but the importance of relationality remains. A longer life-span is correlated with being more relationally-oriented as reflected in speech, thinking, and writing (Pressman & Cohen, 2007).

Positive social engagement confers significant benefits on the health of all individuals. In fact, negative social engagements is comparable to other established risk factors for mortality (on par with ceasing smoking, and exceeds mortality risks associated with obesity and physical inactivity) (Holt-Lunstad et al., 2010). Older persons with strong social relationships possess an average of 55% increase in the likelihood of survival, despite age, gender, health status, and ultimate cause of death (hazard ratios = 1.91 – 1.19, depending on how social relationships were measured) (Holt-Lunstad et al., 2010). Social engagement remains important even into very late adulthood (90–97 years of age) as a determinant of physical health. The number of club memberships and hours spent outside the home predict objective health measures, but not necessarily positive health behaviors (Cherry et al., 2013). Increased social activity, including visiting friends or family, going out to eat, to sporting events, group meetings, church activities, day or overnight trips, and volunteer work, or playing games reduces the risk of disability in performing activities of daily living by as much as 43% for each additional unit of social activity, and 31% for developing a mobility disability (James, Boyle, Buchman, & Bennett, 2011). Subjective well-being is also increased among older persons who provide social support to others, versus those who receive such support, with the exception of receiving support from a spouse or sibling (Thomas, 2010).

Loneliness and social isolation are well documented to increase the risk of morbidity and mortality. As much as 39% of older persons aged 74 years or more reported being lonely, which imparts a 33% greater likelihood of dying for lonely versus nonlonely older adults (Tilvis, Laitala, Routasalo, & Pitkälä, 2011), and a 26% greater likelihood of dying among socially-isolated older adults (Steptoe, Shankar, Demakakos, & Wardle, 2013). Loneliness and social isolation also affect health indirectly through promoting inactivity, smoking and other health-risk behaviors, and directly through increasing blood pressure, C-reactive protein, and fibrinogen levels, all biological markers associated with the development of CVD (Shankar, McMunn, Banks, & Steptoe, 2011). Holt-Lunstad and colleagues (2010) drew a parallel between the health impacts of social isolation and the discovery half a century ago that a lack of human contact among infants in custodial care (orphanages) predicted excess mortality. This single finding altered practices and policies in these settings. Similarly, modern health care could benefit from acknowledging this single, well-documented phenomenon: "Social relationships influence the health outcomes of adults" (Holt-Lunstad et al., 2010, p. 14). The effects of relational connection on health appears to be general, as effects are consistent despite gender, age, cause of death, and health status, suggesting that efforts to reduce relational disconnection and disintegration should be integrated into care at every stage in life.

Interventions to Promote Relational Health

Intervening to improve social engagement, relational capacity, or natural social networks is complex and requires careful consideration of individual circumstances and contexts (Cohen & Janicki-Deverts, 2009). Attempts to reduce social isolation and loneliness include group or one-to-one interventions, and participatory or nonparticipatory interventions. Some interventions provide activities and some instrumental support, and interventions with a theoretical basis may be more effective than those without, as are interventions that provide social activity or support within a group setting that encourages active participation (Dickens, Richards, Greaves, & Campbell, 2011). Windle, Francis, and Coomber (2011) note the use of Community Navigators and emphasize the importance of befriending, mentoring, and social group activities, with fair to good outcomes among most programs.

Exploiting the natural proclivity for health attitudes and behaviors to spread may be an effective approach to improve social ties. For instance, it has been shown that the risk for obesity increases significantly for friends and family of an obese individual (Christakis & Fowler, 2007). Similar patterns are observed in smoking habits within networks (Christakis & Fowler, 2008), alcohol use (Rosenquist, Murabito, Fowler, & Christakis, 2010), happiness spreading through social networks (Fowler, Christakis,

Steptoe, & Roux, 2009), and divorce (McDermott, Fowler, & Christakis, 2013). Policies such as the Health and Human Services Healthy Marriage Initiative, National Scientific Council on the Developing Child, Keeping Children and Families Safe Act, and Individuals with Disabilities Education Act may also impact effective relational engagement (Shonkoff, Boyce, & McEwen, 2009; Umberson & Montez, 2010).

Interventions often aim to provide something to individuals in distress; however, providing opportunities for giving help to others may be an innovative and mutually beneficial approach to improving health for the giver of help through better social engagement. Help given to others is a better predictor of health and well-being than are measures of social engagement or received social support (Poulin et al., 2013). The ability to contribute to one's social network provides unique psychosocial benefits. It enhances a sense of meaning and mattering, and acts as a unique stress buffer that distinguishes it from other kinds of social interactions. The act of giving to others triggers an emotional state of compassion, and the physiological state of the caregiving behavioral system (Konrath, 2014; Oman, 2007; Poulin et al., 2012).

Reappraisal is a powerful tool for adaptive coping to stressful relationships and events. Reappraisal is a process of changing one's thoughts and feelings about their situation. The process begins with allowing the disclosure of feelings about the situation and validation of those feelings. Then guided reflection on the feelings and goals attempts to facilitate a revised view of the situation, rather than attempting to solve the problem. Reappraisal reduces stress and physiological activation long term through actively engaging the problem to arrive at a revised understanding of it (Priem & Solomon, 2009). Reappraisal integrates bodily sensations with external sensory information and knowledge of a situation (Barrett, 2006). With conscious attention and intention, sympathetic activation that is automatically appraised as a threat may be reconceptualized as a challenge. This reconceptualization is a cognition that alters the downstream physiological response into more positive cardiovascular activity that builds physiological toughness. Reappraisal is a centerpiece of cognitive–behavioral therapy, which has a long and well-documented legacy in effective coping (Jamieson, Mendes, & Nock, 2013).

Activities that promote self-understanding, insight, clarity, and exploration of interpersonal relational dynamics can improve social efficacy, motivation for engagement, and empathy. Expressive writing is a powerful technique to accomplish the above outcomes. Writing expressively about a relationship breakup resulted in fewer upper respiratory illnesses, less tension and fatigue, and lower levels of intrusive thoughts and social avoidance behaviors among a cohort of undergraduate students (Lepore & Greenberg, 2002). Pennebaker (1985) found that failure to express thoughts and feelings about a stressful event heightens the probability of obsessing about the event, as well as the probability of illness, with the act of confiding or otherwise translating traumatic events into language, reducing autonomic activity and disease rates. Narration fosters relational connection, allowing diagnosis and treatment to occur on a more profound level. Too, the very act of translating experience into language, either verbal or written, imparts improved biological and mental health through the construction of meaning and understanding of experiences, and through psychophysiological alterations (Adler, 1997; Pennebaker, 1985, 2003). Transforming the amorphous experience of being sick, for example, into a narrative makes one's experience more manageable by organizing it into a chronological sequence of events linked by causal factors (Adler, 1997). The therapeutic potential of narration is realized when the illness or traumatic experience has been organized coherently, makes more sense to the author, and has been mutually processed through engagement with another individual (Adler, 1997). Thus, in a clinical situation, by allowing patients to tell their stories and give context to their illness, not only does the clinician gain a more well-rounded view of the patient, but healing may have already begun even before a diagnosis has been determined. The belief that someone important is listening and cares is healing for body and mind (Adler, 2002), and when caregivers see that their attention has instilled a sense of personal value in a patient who feels isolated and useless, meaning and purpose are added to the lives of the patient and caregiver.

Some have explored the importance of the listener to the quality of the voice that emerges (Adler, 1997; Miller, 1986). Jordan (1997) reported that the expectation that someone will listen and make an effort to understand greatly enhances the clarity and sureness of the message presented. If the listener does not really wish to know the speaker's experience, the speaker may become confused and suffer a decrease in clarity, distinctness, or focus about her experience. With an empathic response, one's experience comes into focus, and without it, anxiety may arise from a sense that one's own reality will blur. We achieve a sense of personal integration through relatedness with others, and it is this integration that provides a sense of well-being (Jordan, 1997).

Growth is achieved through integration. Integration can be described as embracing differences, while at the same time looking for points of connection or linkages both within one's self and between individuals, and constitutes the fundamental component that provides a sense of well-being (Siegel, 2010). Integration is achieved through the processes of insight (looking within one's self and honoring conflicting experiences and promoting new pathways of understanding) and empathy (understanding the experiences of another person), and is the basis for developing secure attachments and enjoying healthy relationships with others (Siegel, 2010). Using a step-by-step process termed "mindsight," integrating mental, emotional, or behavioral *rigidity* on the one hand, and *chaos* on the other, can yield a flexible, cohesive flow that is adaptable to biological and relational perturbations to create well-being (Siegel, 2006).

All relationships are punctuated by disconnections and misunderstandings, and intensity of feeling and powerful conflict is frequently an aspect of relational growth and healing. Connecting in a real and growth-enhancing way with others is not always easy, nor harmonious or comfortable, but there is a powerful force behind the movement toward connection that includes a desire to contribute to others and serve something greater than "the self" (Jordan, Hartling, & Walker, 2006, p. 6). Disconnections can, in fact, facilitate growth when they are redirected toward connection. The process of connection–disconnection–reconnection is a primary pathway of growth in situations of mutual responsiveness (Jordan, 2009). Conflict is inevitable: it is the source of all growth, and an absolute necessity if one is to be alive (Miller, 1986, p. 125). One deals with conflict by making and holding connections between apparent opposites. Acknowledging and naming differences furthers the development of individuals in conflict, and the paradox is that people can tolerate diversity and difference by becoming more connected. Being able to hold conflict within connection enables us to define and understand ourselves and our differences from others (Fedele, 2004, p. 205). Waging good conflict, according to Miller (1986), entails respectful engagement with others while maintaining one's integrity with confidence and hope.

In the midst of intense conflictual struggle, it may be helpful to find "one true thing" that can be said or shared (Jordan, 2009). Sometimes, this one truth can shift an experience from disconnection to "conflict in connection" (Fedele, 2004), with the ultimate goal of improved health.

References

Adler, H. M. (1997). The history of the present illness as treatment: Who's listening, and why does it matter? *Journal of the American Board of Family Practice, 10*(1), 28–35.

Adler, H. M. (2002). The sociophysiology of caring in the doctor-patient relationship. *Journal of General Internal Medicine, 17*(11), 874–881.

Adler, H. M. (2007). Toward a biopsychosocial understanding of the patient-physician relationship: An emerging dialogue. *Journal of General Internal Medicine, 22*(2), 280–285.

Axelrod, R., & Hamilton, W. D. (1981). The evolution of cooperation. *Science, 211*(4489), 1390–1396.

Barrett, L. F. (2006). Solving the emotion paradox: Categorization and the experience of emotion. *Personality and Social Psychology Review, 10*, 20–46.

Bartz, J. A., Zaki, J., Bolger, N., & Ochsner, K. N. (2011). Social effects of oxytocin in humans: Context and person matter. *Trends in Cognitive Sciences, 15*(7), 301–309.

Baumgartner, T., Heinrichs, M., Vonlanthen, A., Fischbacher, U., & Fehr, E. (2008). Oxytocin shapes the neural circuitry of trust and trust adaptation in humans. *Neuron, 58*(4), 639–650.

Bennett, D. A., Schneider, J. A., Tang, Y., Arnold, S. E., & Wilson, R. S. (2006). The effect of social networks on the relation between Alzheimer's disease pathology and level of cognitive function in old people: A longitudinal cohort study. *Lancet Neurology, 5*(5), 406–412.

Blum, R. W., Bastos, F. I. P. M., Kabiru, C., & Le, L. C. (2012). Adolescent health in the 21st century. *Lancet, 379*(9826):1567–1568.

Boston, G. (2006). Women in midlife look for happiness in new ways of expression. *World and I, 21*(2), 17.

Brechwald, W. A., & Prinstein, M. J. (2011). Beyond homophily: A decade of advances in understanding peer influence processes. *Journal of Research on Adolescence, 21*(1), 166–179.

Cacioppo, J. T., Hawkley, L. C., Norman, G. J., & Berntson, G. G. (2011). Social isolation. *Annals of the New York Academy of Sciences, 1231*(1), 17–22.

Carboni, I., & Gilman, R. (2012). Brokers at risk: Gender differences in the effects of structural position on social stress and life satisfaction. *Group Dynamics: Theory, Research, and Practice, 16*(3), 218.

Carstensen, L. L., Mikels, J. A., & Mather, M. (2006). Aging and the intersection of cognition, motivation, and emotion. *Handbook of the Psychology of Aging, 6*, 343–362.

Casey, B. J., Getz, S., & Galvan, A. (2008). The adolescent brain. *Developmental Review, 28*(1), 62–77.

Charles, S. T., & Carstensen, L. L. (2010). Social and emotional aging. *Annual Review of Psychology, 61*, 383–409.

Charles, S. T., & Piazza, J. R. (2007). Memories of social interactions: Age differences in emotional intensity. *Psychology and Aging, 22*(2), 300.

Cherry, K. E., Walker, E. J., Brown, J. S., Volaufova, J., LaMotte, L. R., Welsh, D. A., & Frisard, M. I. (2013). Social engagement and health in younger, older, and oldest-old adults in the Louisiana Healthy Aging Study. *Journal of Applied Gerontology, 32*(1), 51–75.

Christakis, N. A., & Fowler, J. H. (2007). The spread of obesity in a large social network over 32 years. *New England Journal of Medicine, 357*(4), 370–379.

Christakis, N. A., & Fowler, J. H. (2008). The collective dynamics of smoking in a large social network. *New England Journal of Medicine, 358*(21), 2249–2258.

Cohen, S. (2004). Social relationships and health. *American Psychologist, 59*(8), 676.

Cohen, S., Doyle, W. J., Skoner, D. P., Rabin, B. S., & Gwaltney, J. M. (1997). Social ties and susceptibility to the common cold. *Journal of the American Association, 277*(24), 1940–1944.

Cohen, S., & Janicki-Deverts, D. (2009). Can we improve our physical health by altering our social networks? *Perspectives on Psychological Science, 4*(4), 375–378.

Cohen, S., & Lemay, E. P. (2007). Why would social networks be linked to affect and health practices? *Health Psychology, 26*(4), 410.

Cohen, S. D., Sharma, T., Acquaviva, K., Peterson, R. A., Patel, S. S., & Kimmel, P. L. (2007). Social support and chronic kidney disease: An update. *Advances in Chronic Kidney Disease, 14*(4), 335–344.

Comfort, A. (1979). *I and that: Notes on the biology of religion.* New York, NY: Crown.

Costa, J. T. (2013). Hamiltonian inclusive fitness: A fitter fitness concept. *Biology Letters, 9*(6), 20130335.

Cozolino, L. J. (2006). *The neuroscience of human relationships: Attachment and the developing social brain.* New York, NY: Norton.

Davis, E. P., Glynn, L. M., Waffarn, F., & Sandman, C. A. (2011). Prenatal maternal stress programs infant stress regulation. *Journal of Child Psychology and Psychiatry, 52*(2), 119–129.

Delanoë, D., Hajri, S., Bachelot, A., Mahfoudh Draoui, D., Hassoun, D., Marsicano, E., & Ringa, V. (2012). Class, gender and culture in the experience of menopause. A comparative survey in Tunisia and France. *Social Science & Medicine, 75*(2), 401–409.

De Vogli, R., Chandola, T., & Marmot, M. G. (2007). Negative aspects of close relationships and heart disease. *Archives of Internal Medicine, 167*(18), 1951.

Dickens, A. P., Richards, S. H., Greaves, C. J., & Campbell, J. L. (2011). Interventions targeting social isolation in older people: A systematic review. *BMC Public Health, 11*(1), 647.

Dickerson, S. S., Kemeny, M. E., Aziz, N., Kim, K. H., & Fahey, J. L. (2004). Immunological effects of induced shame and guilt. *Psychosomatic Medicine, 66*(1), 124–131.

Dictionary.com Unabridged. (2013). *Based on the Random House Dictionary.* Random House. Retrieved from Dictionary.com website: http://dictionary.reference.com/browse/relationship

Engert, V., Khalili-Mahani, N., Dedovic, K., Buss, C., Wadiwalla, M., & Pruessner, J. C. (2010). Investigating the association between early life parental care and stress responsivity in adulthood. *Developmental Neuropsychology, 35*(5), 570–581.

Entringer, S., Buss, C., Swanson, J. M., Cooper, D. M., Wing, D. A., Waffarn, F., & Wadhwa, P. D. (2012). Fetal programming of body composition, obesity, and metabolic function: The role of intrauterine stress and stress biology. *Journal of Nutrition and Metabolism, 2012,* 632548.

Entringer, S., Buss, C., & Wadhwa, P. D. (2010). Prenatal stress and developmental programming of human health and disease risk: Concepts and integration of empirical findings. *Current Opinion in Endocrinology, Diabetes, and Obesity, 17*(6), 507.

Entringer, S., Epel, E. S., Lin, J., Buss, C., Shahbaba, B., Blackburn, E. H., & Wadhwa, P. D. (2013). Maternal psychosocial stress during pregnancy is associated with newborn leukocyte telomere length. *American Journal of Obstetrics and Gynecology, 208*(2), 134-e1.

Entringer, S., Kumsta, R., Hellhammer, D. H., Wadhwa, P. D. & Wüst, S. (2009). Prenatal exposure to maternal psychosocial stress and HPA axis regulation in young adults. *Hormones and Behavior, 55*(2), 292–298.

Entringer, S., Kumsta, R., Nelson, E. L., Hellhammer, D. H., Wadhwa, P. D., & Wüst, S. (2008). Influence of prenatal psychosocial stress on cytokine production in adult women. *Developmental Psychobiology, 50*(6), 579–587.

Fagundes, C. P., Lindgren, M. E., & Kiecolt-Glaser, J. K. (2013). Psychoneuroimmunology and cancer: Incidence, progression, and quality of life. In B. I. Carr & J. Steel (Eds.), *Psychological aspects of cancer* (pp. 1–11). New York, NY: Springer.

Fedele, N. (2004). Relationships in groups: Connection, resonance, and paradox. In J. V. Jordan, M. Walker & L. M. Harting (Eds.), *Complexity of connection.* New York, NY: Guilford Press.

Fishbane, M. (2001). Relational narratives of the self. *Family Process, 40*(3), 273–291.

Fowler, J. H., Christakis, N. A., Steptoe, A., & Roux, D. (2008). Dynamic spread of happiness in a large social network: Longitudinal analysis of the Framingham Heart Study social network. *British Medical Journal,337*:a2338.

Fredrickson, B. L. (2004). The broaden-and-build theory of positive emotions. *Philosophical Transactions-Royal Society of London Series B Biological Sciences, 359*(1449) 1367–1378.

Fung, H. H., Stoeber, F. S., Yeung, D. Y. L., & Lang, F. R. (2008). Cultural specificity of socioemotional selectivity: Age differences in social network composition among Germans and Hong Kong Chinese. *Journals of Gerontology Series B: Psychological Sciences and Social Sciences, 63*(3), P156–P164.

Gekle, M., & Grossmann, C. (2009). Actions of aldosterone in the cardiovascular system: The good, the bad, and the ugly? *Pflügers Archiv: European Journal of Physiology, 458*(2), 231–246.

Gouin, J. P., Carter, C. S., Pournajafi-Nazarloo, H., Glaser, R., Malarkey, W. B., Loving, T. J., & Kiecolt-Glaser, J. K. (2010). Marital behavior, oxytocin, vasopressin, and wound healing. *Psychoneuroendocrinology, 35*(7), 1082–1090.

Gouin, J. P., Carter, C. S., Pournajafi-Nazarloo, H., Malarkey, W. B., Loving, T. J., Stowell, J., & Kiecolt-Glaser, J. K. (2012). Plasma vasopressin and interpersonal functioning. *Biological Psychology, 91*(2), 270–274.

Gouin, J. P., & Kiecolt-Glaser, J. K. (2011). The impact of psychological stress on wound healing: Methods and mechanisms. *Immunology and Allergy Clinics of North America, 31*(1), 81–93.

Häfner, S., Baumert, J., Emeny, R. T., Lacruz, M. E., Bidlingmaier, M., Reincke, M., & Ladwig, K. H. (2012). To live alone and to be depressed, an alarming combination for the renin–angiotensin–aldosterone-system (RAAS). *Psychoneuroendocrinology, 37*(2), 230–237.

Hatzenbuehler, M. L. (2011). The social environment and suicide attempts in lesbian, gay, and bisexual youth. *Pediatrics, 127*(5), 896–903.

Hawkley, L. C., & Cacioppo, J. T. (2010). Loneliness matters: A theoretical and empirical review of consequences and mechanisms. *Annals of Behavioral Medicine, 40*(2), 218–227.

Hirschman, E. C. (1994). Consumers and their animal companions. *Journal of Consumer Research, 20,* 616–632. doi:10.1086/209374

Holt-Lunstad, J., Smith, T. B., & Layton, J. B. (2010). Social relationships and mortality risk: A meta-analytic review. *PLoS Medicine, 7*(7), e1000316.

House, J. S., Landis, K. R., & Umberson, D. (1988). Social relationships and health. *Science, 241*(4865), 540–545.

Immordino-Yang, M. H., & Damasio, A. (2007). We feel, therefore we learn: The relevance of affective and social neuroscience to education. *Mind, Brain, and Education, 1*(1), 3–10.

Jack, D. C. (1991). *Silencing the self: Women and depression.* Cambridge, MA: Harvard University Press.

Jack, D. C. (1999). Silencing the self: Inner dialogues and outer realities. In T. Joiner & J. C. Coyne (Eds.), *The interactional nature of depression: Advances in interpersonal approaches* (pp. 221–246). Washington, DC: American Psychological Association.

Jack, D. C., & Dill, D. (1992). The silencing the self scale: Schemas of intimacy associated with depression in women. *Psychology of Women Quarterly, 16*, 97–106.

James, B. D., Boyle, P. A., Buchman, A. S., & Bennett, D. A. (2011). Relation of late-life social activity with incident disability among community-dwelling older adults. *Journals of Gerontology Series A: Biological Sciences and Medical Sciences, 66*(4), 467–473.

Jamieson, J. P., Mendes, W. B., & Nock, M. K. (2013). Improving acute stress responses the power of reappraisal. *Current Directions in Psychological Science, 22*(1), 51–56.

Jamieson, J. P., Nock, M. K., & Mendes, W. B. (2012). Mind over matter: Reappraising arousal improves cardiovascular and cognitive responses to stress. *Journal of Experimental Psychology: General, 141*(3), 417.

Jaremka, L. M., Glaser, R., Malarkey, W. B., & Kiecolt-Glaser, J. K. (2013). Marital distress prospectively predicts poorer cellular immune function. *Psychoneuroendocrinology, 38*(11), 2713–2719.

Jaremka, L. M., Lindgren, M. E., & Kiecolt-Glaser, J. K. (2013). Synergistic relationships among stress, depression, and troubled relationships: Insights from psychoneuroimmunology. *Depression and Anxiety, 30*(4), 288–296.

Jordan, J. V. (1986). *The meaning of mutuality.* Wellesley, MA: Stone Center for Developmental Services and Studies, Wellesley College.

Jordan, J. V. (1997). Relational development: Therapeutic implications of empathy and shame. In J. V. Jordan (Ed.), *Women's growth in diversity* (pp. 138–161). New York, NY: Guilford Press.

Jordan, J. V. (1997). *Women's growth in diversity: More writings from the Stone Center.* New York, NY: Guilford Press.

Jordan, J. V. (2000). The role of mutual empathy in relational/cultural therapy. *Journal of Clinical Psychology, 56*(8), 1005–1016.

Jordan, J. V. (2009). *Introduction to relational-cultural theory* (Oral). Wellesley, MA: Stone Center at Wellesley College.

Jordan, J. V., & Hartling, L. M. (2002). The development of relational-cultural theory (article adapted from "New developments in Relational-Cultural Theory"). In M. Ballou & L. S. Brown (Eds.), *Rethinking mental health disorders: Feminist perspectives* (pp. 48–70). New York, NY: Guilford Press.

Jordan, J. V., Hartling, L. M., & Walker, M. (2006). *The complexity of connection: Writings from the Stone Center's Jean Baker Miller Training Institute.* New York, NY: Guilford Press.

Jordan, J. V., Kaplan, A., Miller, J. B., Stiver, I., & Surrey, J. (1991). *Women's growth in connection: Writings from the Stone Center.* New York, NY: Guilford Press.

Jordan, J. V., Surrey, J., & Kaplan, A. (1991). Women and empathy: Implications for psychological development and psychotherapy. In J. V. Jordan, A. G. Kaplan, J. B. Miller, I. P. Stiver & J. L. Surrey (Eds.), *Women's growth in connection.* New York, NY: Guilford Press.

Jordan, J. V., & Walker, M. (2006). Introduction. In J. V. Jordan, M. Walker & L. M. Hartling (Eds.), *The complexity of connection* (pp. 1–8). New York, NY: Guilford Press.

Kamiya, Y., Timonen, V., Romero-Ortuno, R., & Kenny, R. (2013). Back to basics or into a brave new world? The potential and pitfalls of biomarkers in explaining the pathways between social engagement and health. In *Applied demography and public health* (pp. 313–336). Netherlands: Springer.

Kaplan, A. (1986). The "self-in-relation": Implications for depression in women. *Psychotherapy, 23*(2), 234–242.

Karelina, K., & DeVries, A. C. (2011). Modeling social influences on human health. *Psychosomatic Medicine, 73*(1), 67–74.

Keller, A., Litzelman, K., Wisk, L. E., Maddox, T., Cheng, E. R., Creswell, P. D., & Witt, W. P. (2012). Does the perception that stress affects health matter? The association with health and mortality. *Health Psychology, 31*(5), 677.

Kemeny, M. E. (2009). Psychobiological responses to social threat: Evolution of a psychological model in psychoneuroimmunology. *Brain Behavior and Immunity, 23*(1), 1–9.

Kemp, A. H., Quintana, D. S., Kuhnert, R. L., Griffiths, K., Hickie, I. B., & Guastella, A. J. (2012). Oxytocin increases heart rate variability in humans at rest: Implications for social approach-related motivation and capacity for social engagement. *PLoS One, 7*(8), e44014.

Kiecolt-Glaser, J.K., Gouin, J.P., & Hansoo, L. (2010). Close relationships, inflammation, and health. *Neuroscience & Biobehavioral Reviews, 35*(1), 33–38.

Kiecolt-Glaser, J. K., Loving, T. J., Stowell, J. R., Malarkey, W. B., Lemeshow, S., Dickinson, S. L., & Glaser, R. (2005). Hostile marital interactions, proinflammatory cytokine production, and wound healing. *Archives of General Psychiatry, 62*(12), 1377–1384.

Kiecolt-Glaser, J. K., McGuire, L., Robles, T. F., & Glaser, R. (2002). Psychobiological factors in health—Emotions, morbidity, and mortality: New Perspectives from Psychoneuroimmunology. *Annual Review of Psychology, 53*, 83.

Kingston, D., Sword, W., Krueger, P., Hanna, S., & Markle-Reid, M. (2012). Life course pathways to prenatal maternal stress. *Journal of Obstetric, Gynecologic, & Neonatal Nursing, 41*(5), 609–626.

Kivimäki, M., Virtanen, M., Elovainio, M., Kouvonen, A., Väänänen, A., & Vahtera, J. (2006). Work stress in the etiology of coronary heart disease—A meta-analysis. *Scandinavian Journal of Work, Environment & Health, 32*(6), 431–442.

Konrath, S. (2014). The power of philanthropy and volunteering. *Wellbeing: A Complete Reference Guide, Interventions and Policies to Enhance Wellbeing, 6*, 387.

Lakey, B., & Orehek, E. (2011). Relational regulation theory: A new approach to explain the link between perceived social support and mental health. *Psychological Review, 118*(3), 482.

Lastra, G., Dhuper, S., Johnson, M. S., & Sowers, J. R. (2010). Salt, aldosterone, and insulin resistance: Impact on the cardiovascular system. *Nature Reviews Cardiology, 7*(10), 577–584.

Leopold, J. A., Dam, A., Maron, B. A., Scribner, A. W., Liao, R., Handy, D. E., & Loscalzo, J. (2007). Aldosterone impairs vascular reactivity by decreasing glucose-6-phosphate dehydrogenase activity. *Nature Medicine, 13*(2), 189–197.

Lepore, S. J., & Greenberg, M. A. (2002). Mending broken hearts: Effects of expressive writing on mood, cognitive processing, social adjustment and health following a relationship breakup. *Psychology and Health, 17*(5), 547–560.

Levenson, R. W., & Gottman, J. M. (1983). Marital interaction: Physiological linkage and affective exchange. *Journal of Personality and Social Psychology, 45*(3), 587–597.

Littrell, J. (2008). The mind-body connection: Not just a theory anymore. *Social Work in Health Care, 46*(4), 17–37.

Lock, M. (1993). Encounters with aging: Mythologies of menopause in Japan and North America. Berkeley: University of California.

Lock, M. (2002). Symptom reporting at menopause: A review of cross-cultural findings. *Journal of the British Menopause Society, 8*(4), 132e136.

Lock, M. (2007). Conclusion. In F. Saillant & S. Genest (Eds.), *Medical anthropology: Regional perspectives and shared concerns* (pp. 267–287). Malden, MA: Blackwell.

Locker, T. K., Heesacker, M., & Baker, J. O. (2012). Gender similarities in the relationship between psychological aspects of disordered eating and self-silencing. *Psychology of Men & Masculinity, 13*(1), 89.

Marin, T. J., Martin, T. M., Blackwell, E., Stetler, C., & Miller, G. E. (2007). Differentiating the impact of episodic and chronic stressors on hypothalamic-pituitary-adrenocortical axis regulation in young women. *Health Psychology, 26*(4), 447.

Markham, C. M., Lormand, D., Gloppen, K. M., Peskin, M. F., Flores, B., Low, B., & House, L. D. (2010). Connectedness as a predictor of sexual and reproductive health outcomes for youth. *Journal of Adolescent Health, 46*(3), S23–S41.

Marmot, M., & Wilkinson, R. (Eds.). (2009). *Social determinants of health.* Oxford, UK: Oxford University Press.

McDermott, R., Fowler, J. H., & Christakis, N. A. (2013). Breaking up is hard to do, unless everyone else is doing it too: Social network effects on divorce in a longitudinal sample. *Social Forces, 92*(2), 491–519.

McEwen, B. S. (2003). Interacting mediators of allostasis and allostatic load: Towards an understanding of resilience in aging. *Metabolism: Clinical and Experimental, 52*(10), 10–16.

McEwen, B. S. (2007). Physiology and neurobiology of stress and adaptation: Central role of the brain. *Physiological Reviews, 87*(3), 873–904.

McEwen, B. S. (2010). Stress, sex, and neural adaptation to a changing environment: Mechanisms of neuronal remodeling. *Annals of the New York Academy of Sciences, 1204*, 38–59.

McMunn, A., Bartley, M., Hardy, R., & Kuh, D. (2006). Life course social roles and women's health in mid-life: Causation or selection? *Journal of Epidemiology and Community Health, 60*(6), 484–489.

Mednick, S. C., Christakis, N. A., & Fowler, J. H. (2010). The spread of sleep loss influences drug use in adolescent social networks. *PLoS One, 5*(3), e9775.

Miller, G. E., & Chen, E. (2010). Harsh family climate in early life presages the emergence of a proinflammatory phenotype in adolescence. *Psychological Science, 21*(6), 848–856.

Miller, G. E., Rohleder, N., & Cole, S. W. (2009). Chronic interpersonal stress predicts activation of pro- and anti-inflammatory signaling pathways 6 months later. *Psychosomatic Medicine, 71*(1), 57–62.

Miller, J. B. (1986). *What do we mean by relationships? Work in progress.* Wellesley, MA: Stone Center for Developmental Services and Studies, Wellesley College.

Miller, J. B. (2008). Connections, disconnections, and violations. *Feminism Psychology, 18*(3), 368–380.

Miller, J. B., & Stiver, I. (1997). How do connections lead to growth? In J. B. Miller & I. P. Stiver (Eds.), *The healing connection: How women form relationships in therapy and in life.* Boston, MA: Beacon Press.

Millstein, S. G., & Halpern–Felsher, B. L. (2002). Judgments about risk and perceived invulnerability in adolescents and young adults. *Journal of Research on Adolescence, 12*(4), 399–422.

Myers, D. C. (1999). Close relationships and quality of life. D. Kahneman, E. Diener & N. Schwarz (Eds.), *Well-being: Foundations of hedonic psychology,* (pp. 374–391). New York, NY: Russell Sage Foundation.

Oman, D. (2007). Does volunteering foster physical health and longevity? In S. G. Post (Ed.), *Altruism and health* (pp. 15–32). New York, NY: Oxford Press.

Orth-Gomér, K., Wamala, S. P., Horsten, M., Schenck-Gustafsson, K., Schneiderman, N., & Mittleman, M. A. (2000). Marital stress worsens prognosis in women with coronary heart disease: The Stockholm Female Coronary Risk Study. *Journal of the American Medical Association, 284*(23), 3008–3014.

Palchykov, V., Kaski, K., Kertész, J., Barabási, A. L., & Dunbar, R. I. (2012). Sex differences in intimate relationships. *Scientific Reports,* article number: 370, doi: 10.1038/srep00370.

Parkes, A., Henderson, M., Wight, D., & Nixon, C. (2011). Is parenting associated with teenagers' early sexual risk-taking, autonomy and relationship with sexual partners? *Perspectives on Sexual and Reproductive Health, 43*(1), 30–40.

Pennebaker, J. (1985). Traumatic experience and psychosomatic disease: Exploring the roles of behavioural inhibition, obsession, and confiding. *Canadian Psychology, 26*(2), 82–95.

Pennebaker, J. (2003). Telling stories: The health benefits of disclosure. In *Social and cultural lives of immune systems.* New York, NY: Routledge.

Pettit, G. S., Erath, S. A., Lansford, J. E., Dodge, K. A., & Bates, J. E. (2011). Dimensions of social capital and life adjustment in the transition to early adulthood. *International Journal of Behavioral Development, 35*(6), 482–489.

Pluess, M., & Belsky, J. (2011). Prenatal programming of postnatal plasticity? *Development and Psychopathology, 23*(01), 29–38.

Porges, S. W. (1996). Physiological regulation in high-risk infants: A model for assessment and potential intervention. *Development and Psychopathology, 8*(01), 43–58.

Poulin, M. J., Brown, S. L., Dillard, A. J., & Smith, D. M. (2013). Giving to others and the association between stress and mortality. *American Journal of Public Health, 103*(9), 1649–1655.

Poulin, M. J., Holman, E. A., & Buffone, A. (2012). The neurogenetics of nice receptor genes for oxytocin and vasopressin interact with threat to predict prosocial behavior. *Psychological Science, 23*(5), 446–452.

Pressman, S. D., & Cohen, S. (2007). Use of social words in autobiographies and longevity. *Psychosomatic Medicine, 69*(3), 262–269.

Priem, J. S., & Solomon, D. H. (2009). Comforting apprehensive communicators: The effects of reappraisal and distraction on cortisol levels among students in a public speaking class. *Communication Quarterly, 57*(3), 259–281.

Pujazon-Zazik, M., & Park, M. J. (2010). To tweet, or not to tweet: Gender differences and potential positive and negative health outcomes of adolescents' social Internet use. *American Journal of Men's Health, 4*(1), 77–85.

Repetti, R. L., & Taylor, S. E., & Seeman, T. E. (2002). Risky families: Family social environments and the mental and physical health of offspring. *Psychological Bulletin, 128*(2), 330–366.

Reyna, V. F., & Farley, F. (2006). Risk and rationality in adolescent decision making implications for theory, practice, and public policy. *Psychological Science in the Public Interest, 7*(1), 1–44.

Rice, F., Harold, G. T., Boivin, J., Van den Bree, M., Hay, D. F., & Thapar, A. (2010). The links between prenatal stress and offspring development and psychopathology: Disentangling environmental and inherited influences. *Psychological Medicine, 12*(2), 335.

Riess, H., & Marci, C. (2007). The role of neurobiology and physiology of empathy in enhancing the patient-doctor relationship. *Medical Encounter, 21*(3), 38–39.

Rifkin-Graboi, A., Bai, J., Chen, H., Hameed, W. B. R., Sim, L. W., Tint, M. T., & Qiu, A. (2013). Prenatal maternal depression associates with microstructure of right amygdala in neonates at birth. *Biological Psychiatry, 74*(11), 837–844.

Robinson, M., Mattes, E., Oddy, W. H., Pennell, C. E., van Eekelen, A., McLean, N. J., & Newnham, J. P. (2011). Prenatal stress and risk of behavioral morbidity from age 2 to 14 years: The influence of the number, type, and timing of stressful life events. *Development and Psychopathology, 23*(2), 507.

Roisman, G. I., Booth-LaForce, C., Cauffman, E., & Spieker, S. (2009). The developmental significance of adolescent romantic relationships: Parent and peer predictors of engagement and quality at age 15. *Journal of Youth and Adolescence, 38*(10), 1294–1303.

Rosen, W., Walker, M., & Jordan, J. V. (2000). *Shame and humiliation: From isolation to relational transformation.* Wellesley, MA: Stone Center.

Rosenquist, J. N., Murabito, J., Fowler, J. H., & Christakis, N. A. (2010). The spread of alcohol consumption behavior in a large social network. *Annals of Internal Medicine, 152*(7), 426–433.

Rueckert, L., & Naybar, N. (2008). Gender differences in empathy: The role of the right hemisphere. *Brain and Cognition, 67*(2), 162–167.

Russ, T. C., Stamatakis, E., Hamer, M., Starr, J. M., Kivimäki, M., & Batty, G. D. (2012). Association between psychological distress and mortality: Individual participant pooled analysis of 10 prospective cohort studies. *British Medical Journal, 345*, e4933.

Sandman, C. A., Davis, E. P., Buss, C., & Glynn, L. M. (2012). Exposure to prenatal psychobiological stress exerts programming influences on the mother and her fetus. *Neuroendocrinology, 95*(1), 8–21.

Sapolsky, R. M. (2004). *Why zebras don't get ulcers: The acclaimed guide to stress, stress-related diseases, and coping-now revised and updated.* New York, NY: Holt Paperbacks..

Sapolsky, R. M. (2007). Stress, stress-related disease, and emotional regulation. In J. J. Gross (Ed.), *Handbook of emotion regulation* (pp. 606–615). New York, NY: Guilford Press.

Sawyer, S. M., Afifi, R. A., Bearinger, L. H., Blakemore, S. J., Dick, B., Ezeh, A. C., & Patton, G. C. (2012). Adolescence: A foundation for future health. *Lancet, 379*(9826), 1630–1640.

Schore, A. N. (2001). Effects of a secure attachment relationship on right brain development, affect regulation, and infant mental health. *Infant Mental Health Journal, 22*(1–2), 7–66.

Seeman, T. E. (2000). Health promoting effects of friends and family on health outcomes in older adults. *American Journal of Health Promotion, 14*, 362–370.

Seyfarth, R. M., & Cheney, D. L. (2012). The evolutionary origins of friendship. *Annual Review of Psychology, 63*, 153–177.

Shalev, S. (2008). *A sourcebook on solitary confinement.* Available at SSRN 2177495.

Shankar, A., McMunn, A., Banks, J., & Steptoe, A. (2011). Loneliness, social isolation, and behavioral and biological health indicators in older adults. *Health Psychology, 30*(4), 377.

Shonkoff, J. P., Boyce, W. T., & McEwen, B. S. (2009). Neuroscience, molecular biology, and the childhood roots of health disparities: Building a new framework for health promotion and disease prevention. *Journal of American Medical Association, 301*(21), 2252–2259.

Shulman, E. P., & Cauffman, E. (2014). Deciding in the dark: Age differences in intuitive risk judgment. *Developmental Psychology, 50*(1), 167.

Siegel, D. J. (2006). An interpersonal neurobiology approach to psychotherapy. *Psychiatric Annals, 36*(4), 248.

Siegel, D. J. (2010). *Mindsight: The new science of personal transformation.* New York, NY: Random House LLC.

Singh, M., & Singh, G. (2006). A study on family and psychosocial health status of middle-aged working women of Varanasi City. *Internet Journal of Third World Medicine, 3*(2), 2–4.

Slavich, G. M., O'Donovan, A., Epel, E. S., & Kemeny, M. E. (2010). Black sheep get the blues: A psychobiological model of social rejection and depression. *Neuroscience & Biobehavioral Reviews, 35*(1), 39–45.

Smith, P. S. (2006). The effects of solitary confinement on prison inmates: A brief history and review of the literature. *Crime and Justice, 34*(1), 441–528.

Smolak, L. (2010). Gender as culture: The meanings of self-silencing in women and men. In D. C. Jack & A. Ali (Eds.), *Silencing the self across cultures: Depression and gender in the social world* (pp.129–147). New York, NY: Oxford University Press.

Spear, L. P. (2013). Adolescent neurodevelopment. *Journal of Adolescent Health, 52*(2), S7–S13.

Stehr, C. B., Mellado, R., Ocaranza, M. P., Carvajal, C. A., Mosso, L., Becerra, E., & Fardella, C. E. (2010). Increased levels of oxidative stress, subclinical inflammation, and myocardial fibrosis markers in primary aldosteronism patients. *Journal of Hypertension, 28*(10), 2120–2126.

Steptoe, A., & Kivimäki, M. (2012). Stress and cardiovascular disease. *Nature Reviews Cardiology, 9*(6), 360–370.

Steptoe, A., Shankar, A., Demakakos, P., & Wardle, J. (2013). Social isolation, loneliness, and all-cause mortality in older men and women. *Proceedings of the National Academy of Sciences, 110*(15), 5797–5801.

Strating, M. M., Suurmeijer, T. P., & Van Schuur, W. H. (2006). Disability, social support, and distress in rheumatoid arthritis: results from a thirteen-year prospective study. *Arthritis Care & Research, 55*(5), 736–744.

Suchman, A. L., & Matthews, D. A. (1988). What makes the patient-doctor relationship therapeutic? Exploring the connexional dimension of medical care. *Annals of Internal Medicine, 108*(1), 125–130.

Surrey, J. L. (1991). Self-in-relation: A theory of women's development. In J. V. Jordan, A. G. Kaplan, J. B. Miller, I. P. Stiver & J. L. Surrey (Eds.), *Women's growth in connection* (pp. 51–66). New York, NY: Guilford Press.

Tauber, A. (2000). Moving beyond the immune self? *Seminars in Immunology, 12*(3), 241–248.

Taylor, S. E. (2011). Tend and befriend theory. In P. A. M. Van Lange, A. W. Kruglanski & E. T. Higgins (Eds.), *Handbook of theories of social psychology: Collection* (Vol. 1 & 2, p. 32). Thousand Oaks, CA: Sage Publications, Inc.

Taylor, S. E., Saphire-Bernstein, S., & Seeman, T. E. (2010). Are plasma oxytocin in women and plasma vasopressin in men biomarkers of distressed pair-bond relationships? *Psychological Science, 21*(1), 3–7.

Thomas, P. A. (2010). Is it better to give or to receive? Social support and the well-being of older adults. *Journals of Gerontology Series B: Psychological Sciences and Social Sciences, 65*(3), 351–357.

Thompson, R. R., George, K., Walton, J. C., Orr, S. P., & Benson, J. (2006). Sex-specific influences of vasopressin on human social communication. *Proceedings of the National Academy of Sciences, 103*(20), 7889–7894.

Tilvis, R. S., Laitala, V., Routasalo, P. E., & Pitkälä, K. H. (2011). Suffering from loneliness indicates significant mortality risk of older people. *Journal of Aging Research*, Article ID: 534781, 5 pages.

Troxel, W. M., Buysse, D. J., Matthews, K. A., Kravitz, H. M., Bromberger, J. T., Sowers, M., & Hall, M. H. (2010). Marital/cohabitation status and history in relation to sleep in midlife women. *Sleep, 33*(7), 973.

Tsakos, G., Sabbah, W., Chandola, T., Newton, T., Kawachi, I., Aida, J., & Watt, R. G. (2013). Social relationships and oral health among adults aged 60 years or older. *Psychosomatic Medicine, 75*(2), 178–186.

Uchino, B. (2006). Social support and health: A review of physiological processes potentially underlying links to disease outcomes. *Journal of Behavioral Medicine, 29*(4), 377–387.

Uchino, B. N., Bosch, J. A., Smith, T. W., Carlisle, M., Birmingham, W., Bowen, K. S., & O'Hartaigh, B. (2013). Relationships and cardiovascular risk: Perceived spousal ambivalence in specific relationship contexts and its links to inflammation. *Health Psychology, 32*(10), 1067.

Umberson, D., & Montez, J. K. (2010). Social relationships and health: A flashpoint for health policy. *Journal of Health and Social Behavior, 51*(1 Suppl.), S54–S66.

Vaillant, G. E. (2012). *Triumphs of experience: The men of the Harvard Grant Study*. Cambridge, MA: Belknap Press of Harvard University Press.

Voellmin, A., Entringer, S., Moog, N., Wadhwa, P. D., & Buss, C. (2013). Maternal positive affect over the course of pregnancy is associated with the length of gestation and reduced risk of preterm delivery. *Journal of Psychosomatic Research, 75*(4), 336–340.

Waite, L. J., & Harrison, S. C. (1992). Keeping in touch: How women in mid-life allocate social contacts among kith and kin. *Social Forces, 70*(3), 637–654.

Wanic, R., & Kulik, J. (2011). Toward an understanding of gender differences in the impact of marital conflict on health. *Sex Roles, 65*(5–6), 297–312.

Ward, T., Scheid, V., & Tuffrey, V. (2010). Women's mid-life health experiences in urban UK: An international comparison. *Climacteric, 13*(3), 278–288.

Wilce, J. M. (2003). *Social and cultural lives of immune systems*. London, UK: Routledge.

Windle, K., Francis, J., & Coomber, C. (2011). Preventing loneliness and social isolation: Interventions and outcomes. Social Care Institute for Excellence Research Briefing, ID: 39, 5 pages.

Wohlgemuth, E., & Betz, N. E. (1991). Gender as a moderator of the relationships of stress and social support to physical health in college students. *Journal of Counseling Psychology, 38*(3), 367.

Wrzus, C., Hänel, M., Wagner, J., & Neyer, F. J. (2013). Social network changes and life events across the life span: A meta-analysis. *Psychological Bulletin, 139*(1), 53.

Wüst, S., Entringer, S., Federenko, I. S., Schlotz, W., & Hellhammer, D. H. (2005). Birth weight is associated with salivary cortisol responses to psychosocial stress in adult life. *Psychoneuroendocrinology, 30*(6), 591–598.

Yancey, A. K., Grant, D., Kurosky, S., Kravitz-Wirtz, N., & Mistry, R. (2011). Role modeling, risk, and resilience in California adolescents. *Journal of Adolescent Health, 48*(1), 36–43.

Zender, R., & Olshansky, E. (2012). The biology of caring researching the healing effects of stress response regulation through relational engagement. *Biological Research for Nursing, 14*(4), 419–430.

Chapter 17

Promoting Healthy Sleep

Joan L. F. Shaver

Introduction: Healthy Sleep as Essential for Wellness

Sleep has been studied intensively for the last 40 or so years with unequivocal evidence that it is essential to health and wellness. Sleep deficit or loss has been associated with all manner of negative consequences, most particularly related to mental (neurocognitive) competence, emotional state, physical performance, and metabolism. Loss of sleep is a stressor, evident in higher levels of stress hormones such as epinephrine or cortisol with detrimental immune effects. As a result, chronically sleep-deficient people are vulnerable to accidental injury, infection, and poor recovery as well as mental and physical illness. Across studies of sleep, negative outcomes have led sleep scientists to recommend that it is optimum for most people to get between 7 and 9 hours of sleep and to sleep the number of hours that allow one to awaken refreshed and have sustained energy and alertness while awake.

After a good night's sleep, people say they learn better and remember more. Scientists and artists claim that creative insights often come during or after good sleep. Lack of sleep is associated with slower thinking, difficulties focusing and paying attention, as well as with confusion, poor decision making and a greater tendency to engage in risky behaviors. Emotionally, inadequate or poor sleep makes one irritable and withdrawn or depressed. Physically, sleep deficit makes one feel tired and slows reaction times, making sleep deprivation as powerful as being drunk while driving vehicles. Thus, not getting a good night's sleep can be dangerous—to sleep-deprived zombies and those around them!

The aims of this chapter are to

1. Describe the human ecology of sleep
2. Describe the stages and cycles of healthy sleep
3. Present methods to assess sleep and screen for disorders of sleep
4. Present various approaches to enhancing healthy sleep
5. Describe how sleep is affected at various stages of a woman's life span
6. Describe variations of sleep in the context of mental and physical disturbances

Emerging evidence indicates that sleep is a powerful regulator of appetite, energy use, and body weight, and too little sleep makes us prone to obesity and diabetes-like status (provokes insulin-resistance). During sleep, a rise in a suppressor of appetite (leptin) is observed in concert with a drop in a stimulator of appetite (grehlin). Inadequate sleep shifts from appetite suppression and toward stimulation, making people more likely to eat more food and foods that are high in calories and carbohydrates, thus raising the likelihood of being overweight or obese. Moreover, with sufficient sleep loss, cellular glucose resistance and blood glucose levels resembling a diabetes-like state emerge (Van Cauter, 2011).

There appears to be truth to the old adage "I need my beauty sleep." With enduring sleep loss, detrimental skin outcomes occur, including the hastening of wrinkles and worsening of acne. Skin sensitivities and irritations signal that skin has become less protective against the effects of environmental chemicals and pollutants. Abstract data from a study titled "Effects of Sleep Quality on Skin Aging and Function" showed that women who did not sleep well exhibited more signs of skin aging, including fine lines, uneven pigmentation, and reduced skin elasticity. Moreover, those who enjoyed quality sleep recovered more quickly from a UV light challenge to the skin (Oyetakin-White et al., 2013). Sleep debt negatively affects collagen production, and therefore the scaffolding within skin tissue that helps maintain shape and firmness, seals in moisture (hydrates), and promotes elasticity (Kahan, Andersen, Tomimori, & Tufik, 2010). Importantly, sleep protects against UV damage and skin breakdown changes that make one vulnerable to bacterial invasion (e.g., acne).

Insights into the Human Health Ecology of Sleep

Sleep can be profiled as largely influenced by three interfacing ecological (person/environment) components (see Fig. 17.1). These three components include sleep drive factors, sleep timing factors, and facilitators and inhibitors of sleep. Healthy sleep is composed of sleep and waking behaviors oscillating in a predictable manner relative to one another, generally on a regular 24-hour (circadian) basis. Inherently, a sleep drive (homeostatic) component is coordinated by changes over time to the balance of arousing and sleep-inducing brain biochemicals. The main arousing neurochemicals are norepinephrine, serotonin, acetylcholine, dopamine, histamine, and orexin, while sleep-inducing ones are γ-aminobutyric acid (GABA), glycine, melatonin, and adenosine. Sleep-inducing biochemicals (e.g., adenosine) build over the next 15 to 16 hours from the last sleep episode, producing a progressively growing desire to sleep. The longer one stays awake, the stronger one feels the pressure to sleep. Over the course of sleeping, the sleep drive is rebalanced by waning of the sleep-inducing and a building up of wake-inducing (arousal) biochemicals. Operating synergistically with the sleep drive is an environmental light–dark timing/rhythm component, largely coordinated by the sleep-inducing pineal gland hormone, melatonin, which is suppressed by light (daytime) and released in the dark (nighttime). During night, melatonin is released to reinforce sleep and as the sleep drive dissipates over the course of sleep and one is exposed to the light of day, the timing/rhythm component (reduced melatonin) promotes awakening as well. This synergy allows for consolidated periods of waking, normatively 16 to 17 hours and consolidated bouts of sleeping to occur, optimally 7 to 8 hours for most people. A regular schedule for going to and waking from sleep positions sleep bouts on a consistent portion of the light/dark cycle and is very influential in promoting sleep quality. Staying up late (e.g., on work-/school days) and failing to fully dissipate the sleep drive elements over bouts of sleep cut short by having to get up will impair next-day full alertness. Getting up later on non–work-/school days such as the weekend to compensate interferes with being able to fall asleep until late on the night before going back to work/school, cutting the sleep time

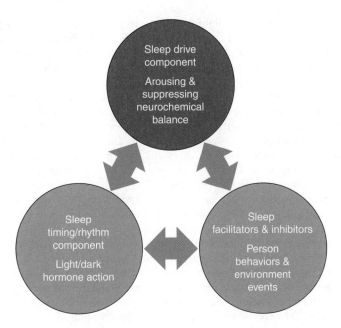

FIGURE 17.1 Key components coordinating the cycle of sleep and wake.

short and impacting energy and alertness as one starts the workweek. Other disruptors of the sleep drive and timing/rhythm synchrony include flying across time zones and performing shift work. A third component encompasses facilitators and inhibitors of sleep that are environmental (e.g., artificial lighting, stressor exposure) and behavioral factors (e.g., engaging in arousing activities, ingestion of caffeine or alcohol). These factors can override or negatively alter the reciprocal synergy of the sleep drive and timing/rhythm interface or on the other hand can be modified for positive effects. Hence, the propensity for poor sleep (insomnia) can be one or a combination of factors such as an inherently weak sleep drive, excessive stress arousal/activation, disruptive schedules, excessive arousal-oriented environment exposure, and/or sleep-interfering behaviors.

Healthy Sleep: Stages and Cycles

Normatively within sleep bouts, adult human physiology oscillates in a relatively predictable cycle through four stages of sleep. A period of non–rapid eye movement (NREM) sleep is followed by a short period of rapid eye movement (REM) sleep before returning to light sleep or even briefly awaking to complete a cycle. The cycle then begins again. Each cycle takes between 60 and 100 minutes and depending on sleep bout duration, a full night of sleep consists of 3 to 6 cycles of sleep. Normatively, sleep begins with transitional sleep (referred to as N1) progressing into light sleep (N2), and then into deep sleep (N3). These three NREM stages make up about 80% to 85% of the total cycle. The remainder (15% to 20%) of a cycle consists of REM sleep. Of note is that early sleep cycles contain proportionately more deep sleep than later cycles. Alternately, REM sleep shows a progressive increase in duration from the first to the last third of the night; the majority recorded in the latter third of the night. While the exact functions of the sleep stages are not known, deep sleep is believed to be crucial to the body and brain restitution and REM sleep has been associated most often with promoting good emotional/mental functions, including memory. While all sleep stages are critical, sleep in the early part of the night is especially important to feeling energetic upon awakening.

Body physiology during the sleep stages also has a predictable pattern. During NREM sleep compared with wake, the breathing and heart rates become slower and regular, blood pressure lowers and stabilizes, and muscle tension relaxes as the brain waves become slower in frequency and deeper in amplitude. During the relatively short period of REM sleep, cardiovascular and breathing signs are erratic; muscle tension approaches paralysis; and the brainwaves look more like wake with mixed frequencies and low amplitude. One thought is that besides preserving or improving mental/emotional function, REM sleep serves to periodically recharge neural circuits and shift brain function away from deep slowing (loss of consciousness), all necessary to preserving consciousness, performance, and neurobehavioral flexibility.

Sleep stages are detected by electrophysiological waveform capture and pattern scoring in a process referred to as polysomnography (PSG). Stages are identified from recorded patterns of brainwaves (electroencephalogram—EEG), facial muscle tension (electro-myogram), and eye movements (electro-oculogram). Standardized scoring conventions are applied to the graphic output, that is, the somnogram, ultimately allowing calculation of how long it takes to fall asleep (sleep latency); the duration of each sleep stage and cycle; type, number, and duration of sleep/brain arousals or awakenings; wake time after sleep onset; total sleep time; and total time in bed—the ratio of the latter two variables constitute sleep efficiency. Generally, breathing, heart rate, and leg movements are monitored so that interferences with sleep patterns due to such disruptors as abnormal breathing (apneas, hypopneas) or body movements are evident. Often considered the "gold standard" for assessing physical sleep patterns, since it reveals the structure of sleep, PSG is time-consuming, technology dependent, and normally done by referral to an accredited sleep center. Many types of insomnia (self-reported poor sleep) do not warrant PSG for diagnosis or treatment, but a prominent source of poor sleep, that is, sleep apnea/hyponea syndrome, does and represents the majority diagnostic service at sleep centers.

Not used extensively in clinical practice but rather in research, a less intrusive and less complex technology to gauge physical sleep patterns are activity monitors. The quantity of sleep and waking over time but not the structure of sleep can be detected with acceptable comparability with PSG. However, accuracy is affected by the extent of quiet resting rather than sleeping, and activity monitors are not suitable for certain types of individuals (e.g., those with tremors or with muscle paralysis).

Clinical Sleep Assessment: Recognizing Insomnia and Sleep Disorders

With increasing recognition of how essential adequate sleep is to overall health and wellness, assessment of sleep in everyday clinical practice becomes vital. In clinical practice or research, sleep quality is mainly detected through recall self-report, often by specific questions or items on health histories, sleep histories, or rating instruments, or concurrent self-report with sleep diaries or sleep logs. However, self-report is prone to participants recalling inaccurately or giving "desired" answers and it depends on their motivation, memory, and concentration. When people are asked to "recall" their sleep quality over a number of days or weeks, they will often report a higher prevalence of problems than when they rate daily (e.g., daily diary). What people report about the quality of their sleep and what is recorded physically do not always match. This is not to imply that either type of data is more "correct" or accurate in reflecting sleep quality but rather that reported and recorded types reveal different dimensions of sleep quality. Like pain, sleep can be viewed as having cognitive/emotional and physiological (sensory) dimensions. In some cases, people's perceptions rather than their physical sleep may need "treatment." Asking women to keep sleep diaries or logs can be enlightening for them and indeed have therapeutic effects on their perceptions of sleep quality. Women might find that they have fewer sleep problems than they thought and monitoring their own sleep can help to reframe how they view their sleep.

Apparently sleep health is not assessed routinely by primary care clinicians. A 2005 poll showed that 7 in 10 respondents (70%) reported that their health care providers (doctors) had never asked them about their sleep, while 29% reported that they had done so (National Sleep Foundation, 2005). Most people do not seek treatment for sleep problems, although when older adults identified from 11 primary care sites were specifically questioned, 69% reported one sleep indicator of insomnia and 40% reported two or more (Reid et al., 2006). When sleep-related disorders are suspected (e.g., sleep apnea, narcolepsy, limb movement disorders such as periodic leg movements, or sleep parasomnias such as sleep walking), patients are best referred to sleep centers or specialists for diagnosis and management. As an aside, these conditions are technically not sleep disorders but rather neurologically invoked disorders with signs that manifest like, during or close to sleep bouts.

Evident by self-report of inadequate, insufficient, or unrefreshing sleep, insomnia is the most common sleep issue for women or men. Estimates are that about one-third to one-half of the population report insomnia, with about 10% to 15% reporting accompanying distress or wake time impairment due to poor sleep (general insomnia disorder). Estimates indicate that 10% to 20% of people have insomnia as a specific sleep disorder (Buysse, 2013). Women are more likely than men to report sleep difficulties, although this might partly be a function of women being more open to perceiving and/or reporting their symptoms. In the 2005 poll, more women than men reported symptoms of insomnia at least a few nights a week (57% vs. 51%) and were more likely to report daytime sleepiness (National Sleep Foundation, 2005).

For only a fraction of people reporting insomnia, is it considered a primary disorder, as more often insomnia is seen as a consequence of sleep-disrupting circumstances. Commonly reported vulnerability factors include being female, older in age, and comorbid contexts (medical, psychiatric, medication, and substance use). The diagnostic criteria for insomnia are listed in Table 17.1.

Part of any overall health/wellness assessment should include sleep quality. According to a clinical guideline for assessing (diagnosing) sleep problems (Schutte-Rodin, Broch, Buysse, Dorsey, & Sateia, 2008), recommended initial assessment should begin with two key questions (rating in brackets) as seen in Table 17.2. Adapted from a prior paper, Table 17.3 represents a potential short assessment to detect insomnia, sleep disordered breathing, or other key sleep related disorders (Shaver & Zenk, 2000).

A number of other instruments for assessing healthy sleep and recognizing insomnia include many of the aforementioned criteria. One example is the Insomnia Symptom Questionnaire (ISQ), which is a 13-item self-administered rating scale. Recent validation of the tool showed it should be effective for insomnia screening in primary care (Gagnon, Belanger, Ivers, & Morin, 2013; Toward Optimized Practice Program, 2007). Often used in research and sometimes in clinical practice, another popular measure for recalling sleep quality over the last month is the 19-item Pittsburgh Sleep Quality Index (PSQI)

TABLE 17.1	**The International Classification of Sleep Disorders**

A. Difficulty initiating or maintaining sleep or waking up too early or sleep that is chronically nonrestorative or poor in quality
B. Occurs despite adequate opportunity and circumstances for sleep
C. At least one of the following wake time factors is reported by the patient:
   1. Fatigue or malaise
   2. Daytime sleepiness
   3. Attention, concentration, or memory impairment
   4. Social or vocational dysfunction or poor school performance
   5. Mood disturbance or irritability
   6. Motivation, energy, or initiative reduction
   7. Proneness for errors/accidents at work or while driving
   8. Tension, headaches, or gastrointestinal symptoms in response to sleep loss
   9. Concerns or worries about sleep

Reprinted with permission from Schutte-Rodin, S., Broch, L., Buysse, D., Dorsey, C., & Sateia, M. (2008). Clinical guideline for the evaluation and management of chronic insomnia in adults. Clinical Sleep Medicine, 4(5), 487–504.

(plus 5 items answered by a bed partner). The maximum score is 21, and in comparison with PSG, a score over 5 has been found to accurately identify poor sleep with high sensitivity (90%) and specificity (87%). The PSQI is often used to monitor sleep quality associated with mood and other medical disorders (Buysse, Reynolds, Monk, Berman, & Kupfer, 1989; Schutte-Rodin et al., 2008).

Insomnia is most often seen as a symptom associated with other factors, but in its primary form is considered a sleep disorder. Table 17.4 indicates the International Classification of Sleep Disorders (ICSD-2) insomnia classification (American Academy of Sleep Medicine, 2005). Three types of primary insomnia are classified with the remaining insomnia types associated with other contexts.

Insomnia-associated factors that combine to reach a threshold whereby clinical manifestations are evident have been viewed as *predisposing*, *precipitating*, and *perpetuating*. Predisposing factors may be relatively nonmodifiable such as age, genetics, or unspecified physiologic function. As seen in Table 17.4 ICSD-2 classifications, precipitating and perhaps perpetuating factors can include, for example, stressful life events, mental

TABLE 17.2	**A Clinical Guideline for Assessing Sleep Problems***

1. How would you rate the quality of your sleep?
   Very Good (=0), Good (=1), Somewhat (=2), Poor (=3), Very Poor (=4)

2. How much does your sleep quality affect your daytime function?
   Not at all (=0), Somewhat (=1), Quite a bit (=2), A Great Deal (=3)

If the score is greater than or equal to 5, a more comprehensive self-reported assessment for insomnia is warranted

*This table represents a potential short assessment to detect insomnia, sleep disorders breathing, and other key sleep-related disorders.

Adapted from Shaver, J. L., & Zenk, S. N. (2000). Sleep disturbance in menopause. Journal of Women's Health and Gender-based Medicine., 9(2), 109–118.

TABLE 17.3	Short Screening for Insomnia and Sleep-Related Disorders

A. Of the following, when taking adequate time to sleep, check any that you experience:
_____ Take too long to fall asleep
_____ Wake up too often
_____ Difficult to fall back to sleep if awakened
_____ Awaken too early—can't return to sleep
_____ Awaken feeling tired
_____ Feel excessively tired much of day
Any of the above indicates insomnia
B. Check any of the following that you know applies to you:
_____ Loud, heavy snoring most nights (patient or partner report)
_____ Pauses in breathing (patient or partner testimony)
_____ Wake with a headache
Clinician note: Overweight? Y/N   High blood pressure? Y/N
Any combination of excessive daytime sleepiness from Part A with factors in B should raise suspicion of possible sleep-related breathing disorder. For more intensive assessment, see STOP–BANG assessment on page 330.
C. Check any of the following that describes what you experience:
_____ Sudden, unintentional attacks of sleep in the day
_____ Awaken from sleep feeling paralyzed
_____ Feel, see, or hear things when falling asleep or awakening
_____ Many jerking movements of legs during sleep (patient or partner testimony)
_____ Uncomfortable crawly sensations in the legs prior to bedtime that are relieved by walking, moving, or massage
Any of the factors in C indicates possible narcolepsy or restless leg/periodic muscle movement disorders.

or physical disorders, or substance use. Behaviorally, insomnia can be precipitated and perpetuated by engaging in what is referred to as negative thinking (racing mind) and poor sleep hygiene, including adoption of an irregular sleep–wake schedule, use of caffeine or alcohol.

Often accompanying insomnia is daytime sleepiness, which when severe, impairs performance of daily activities, be they mental, physical, or both. A commonly used self-report instrument to judge daytime sleepiness is the Epworth Sleepiness Scale. People rate their tendency for dozing or falling asleep (no, slight, moderate, high chance), in the daytime when performing eight activities: (1) sitting and reading, (2) watching TV, (3) sitting inactive in public place (e.g., in a meeting), (4) passenger in a car without a break, (5) lying down to rest in afternoon, (6) sitting and talking to someone, (7) sitting after lunch (no alcohol), and (8) in car stopped a few minutes in traffic (Johns, 1991). From a possible total score of 24, a score of ≥10 warrants further targeted assessment to uncover the contributors to excessive wake time sleepiness.

Therapies for Better Sleep (Preventing or Treating Insomnia)

Therapies for preserving and promoting healthy sleep or treating insomnia are generally a combination of sleep medications and behavioral strategies, the latter being the preferred mainstay for long-term promotion of healthy sleep. While sleeping medications play a role in treating insomnia, they remain best used for breaking the cycle of poor sleep on an episodic basis except perhaps for severe, persistent primary insomnia. Rather than the traditional benzodiazepines, newer forms of sleeping medications (e.g., zolpidem/ Ambien) are shorter acting, in some cases have fewer residual daytime side effects and are being used for longer times with persistent insomnia. In the context of sleep-disrupting circumstances where insomnia is not primary, paramount is a focus on treatment of key disruptors, for example, pain or hot flashes, in concert with specific cotreatment of insomnia. Besides inherent person behaviors that influence sleep drive and timing rhythm

TABLE 17.4	Types and Features of Insomnia as Specific Disorders
Types of Insomnia	**Features**
Primary Insomnias	
Psychophysiological insomnia	Heightened arousal (cognitive, emotional, physiological—e.g., racing thoughts, higher body temperature, metabolism, muscle tension)
Paradoxical insomnia	Insomnia reported severity exceeds any objective evidence. Has been called sleep misperception insomnia
Idiopathic insomnia	Persistent insomnia with insidious onset from childhood, no precipitating or perpetuating factors evident
Insomnia Associated with Other Conditions/Situations	
Adjustment (acute) insomnia	Identifiable situational stressor, expected to be short term, and insomnia resolves when stress situation dissipates
Insomnia due to mental disorder	Insomnia emergence in the course of psychiatric and mental health disorders
Insomnia due to medical condition	Medical disorder or other physiological factor invokes insomnia that is marked by excess distress and/or warrants separate or additional clinical attention, includes sleep-related disorders of breathing or movement, or circadian rhythm disorders, among others
Insomnia due to drug or substance use	Insomnia invoked with use of a prescription medication, recreational drug, caffeine, alcohol, food, or environmental toxin
Insomnia not due to substance or known physiological condition, unspecified	Two types of insomnia that cannot be classed in the other types but thought to be associated with mental disorders, psychological factors, behaviors, medical disorders, physiological states, or substance use or exposure and warrant further evaluation
Physiological (organic) insomnia, unspecified	
Behavior-Induced Insomnia	
Inadequate sleep hygiene	Failure to engage in sleep-promoting behaviors or engaging in sleep-preventing behaviors such as irregular sleep scheduling, using alcohol, caffeine, or nicotine

Adapted from American Academy of Sleep Medicine. (2005). International classification of sleep disorders: Diagnostic and coding manual (2nd ed.). Westchester, IL: Author.

physiology, a number of environmental exposures and cognitive behavioral choices can be modified to therapeutically influence sleep health. The spectrum of behavioral therapies can be classed into four "R" categories: (1) ritualizing or routinizing for sleep preparation, (2) regularizing the sleep/wake cycle, (3) relaxing to modulate arousal, and (4) resisting sleep-interfering behaviors, described in detail next.

Behavioral Therapies

1. As a matter of routine, a bedtime *ritual* (e.g., brush teeth, have a cup of warm liquid, read for 15 minutes) is recommended along with lying down in a quiet, dark, and comfortable environment, preferably when feeling sleepy (ready to sleep). For insomnia, a reinforcing or conditioning behavioral therapy for sleep readiness is *stimulus control*. Health coaching instructions include to lie down only when sleepy to try to fall asleep; if not asleep in 10 or so minutes, get up and go elsewhere and engage in relaxing or relatively boring activity; and when drowsy, lie down in bed. If not able to fall asleep within 10 minutes, the scenario is repeated. This is to reinforce lying down to sleep with feeling drowsy or sleepy.

2. How *regular* the sleep bouts occur in relation to the light/dark cycle influences sleep quality. One reason is that consolidated sleep is positively influenced by falling asleep on the falling portion of the circadian body temperature curve, that is, a few hours after the peak (around 4 p.m.). Individuals are asked to identify an optimal nighttime sleep duration to feel well and then to go to bed and to arise at a consistent time every day. Regardless of the chosen bedtime, *most* important is to arise at a consistent time every day.

3. For persistent insomnia, in order to preserve or reestablish consistent sleep bouts relative to day/night timing, women can benefit from learning a behavioral technique called *sleep restriction*. The steps are that individuals (1) identify the current duration of their consolidated nighttime sleep, for example, 4 hours; (2) choose a consistent time to arise, for example, 7 a.m., every day; (3) go to bed only at a time in close proximity to the identified sleep duration, for example, at 2:45 a.m.; (4) maintain this schedule to achieve the designated duration, for example, 4 hours, of consolidated sleep for 1 week, after which; (5) move the bedtime to be earlier by 15 to 30 minutes, for example, to 2:30 a.m., and adopt the revised scheduling until a week of slightly longer nighttime sleep is achieved. This incremental routine (steps 3 to 5) is repeated with progressive movement of bedtime to an earlier time until gradually the duration of consistently achieved consolidated sleep is 7 to 8 hours. During sleep restriction, excess daytime napping is curtailed.

4. In order to shift from a state of sleep-interfering, hyperemotional arousal (often driven by negative thoughts about poor sleep health or accelerated worry about life's challenges) to a state that is more sleep-inducing, a variety of techniques is recommended. The goal is to engage the mind to achieve a bodily state of "deep *relaxation*." Like the wellness-promoting effects of exercise, this behavioral technique requires the discipline for repetitive practice. Four fundamental requirements of mindfully creating relaxation are (1) dedicated *time* for consistent, repetitive use (e.g., 15 minutes, two times per day); (2) a quiet, undisturbed, *tranquil environment*; (3) assumption of a *comfortable posture or specific movements*; and (4) *concentration* on a pleasant, neutral, tranquil, rhythmic focus (to clear the mind of intrusive thoughts and enhance bodily awareness). A number of approaches, including progressive muscle relaxation, creative imagery, meditation, deep breathing, or other movement

modalities such as yoga or tai chi may be self-learned and practiced individually from video or audio recordings or printed instructions or learned through personal coaching or group classes.

5. In the realm of *resisting* or avoiding sleep jeopardizing behaviors, alternatively referred to as performing good sleep hygiene, people can be counseled in relation to lifestyle factors such as eating, drinking beverages, and exercising. Recommended is to avoid heavy meals, particularly high-fat meals, near bedtime but to have a light snack that includes some carbohydrate and protein, perhaps in the form of a warm drink such as milk. The rationale for effect is based on promoting the transfer of amino acids (e.g., tryptophan) across the blood–brain barrier to facilitate synthesis of biochemicals (e.g., serotonin) known to promote sleep. Foods high in tryptophan include nuts and seeds, bananas, honey, and eggs. Ingesting substances with caffeine such as coffee, tea, colas, and chocolate interfere with sleep in most individuals, although the stimulating effects vary across people. Found in coffee, tea, soft drinks, energy drinks, and medications, caffeine is an adenosine-receptor antagonist (Porkka-Heiskanen, Zitting, & Wigren, 2013) and has a half-life of 3 to 7 hours (Cheek, Shaver, & Lentz, 2004). While alcohol often is taken to self-medicate for poor sleep and potentially helps falling asleep, PSG sleep stages are disturbed and people often awaken feeling unrefreshed. Thus, alcohol is to be avoided when sleep quality is persistently a problem. While timing of strenuous exercise in relation to sleep is somewhat controversial, most experts recommend it be curtailed close to bedtime but occur within 3 to 6 hours of bedtime. As the rise in body temperature that accompanies exercise falls upon cessation of exercise, a sleep-inducing effect is thought to occur. Indeed, a warm bath or warming the feet prior to bedtime also promotes a steeper drop in body temperature that has been associated with a shorter latency to sleep.

A bundling of therapeutic principles and techniques into an approach called *cognitive–behavioral therapy for insomnia* (CBT-I) has proven effective for persistent insomnia (Williams, Roth, Vatthauer, & McCrae, 2013). CBT-I is generally administered in a five- or six-session series with an expert coach or guide. Incorporated into the sessions are belief and behavioral restructuring and skill building related to general sleep knowledge; sleep medication withdrawal; stimulus control techniques; sleep regularizing through scheduling (sleep restriction); relaxation; and sleep hygiene techniques (Williams et al., 2013).

Sleep Medications

Nonbenzodiazepine *prescription sleep medications* have gained popularity over traditionally used benzodiazepines. Comparatively, most are short-acting and pose less risk of tolerance, dependence, or hangover effects. Like benzodiazepines, most act through GABA-receptor mechanisms. However, prescription sleeping medications remain recommended for long-term use only in circumstances of persistent and severe insomnia that is not improved by behavioral interventions. Short-term use is generally to break a cycle of insomnia precipitated by environmental circumstances, for example, major life event, sleep-interfering symptoms flare. Sometimes, antidepression tricyclic amine medications such as amitriptyline (Elavil) or doxepin (Sinequan), in doses lower than used in treatment of depressed mood, are prescribed to help sleep. People taking sleep medications generally should be counseled to (1) take medication in the prescribed dosage, times (most should be taken 30 minutes before sleep time), and duration (often 7 to 10 days); (2) take only when sufficient time (7 to 8 hours.) is available for sleep; (3) if awaken groggy, refrain from driving; (4) report side effects to health care provider, for example, unusual depressed/anxious mood, stomach/muscle cramps, vomiting, sweating, shakiness; and (5) reduce the dose gradually when halting treatment. Examples of prescribed sleep medications are summarized in Table 17.5.

In general, self-medicating with *over-the-counter (OTC) drugs* for insomnia (e.g., Nytol, Sominex, Compoz, Sleep-Eze, or Unisom) is not recommended for other than

TABLE 17.5	Examples of Common Prescription Sleep Medications	
Medication	**Cautions**	**Considerations**
Nonbenzodiazepine Medications to Fall Asleep		
Eszopiclone (Lunesta) (cylopyrrolone— GABAergict)	History of drug or alcohol abuse, depression, lung disease, or metabolic	Helps people fall asleep and stay asleep for 7–8 hours. May be used for a longer period of time than zolpidem or zaleplon
		High-fat meals may slow absorption—less effective
		Sudden stopping—symptoms of withdrawal, e.g., anxiety, unusual dreams, nausea and vomiting
Zaleplon (Sonata) (pyrazolopyridine— GABAergic)	Pregnant or breast-feeding	Shortest action—helps people fall asleep but not stay asleep
	History of depression, liver or kidney disease, or respiratory conditions	May interact with other medications
	Severe liver problems	Can be habit-forming
		High-fat meals may slow absorption—less effective
		Very short-acting, can be taken in the middle of the night following precautions
Zolpidem (Ambien, and Ambien CR) (imidazopridine— GABAergic)	History of depression, liver or kidney disease, or respiratory conditions	Regular form—helps people fall asleep but some people have trouble staying asleep. May become less effective over time
		Sleep behaviors, such as sleep-driving and sleep-eating may occur. Extended release form may be used for longer period of time than regular form
Ramelteon (Rozerem) (melatonin receptor agonist)	Pregnant or breast-feeding	Rozerem can be prescribed for long-term use—no evidence of dependence. May interact with alcohol
	History of kidney or respiratory problems, sleep apnea, or depression	High-fat meals may slow absorption—less effective
	Liver disease	

(continued)

TABLE 17.5	Examples of Common Prescription Sleep Medications *(continued)*	
Medication	**Cautions**	**Considerations**
Benzodiazepine Sleep Medications		
Triazolam (Halcion) (benzodiazepine— GABAergic)	Pregnant or breast-feeding	Recommended to take with or without food, usually once nightly, 30 minutes before bedtime. May interact with grapefruit juice, alcohol, many medications
	History of drug abuse, depression, or respiratory conditions	Can be habit-forming. Seldom prescribed by sleep specialists
		Drug must be stopped gradually
Estazolam (benzodiazepine— GABAergic)	Pregnant, breast-feeding, older adults	May interact with many other medications
		May not work as well over extended periods
		Can be habit-forming
Temazepam (Restoril) (benzodiazepine— GABAergic)	History of severe depression, substance abuse, lung disease, or kidney or liver conditions	May interact with alcohol and many medications
	Pregnant or breast-feeding	May not work as well over extended periods
		Can be habit-forming

Adapted from http://www.mayoclinic.org/diseases-conditions/insomnia/in-depth/sleeping-pills/ART-20043959.

mild, situation-driven insomnia. Most OTC sleep preparations contain antihistamines that act to block the arousing effects of histamine. Side effects can include dry mouth, dizziness, daytime sleepiness, and cognitive impairments. Women who are pregnant or breast-feeding should be counseled not to take and older adults guided to exercise caution (Gulyani, Salas, & Gamaldo, 2012).

The hormone melatonin is available OTC for insomnia. Naturally produced by the pineal gland, it coordinates the timing component of sleep regulation. While there has been a belief that melatonin levels decrease with age, comparison of younger and older adults has indicated that this is not so. As a supplement, melatonin is believed to reset the body's clock, and therefore reduce sleep/wake problems associated with jet lag or shift work, but this remains in debate. In some people, side effects from melatonin include altered heart rhythm, blood pressure, GI motility, and glucose metabolism (Gulyani et al., 2012). Melatonin has inhibiting effects on ovarian function and vasoconstrictor properties. Therefore, taking it for insomnia, particularly in the context of cardiovascular disease or vulnerability requires caution.

Integrative Therapies for Sleep

Solid evidential support for insomnia-modulating effects of common integrative therapies has yet to be generated. In a rigorous systematic review, supportive evidence for insomnia reduction was reported for acupressure, tai chi, and yoga (Sarris & Byrne, 2011). Lacking or too weak to meet the design/methods criteria for review inclusion were any studies of homeopathy, massage, or aromatherapy. Weak and unsupportive evidence was found for herbal therapies such as valerian.

However, hypnotic- or sedative-type herbals are known to have GABAergic-, melatonergic-, and adenosine-receptor modulation properties, all of which are mechanisms influential in sleep regulation (Sarris, Panossian, Schweitzer, Stough, & Scholey, 2011). Therefore, despite marginal to no current evidence of therapeutic effects beyond placebo, further rigorous studies of sleep-promoting herbs have the potential for positive effects on healthy sleep. It might be remembered that findings of no differences from placebo can represent some level of therapeutic gain through positive outcome expectations of patients. If not harmful, their use need not be discouraged. Common plant substances for which there are healthy sleep promotion claims include valerian (*Valeriana* spp.), for which the optimum dose is said to be 450 mg of valerian in aqueous extract. A suggestion is to pour boiling water over teaspoons of valerian root, infuse for 15 minutes and drink before bedtime (with lemon balm). Chamomile (*Matricaria recutita*) or passionflower (*Passiflora app*) as a tea sipped 30 minutes before sleep is believed to promote sleep. Lavender *oil* has been shown to depress the central nervous system and prime for sleep. Lavender can be inhaled as an aroma (e.g., during a bath or placed near a pillow) or taken as lavender tea before bedtime. Kava (*Piper methysticum*) is a common beverage ingredient in the South Seas and has substances to promote muscle relaxation and anxiety reduction, thereby promoting sleep.

Unique Features of Sleep over the Life span of Women

Sleep in Childhood and Puberty

Over the course of development from infancy to adulthood, there is a gradual but striking increase in both slow-wave sleep (SWS) and REM sleep in the context of a reduction in total sleep time, both at night and during the day (scheduled napping reduces mostly between 18 months and 5 years of age) (Owens, 2008). In infants, sleep is normally consolidated (ability to sleep for continuous time during the night) starting between 6 and 12 weeks of age. The majority of infants sleep through the night by 9 months of age. Through early childhood, nighttime awakenings are common, but important in indicating healthy sleep is not so much the awakenings but whether the child can return to sleep without intervention. Although influenced by ethnic/racial differences, most children are no longer napping by 5 years of age (Galland, Taylor, Elder, & Herbison, 2012). Nighttime sleep durations are highly variable across age groups but are gradually lessened as children get older through a shift to later bedtimes and scheduled arising times, governed by attending school and other scheduled activities. Research shows that older adolescents function best with the same amount of sleep as preadolescents but circumvent this need by staying up late and frequently adopt an adult pattern of only 7 or fewer hours of sleep during week nights (Vallido, Peters, O'Brien, & Jackson, 2009) and sleeping longer on the weekend days to compensate for sleep loss during the week. Differences between girls and boys are not clear, although girls have been found to reduce their nighttime sleep duration at an earlier age and were seen to waken earlier than boys during the week (a guess being because of longer grooming activities), and girls have been observed to sleep longer on weekends as compensation (Vallido, Jackson, & O'Brien, 2009).

Although largely understudied and apart from biological age, both onset of puberty and menstruation (menarche) have been associated with sleep changes. Although maturation rates vary across ethnic/racial groups, over the last several decades, onset of puberty has been dropping at a faster rate than onset age of menarche. Currently girls get their first periods a few months earlier than girls 40 years ago, with the average age now said to be 12.6 (White non-Hispanic) and 12.1 (African descent) years but begin breast development 1 to 2 years earlier (Steingraber, 2007). Age of breast stage 2 onset was seen to vary from 8.8 years (African American) to 9.3 years (Hispanic) to 9.7 years (White non-Hispanic and Asian) (Biro et al., 2013). Likely to have indirect sleep health effects, earlier puberty maturation has been associated with psychosocial vulnerabilities such as lower self-esteem, depression proneness, and risky behavior engagement but also with reproductive system cancers, especially breast, ovarian, and endometrial cancers, as well as high insulin and high blood pressure (Biro et al., 2013; Steingraber, 2007).

In American girls, the onset of menarche has been associated with delayed bedtimes with the impact of hormonal changes, for example, melatonin and luteinizing hormones, apparently having a more profound effect than psychosocial factors (Vallido, Jackson, et al., 2009). Reduced total sleep time appears to be related to later pubertal stage. In girls, but not boys, a more advanced pubertal status, even in the context of reported sufficient sleep, was correlated with being prone to insomnia and daytime tiredness. More girls (20.5%) than boys (6.5%) of adolescent age reported daytime sleepiness, fatigue, and reduced energy (ter Wolbeek, van Doornen, Kavelaars, & Heijnen, 2006). At question is whether fatigue might be due to coincidental emotional or somatic distress with stress-immune physiological function. However, in a study of adolescents with and without fatigue, neither stress hormones nor immune indicators showed differences (ter Wolbeek, van Doornen, Coffeng, Kavelaars, & Heijnen, 2007; ter Wolbeek, van Doornen, Kavelaars, et al., 2007).

Poor sleep poses a challenge to emotional regulation and cognitive performance, which for teen girls can impair school performance and interpersonal relationships with parents and peers. Thus, many aspects of wellness for adolescent girls are influenced by the quality of their sleep or vice versa. After the mid-teen years, females over their adult life are more prone to report psychological distress and sleep difficulties. How much of this vulnerability could be evident in the teen years is not clear. Especially prone to sleep difficulties are females who express depressive, anxious, or somatic symptoms as well as females exposed to current or past sexual abuse. Moreover, females are more likely than males to report taking psychoactive drugs to increase daytime alertness or help them sleep.

Sleep during the Reproductive Years

Insomnia and other symptoms can appear or are worsened during periods of natural fluctuations in hypothalamic–pituitary–ovarian (HPO)–axis hormones, that is, with menstruation, pregnancy, and menopause. Most attempts to link ovarian hormone blood concentrations with symptoms such as depressed mood or insomnia have failed to provide convincing evidence of a link. However, rather than absolute deficits or surfeits of hormones, the link is likely to be with speed (rapid) or erratic pattern of hormone changes (Shaver, 2010). For most women, no or mild symptoms are noticed at the time of reproductive hormone fluctuations or change, but a subset of women appear to be particularly sensitive to these hormone variations and suffer cyclical or enduring symptoms over the course of menstrual cycles, pregnancy, and menopause transition.

Across the *menstrual cycle*, studies of sleep in healthy adult women show little evidence of primarily menstrual cycle-related sleep disturbances, although some subtle changes in sleep microstructure have been noted during the luteal phase, which represents progesterone exposure and ultimately estrogen and progesterone withdrawal. When sleep disturbance is noted, it is mostly around the time of menstruation (premenstrual week and early bleeding days) when there is rapid reduction in hormone levels. In national polling, roughly one-quarter to one-third of menstruating women reported perimenstrual sleep disturbances, often attributed to cramps, bloating, and headaches (Lee, Baker, Newton, & Ancoli-Israel, 2008). Given the relative high cost and complexity of measurement, few studies have used physical sleep assessment and those that have demonstrate at best only slight changes in PSG recordings (Lee et al., 2008). Women who are noticeably more likely to report menstrual-related sleep disturbance include those with severe premenstrual syndrome (PMS) and premenstrual dysphoric disorder (PMDD). It is to be noted that compared with age- and weight-matched controls, women with polycystic ovarian syndrome (PCOS), often have irregular or absent menstrual cycles, are obese and show insulin-resistance, and are prone to sleep-disordered breathing (SDB), that is, 30 to 40 times more likely.

In summary, sleep is likely to remain robust across menstrual cycles in healthy women who normally experience refreshing sleep. For women who experience perimenstrual sleep disturbances, treatments to modulate uncomfortable symptoms such as cramps are likely to improve or restore good sleep. Behavioral sleep-promoting strategies are recommended as well.

In *pregnancy and postpartum periods*, a variety of factors can impact sleep, including hormone effects and discomforts from the growing fetus. Sleep changes have been observed by near end of the first trimester. Even in healthy pregnant women, night wake time doubles from a normal of ≤5% before pregnancy to 10% in the third trimester. NREM sleep shows more light sleep and awakenings and less deep sleep, although REM sleep stays relatively stable (Lee & Kryger, 2008). Awakenings are often driven by bodily sensations, for example, need to urinate, back ache, or sometimes leg cramps. Important to rule out as sleep disruptors are restless legs syndrome (RLS), nocturnal periodic leg movements, nocturnal esophageal reflux, or SDB.

Often beginning toward bedtime and preventing induction of sleep, RLS is manifested by an overwhelming urge to move the legs, which can be ameliorated by walking (see more RLS detail on page 330). By the end of the third trimester, RLS occurs in as many as 27% of women (Okun, Roberts, Marsland, & Hall, 2009). RLS that first appears in pregnancy has been associated with increased vulnerability to RLS manifestations outside of being pregnant and with ensuing pregnancies (Jones, 2013).

By the third trimester and possibly heralding SDB or pregnancy-induced high blood pressure, the prevalence of snoring during sleep goes up by 3 to 6 times, from 5% to anywhere from 15% to 30% (Beebe & Lee, 2007; Okun et al., 2009). Possible contributors to snoring include upper airway edema, largely from increased blood volume and pregnancy hormonal effects on blood vessels and capillaries. Aside from being linked to excessive weight gain or obesity and smoking, snoring during pregnancy portends to lower infant Apgar scores at birth and an elevated risk of fetal growth retardation. Since serious SDB in pregnancy can be alleviated with ventilator-delivered continuous positive airway pressure (CPAP) breathing, early referral to a sleep specialist is essential to avoid threats to placental perfusion and healthy fetal growth (Beebe & Lee, 2007).

Shortened sleep (sleep loss) is frequent prior to delivery and raises the possibility of negative outcomes. In the 5 days prior to delivery, sleep time has been seen to be shortened (from 7.5 to 4.5 hours per night) and wake time lengthened (from 15% to 30%) (Beebe & Lee, 2007). Importantly, cumulative sleep loss may invoke longer labors and negative delivery outcomes. In one study of healthy uncomplicated pregnancies, compared with women getting ≥7 hours of sleep per night, women getting ≤6 hours in the 3 weeks prior to delivery, averaged longer labors by about 12 hours and had 4.5 times the rate of cesarean births (Lee & Gay, 2004).

For women who are postpartum, sleep is often disrupted by a variety of factors, most particularly related to the hormone balance returning back to prepregnancy status and the new-found demands of infant care. Postpartum sleep is reportedly deeper and longer for women who are breast-feeding as compared with those who are not. This is perhaps a result of nighttime prolactin secretion patterns, infant closeness with less need for maternal arousal to prepare for feedings, or closer synchrony of infant to maternal sleep and wake durations, among other possibilities (Lee et al., 2008). Most women get past this period and can be coached into taking every opportunity as they arise to juggle childcare demands with engaging in relaxed wakefulness or napping and practicing strong sleep hygiene behaviors.

In summary, maintaining healthy sleep in pregnancy can be a challenge due to the profound physiological changes that naturally occur. Sleep tends to become lighter, somewhat more fragmented and shortened. For most women, the effects on sleep are accommodated without negative outcomes and mostly adequate sleep can be maintained by alleviation of bodily discomforts, and adopting periods of relaxation or napping frequently across the day. For women who are prone to severe snoring or the manifestations of sleep-related disorders such as RLS or SDB, more rigorous assessment and referrals to specialists are necessary in order to improve sleep and prevent any negative consequences for labor, delivery, and neonatal growth and development. In the postpartum period, maternal sleep disruption is prevalent in women who are sensitive to reproductive hormone levels (which are returning to prepregnancy levels) and due to infant care demands. Breast-feeding should be encouraged for a variety of health reasons, including for better maternal sleep.

The menopausal transition impacts sleep health for many women. Compared with women in premenopause stage, more women report sleep disturbances when in peri- or postmenopause stages. However, at issue is whether to view the sleep changes as attributable to reproductive system, brain, or general aging (Shaver, 2010). In men and women (studied mostly in late postmenopause), the amount of physically recorded (PSG) deep sleep (stages 3 and 4) declines with age. One possible confounder is that the electroencephalographic high amplitude waves set as the standard for scoring PSG deep sleep (historically based on normative sleep in younger people) are diminished (due to brain aging) and fall below the scoring threshold. However, in women compared with men, slow-wave (deep) sleep appears to remain more robust and there is a shorter latency to REM sleep. With aging, sleep appears to get lighter and less stable, with more waking episodes during the night. Waking is most likely to occur at the end of sleep cycles and contributes to older adults often reporting that they wake up every hour or hour and a half or so. If able to return to sleep fairly rapidly, people likely are not losing much sleep time and this pattern need not be a reason for concern. Explaining this dynamic can help older adults to feel more satisfied with their sleep.

In transition to menopause, women show vulnerability to a cluster of symptoms that includes sleep disturbances (insomnia), vasomotor symptoms (VMS) such as hot flashes and night sweats, and depressed mood. Clarity of the relationship among these symptoms remains elusive (Shaver, 2009). While more midlife women report sleep disturbances throughout the menopause transition than when in premenopause, menopause status (usually judged by HPO–axis hormone levels and/or irregular menstrual bleeding) does not appear to negatively impact physical sleep in most women, except in the context of

VMS. As discussed elsewhere, early work showed that midlife women reporting insomnia were not distinguished by menopause status. Ignoring menopause status, two groups with insomnia (reported poor sleep) were apparent. One insomnia group exhibited poor physical sleep (PSG), and in spite of reporting insomnia, the other group exhibited normative physical sleep patterns. Compared with midlife women reporting no insomnia (comparative control group), women with insomnia but normative physical sleep had higher life strain and psychological distress scores, but VMS were not elevated. Also compared with the control group, women with insomnia plus poor recorded sleep (lower sleep efficiency) showed higher VMS, while life strain and psychological distress scores were not elevated (Shaver, 2009). These observations suggested that some midlife women with insomnia have varying contributing factors, and as a result, some should be treated for VMS to improve sleep while others should be treated for elevated strain and emotional distress.

Late menopausal transition stage, particularly when VMS are persistent, conveys vulnerability to depressed mood. Sleep and depressed mood are closely connected as briefly discussed in the next section. In premenopause women with no history of depression prior to menopause and followed over time, depressed mood scores were quadrupled and a depression diagnosis was 2.5 times more likely to occur during menopause transition (Shaver, 2009). Women vulnerable to depression at times of significant hormone fluctuations show excess vulnerability to depression in menopause transition (Shaver, 2010). Treating serious insomnia for women in late menopause/early postmenopause stages in order to prevent or reduce depressed mood is highly recommended.

To sum up, during transition to and after menopause, some women are vulnerable to the symptom cluster of poor sleep and depressed mood, the majority of evidence suggesting this occurs mostly in the context of VMS. Whether there is a linear relationship between these symptoms whereby one precedes the other is not clear. Since the regulation of sleep, mood, and body temperature is known to involve common central neurochemicals (e.g., serotonin, adrenalin) and brain areas, more likely is that they are concurrent manifestations of common underlying physiological pathways affected by erratic HPO fluctuations during reproductive aging. Since a variety of social determinants for these symptoms have been uncovered, how women express their symptoms will be modulated by environmental exposures. Hence, women will vary in the configuration of factors that contribute to their clinical profile. The contributors may be biological (e.g., pattern of HPO–axis hormone fluctuations, menopausal stage, or genetic propensity) or psychosocial (e.g., life strain, social milieu, or emotiveness). This makes clinical assessment complex, but striving to comprehensively assess key contributors that are both biological and psychosocial is essential to therapy planning.

Sleep in the Context of Mental and Physical Disturbances

Depression

An almost ubiquitous core manifestation of depression is poor sleep (insomnia). Longitudinal studies across the adult age span indicate that insomnia can precede initial and recurring major depression episodes, leading to the postulate that treatment of persistent insomnia could prevent the onset of depressive episodes. Moreover, excess depressed mood has been observed in people with sleep disorders (SDB, narcolepsy, delayed sleep phase, periodic leg movement, and RLS) (Shaver, 2009). Depressed mood is another multifaceted condition that is underrecognized in clinical practice. More than half of people who are depressed when they present for health care only report somatic symptoms, particularly somatic pain in some part of the body. Not yet adequately studied are medications and behavioral or combined therapies aimed at concurrently ameliorating depression and insomnia.

Medical Conditions, Tissue Injury, and Sleep

Almost every medical condition, that is, respiratory, endocrine, renal, cardiovascular, infectious, and neurological diseases, has been associated with sleep disturbances (Dikeos & Georgantopoulos, 2011). Sleep associated with major medical conditions emanates from a variety of complex factors, usually some combination of pathophysiologic mechanisms, symptoms, medications, mood state, and underlying systemic stress-immune and metabolic activation. In general, sleep disturbances will be improved by determining the medical condition or other specific contributors and modifying them. However, often overlooked is that the medical condition context can be superimposed on inherently poor sleep, and therefore, sleep quality assessment and sleep medicinal and behavioral modalities are warranted as adjunctive to direct medical condition treatments.

Pathophysiological sleep disruptors, for example, with cardiovascular or pulmonary conditions, can take the form of tissue oxygen desaturation episodes. Symptoms are most particularly pain, disturbed sleep, such as postinjury (surgical, trauma) pain, or cancer, arthritic, gastrointestinal, or peripheral neuropathic pain. Neurocognitive impairments, for example, psychiatric disorders, stroke, dementias, indicate direct brain pathophysiology and jeopardy of normal sleep regulation. Many medications, most particularly sedative and analgesic combinations, and other cardiovascular, gastric-protective, antiasthma, antiinfective, antidepressant, and anticonvulsant drugs, are known through central actions to disturb the normative patterns of physical sleep. As mentioned, sleep disturbances can be precipitated or perpetuated by mood states such as depression or anxiety, and since such mood changes are evident with many chronic medical conditions, they could be reinforcing sleep disturbances.

There is growing appreciation that many diseases and illnesses have multiple manifestations, including clusters of symptoms that are derived from common underlying alterations in stress-immune pathways. Much attention is being paid to cytokines, which act to coordinate what is a protective bodily response to ensure healing and recovery from episodic challenges but which can become enduring or chronic as a low-grade inflammatory activation. Cytokines are immune system signaling proteins acting as messengers and are expressed by various cell types, including macrophages, lymphocytes, vascular endothelial cells, smooth muscle cells, adipose tissue, and neurons and classed as pro- or anti-inflammatory (Dantzer, 2009). Emotional stress or tissue infection/injury evokes a higher-than-normal set of circulating pro-inflammatory cytokines, such as interleukin (IL)-1β, IL-1RA, IL-2, tumor necrosis factor-α (TNF-α), C-reactive protein (CRP), and interferon-γ (IFN-γ), among others. Peripheral tissue cytokine release and afferent nerve activity provoke brain cytokine release (Dimsdale & Dantzer, 2007) to activate the stress hypothalamus/pituitary/adrenal (HPA) axis with ultimate increases in glucocorticoids, that is, cortisol. As well, pro-inflammatory cytokines promote brain release of epinephrine, dopamine, and serotonin (Irwin, 2011), all neuromodulators of behavior and symptoms, particularly sleep, pain, and mood. Increasingly evident is that low-grade (sub-clinical) inflammatory activation underlies the emergence of symptoms and chronic conditions. Of note is that inflammatory activation has been documented in conditions ranging from chronic heart failure and progressive neurodegeneration to obesity and aging (Dantzer & Kelley, 2007). Certain indicators such as IL-6 and CRP, when elevated, showed predictive power for later life morbidity and mortality (Steptoe, Hamer, & Chida, 2007).

Interestingly, women are seen to have a more robust immune mechanism than men, which helps women to recover from hemorrhage and trauma, perhaps protective in the context of childbirth. However, women are more vulnerable than men to having conditions with strong autoimmune components such as systemic lupus erythematosus or Sjogren syndrome (women 7 to 10 times are more likely) (Darnall & Suarez, 2009). Hindering the understanding of stress and immune linkage differences between women and men, rarely seen in the literature is differential gender analysis or an accounting for women's reproductive/menstrual status. However, evidence supports the idea that stress and inflammatory activation patterns differ in men and women as a function of type of stressor, and the types of emotions elicited (Darnall & Suarez, 2009). Much more rigorous study is needed to generate knowledge that is applicable to clinical practice.

Too little sleep is a stressor, seen in accompanying signs of bodily stress activation, for example, excess levels of epinephrine, cortisol, and other stress hormones. At a tissue and cellular level, in the face of sleep loss, the release of proteins (e.g., CRP) and pro-inflammatory cytokines is evident. This represents a tip in the balance toward systemic inflammatory activation, and therefore, vulnerability to infection, inflammatory conditions, and chronic diseases.

Chronic Pain and Fatiguing Conditions

With higher prevalence in women than men and associated with debilitating fatigue and poor sleep quality are a set of syndromes (e.g., fibromyalgia [FM], irritable bowel [IB]) characterized by widespread or regional pain (Shaver, 2008). For example, FM is estimated to affect at least 1% to 3% of the adult population and five to nine times more common in women. IB prevalence ranges from 3% to 20%, with two to four times more women affected than men. These multisymptom conditions include FM, chronic fatigue syndrome (CFS), IB syndrome, chronic pelvic pain (CPP), idiopathic back pain, temporomandibular joint disorder, multiple chemical sensitivity, headache (tension, migraine, and mixed), primary dysmenorrhea, interstitial cystitis or painful bladder syndrome, myofascial pain syndrome/regional tissue pain syndrome, and RLS/periodic leg movement in sleep disorder. Because no clear pathological but rather functional indicators are present, these conditions have been labeled as functional somatic syndromes, multisymptom illnesses, or central sensitivity syndromes (CSSs). Upon comprehensive assessment, it is common for women to meet criteria for more than one CSS. Important to diagnosis is the exclusion of other pathology-defined medical diagnoses (Smith, Harris, & Clauw, 2011).

Pain, fatigue, and sleep difficulties are highly correlated with each other and linked in reciprocal and reinforcing ways. People in chronic pain report more wakefulness, that is, fewer hours of sleep, longer times to fall asleep, more and longer nighttime awakenings, and as expected overall perceptions of poor or unrefreshing or what is called *nonrestorative* (i.e., wake up tired) sleep (Shaver, 2008). Even compared with people with arthritis, people with FM report more difficulty falling and staying asleep, fewer hours of sleep, and taking more sleep medications. An almost ever-present dimension is waking up feeling tired or unrefreshed (Shaver, 2008). Sleep recordings (PSG) in people with chronic pain tend to show a pattern of modestly lighter and less-consolidated (more fragmented) sleep with more wakefulness and arousals but the extent of disruption from normative patterns does not seem to match the intensity of subjective poor sleep reports. Compared with controls with no painful conditions, people with FM generally show more wake (longer sleep latency, and wake after sleep onset), somewhat lighter sleep with less deep sleep and higher fragmentation, particularly in the early part of the night. The documented sleep disturbances associated with the CSSs are similar to those sleep disturbances seen in people with chronic primary insomnia. While sleep biomarkers of fragmented, nonrestorative sleep, for example, α-wave intrusion into sleep, sleep spindles and EEG power have been sought, no definite marker is yet available for use in clinical practice (Shaver, 2008).

Pain and sleep have a reciprocal relationship such that pain interferes with sleep regulation and poor sleep can instigate or amplify pain. When pain and sleep are carefully tracked in relation to one another, more wake time pain results in poor sleep reports and poor sleep results in reports of more wake time pain symptoms. When healthy people are sleep-deprived, particularly of deep sleep, somatic symptoms emerge, especially increased musculoskeletal discomfort (Shaver et al., 1997). It has been argued that disrupted sleep continuity or consolidation is more important than shorter sleep duration in creating perceptions of nonrestorative sleep. The reciprocal dynamics between sleep and pain portend that both sleep quality and pain patterns should be concurrently assessed and symptom treatment for both is likely to invoke synergistic reduction or relief in both domains.

Central to the pathophysiology across CSSs is pain hypersensitivity or sensitization and altered stress-immune regulation. Women with CSSs show lower pain thresholds and more and longer-lasting pain when a pain-producing stimulus is applied (hyperalgesia), and they express pain in response to stimuli that would not normally be painful (allodynia). Moreover, with brain imaging, altered blood flow or neuronal activity within brain pain-related areas is seen. Excessive or constant pain signals (neuronal or biochemical) from peripheral tissues hyperexcite central neurons, provoke spontaneous nerve activity, and expand neuronal receptive fields, among other changes (Shaver, 2008). At least partially influential in sensitizing central pain processing mechanisms is the aforementioned cytokine-induced stress/immune inflammatory activation with changes to neurochemicals such as serotonin, epinephrine, and dopamine—important to sleep, pain and mood regulation. Pro-inflammatory cytokines such as IL-1, IL-6, and others show higher-than-normative levels in CSSs such as FM and IB.

While a belief has been that psychiatric disorder, especially major depression, accompanies or is part of the CSSs, this is perhaps a bias derived from small group and biased sampling from tertiary care, not blinding raters and nonstandard diagnostic interviews. With strong study designs, no excess vulnerability to psychiatric diagnoses has proved evident, although it is estimated that 25% to 33% of patients with FM who present for health care have major depression (Shaver, 2008).

Women with CSSs can often pinpoint a particular stressor, for example, severe emotional stress, infections or injury, believed to precipitate the "clinical" breakthrough, that is, the obvious presence of manifestations. Preclinical factors found to predispose and perpetuate CSSs in women involve high exposure to negative life events, including sexual, physical, or emotional abuse; and a highly driven lifestyle, that is, engaging in excessively active mental and or physical activities (Shaver, 2008).

Sleep-Related Disorders

Two common sleep-related disorders are SDB and sleep-related movement disorders. Difficulty breathing during sleep can be a major life-threatening phenomenon and is a topic of considerable biomedical diagnostic and treatment effort and study. Women compared with men have lower susceptibility, at least in younger ages, and exhibit some different manifestations. Difficulties with aberrant or exaggerated sleep-related movements have major life-quality threatening dimensions, and women have more susceptibility than men.

SDB is classified on a spectrum from increased upper airway resistance, evident as snoring, through to hypopneas (airflow reductions) and apneas (airflow cessation) (Shaver, 2013). Airflow reductions appear as powerful a threat to health status as apneas, therefore clinical assessment is aimed at identifying the sleep apnea/hypopnea syndrome (SAHS). Airflow can be detected as temperature changes during breathing with an oral or nasal thermistor or abdominal or chest wall excursion monitoring with a pneumotachograph. Apneas are recognized by nearly zero airflow or no chest excursion for at least 10 seconds or more during sleep. When airflow or chest excursion shows a drop to ≤70% of normal for at least 10 seconds, hypopneas are said to occur. A sleep apnea/hypopnea index (AHI) or respiratory disturbance index (RDI) is calculated by summing the number of apnea and hypopnea episodes per hour. Snoring (increased efforts to breath) is often reported and is considered an indicator for suspecting SAHS. When increased efforts to breathe do not meet criteria for apneas or hypopneas, upper airway resistance syndrome (UARS) is said to exist. Airway resistance changes can be detected by inserting an esophageal balloon with a pressure transducer in the lower third of the esophagus (Shaver & Zenk, 2000).

Frequent or lengthy episodes of apnea or hypopnea can lead to profound disturbances in sleep patterns and arterial blood gases. Episodes are often associated with brain-pattern arousals seen on the polysomnograph and varying levels of oxygen desaturation as seen through finger pulse oximetry. Obstruction of the airways leads to repeat inspiratory efforts until arousal from sleep occurs to reestablish a patent airway. A high frequency of sleep disruptions and brain arousals constitutes fragmented sleep and leads to reports of excessive daytime sleepiness.

Women are less susceptible than men to SDB at any age. For example, from a random sample of employed men and women 30 to 60 years old, extrapolated estimates were that 2% of midlife women and 4% of midlife men in the workforce meet the minimal diagnostic criterion of SAHS (RDI ≥15 and daytime sleepiness) (Shaver & Zenk, 2000). Mostly derived from studies of men, key indications for SDB are

- Loud snoring
- Excessive daytime sleepiness
- Insomnia
- Frequently witnessed apneas
- Obesity (especially nape of the neck)
- Increased propensity for vehicle and work-related accidents

Commonly present are the physical features of a large neck circumference and a crowded oropharynx, although in nonobese patients, abnormal posterior positioning of one or both jaws, a high-arched narrow palate, enlarged tongue or tonsils, temporomandibular joint abnormalities, or chronic nasal obstruction are associated. Either as consequences of or as contributors to SDB, frequently coexisting conditions are systemic hypertension, heart arrhythmias, and possibly myocardial ischemia and infarction.

In both men and women, SDB remains underrecognized but likely more so for women because they deviate from men in their presenting symptoms and women often do not have a bed partner to confirm snoring or breathing difficulties. Women appear similar to men in reporting loud snoring and daytime sleepiness for a given RDI, but are less likely to report restless sleep or witnessed apneas and more likely to report morning fatigue and morning headache (Shaver, 2013). Women and men with SAHS show similar pulmonary function, respiratory distress, and nocturnal desaturation patterns, although women show fewer completely occluded breathing events and have apneas of shorter mean and maximum duration than men. These differences in upper airway occlusion and apnea duration are suggestive of gender differences in upper airway physiology or respiratory control (Shaver & Zenk, 2000).

Originally derived for preoperative screening for obstructive sleep apnea (OSA) and growing in popularity for *general SAHS screening* is the STOP–BANG assessment (Chung et al., 2008). This has four questions coupled with four objective measures. The four STOP questions are S = Do you snore loudly (louder than talking or loud enough to be heard through closed doors)?; T = Do you often feel tired, fatigued, or sleepy during the daytime?; O = Has anyone observed you stop breathing during your sleep?; and P = Do you have or are you being treated for high BP? The four BANG measures are B, BMI, ≥ 28 kg/m^2; A, aged, ≥ 50 years; N, neck circumference ≥ 17 inches for men or ≥ 16 inches for women; and G, male gender. A high risk of OSA is judged to be present if three or more items are affirmed. In a general population referred for PSG assessment, STOP–BANG had a sensitivity of 86.1% for mild OSA, 92.8% for moderate OSA, and 95.6% for severe OSA (Chung et al., 2008).

RLS and *periodic limb movement disorder* (PLMD) are sleep-related neurological disorders associated with poor sleep. As reviewed by Thomas and Watson (2008), RLS increases with age, and occurs in twice as many women as in men (9.0% to 10.8% vs. 5.4% to 5.8%). Sleep disturbances include delayed sleep onset (e.g., more than 30 minutes), multiple awakenings (e.g., three or more times), shortened sleep duration (e.g., 4 to 5 hours/night), and a reduction in sleep efficiency. Insomnia is the main reason for seeking treatment. Four diagnostic criteria for RLS include (1) an urge to move the legs, usually accompanied or caused by uncomfortable and unpleasant sensations in the legs; (2) worsening during periods of rest or inactivity; (3) worse or only appears in the evening or night; and (4) partial or total relief by movement, at least as long as the activity continues (Thomas, 2008). Besides insomnia, RLS has been associated with depressed mood, morning headache, and muscle and joint pain; and can coexist with heart disease. Accompanying RLS in about 80% of people is PLMD. This refers to involuntary movements of rhythmic extension of the big toe and dorsiflexion of the ankle, with occasional flexion of the knee and hip during sleep, usually in association with reports of insomnia.

Contributors to RLS/PLMD in women are believed to be anemia, low iron or folate levels, and genetic or familial problems with dopamine and iron metabolism (Lee et al., 2008). As mentioned, RLS emerges in pregnancy in up to nearly 30% of women (Okun et al., 2009). A strong relationship was found between RLS and VMS in midlife women, but neither RLS nor PLMD have been responsive to estrogen therapy. While not yet definitive, RLS and PLMD may be related to stress hormone changes and particularly down regulation within the dopaminergic system. Of note is that iron is critical to dopaminergic function, and people manifesting RLS tend to have low serum iron (in storage form, ferritin). Women prone to heavy menstruation or excessive bleeding in menopause transition may be vulnerable. Iron deficiency can result from or be amplified by vegetarian diets. Therefore, RLS prevention or treatment warrants attention to an adequate dietary intake of iron (and folate and prenatal vitamins in pregnancy), avoidance of antihistamines, caffeine, nicotine, and alcohol. Of help symptomatically may be mental-alerting activities and sensory input that counters the unpleasant sensations such as light massage or warm baths (Thomas, 2008). Pharmacologically, dopamine agonists, such as ropinirole and pramipexole, usually help achieve relief.

Summary

In summary, healthy sleep is critical to overall wellness. Falling asleep promptly when desired, staying asleep, or quickly falling back to sleep if awakened to achieve 7 to 8 hours of consolidated sleep and awakening feeling refreshed are the hallmarks of healthy sleep. Sleep that is perceived as poor (i.e., insomnia) might be inherent and enduring or be due to a variety of contributors (e.g., high exposure to life stress events or medical disorders) that can be episodic or enduring. Multisymptom medical disorders incorporating persistent pain and/or depressed mood such as CCSs (e.g., FM or IB, migraine headache) have insomnia as a prominent comanifestation. Of concern in all patients is recognizing sleep-related disorders, especially RLS or periodic leg movements during sleep and those worthy of referral to sleep specialists such as narcolepsy and parasomnias. Over the course of their lifetimes, women who apparently have heightened sensitivity will perceive insomnia at times of significant HPO hormonal fluctuations, such as with the menstrual cycle, pregnancy, or menopausal transition. Comprehensive assessment of sleep quality involves documenting sleep patterns, associated manifestations, the medical disease and treatments context, reproductive age and status, and sleep-related lifestyle and behavioral dimensions. The mainstays for long-term promotion of healthy sleep where insomnia is primary are behavioral strategies with judicious use of sleep medications. Where insomnia is secondary to other conditions and circumstances, treatment of sleep-interfering factors (e.g., pain or breathing disorders) will improve sleep. Sleep therapies, be they pharmacologic or behavioral, can be effective adjuncts to any therapies aimed at improving overall health and wellness.

References

American Academy of Sleep Medicine. (2005). *International classification of sleep disorders: Diagnostic and coding manual* (2nd ed.). Westchester, IL: Author.

Beebe, K. R., & Lee, K. A. (2007). Sleep disturbance in late pregnancy and early labor. *Journal of Perinatal Neonatal & Nursing, 21*(2), 103–108. doi:10.1097/01.jpn.0000270626.66369.26

Biro, F. M., Greenspan, L. C., Galvez, M. P., Pinney, S. M., Teitelbaum, S., Windham, G. C., . . . Wolff, M. S. (2013). Onset of breast development in a longitudinal cohort. *Pediatrics, 132*(6), 1019–1027. doi:10.1542/peds.2012-3773

Buysse, D. J. (2013). Insomnia. *JAMA, 309*(7), 706–716.

Buysse, D. J., Reynolds, C. F., 3rd, Monk, T. H., Berman, S. R., & Kupfer, D. J. (1989). The Pittsburgh Sleep Quality Index: A new instrument for psychiatric practice and research. *Psychiatry Research, 28*(2), 193–213.

Cheek, R. E., Shaver, J. L. F., & Lentz, M. J. (2004). Variations in sleep hygiene practices of women with and without insomnia. *Research in Nursing and Health, 27*, 225–236.

Chung, F., Yegneswaran, B., Liao, P., Chung, S. A., Vairavanathan, S., Islam, S., . . . Shapiro, C. M. (2008). STOP questionnaire: A tool to screen patients for obstructive sleep apnea. *Anesthesiology, 108*(5), 812–821. doi:10.1097/ALN.0b013e31816d83e4

Dantzer, R. (2009). Cytokine, sickness behavior, and depression. *Immunology and Allergy Clinics of North America, 29*(2), 247–264. doi:10.1016/j.iac.2009.02.002

Dantzer, R., & Kelley, K. W. (2007). Twenty years of research on cytokine-induced sickness behavior. *Brain Behavior and Immunity, 21*(2), 153–160. doi:10.1016/j.bbi.2006.09.006

Darnall, B. D., & Suarez, E. C. (2009). Sex and gender in psychoneuroimmunology research: Past, present and future. *Brain Behavior and Immunity, 23*(5), 595–604. doi:10.1016/j.bbi.2009.02.019

Dikeos, D., & Georgantopoulos, G. (2011). Medical comorbidity of sleep disorders. *Current Opinion Psychiatry, 24*(4), 346–354. doi:10.1097/YCO.0b013e3283473375

Dimsdale, J. E., & Dantzer, R. (2007). A biological substrate for somatoform disorders: Importance of pathophysiology. *Psychosomatic Medicine, 69*(9), 850–854. doi:10.1097/PSY.0b013e31815b00e7

Gagnon, C., Belanger, L., Ivers, H., & Morin, C. M. (2013). Validation of the insomnia severity index in primary care. *Journal of the American Board of Family Medicine, 26*(6), 701–710. doi:10.3122/jabfm.2013.06.130064

Galland, B. C., Taylor, B. J., Elder, D. E., & Herbison, P. (2012). Normal sleep patterns in infants and children: A systematic review of observational studies. *Sleep Medicine Review, 16*(3), 213–222. doi:10.1016/j.smrv.2011.06.001

Gulyani, S., Salas, R. E., & Gamaldo, C. E. (2012). Sleep medicine pharmacotherapeutics overview: Today, tomorrow, and the future (Part 1: Insomnia and circadian rhythm disorders). *Chest, 142*(6), 1659–1668. doi:10.1378/chest.12-0465

Irwin, M. R. (2011). Inflammation at the intersection of behavior and somatic symptoms. *Psychiatric Clinics of North America, 34*(3), 605–620. doi:10.1016/j.psc.2011.05.005

Johns, M. W. (1991). A new method for measuring daytime sleepiness: The Epworth Sleepiness Scale. *Sleep, 14*(6), 540–545.

Jones, C. R. (2013). Diagnostic and management approach to common sleep disorders during pregnancy. *Clinical Obstetrics and Gynecology, 56*(2), 360–371.

Kahan, V., Andersen, M. L., Tomimori, J., & Tufik, S. (2010). Can poor sleep affect skin integrity? *Medical Hypotheses, 75*(6), 535–537. doi:10.1016/j.mehy.2010.07.018

Lee, K. A., Baker, F. C., Newton, K. M., & Ancoli-Israel, S. (2008). The influence of reproductive status and age on women's sleep. *Journal of Women's Health (Larchmt), 17*(7), 1209–1214. doi:10.1089/jwh.2007.0562

Lee, K. A., & Gay, C. L. (2004). Sleep in late pregnancy predicts length of labor and type of delivery. *American Journal of Obstetrics Gynecology, 191*(6), 2041–2046. doi:10.1016/j.ajog.2004.05.086

Lee, K. A., & Kryger, M. H. (2008). Women and sleep. *Journal of Womens Health (Larchmt), 17*(7), 1189–1190. doi:10.1089/jwh.2007.0574

National Sleep Foundation. (2005). *2005 sleep in America poll.* Arlington, VI: Author.

Okun, M. L., Roberts, J. M., Marsland, A. L., & Hall, M. (2009). How disturbed sleep may be a risk factor for adverse pregnancy outcomes. *Obstetrical Gynecological Survey, 64*(4), 273–280. doi:10.1097/OGX.0b013e318195160e

Oyetakin-White, P., Koo, B., Matsui, M. S., Yarosh, D., Cooper, K. D., & Baron, E. D. (2013). Effects of sleep quality on skin aging and function. *Journal of Investigative Dermatology, 133*(Suppl), S126.

Owens, J. (2008). Classification and epidemiology of childhood sleep disorders. *Primary Care, 35*(3), 533–546, vii. doi:10.1016/j.pop.2008.06.003

Porkka-Heiskanen, T., Zitting, K. M., & Wigren, H. K. (2013). Sleep, its regulation and possible mechanisms of sleep disturbances. *Acta Physiologica (Oxford, England), 208*(4), 311–328. doi:10.1111/apha.12134

Reid, K. J., Martinovich, Z., Finkel, S., Statsinger, J., Golden, R., Harter, K., & Zee, P. C. (2006). Sleep: A marker of physical and mental health in the elderly. *American Journal of Geriatric Psychiatry, 14*(10), 860–866. doi:10.1097/01.JGP.0000206164.56404.ba

Sarris, J., & Byrne, G. J. (2011). A systematic review of insomnia and complementary medicine. *Sleep Medicine Review, 15*(2), 99–106. doi:10.1016/j.smrv.2010.04.001

Sarris, J., Panossian, A., Schweitzer, I., Stough, C., & Scholey, A. (2011). Herbal medicine for depression, anxiety and insomnia: A review of psychopharmacology and clinical evidence. *European Neuropsychopharmacology, 21*(12), 841–860. doi:10.1016/j.euroneuro.2011.04.002

Schutte-Rodin, S., Broch, L., Buysse, D., Dorsey, C., & Sateia, M. (2008). Clinical guideline for the evaluation and management of chronic insomnia in adults. *Journal of Clinical Sleep Medicine, 4*(5), 487–504.

Shaver, J. L. (2008). Sleep disturbed by chronic pain in fibromyalgia, irritable bowel, and chronic pelvic pain syndromes. *Sleep Medicine Clinics, 3,* 47–60.

Shaver, J. L. (2009). The interface of depression, sleep, and vasomotor symptoms. *Menopause, 16*(4), 626–629. doi:10.1097/gme.0b013e3181a9c54f

Shaver, J. L. (2010). Sleep difficulties: Due to menopause status, age, other factors, or all of the above? *Menopause, 17*(6), 1104–1107. doi:10.1097/gme.0b013e3181fbbae1

Shaver, J. L. (2013). Sleep during perimenopause. In C. Kushida (Ed.), *The encyclopedia of sleep* (Vol. 2, pp. 680–684). Waltham, MA: Academic Press.

Shaver, J. L., Lentz, M., Landis, C. A., Heitkemper, M. M., Buchwald, D. S., & Woods, N. F. (1997). Sleep, psychological distress, and stress arousal in women with fibromyalgia. *Research in Nursing & Health, 20*(3), 247–257. doi:10.1002/(SICI)1098-240X(199706)20:3<247::AID-NUR7>3.0.CO;2-I

Shaver, J. L., & Zenk, S. N. (2000). Sleep disturbance in menopause. *Journal of Women's Health and Gender-based Medicine, 9*(2), 109–118.

Smith, H. S., Harris, R., & Clauw, D. (2011). Fibromyalgia: An afferent processing disorder leading to a complex pain generalized syndrome. *Pain Physician, 14*(2), E217–E245.

Steingraber, S. (2007). *The falling age of puberty in US girls: What we know, what we need to know.* San Francisco, CA: Breast Cancer Fund.

Steptoe, A., Hamer, M., & Chida, Y. (2007). The effects of acute psychological stress on circulating inflammatory factors in humans: A review and meta-analysis. *Brain Behavior and Immunity, 21*(7), 901–912. doi:10.1016/j.bbi.2007.03.011

ter Wolbeek, M., van Doornen, L. J., Coffeng, L. E., Kavelaars, A., & Heijnen, C. J. (2007). Cortisol and severe fatigue: A longitudinal study in adolescent girls. *Psychoneuroendocrinology, 32*(2), 171–182. doi:10.1016/j.psyneuen.2006.12.003

ter Wolbeek, M., van Doornen, L. J., Kavelaars, A., & Heijnen, C. J. (2006). Severe fatigue in adolescents: A common phenomenon? *Pediatrics, 117*(6), e1078–e1086. doi:10.1542/peds.2005-2575

ter Wolbeek, M., van Doornen, L. J., Kavelaars, A., van de Putte, E. M., Schedlowski, M., & Heijnen, C. J. (2007). Longitudinal analysis of pro- and anti-inflammatory cytokine production in severely fatigued adolescents. *Brain Behavior and Immunity, 21*(8), 1063–1074. doi:10.1016/j.bbi.2007.04.007

Thomas, K., & Watson, C. B. (2008). Restless legs syndrome in women: A review. *Journal of Women's Health, 17*(5), 859–868. doi:0.1089/jwh.2007.0515

Toward Optimized Practice Program. (2007). *Adult insomnia: Assessment to diagnosis.* Edmonton, Canada: Alberta College of Family Physicians.

Vallido, T., Jackson, D., & O'Brien, L. (2009). Mad, sad and hormonal: The gendered nature of adolescent sleep disturbance. *Journal of Child Health Care, 13*(1), 7–18. doi:10.1177/1367493508098377

Vallido, T., Peters, K., O'Brien, L., & Jackson, D. (2009). Sleep in adolescence: A review of issues for nursing practice. *Journal of Clinical Nursing, 18*(13), 1819–1826. doi:10.1111/j.1365-2702.2009.02812.x

Van Cauter, E. (2011). Sleep disturbances and insulin resistance. *Diabetic Medicine, 28*(12), 1455–1462. doi:10.1111/j.1464-5491.2011.03459.x

Williams, J., Roth, A., Vatthauer, K., & McCrae, C. S. (2013). Cognitive behavioral treatment of insomnia. *Chest, 143*(2), 554–565. doi:10.1378/chest.12-0731

Chapter 18

Peaceful Dying

JoAnne Reifsnyder

"Death is not what it used to be" (Field & Cassel, 1997).

L aurie is a 38-year-old woman who, on a routine visit to her gynecologist, mentioned that she had noticed abdominal fullness and occasional abdominal discomfort, as well as a feeling of early satiety when she was eating. She reported that she had had these symptoms on and off for as long as 9 months previous to her visit, and assumed that her fatigue and vague symptoms stemmed from a demanding job and caring for three children as a single mom. In the past several weeks, her abdominal discomfort had been unrelenting, her abdomen seemed swollen to her, and she reported that she had lost weight. Following numerous studies, Laurie was diagnosed with stage IV ovarian cancer. She underwent cytoreductive surgery followed by 6 months of chemotherapy. She was exhausted by the treatment, but recovered her energy and was able to return to work after completing the chemotherapy. Laurie's disease recurred within 6 months of completing initial treatment, and she was found to have metastases to the bone, liver, and brain. She underwent second-line chemotherapy. Laurie developed significant pain and periodic bouts of nausea and vomiting. During her last hospital stay for treatment of a malignant bowel obstruction, Laurie's physician asked the palliative care team to initiate conversation about goals of care and advance care planning with Laurie and her family. The palliative care Nurse Practitioner and chaplain met with Laurie, her mother, and her sister. Laurie completed a living will and durable power of attorney designation, and decided to enroll in hospice. Laurie died 3 weeks later on home hospice, surrounded by her friends and family.

Life expectancy, causes of death, locations where dying and death occur, involvement of family caregivers, the trajectories of terminal illnesses and processes of dying have changed dramatically in the past 100 years. The greatest changes have taken place in more recent decades as the use of technology to cure previously fatal illnesses and to prolong life has become ubiquitous in our approach to health-care delivery. Death is indeed not what it used to be. As the population in the United States and other developed countries ages, as new discoveries to prolong life come to market, and as economic pressures on the health-care system driven by the aging population come to bear, we can anticipate that death is not likely to be in the coming decades what it is today. This chapter explores the evolution of approaches to assure peaceful dying and to accelerate the integration of palliative care in the United States. Further, the chapter highlights particular issues that women face as recipients of care when facing terminal illness, as the customary informal caregivers to ill family members, and as bereaved survivors when a spouse, partner, or child dies.

It may seem that a chapter on dying does not fit with a book on women's wellness across the life span. However, since dying is part of the lifecycle, the intent is to approach dying as a normal process and emphasize how to promote the health of those who mourn the dying and make the death experience as comfortable as possible. In the primary care setting, health-care providers are in excellent positions to discuss advance directives (ADs) with their patients, encouraging them to plan ahead and to make their wishes known regarding how they want to be treated at the end of life.

Dying and Death in the United States

In little more than a century, illness, dying, and death have transformed in significant ways, and as will be explored, not all of these profound changes are viewed as positive. In the early part of the last century, most Americans died from acute, communicable diseases. Maternal death during childbirth was common—as high as 7 to 9 deaths for every 1,000 live births (Centers for Disease Control [CDC], 1999), of which 40% was attributed to sepsis and the remaining deaths associated with hemorrhage and toxemia (CDC, 1999). Approximately 100 infants (per 1,000 live births) died before 1 year of age. Both rates declined dramatically with the discovery and widespread use of antibiotics, improved obstetrical care, access to health care, education, and improved standard of living (CDC, 1999). In 1900, pneumonia, tuberculosis, and diarrhea/enteritis were ranked as the first through third causes of death, respectively (CDC, 2009) and life expectancy for an adult was just 48 years for males and 51 years for females (Arias, 2011). Most deaths took place at home with family in attendance and acting as the primary caregivers. Medical science had little to offer the dying person. By the mid-1940s, penicillin had become widely available, saving lives and ushering in a new era of disease treatment (Jones, Podolsky, & Greene, 2012).

The average life expectancy for a child born in 2010 is 81.3, 78, and 83.8 respectively for Whites, Blacks, and Hispanics (Murphy, Xu, & Kochanek, 2013). Along with longevity has come the burden of chronic illness. An analysis of 2010 data from the National Health Interview Survey revealed an increasing trend in the presence of multiple chronic conditions (MCCs) in the years 2001 to 2010. The study authors reported that one-quarter of Americans have one chronic condition and another quarter have MCCs (Ward & Schiller, 2013). In the same study, analysis of gender differences revealed that women are more likely than men to have MCCs in age cohorts 18 to 44 and 45 to 65. In the older adult population, women were less likely than men to have four or more chronic conditions (Ward & Schiller, 2013).

In contrast to the last century, most older Americans today live with one or more chronic illnesses and death most often follows a long period of decline and functional dependence. Causes of death have shifted from infectious diseases to heart disease, cancer, non–infectious respiratory diseases, and cerebrovascular disease (Jones et al., 2012). Often considered a disease more closely associated with males, heart disease is the leading cause of death for Caucasian and African American women (24%), followed by breast cancer (21%). By 2020, an estimated 50% of the US population is projected to have at least one chronic condition ("Tackling the burden of chronic diseases in the USA," 2009). Most chronic illnesses are related to lifestyle choices and circumstances—poor nutrition, sedentary lifestyle, smoking, and stress contribute to obesity, hypertension and heart disease, and many cancers. Fully two-thirds of all deaths in the United States of America are attributable to one of five chronic disorders: cancer, chronic obstructive pulmonary disease (COPD), diabetes, heart disease, and stroke ("Tackling the burden of chronic diseases in the USA," 2009). These trends have important implications for wellness and illness, how Americans live, and how they die. Particularly troublesome is the reality of the end of life—most older Americans do not die from cancer (22%), where the trajectory and decline is better understood and anticipated. Instead, most die after a period of slow decline marked by acute exacerbations and plateaus, leading to uncertainty about prognosis and in turn, uncertainty about when to engage in advance care planning (Agency for Healthcare Research Quality [AHRQ], 2003).

During the 20th century, place of death shifted from home to institutions (hospitals and nursing homes), where an estimated 70% of deaths now take place (Meier, Isaacs, & Hughes, 2010). By 1998, the nursing home had surpassed hospitals as location of death for most decedents. Although most Americans express a preference for death at home, far fewer deaths take place at home, and family members are geographically distant and unable to participate in care to a loved one who is ill. At the same time, medical intervention has become increasingly technologically sophisticated, and many persons with advanced illness and their families find themselves facing the care/cure dichotomy embedded in the lure of aggressive medical intervention. While modern health care has enabled countless individuals to live longer, healthier lives, the reality remains that each of us must die. Technology is amoral—it is external to issues of "right" or "wrong"—those issues are left to health-care professionals, ethicists, families. The use of technology in the service of prolonging life in people with serious, progressive illness is the subject of ongoing ethical debate.

Emergence of Approaches to Improving Care of the Dying

By the 1960s, as hospitals had become the more common location of death, talking about death had become taboo and a grassroots movement to provide more humane, person-focused care at the end of life began to take hold. Gaps in care for the dying were becoming more apparent—notably, between denial of death in society and the reality that those facing death must accept, and between technological research and patient-centered care (Wentzel, 1981). Sociologists Glaser and Strauss published the first study of dying in hospitals in 1965. In *Awareness of Dying*, Glaser and Strauss observed and described four principal "awareness contexts"—ways in which "pretense" about dying was maintained by professional caregivers, family members, and patients themselves. Importantly, they observed that most patients had "closed awareness," meaning that professional caregivers knew that the patient was dying but the patient did not (Glaser & Strauss, 1965).

Elisabeth Kubler-Ross's seminal work, *On Death and Dying*, was published just a few years later in 1969. The interviews with dying people in which she placed students at the Chicago Theological Seminary were unprecedented at that time. This project revealed important insights into the connectedness that seriously ill people desired as they were approaching the end of life and the assumptions that health-care providers made with regard to those preferences. Kubler-Ross's research with terminally ill patients inspired her description of five stages of normal grief that terminally ill persons experience as they are approaching death, namely, denial, anger, bargaining, depression, and acceptance. The model has since been applied to other grief situations, including the grief experiences of children living through divorce.

Hospice and the Good Death

Development of the modern hospice movement is attributed to British physician, Dame Cicely Saunders. Saunders visited the United States in 1963 to lecture about her work with terminally ill cancer patients at St. Joseph's Hospice in London. She described her vision for St. Christopher's Hospice, which would later be founded in 1967. Historian Dr. Joy Buck observed that

> Saunders' initial visit (to the United States) came at a critical point in the history of the United States. Because of a variety of social, economic and political factors, care for the dying had moved from home to hospital, and with that move, control over care decisions was transferred from the individual and family (to) medical professionals. (Buck, 2011, p. 536)

Saunders was a visionary leader and change agent, whose focus on dignity and person-centered care sparked a transformation in how dying was viewed and how dying people received care. Her example taught that dying could be as growthful and meaningful a phase in life as any other, and that pain and symptom management coupled with psychosocial and spiritual support of both patient and family could assure that while loss of a beloved would always be painful, the process of dying did not have to be. By 1974, Florence Wald, Dean of the School of Nursing at Yale University, who had been profoundly impacted by meeting Saunders and learning about her vision for specialized care of the dying, founded Connecticut Hospice, the first hospice in the United States. (National Hospice and Palliative Care Organization [NHPCO], 2012).

The word "hospice" is derived from the Latin word "hospitium," which refers to a way station for weary religious pilgrims (Hospice Foundation of America, 2014). As it developed in the United States, hospice grew not as a place but an approach to care. Hospice is both a philosophy of care that guides and an approach to care of the dying and an organized care delivery system (National Consensus Project [NCP] for Quality Palliative Care, 2013). First launched in the United States in 1974, hospice was in its earliest days a spiritually based, grassroots movement to improve care of the dying. Early hospice pioneers were motivated by the disconnectedness of institutional death, where symptoms were often poorly managed and where family and other loved ones were more spectator to the dying process than participants. As a philosophy, hospice focuses on optimizing quality of life and comfort, where terminally ill individuals can be surrounded by the persons and objects that have been most meaningful in their lives. Originally conceived as a way to support more natural, home-based care and death, hospice's focus on creating a home-like setting for dying has extended to every setting where seriously ill patients receive care—home, freestanding hospice facilities, nursing homes, and hospitals (NHPCO, 2013a). Hospice care neither hastens death, nor does it prolong dying. Instead, hospice care holds central a realism about death (Wentzel, 1981), and in that context, hospice professionals support both patient and loved ones to live fully, to explore what is most important to them, and to connect values and preferences with choices about medical treatment.

Hospice care is provided by an interdisciplinary team (IDT) that includes nurses, physicians, social workers, therapists (speech/language, occupational, physical), spiritual advisors/chaplains, personal caregivers (homemakers and health aides), grief counselors, and trained volunteers (Fig. 18.1). The *patient and family* are considered the unit of care, and hospice interventions therefore support both patient comfort and quality of life as well as caregiver and family coping skill, dealing with anticipatory grief, and adjustment to loss. Hospice care is not a replacement for informal caregivers in the home, but rather, the hospice IDT supports and supplements informal caregivers to meet the patient's needs for care and comfort as well as caregiver and family needs for respite from physical caregiving and emotional/spiritual support. The hospice IDT will assist the family or community of caregivers to designate a "primary caregiver"—a person who will serve as the main conduit for communication and decision making. As an example, the hospice team caring for a dying mother would support the primary caregiver (be that person her husband, partner, parent, son/daughter, friend, etc.) to learn caregiving interventions and to cope with the ongoing burdens of caregiving. The chaplain or grief counselor engages with the patient and family as early in the hospice episode as possible, so that existential

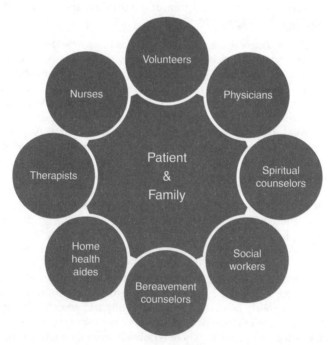

FIGURE 18.1 Hospice interdisciplinary team. From National Hospice and Palliative Care Organization. (2013). *NHPCO's hospice facts and figures. Hospice care in America.* Retrieved from www.nhpco. org/sites/default/files/public/Statistics_Research/2012_Facts_Figures.pdf

and practical concerns can be addressed—such as the "why" of suffering and grieving/coping with loss by children and other loved ones.

Hospice Utilization and Payment

Prior to 1983, hospice care was provided by hospital-based hospice programs, home care–affiliated hospice programs and independent hospice organizations, like Connecticut Hospice (Buck, 2011). There was little research evidence to support practice and little standardization of systems, processes, and interventions. In 1982, Congress authorized the Medicare Hospice Benefit, a significant expansion of the Medicare program that was enacted as an alternative to cure-focused care, intended to improve the quality of end-of-life care and to curb costs associated with aggressive end-of-life intervention. Policy-makers had concluded that enrollment in hospice at the end of life could prevent undesired and unnecessary hospital admission. Payment was, and continues to be, prospective—that is, the Medicare-certified hospice program receives a daily lump sum or "per diem," out of which the hospice pays for the services of the IDT, and supplies equipment and drugs/biologicals for palliation of the terminal diagnosis. Originally, the benefit was structured to cover no more than 210 days of Medicare-reimbursed hospice services in a beneficiary's lifetime, and hospices were tasked with evaluating progression of illness and need for continued services prior to initiation of a new "benefit period." The lifetime limit was amended in 1990, when Congress authorized a final "open-ended" benefit period and eliminated entirely in 1997 when Congress authorized unlimited 60-day benefit periods (Hospice Association of America, 2014).

Coverage of hospice by Medicare ushered in a new era of both standardization and growth. In 1985, just a few years after the benefit was authorized, there were 158 Medicare-certified hospice programs. By 2012, the NHPCO reported that there were 5,500 hospice programs operating in all 50 states as well as the District of Columbia, Guam, Puerto Rico, and the US Virgin Islands (NHPCO, 2013b). Most state medical assistance programs (Medicaid) and commercial insurance plans cover hospice services.

Eligibility for hospice coverage under Medicare is determined by the patient's physician and by the hospice medical director. In order to be eligible, the patient must be entitled to Medicare Part A benefits and must be "certified" by her/his physician and the hospice medical director as being terminally ill. At the time of publication of this book, advance practice nurses (nurse practitioners) who may be serving as the patient's primary care provider are nonetheless not authorized to certify terminal illness for eligibility under Medicare hospice regulations. For purposes of the Medicare Hospice Benefit, "terminally ill" is defined as having a likely life expectancy of 6 months or less if the disease follows its natural, expected course (DHHS, 2013). Additionally, the beneficiary must sign a waiver of standard Medicare benefits for coverage of the terminal illness, electing instead to have hospice cover the illness. The beneficiary retains standard Medicare coverage under her/his preexisting Medicare indemnity (fee for service) or Medicare Advantage plan (managed Medicare) for treatment of illnesses/conditions other than the terminal illness. Most state Medicaid and commercial benefits have followed the Medicare regulatory standards for program eligibility.

The aforementioned caveats in Medicare coverage for hospice are important, in that they limit hospice coverage to those who are no longer pursuing aggressive, disease-remitting treatment for a terminal illness. The implications of these regulatory guidelines have intensified, as the availability of high technology (and high cost) treatments to manage symptoms and in some cases, to extend life, have become more available. Decisions to withdraw from disease-remitting treatment, opting for palliation alone, often occur late in a disease trajectory. Hospice advocates argue that persons with life-threatening illness would benefit from earlier hospice care, concurrent with disease-remitting treatment. Hospice advocates have further argued that eligibility criteria do not fit the needs of terminally ill children and their families, as a child's life-threatening illness may follow long and variable patterns, throughout which hospice services and supports are needed.

Consider again the case of Laurie, a 38-year-old single mother of three children who elected to enroll in hospice when she was just 3 weeks from death. While hospice can (and did) provide Laurie and her family with invaluable services and support, the reality of ineligibility during treatment of her advanced ovarian cancer meant that she, her children, and her extended family were tasked with coping without the guidance and support of an expert IDT. In other words, Laurie's medical care was episodic, timed, and delivered according to treatment intervals and disease exacerbations. Concurrent hospice care would have supported Laurie's symptom management, emotional cycles, and current emotional needs of and future plans for her children.

The Medicare Hospice Benefit is structured as four levels of care that may be applied at different points in the hospice episode to assure that the patient's and family's needs are met. These four levels are routine, continuous, general inpatient, and inpatient respite care (Table 18.1). The "routine home care" level is the most common, accounting for 96.5% of hospice days in 2012 (NHPCO, 2013b). Under the routine home care level, the patient receives intermittent visits from members of the IDT at the location where

TABLE 18.1	Levels of the Medicare Hospice Benefit	
Level	**Purpose**	**Services provided**
Routine home care	Support the patient in a home or home-like setting to assure quality of life in all dimensions	Interdisciplinary team (intermittent) Supplies Equipment Drugs/Biologicals
Continuous care	Enable the patient to remain at home by providing additional, continuous nursing support until crisis subsides	Routine home care plus continuous nursing care at home until period of crisis stabilizes. Must be primarily provided by licensed nurses
General inpatient care	Treat exacerbation of symptoms that cannot be managed effectively at home/in home-like setting	Treatment of symptoms under contract with an inpatient acute facility or skilled nursing facility
Inpatient respite care	Relieve home caregiver on an occasional basis	Routine home care services in an inpatient setting, most often a skilled nursing/long-term care facility for up to 5 days on an occasional basis

Data from National Hospice and Palliative Care Organization. (2013). NHPCO's facts and figures. Hospice care in America. Retrieved from http://www.nhpco.org/sites/default/files/public/Statistics_Research/2013_Facts_Figures. pdf; United Sates Department of Health and Human Services, Centers for Medicare and Medicaid Services. (2013). Medicare hospice benefits. Retrieved from http://www.medicare.gov/pubs/pdf/02154.pdf

she/he resides. The hospice team assesses the need for and provides disposable supplies (e.g., wound dressings), durable medical equipment (e.g., hospital beds and commodes) and drugs/biologicals for palliation of the terminal illness (e.g., analgesics, laxatives, antiemetics). The location for routine home care is most often a private residence, but since 1989 hospices have provided hospice services in nursing homes (see next section). Hospices also provide continuous nursing care in the home for brief periods of crisis. An example would be new onset of seizure activity from brain metastases, requiring monitoring and medication management until the patient is stabilized. Two levels of inpatient care may be provided: general inpatient care (GIP) and inpatient respite care. The GIP level is provided either in an acute care setting or a skilled nursing facility with which the hospice has a contractual agreement. GIP care provides for treatment of a symptom exacerbation that cannot be effectively treated at home. The inpatient respite level of the benefit allows for occasional facility-based care that is provided to relieve the primary caregiver(s) at home (Box 18.1).

Box 18.1 Ten Components of Quality Hospice Care

Patient and Family-Centered Care–Providing care and services that are responsive to the needs and exceed the expectations of those we serve

Ethical Behavior and Consumer Rights–Upholding high standards of ethical conduct and advocating for the rights of patients and their family caregivers

Clinical Excellence and Safety–Ensuring clinical excellence and promoting safety through standards of practice

Inclusion and Access–Promoting inclusiveness in our community by ensuring that all people–regardless of race, ethnicity, color, religion, gender, disability, sexual orientation, age, or other characteristics–have access to our programs and services

Organizational Excellence–Building a culture of quality and accountability within our organization that values collaboration and communication and ensures ethical business practices

Workforce Excellence–Fostering a collaborative, interdisciplinary environment that promotes inclusion, individual accountability and workforce excellence, through professional development, training, and support to all staff and volunteers

Standards–Adopting the NHPCO Standards of Practice for Hospice Programs and/ or the National Consensus Project's Clinical Practice Guidelines for Quality Palliative Care as the foundation for an organization

Compliance with Laws and Regulations–Ensuring compliance with all applicable laws, regulations, and professional standards of practice, and implementing systems and processes that prevent fraud and abuse

Stewardship and Accountability–Developing a qualified and diverse governance structure and senior leadership who share the responsibilities of fiscal and managerial oversight

Performance Measurement–Collecting, analyzing, and actively using performance measurement data to foster quality assessment and performance improvement in all areas of care and services

Reprinted with permission from National Hospice and Palliative Care Organization. (2013). NHPCO's facts and figures. Hospice care in America. Retrieved from http://www.nhpco.org/sites/default/files/public/Statistics_Research/2013_Facts_Figures.pdf

Hospice in the Nursing Home

More than 1.4 million Americans reside in nursing homes, and women constitute a significant majority of residents at more than two-thirds of the nursing home population (Centers for Medicare and Medicaid Services [CMS], 2012). Approximately one-quarter of Medicare decedents die in nursing home settings (National Center for Health Statistics, 2011), and that number is even higher for white decedents (30%) and for decedents with dementia (Mitchell, Teno, Miller, & Mor, 2005). Aging of the population and prevalence of dementia are key factors that will impact nursing home as location of end-of-life care and death in the coming years. Nursing home expenditures are projected to accelerate through 2019, with the bulk of the spending falling on Medicare and Medicaid. Prevalence and under treatment of nursing home residents with pain (2010) and non–pain symptoms (Rodriquez, Hanlon, Perera, Jaffe, & Sevick, 2010) have been documented, and hospitalization of residents at the end of life is common.

Following the Omnibus Budget Reconciliation Act (OBRA) of 1989, barriers to providing hospice care in nursing homes were removed (Stevenson & Bramson, 2009) and the penetration of hospice care in nursing homes has risen steadily. While experts cite the benefits of hospice enrollment for nursing home residents, such as reduced hospital readmission, better pain and symptom management and decreased use of restraints, intravenous therapy, and feeding tubes, under 20% of nursing home residents were enrolled in hospice in 2009 (NHPCO, 2013a). Both hospice and non–hospice palliative care (discussed in a subsequent section) hold promise for improving care coordination and care management for nursing home residents. With its focus on communication, realism about the end of life, and support to family, hospice has great potential to expand its expert and compassionate guidance to nursing home residents, their families, and their nursing home–based caregivers (physicians, social workers, nurses, nurse aides, others).

Profile of Hospice Patients

For various reasons, including consumer demand; the availability of Medicare, Medicaid, and commercial insurance coverage of hospice services; and efforts of hospice and palliative care professionals, the use of hospice in the United States has grown steadily year over year. For 2011, NHPCO estimated that 1.65 million patients received services from hospice, representing 44.6% of all deaths in the United Sates (NHPCO, 2012). Most hospice decedents are Medicare beneficiaries (83.7%), female (56.4%), and over the age of 65 (84.5%) (NHPCO, 2013b). By far, the majority of hospice decedents are White/Caucasian (81.5%) (NHPCO, 2013b). When hospice first developed in the United States, most patients had a primary (terminal) diagnosis of cancer, but in recent years noncancer diagnoses including dementia, heart disease, and pulmonary disease comprise more than 60% of primary hospice diagnoses. The shift in diagnosis has had an impact on time of referral as well as length of stay on hospice. While cancer patients, like Laurie, are often referred late in the disease process after disease-remitting treatment has concluded, their terminal trajectory once enrolled in hospice tends to be more predictable. Clinicians often associate hospice use with a cancer diagnosis, and hesitate to refer other patients with serious illness who could benefit from hospice. Many clinicians would argue that the dementia or heart failure disease course is unpredictable, leading to late (or no) referral. In one study, researchers found that physicians reported discussing hospice with 46% of their oncology patients but just 10% and 7% with COPD and heart failure patients, respectively (Thomas, O'Leary, & Fried, 2009). Further, physicians tend to overestimate life expectancy (Christakis & Lamont, 2000; Krishnan et al., 2013; Mitchell et al., 2009) and misperceive patients' desire for aggressive treatment if they have not specifically discussed patient preferences. In a study of veterans with COPD, physicians were more likely to err on predictions of patient preferences to forgo treatment under end-of-life circumstances (Downey, Au, Curtis, & Engelberg, 2013). At the same time, patients with noncancer diagnoses appropriately referred to hospice can indeed experience a plateau or even improvement, making them ineligible for hospice if their prognosis (life expectancy) is deemed to have changed. In sum, the rules around hospice eligibility and the realities of complex chronic illness conflict, and some would argue, are completely incompatible. One solution that has emerged is concurrent care, that is, providing hospice care in addition to life-extending treatment for patients with serious illness. Another is non–hospice palliative care, described in the next section.

Palliative Care

Palliative care can be thought of as the overarching umbrella that contains hospice care as a specific application of its goals and tenets. While all hospice care is palliative in nature, not all palliative care takes place at end of life or in a hospice setting. Further, palliative care is conceived more broadly as "patient and family care that optimizes quality of life by anticipating, preventing and treating suffering" (NCP for Quality Palliative Care, 2013, p. 9), contributing as meaningfully to the overall quality of care for patients who have been recently diagnosed with life-threatening illness as it does for patients who are battling disease and those who are approaching the end of life. Because of *policy* decisions made in the late 1970s and early 1980s that led to narrow eligibility criteria for hospice-provided palliative care, non–hospice palliative care has evolved as a broadened application of hospice concepts and practices across the entire serious illness/disease trajectory and all settings where care is provided—from hospital to nursing home to outpatient/ambulatory settings to home care (see Box 18.2). Like hospice care, palliative care is delivered by an IDT that may comprise nurses, physicians, social workers, and chaplains.

Box 18.2 World Health Organization Definition of Palliative Care

". . . an approach that improves the quality of life of patients and their families facing the problem [sic] associated with life-threatening illness, through the prevention and relief of suffering by means of early identification and impeccable assessment and treatment of pain and other problems, physical, psychosocial and spiritual."

PALLIATIVE CARE

- Affirms life and regards dying as a normal process
- Intends neither to hasten nor to postpone death
- Uses a team approach to address the needs of patients and their families, including bereavement counseling if indicated

Hall, S., Petkova, H., Tsouros, A. D., Costantini, M., & Higginson, I. J. (2011). *Palliative care for older people: Better practices* (p. 6). Copenhagen, Denmark: WHO Regional Office for Europe. Retrieved from http://www.euro.who.int/en/publications/abstracts/palliative-care-for-older-people-better-practices

The IDT collaborates and communicates with other care providers in the setting. Unlike hospice care in the United States, palliative care can be offered concurrently with disease-remitting treatment beginning at the time of diagnosis (NCP for Quality Palliative Care, 2013). Also unlike hospice, palliative care has no dedicated reimbursement stream. Rather, palliative care developed and has been sustained through a combination of philanthropic support, government grants, and practitioner billing for services such as advance practice nurse and physician consults and licensed social worker direct reimbursement.

Palliative care programs are present in more than 1,600 hospitals representing greater than 65% of all US hospitals (CAPC, 2012). Teams contribute to timely assessment of patient and family needs, family conferences to support decision making about goals for care and adjuncts to the medical plan of treatment that supports pain and symptom management as well as interventions to relieve emotional suffering. Palliative care is recognized as a medical subspecialty and an advanced certification for all members of the nursing team. Despite the growth and contribution of palliative care, it remains underutilized and misunderstood. Often confused with hospice or associated only with end-of-life care, the advance care planning, medical coordination, and psychosocial support provided by palliative care teams are increasingly deemed to be critical attributes of emerging population health initiatives (Verret & Rohloff, 2013). In a landmark study, Temel et al. (2010), found that patients with advanced non–small cell lung cancer randomized to early palliative care plus standard oncology care had significant improvements in quality of life and mood, less aggressive care at the end of life and *longer survival* compared with those who received standard oncology care alone (Temel et al., 2010). Further, both palliative care (Kelley, Deb, Qingling, Aldridge Carlson, & Morrison, 2013; Morrison et al., 2008) and hospice have been shown to improve outcomes and to decrease overall costs of care at the end of life (Kelley et al., 2013; Pyenson, Connor, Fitch, & Kinzbrunner, 2004).

Advance Care Planning

Advance care planning is widely viewed as an essential contributor to assuring a good death. That is, a person who has both reflected on his or her values and preferences and has communicated those, orally and in writing, is more likely to have his or her wishes fulfilled as serious illness and end of life unfold. The advance directive (AD) commonly contains two components, namely a treatment directive (also called a living will) and a proxy directive (also called a durable power of attorney, or legally authorized representative). The public debate over ADs was sparked by important cultural/sociological events, including the shift in location of death from home to hospital in the mid-20th century, as well as several landmark court cases that cast a spotlight on questions pertaining to the end of life: When is a life not worth living? Who decides? When can treatment be refused? When can treatment be withdrawn? In particular, is the case of Karen Ann Quinlan, a young woman who in 1976 lapsed into what was thought to be a persistent vegetative state. Her parents' request to the hospital to discontinue her ventilator sparked a right-to-die debate and ultimately led to development of hospital-based ethics committees. In 1983, another young woman by the name of Nancy Beth Cruzan was critically injured in an automobile crash. Her parents petitioned the state of Missouri to remove her feeding tube and allow her to die, arguing that Nancy would not have wanted to be kept alive in her current condition. Ultimately, the United States Supreme Court ruled that states could require clear and convincing evidence of a patient's wishes when she could not speak for herself, ushering in new regulations to support patient participation in end-of-life care decisions and to document those decisions. The Patient Self Determination Act (PSDA) of 1990 requires all health-care facilities that receive Medicare or Medicaid funding (which is a majority) to inform patients of their rights to make health-care decisions, including the right to create an AD. Importantly, neither federal nor state regulations *require* any individual to participate in or document advance care planning.

Despite the availability of standard AD forms in every state and PSDA regulatory guidance, most Americans have not documented their wishes in any formal manner (AHRQ, 2003). While most American adults report having given at least some consideration to their wishes for medical treatment at the end of life, 27% report that they have not given this topic any consideration at all, 25% of those over the age of 75 have given little thought to the topic, and 22% of those over the age of 75 have not communicated wishes orally or in writing (Pew, 2013). Those with higher education and income are more likely than less educated and lower income persons to have communicated their wishes, and Whites are more likely than Blacks or Hispanics to have done so. Those who have not communicated their wishes are more likely to want everything possible done to extend their lives if facing serious illness (Pew, 2013). Among older adults, factors predicting AD completion include perceptions that ADs might mitigate end-of-life suffering, having undergone major surgery and having received information about ADs or having been asked to complete one (Alano et al., 2010). In this study, the researchers also found that increasing age, education, and female gender were associated with AD completion (Alano et al., 2010). An interesting question for further research is whether older women's likelihood to have been a caregiver to a family member at the end of life influences their own values or actions concerning end-of-life care. Finally, the youngest adults (18 to 49) are less likely to have communicated preferences and are more likely to request continuation of treatment in serious illness. While this last finding is not surprising given the developmental tasks of young adulthood, some of the most difficult and public end-of-life decisions have involved young adults who had not communicated their wishes (e.g., Quinlan, Cruzan, mentioned earlier, as well as Terri Schiavo). All adults with decision capacity need to be encouraged by their health-care providers, and indeed, their older family members, to clarify their preferences and make these known.

Of equal importance to documenting preferences at a specific point in time is the *ongoing communication* between health-care providers and patients/families. Advance care planning at its best is not a document, but an ongoing dialogue that considers both the foundational values of the patient and the emerging circumstances of illness or end-of-life trajectory. For any of us, predicting what we would prefer under circumstances not yet known—future pain and other symptoms, fears of the unknown, and value still apparent in a life of diminished quality—is a particular conundrum. Under any circumstances, facilitating conversations when the patient is still capable of participating is paramount, and for many families, hardest to translate to action. Research has shown that clinicians delay conversations about advance care planning and that neither physicians nor family members are especially accurate in predicting patient preferences even when known in advance, both groups typically erring in favor of over treatment (AHRQ, 2003). Americans are especially death-averse, preferring instead to avoid painful conversations about the end of life as a strategy to retain "hope." Yet research indicates that patients want to engage in conversations (AHRQ, 2003). These findings have implications for primary care providers, who are in a position to talk with patients about ADs well before patients are actually at the end of life.

Patients with complex chronic illness experience exacerbations and plateaus in illness and recovery, with slow, steady decline across a longer trajectory than a person with advanced cancer (the terminal illness on which hospice care was modeled). Their underlying illness cannot be cured, and the absence of any "bright line" between declining and dying combined with confusion about the intent of palliative care (specifically understanding that it is not solely for the "dying") is viewed as barriers to advance care planning and appropriate palliative care. Palliative care experts can engage as early as time of diagnosis, and conceptualize hope differently, seeing the possibility for reframing hope in ways that realistically match the patient's circumstances and provide sustenance in dire circumstances—instead of hope for cure, hope may be reframed as preserving meaning, communicating with others, involving fellow "travelers" and changing focus (Olsson, Östlund, Strang, Jeppsson Grassman, & Friedrichsen, 2010). Palliative care experts are especially suited to guiding such conversations via a family meeting to clarify the patient and family's understanding of and preference for goals given the treatment and care options, and likewise, hospice experts are uniquely qualified to support patients and families with existential questions and with maintaining hope. Communication of goals of care and preferences about health-care settings is especially important, but to date has relied heavily on transmission of written documents. By leveraging technology, new opportunities are emerging for electronic registry of ADs and facilitated sharing of those documents via integrated electronic health-care records.

Gender may have an important association with preferences for advance care planning, although the research findings to date have been equivocal. Most studies, to date, report that women generally prefer less aggressive care in terminal illness (Bookwala et al., 2001; Miesfeldt et al., 2012). In a small, hypothesis-generating study that included Americans of European, Mexican, and African ethnicity, researchers found that gender subcultures within ethnic identities are distinct. For example, the research team identified that men's end-of-life wishes primarily address functional outcome, whereas women were additionally concerned about where they would die, the impact on family dynamics and economics, past illness experiences, and personal views about life and death. Regardless of culture, women viewed the health-care system as empowering patients (men felt disempowered and fearful) and anticipated that they will be respected by the team and benefit from it (Perkins, Cortez, & Hazuda, 2004). The authors suggest that clinician understanding of "layered cultures," within which ethnicity is important (and arguably better understood), while gender differences may be less well understood and provide important insight to advance care planning with women. In a larger study, Bookwala et al. (2001), examined gender differences in life-sustaining treatment preferences and end-of-life values in a sample of older adult outpatients. Using hypothetical case scenarios, they found that women exhibited significantly lower overall preference for life-sustaining treatments, even when asked to consider absence of a serious condition—that is, in the context of their current health. Women also were found to express lower desire for life-sustaining treatment when considering cognitive impairment (Alzheimer disease, for example) or coma. Finally, in terms of end-of-life values, women expressed a stronger desire to have a dignified death when compared with men. The researchers suggested that while both women and men consider values important in end-of-life decision making, they may differ in *how* they consider and weight their values (Bookwala et al., 2001). In a study of psychosocial influences on end-of-life care planning among adults age 64 to 65, Carr and Khodyakov (2007) found that encounters with the health-care system in the prior year and having survived the painful death of a loved one were significant predictors of end-of-life planning. This latter finding is particularly germane to the experience of women, whose husbands frequently predecease and who commonly assume caregiving roles for other family members at the end of life. While more research is needed, taken together these findings point to the need for greater attention to women's unique experiences and considerations in advance care planning.

Decision making for loved ones in the absence of clear directives is challenging, and decision making for minors who are not legally recognized as having decision authority is particularly difficult and indeed painful for parents and other caregivers. Little is known about the preferences of adolescents and young adults regarding end-of-life care. While the number of deaths among people age 15 to 34 is relatively small when compared with older age cohorts, the circumstances underlying terminal illness and promotion of peaceful dying are no less important. Not only is broaching the topic of death difficult when the patient is a young person, the tools available to assist with carrying out and documenting preferences are not suited to young people, either because adolescents are legally not recognized as decision makers in their own care, not having reached the age of majority, or because the tools are geared more toward older adults' needs. In a study examining patient-perceived usefulness of an adapted advance care planning guide, Wiener et al. (2012), found that adolescents and young adults wanted to be able to consider and document treatment choices, their care preferences, information they would like friends and family to know and how they would like to be remembered. The authors proposed the use of an advance care planning document developed specifically for adolescents and young adults, "Voicing my Choices" (Aging with Dignity, 2013).

Caregivers to the Dying

The physical burden of caregiving at the end of life inevitably falls on the shoulders of family members. As discussed, home hospice care is available to supplement care provided by family but not to replace it. Even when a loved one is approaching the end of life in a nursing home or hospice inpatient facility, or when a medically fragile child is being supported at home with 24-hour nursing care, the physical burden is still present and emotional burden, in some ways, might be even greater. The decision to place a dying loved one in an institutional setting of any kind is complicated by a sense of failure, loss, fear, and profound sorrow. Further, while providing care at home to a dying loved one is an ever-present physical and emotional challenge, spending long hours away from home (and other family members) to attend to the needs of the inpatient can be equally taxing. We know that women—mothers, spouses, daughters, and sisters—provide the majority of informal caregiving to dying loved ones; 72% of primary caregivers to the terminally ill are women (The Commonwealth Fund, 1999). Family caregiving has enormous quality-of-life and economic implications. The economic value of "informal caregiving" (that provided by unpaid family and friends) is estimated at $375 billion annually—nearly twice that spent on home health and nursing home care combined (Caregiver Action Network, 2009). Women caregivers are 2½ times more likely to live in poverty, and caregivers report poorer self-care and overall health, greater depression, and stress (Hebert & Schulz, 2006). The Rosalynn Carter Institute (RCI), formed in 1987 to provide leadership around home and community services and caregiving, published a set of recommendations that it says are imperative to avert a national caregiving crisis. Among these, the Institute recommends investment in translation of completed research findings to actionable tools and supports for family caregivers, tax and public policy changes that would offset family time devoted to caregiving, and creation of greater flexibility in employment schedules to accommodate home caregiving (RCI for Caregiving, 2012). Caregivers to dying patients report that tailored communication with health-care providers is one the most important and frequently neglected aspects of care (Hebert & Schulz, 2006). These authors recommend that professionals use existing tools to help caregivers build knowledge and coping skills, and that they leverage the IDT to address varied needs of caregivers.

Caregiver Grief, Mourning, and Bereavement

When death is expected and family members have had adequate support to prepare for the aftermath of emotional and practical concerns, loss of a loved one is nevertheless one of the most significant and painful events in our human lifecycles. When the death was unexpected, or when the circumstances surrounding end-of-life care are suboptimal and decisions are contentious, the pain of loss can be even more intense and healthy adaptation can be impeded. Grief, mourning, and bereavement experiences are unique to individuals and are culturally bound.

Often used incorrectly as synonyms, grief and mourning are distinct processes. Grief refers to one's individual, emotional reaction to the anticipation of loss and/or to an actual loss. As the definition suggests, grief reactions are highly personal, and are bound by cultural expectations, family roles and function, communication style, prior experience with loss, circumstances surrounding the death, relationship with person whose death is anticipated (or who has died), and other stresses in the griever's life. Mourning refers to the behavioral *expression* of grief feelings, and may be exhibited by individuals, families, groups, and cultures. While research findings suggest that intrapersonal experiences of *grief* are quite similar across cultures (Cowles, 1996), culturally acceptable (or even expected) mourning rituals vary widely—from stoicism about loss and limited expressions of grief to overt displays of emotion. Finally, bereavement refers to the period of time during which mourning a loss takes place. Health-care providers can support healthy grief and mourning through understanding individuals and families' unique, culturally bound grief experiences and mourning behaviors or rituals.

Caregiver anticipatory grief and mourning commonly commence before the actual death of a loved one, and may persist over a prolonged period when illness is extended (such as with Alzheimer disease and related disorders). Family caregivers experience a range of emotions during the loved one's period of disability and after the death. To illustrate, Waldrop (2007) found that caregivers to terminally ill individuals experienced "heightened responsiveness" during terminal illness care, characterized by anxiety, hostility, and trouble concentrating and remembering. Not surprisingly, patient symptoms and physical caregiving demands heightened caregiver stress. After the death of patients, caregivers experienced "sustained reactivity," in which distress diminished but feelings of loneliness and sadness increased. Importantly, Waldrop (2007) found that emotional responses and reactions were highly influenced by relationships with family and friends. These findings are important, in that they highlight the need for services and systems that honor and effectively support the profound *work* of grief and mourning that could span many months or even years, leading to physical and emotional exhaustion. Women are at particular risk for caregiving-associated stresses, as they are most likely to assume caregiving roles within families (Mackinnon, 2009; Navaie-Waliser, Spriggs, & Feldman, 2002). Research findings indicate that spousal caregivers experience more stress than other caregivers, and that women experience greater distress than men (National Cancer Institute [NCI], 2013). Women are more likely to be influenced by social and cultural pressures to become caregivers and to engage in personal care tasks, and are less likely to obtain formal assistance (NCI, 2013).

Kubler-Ross (1969) first described common emotional reactions to terminal illness and awareness of dying that are applicable to caregiver experiences—both during anticipation of loss and after the death of a loved one. Experience of the five stages of grief described by Kubler-Ross, namely, denial, anger, bargaining, depression, and acceptance, varies among individuals, and in no way do the stages represent an expected progression of emotional processing. On the contrary, the "stages" represent fluid emotional states that may not characterize every person's experience, occur in any defined order, or be resolved by "acceptance" in all cases. Further, patient and family member trajectories of grief and mourning are highly personal—in anticipation of death, the dying person might be angry, a spouse depressed, and an adult child bargaining by seeking multiple treatment opinions. While such discontinuity in emotional reaction and expression is normal, it often heightens stress within a family. Families whose relationships were strained before terminal illness of a family member sometimes experience significant conflict and may need more intensive professional support and intervention. Health-care professionals can support effective transition through phases of grief, mourning, and bereavement through unconditional acceptance, deep listening, and referral to professional grief counselors. Finally, some family members may experience prolonged or *complicated* grief and mourning characterized by feelings of hopelessness, somatic symptoms, or self-destructive behaviors. Such individuals should be referred for professional support and intervention.

Coping with Loss of a Child

Infant and childhood death rates have been dramatically reduced in countries where immunizations, sanitation, and nutritional support are optimal. In developed countries, the most commons causes of infant mortality are birth defects, preterm birth, sudden infant death syndrome, complications of pregnancy, and suffocation (Hoyert & Xu, 2012). Among children aged 1 to 19, the leading cause of death across all age groups is unintentional injuries, followed by congenital and chromosomal abnormalities (aged 1 to 4), malignant neoplasm (aged 5 to 14), and assault (aged 15 to 19) (Michelson & Steinhorn, 2008). The array of causes and location of death (principally hospital) for infants and children is the backdrop for difficult prognostication and emotionally intense and complicated caregiver and clinician decisions.

The principles of palliative care are broadly applicable to care dying children and their parents, siblings, and caregivers. However, pediatric palliative and end-of-life care programs are specifically tailored to the unique ethical issues, communication conflicts and needs, symptom management challenges and grief, mourning and bereavement challenges. Adaptation of standard hospice benefits to the needs of a child is evolving, as children and their parents could benefit from early and continued palliative care, despite the fact that the child's life expectancy may be undetermined. Many pediatric palliative care and hospice programs have developed broad acceptance criteria, reaching out to families whose child has a life-limiting illness or condition and is not expected to survive to adulthood. Such programs also offer ongoing grief counseling and support to families, whose grief during illness of a child and after the child's death may be prolonged and highly variable. One study of bereaved parents found that depressive symptoms persisted in some parents for as long as 18 years after the child's death and that bereaved parents are at high risk for health and marital problems (Rogers, Floyd, Seltzer, Greenberg, & Hong, 2008). Studies indicate that women may grieve more openly than do men after the death of a child, face greater challenges in resuming day-to-day functions, and seek to connect with others to cope with the loss (Welte, 2013). Both women and men are profoundly affected by the loss of a child; gender differences in feelings and expressions of grief point to different needs for support.

More recently, perinatal palliative care has emerged as an approach to supporting women and their partners whose fetuses have been diagnosed with a life-limiting condition. Here too, the principles of palliative care are broadly applicable. Whether the woman and her partner elect to continue or terminate a pregnancy after diagnosis, they value provision of family-centered, interdisciplinary communication and psychosocial support (Wool, 2013). For those families who elect to carry the fetus to term, palliative care professionals provide continuing assessment and comfort measures, permitting time for bonding and adapting to the painful reality of the child's impending death (Wool, 2013). Finally, while a rare condition, recurrent miscarriage can be psychologically and relationally devastating to couples, and has been associated with anxiety, depression, and lowered self-esteem (Serrano & Lima, 2006). In a study of 30 couples with at least three miscarriages, Serrano and Lima (2006) found that women grieved more intensely than their partners. Whether perinatal loss is expected or unexpected, parental grief and suffering should be acknowledged and support and counseling should be offered.

Conclusion

Death is, indeed, not what it used to be. The advent of antibiotics, improvements in sanitation, prenatal care, nutritional improvements and methods for improving safety in high-risk work environments have contributed to increased longevity and quality of life. As Americans live longer, many will develop chronic illnesses and associated functional impairment and need for chronic disease medical management. Yet technological and pharmaceutical breakthroughs allow many children and adults to live healthy, productive lives with illnesses and conditions they would likely not have survived just a century ago. With the ability to prolong life, we now wrestle with complex ethical and emotional issues about when the burdens of medical intervention outweigh the benefits. We cannot change the fact of death; but we can change the manner in which death takes place. Palliative care and hospice have evolved as person- and family-centered, interdisciplinary care models to address psychosocial, physical, and spiritual suffering. Communication is the key to improving end-of-life care. Advance care planning "documents" are necessary, but not sufficient. Advance care planning is an ongoing dialogue between health-care providers and patients that anticipates changes in condition and honors the person's values and preferences. As the principal caregivers to sick and dying children and adults, women are particularly at risk for caregiving-associated stress. Palliative and hospice care provide support to patients and to caregivers during life-threatening illness and after loss of a loved one. Understanding the process of dying and death as a normal part of life is important in order to comprehensively care for women across the life span.

References

Agency for Healthcare Research and Quality. (2003). Advance care planning: Preferences for care at the end of life. *Research in Action*, (12), 1–19.

Aging with Dignity. (2013). *Voicing my choices.* Retrieved from http://www.agingwithdignity.org/voicing-my-choices.php

Alano, G. J., Pezmezaris, R., Tal, J. Y., Hussain, M. J., Jeune, J., Louis, B., . . . Wolf-Klein, J. P. (2010). Factors influencing older adults to complete advance directives. *Palliative and Supportive Care, 8*(3), 267–275.

Arias, E. (2011). United States life tables, 2007. *National Vital Statistics Reports, 59*(9). Retrieved from http://www.cdc.gov/nchs/data/nvsr/nvsr59/nvsr59_09.pdf

Bookwala, J., Copploa, K. M., Fagerlin, A., Ditto, P. H., Danks, J. H., & Smucker, W. D. (2001). Gender differences in older adults' preferences for life-sustaining medical treatments and end-of-live values. *Death Studies, 25*, 127–149.

Buck, J. (2011). Policy and the reformation of hospice. *Journal of Hospice & Palliative Nursing, 13*(65), 535–543.

CAPC. (2012). *Growth of palliative care in US hospitals.* Retrieved from http://www.capc.org/capc-growth-analysis-snapshot-2011.pdf

Caregiver Action Network. (2009). *Caregiving statistics.* Retrieved from http://caregiveraction.org/statistics/

Carr, D., & Khodyakov, D. (2007). End-of-life health care planning among young-old adults: An assessment of psychosocial influences. *The Journal of Gerontology. Series B, Psychological Sciences and Social Sciences, 62*(2), S135–141.

Centers for Disease Control. (1999). Achievements in public health, 1900–1999: Healthier mothers and babies. *Morbidity and Mortality Weekly Report.* Retrieved from http://www.cdc.gov/mmwr/preview/mmwrhtml/mm4838a2.htm

Centers for Disease Control. (2009). *Leading causes of death 1900–1998.* Retrieved from http://www.cdc.gov/nchs/nvss/mortality_historical_data.htm

Centers for Medicare and Medicaid Services. (2012). *Nursing home data compendium* (2012 ed.). Retrieved from http://www.cms.gov/Medicare/Provider-Enrollment-and-Certification/CertificationandComplianc/downloads/nursinghomedatacompendium_508.pdf

Christakis, N. A., & Lamont, E. B. (2000). Extent and determinants of error in physicians' prognoses in terminally ill patients. *Western Journal of Medicine, 172*(5), 310–313.

Commonwealth Fund (1999). *Care for the dying overwhelmingly falls on families, according to first major study in decade with patients and caregivers.* Available at: http://www.commonwealthfund.org/publications/press-releases/1999/sep/care-for-the-dying-falls-overwhelmingly-on-families--according-to-first-major-study-in-decade-with-p

Cowles, K. V. (1996). Cultural perspectives of grief: An expanded concept analysis. *Journal of Advanced Nursing, 23*(2), 287–294.

Downey, L., Au, D. H., Curtis, J. R., & Engelberg, R. A. (2013). Life-sustaining treatment preferences: Matches and mismatches between patients' preferences and clinicians' perceptions. *Journal of Pain and Symptom Management, 46*(1), 9–19.

Field, M. J., & Cassel, C. K. (Eds.). (1997). Approaching death: Improving care at the end of life. Washington, DC: National Academies Press.

Glaser, B.G., & Strauss, A.L. (1965). Awareness of dying. Chicago: Aldine.

Herbert, R.S., & Schulz, R. (2006). Caregiving at the end of life. *Journal of Palliative Medicine, 9*(5), 1174–1187.

Hospice Association of America. (2014). *Hospice: A HAA/NAHC historical perspective.* Retrieved from http://www3.nahc.org/haa/history.html

Hoyert, D. L., & Xu, J. (2012). Deaths: Preliminary data for 2011. *National Vital Statistics Reports, 61*(6). Retrieved from http://www.cdc.gov/nchs/data/nvsr/nvsr61/nvsr61_06.pdf

Jones, D. S., Podolsky, S. H., & Greene, J. A. (2012). The burden of disease and the changing task of medicine. *New England Journal of Medicine, 366*, 2333–2338.

Kelley, A. S., Deb, P., Qingling, D., Aldridge Carlson, M. D., & Morrison, S. (2013). The care span: Hospice enrollment saves money for medicare and improves care quality across a number of different lengths-of-stay. *Health Affairs, 32*, 3551–3561.

Krishnan, M., Temel, J. S., Wright, A. A., Bernacki, R., Selvaggi, K., & Balboni, T. (2013). Predicting life expectancy in patients with advanced incurable cancer: A review. *Supportive Oncology, 11*, 68–74.

Kubler-Ross, E. (1969). On death and dying. New York: Macmillan.

Mackinnon, C. J. (2009). Applying feminist, multicultural and social justice theory to diverse women who function as caregivers in end-of-life and palliative home care. *Palliative and Supportive Care,* 7(4), 501–512.

Meier, D. E., Isaacs, S. L., & Hughes, R. G. (2010). *Palliative care: Transforming the care of serious illness.* San Francisco, CA: Jossey-Bass.

Michelson, K. N., & Steinhorn, D. M. (2008). Pediatric end-of-life issues and palliative care. *Clinical Pediatric Emergency Medicine,* 8(3), 212–219.

Miesfeldt, S., Murray, K., Lucas, L., Chang, C. H., Goodman, D., & Morden, N. E. (2012). Association of age, gender, and race with intensity of end-of-life care for Medicare beneficiaries with cancer. *Journal of Palliative Medicine,* 15(5), 548–554.

Mitchell, S. L., Teno, J. M., Kiely, D. K, Shaffer, M. L., Jones, R. N., Prigerson, H. G., . . . Hamel, M. B. (2009). The clinical course of advanced dementia. *New England Journal of Medicine,* 361, 1529–1538.

Mitchell, S. L., Teno, J. M., Miller, S. C., & Mor, V. (2005). A national study of location of death for older persons with dementia. *Journal of the American Geriatric Society,* 53(2), 299–305.

Morrison, R. S., Penrod, J. D., Cassel, J. B., Caust-Elelnbogen, M., Litke, A., Spragens, L., & Meier, D. E. (2008). Cost savings associated with US hospital palliative care consultation programs. *Archives of Internal Medicine,* 168(16), 1783–1790.

Murphy, S.L., Xu, J., & Kochanek, K.D. (2013). Deaths: Final data for 2010. *National Vital Statistics Reports,* 61(4). Available at: http://www.cdc.gov/nchs/data/nvsr/nvsr61/nvsr61_04.pdf

National Cancer Institute. (2013). Retrieved from http://www.cancer.gov/cancertopics/pdq/supportivecare/caregivers/healthprofessional/page1/All Pages

National Center for Health Statistics (2011). Health, United States, 2010: With special feature on death and dying. Available at: http://www.cdc.gov/nchs/data/hus/hus10.pdf

National Consensus Project for Quality Palliative Care. (2013). *Clinical practice guidelines for quality palliative care* (3rd ed.). Retrieved from http://www.nationalconsensusproject.org/NCP_Clinical_Practice_Guidelines_3rd_Edition.pdf

National Hospice and Palliative Care Organization. (2012). *NHPCO's facts and figures. Hospice care in America.* http://www.nhpco.org/sites/default/files/public/Statistics_Research/2012_Facts_Figures.pdf.

National Hospice and Palliative Care Organization. (2013a). *Hospice action network: Hospice in the nursing home.* Retrieved from http://hospiceactionnetwork.org/get-informed/issues/hospice-in-the-nursing-home/

National Hospice and Palliative Care Organization. (2013b). *NHPCO's facts and figures. Hospice care in America.* Retrieved from http://www.nhpco.org/sites/default/files/public/Statistics_Research/2013_Facts_Figures.pdf

Navaie-Waliser, M., Spriggs, A., & Feldman, P. H. (2002). Informal caregiving: Differential experiences by gender. *Medical Care,* 40(12), 1249–1259.

Olsson, L., Östlund, G., Strang, P., Jeppsson Grassman, E., & Friedrichsen, M. (2010). Maintaining hope when close to death: Insight from cancer patients in palliative home care. *International Journal of Palliative Nursing,* 16(12), 1–6.

Perkins, H.S., Cortez, J.D., & Hazuda, H.D. (2004). Advance care planning: Does patient gender make a difference? *American Journal of Medical Sciences,* 327(1), 25–32.

Pew Research Religion & Public Life Project (2013). *Views on end-of-life medical treatments.* Available at: http://www.pewforum.org/2013/11/21/views-on-end-of-life-medical-treatments/

Pyenson, B., Connor, S., Fitch, K., & Kinzbrunner, B. (2004). Medicare cost in matched hospice and non-hospice cohorts. *Journal of Pain and Symptom Management,* 28(3), 200–210.

Rodriquez, K. L., Hanlon, J. T., Perera, S., Jaffe, E. J., & Sevick, M. A. (2010). A cross-sectional analysis of the prevalence of undertreatment of nonpain symptoms and factors associated with undertreatment in older nursing home hospice/palliative care patients. *American Journal of Geriatric Pharmacotherapy,* 3, 225–232.

Rogers, C. H., Floyd, F. J., Seltzer, M. M., Greenberg, J., & Hong, J. (2008). Long-term effects of the death of a child on parents' adjustment in midlife. *Journal of Family Psychology,* 22(2), 203–211.

Rosalynn Carter Institute for Caregiving. (2012). *Averting the caregiving crisis: An update.* Retrieved from http://www.rosalynncarter.org/UserFiles/File/PositionPaperUpdate3-19-12.pdf

Serrano, F., & Lima, M. L. (2006). Recurrent miscarriage: Psychological and relational consequences for couples. *Psychology & Psychotherapy: Theory, Research & Practice,* 79, 585–594.

Stevenson, D. G., & Bramson, J. S. (2009). Hospice care in the nursing home setting: A review of the literature. *Journal of Pain and Symptom Management,* 38(3), 440–451.

Tackling the burden of chronic diseases in the USA. (2009). *Lancet,* 373(9569), 185.

Temel, J. S., Greer, J. A., Muzikansky, A., Gallagher, E. R., Admane, S., Jackson, V. A., . . . Lynch, T. L. (2010). Early palliative care for patients with metastatic non-small-cell lung cancer. *New England Journal of Medicine*, *363*(8), 733–742.

Thomas, J. M., O'Leary, J. R., & Fried, T. R. (2009). Understanding their options: Determinants of hospice discussion for older persons with advanced illness. *Journal of General Internal Medicine*, *24*(8), 923–928.

US Department of Health and Human Services, Centers for Medicare and Medicaid Services (2013). *Medicare hospice benefits.* Available at: http://www.medicare.gov/Pubs/pdf/02154.pdf

Verret, D., & Rohloff, R. M. (2013). The value of palliative care. *Healthcare Financial Management*, *67*(3), 50–54.

Waldrop, D. P. (2007). Caregiver grief in terminal illness and bereavement: A mixed methods study. *Health & Social Work*, *32*(3), 197–206.

Ward, B. W., & Schiller, J. S. (2013). *Prevalence of multiple chronic conditions among US adults: Estimates from the National Health Interview Survey, 2010.* Retrieved from http://dx.doi.org/10.5888/pcd10.120203

Welte, T. M. (2013). "Gender differences in bereavement among couples after loss of a child: a professionals perspective." *Master of Social Work Clinical Research Papers.* Paper 271. Retrieved from http://sophia.stkate.edu/msw_papers/271

Wentzel, K. (1981). *To those who need it most . . . hospice means hope.* Boston, MA: Charles River.

Wiener, L., Zadeh, S., Battles, H., Baird, K., Ballard, E., Osherow, J., & Pao, M. (2012). Allowing adolescents and young adults to plan their end-of-life care. *Pediatrics*, *130*(5), 1–10.

Wool, C. (2013). State of the science on perinatal palliative care. *Journal of Obstetric, Gynecologic & Neonatal Nursing*, *42*(3), 372–382.

Index

Note: Page number followed by "f" indicate figure; those followed by "t" indicate table; those followed by "b" indicate boxes.

A

AARP, 108, 109, 115
ABC-and-D model, 55–56
Abdominal awareness, 251, 255
Abortion
  induced, 229t, 230
  spontaneous, 38t
Acarbose, 229t, 232
Acceptance, 337, 349
Accreditation Commission for Education in Nursing
  (ACEN), 23t
Accreditation resources, 23t
Acetaminophen, 224, 234t, 236
Acne vulgaris, 49
Actaea racemosa. See Black cohosh
Acupuncture, 83
Acute pain, complementary therapies for, 195
Addictions, influence on women's health, 271
Adipocyte, 136, 137, 138, 139, 150t
Adipocyte hyperplasia, 137
Adipocyte hypertrophy (cell expansion), 137
Adipokines, 138, 139, 150t
Adiponectin, 137, 149, 150t
Adipose tissue, 133, 134, 135, 136, 139, 140, 141, 145–146, 150t
  brown, 137–138
  deposition in bone, 138
  intermuscular, 137
  white, 137
Adolescence, 52, 273, 295–297
  body composition, 143
  conversation tips for parents of, 54–55
  friendship and, 53, 55
  hormonal changes of, 31
  USPSTF recommendations for, 58–60
Adrenarche, 31
Advance care planning, 344–347
Advanced practice registered nurse (APRN),
  21–22, 23t

Adverse Childhood Experience (ACE) study, 273
Advisory Committee on Immunization Practices
  (ACIP), 31, 43, 168
Affordable Care Act, 4, 22, 25, 116
Age-related dementias, 98–99
Aging
  healthy, for women, 96–117
    functional health, 104–105
    health-care systems for, 115–116
    issues and challenges for, 96
    mental health, 97–99
    physical health, 99–104
    promoting body image, self-esteem and
      relationships, 111–117
    promoting healthy behaviors, 105–111
    self-management of chronic conditions,
      116–117
  menopause/older women, 298–299
Air, influence on women's health, 265
Albuterol, 242t, 243
Alcohol, 271
  breast cancer and, 35t
  among older women, 106–107, 117
  preconception counseling and, 40t
  in young women, 44–45
Alignment, 257–258
α-Glucosidase inhibitors, 232
Alprazolam, 234t, 235
Alzheimer's Association, 115
Alzheimer's Disease (AD)
  rates of, 98–99
  Reiki therapy for, 194–195
Ambien. *See* Zolpidem
Ambien CR. *See* Zolpidem
Amenorrhea, 36, 37
American Academy of Nursing (AAN), 21
American Academy of Pediatrics (AAP), 36, 271
American Association of Colleges of Nursing
  (AACN), 20, 23t

355

American Cancer Society (ACS), 33
American College of Obstetrician and Gynecologist (ACOG), 20
American Congress of Obstetricians and Gynecologists (ACOG), 24t, 264, 267
American Dental Association, 162
American Heart Association (AHA), 69
American Insomnia Survey (AIS), 216
American Nurses Association (ANA), 264
American Nurses Credentialing Center (ANCC), 23t
American Society for Reproductive Medicine (ASRM), 264, 267
Amitriptyline (Elavil), 238, 318
Anger, 337, 349
Angiotensin-converting enzyme (ACE), 240
Angiotensin receptor blockers (ARBs), 240
Annotated Mini Mental State Examination (AMMSE), 194
Anorexia nervosa (AN), 174
Anterograde amnesia, 236
Anthropomometry, 135–136
Antiallergy, 243–244
Antianxiety drugs, 234t, 235
Anticoagulants, 239t, 241
Antidepressants, 81–82, 174, 233–235, 234t, 238
Antihistamines, 234t, 236, 243
Antimigraine drugs, 238
Antiplatelet drugs, 241
Antiretroviral (ARV) therapy, 169
Anxiety, 89, 190, 191, 193, 196, 198, 247, 350
    disorders, 79, 81–82
    and older women, 97–98
    risk reduction for, 81
    treatment for, 81–82, 205–209
Apigenin, 212
Apnea/hypopnea index (AHI), 329
Arthritis, 101, 102, 237
Articulation, 255–257
    of spine, 251–252
Aspergillus bacteria, 208
Aspirin, 58t, 101, 234t, 236, 239t, 241
ASSIST (Alcohol, Smoking and Substance Involvement Screening Test), 44
Association of Reproductive Health Professional (ARHP), 24t
Association of Women's Health, Obstetric, and Neonatal Nursing (AWHONN), 21, 24t
Asthma, 142, 242t, 243
Ataxia, 236
Atenolol, 239t, 240
Atorvastatin, 239t, 240
Atypical antidepressant, 235
Autonomy, 287
Awareness of Dying, 336

B
Baby teeth, 159
Bacall, Lauren, 249
Balanchine, George, 249
Bargaining, 337, 349

Beclomethasone, 242t, 243
Behavioral therapies, for insomnia, 317–318
Beige adipocytes, 138
Beige adipose tissue, 138, 150t
Benzodiazepines, 82, 206, 208, 235, 236, 316, 318, 320t
Bereavement, 348–349
Biguanides, 229t, 232
Bill McKibben of 350.org, 267
Bioelectrical impedance analysis (BIA), 134
Birth control pills, 82, 228
Bisphosphonate-related osteonecrosis of jaw (BRONJ), 171
Bisphosphonates, 102, 171, 231
Black cohosh, 214–215
Bladder syndrome, 327
Blood clots, drugs for, 241
Blood pressure, 69–70, 73, 74, 82, 86, 198, 239–240, 291, 312
Body art, 49–51
Body composition, 133–149
    compositional tissues, 136–139
    division of, 133–134
    exercise to enhance, 145–147, 146–147t
    health and, 139–142
        bone health, 141–142
        metabolic syndrome, 140–141
        morbidity and mortality, 140
        sarcopenia, 142
    methods of measuring, 134
    nutrition to enhance, 145–149, 146–147t
    patterns of, 144
    percent body fat, 134–136
    skeletal muscle/lean muscle mass, 139
    study of, 134
    across women's life span, 142–144
        adolescence, 143
        childhood, 143
        prenatal and infancy, 143
        reproductive phase and older women, 143–144
Body image, promoting healthy, 47
    healthy skin, 49
    healthy weight, 47–48
    older women and, 111–112
    sexual identity, healthy, 51–52
Body mass index (BMI), 47–48, 135–136, 135b, 140, 143, 144
Body modification, 49–51
Bone, 37, 143, 144, 171. See also Osteoarthritis; Osteoporosis
    adipose tissue deposition in, 138
    health in older women, 101–102, 141–142
Bone marrow fat, 138, 144
Botox (botulinum toxin type A), 171, 238
Breast cancer, 44, 74–77, 197, 230, 231
    assessment tools for, 36
    familial, 36
    occurrence of, 33
    risk factor for, 34–35t, 74, 75
    risk reduction strategies for, 75

screening for, 78t
sporadic, 36
treatment for, 77
Breast mass, palpation of, 34
Breast pain. *See* Mastalgia
Breast self-awareness, 33–34
Breathe, 251, 253–254
Brief intervention (BI), 45
Brite adipose tissue, 150t
Brite fat, 139
Brown adipose tissue, 137–138, 150t
Buck, Joy, 337
Budesonide, 243
Bulimia nervosa (BN), 174
Bullying, 56–57
Bupropion, 234t, 235
Burning mouth syndrome (BMS)
    prevention/treatment, 167
    symptoms, 166–167
Buspirone, 208

C
Calcium channel blockers, 240
Cancer
    breast. *See* Breast cancer
    cervical. *See* Cervical cancer
    in older women, 102–103
    oral. *See* Oral cancer
    symptom management, 197–198
    therapy, oral health in, 169–170
Captopril, 239t, 240
Cardiac arrhythmia, 224
Cardiovascular disease (CVD), 69–74, 84, 100,
    151t, 291
    diabetes, 72–74
    high cholesterol (hypercholesterolemia), 70
    hypertension as risk factor for, 69–70
    mortality, 140
    in older women, 100–101
    overweight and obesity, 72
    physical inactivity, 71–72
    smoking, 70–71
Cardiovascular drugs, 238–241, 239t
Caregiver(s)
    bereavement, 348–349
    to dying, 347–348
    grief, 348–349
    health promotion related to, 88
    mourning, 348–349
    older women and, 115
    primary, 338
Cataracts, 103, 104
Celecoxib, 234t, 237
Center/abdominal connectivity, finding, 255–258
Centers for Disease Control and Prevention (CDC),
    135, 267
Centers for Medicare and Medicaid Service, 116
Central sensitivity syndromes (CSSs), 327, 328
Certification resources, 23t
Cervical cancer, 46–47, 77

prevention of, 78–79
risk factor of, 78
risk reduction for, 79
screening, 78
signs and symptoms of, 78
treatment for, 79
Cetirizine, 242t, 243, 244
Chamomile (*Matricaria recutita*), for insomnia, 321
Chasteberry, prevention of PMS, 211–213
Chemicals, influence on women's health, 267
Chemosensory perception, 104
Chicago-based Abortion Counseling Service of
    Women's Liberation, 13
Childhood
    body composition, 143
    early, 293–294
        motivation and ability to environment
            care, 272
        susceptibility and vulnerability to risk
            factors, 272
    sleep in, 321–322
Chinese herbal medicine (CHM), 82, 83
Chlamydia, 45. *See also* Sexually transmitted
    infections (STIs)
Chlorhexidine, 173
Cholesterol, 59t
    drugs to lower, 240–241
    high, 70
Chronic conditions, self-management
    of, 116–117
Chronic fatigue syndrome (CFS), 327
Chronic neuropathic pain, drugs for, 238
Chronic pain syndromes
    complementary therapies for, 195
    drugs for, 238
Chronic pelvic pain (CPP), 327
Cimicifuga racemosa. *See* Black cohosh
Citalopram, 233
Clayburgh, Jill, 249
Climate, influence on women's health, 266–267
Clinical breast examination (CBE), 33, 34
Clonazepam, 167
Clopidogrel, 239t, 241
CNS drugs/pain medications, 234t
Cocooning, 43–44
Codeine, 225, 234t, 237
Cognitive aging, 98
Cognitive behavioral therapy (CBT), 194
    for anxiety disorders, 82, 98
    for chronic pain, 195
    for depression, 81
    for insomnia, 318
Cognitive health, older women and, 108
Cohesion, influence on women's health, 271
Combination hormone therapy, 34
Commission on Collegiate Nursing Commission
    (CCNE), 23t
Community actions, for health, 278–279, 278–279t
Community design, influence on women's
    health, 268

Community Navigators, 299
Complementary and alternative medicine (CAM), 203, 204
Complementary therapies
  for Alzheimer's Disease, 194–195
  for anxiety and stress, 193–194
  for cancer symptom management, 197–198
  for depression, 192–193
  for health-care providers, 198–199
  for menopause, 192
  for mood disorders, 192
  for pain, 195–197
  for pediatrics, 190–191
  for posttraumatic stress disorder, 194
  for pregnancy and birth, 190
Complete Streets, 268, 278t
Compositional tissues, 136–139
Compoz, for insomnia, 319
Congressional Caucus on Women's Issues, 15
Connected Kids, 53
Connecticut Hospice, 337, 339
Connor–Davidson Resilience Scale (CD-RISC), 184
Consensus Model for APRN Regulations, 22
Continuous care, Medicare Hospice Benefit, 341
Contraception
  drugs, 223, 228
  long-acting reversible contraceptives, 41–42
Contrology, 249, 252
Conversation tips, for parents of adolescents, 54–55
Coping, with loss of child, 349–350
Coronary heart disease (CHD)
  periodontal disease and, 173
  risk factors for, 70–71, 100, 101
Cortisol, 148, 292, 293
COX-2 selective NSAID, 237
CRAFFT screener, 44
Cranberry, prevention of UTI, 210–211
Creative imagery, for insomnia, 317
Crime Prevention Through Environmental Design, 278t
Crossing the Quality Chasm: A New Health System for the 21st Century, 7
Cytochrome P450 3A4, 206

D
Dabigatran, 239t, 241
D'Amboise, Jacques, 249
Dan, Alice, 15
Daytime sleepiness, 315
Death and dying
  approaches to care, improving, 336–337
  caregivers to, 347–348
  good death, hospice and, 337–339
  peaceful, 334–350
  in United States, 335–336
Deep breathing, for insomnia, 317
Delayed sleep onset, 330
Delirium, 98
Delos Living, 279t
Denial, 337, 349

Dental anatomy, 158–159
Dental caries, 174
Department of Health, Education, and Welfare (DHEW), 20
Depression, 79–81, 292, 337, 349, 350
  anxiety and, 205–209
    kava kava (Piper methysticum), 207–208
    Rhodiola. rosea, 208–209
    St. John's wort (Hypericum perforatum), 205–207
  inflammation and, 291
  insomnia and, 325–326
  older women, 97
  psychotherapy for, 81
  risk factors for, 80
  signs and symptoms of, 80b
  treatment for, 81
Desmethoxyyangonin, 207
Developmental plasticity, 292–293
Diabetes, 72–74
  bone health and, 142
  drugs for, 231–233
  periodontal disease and, 172–173
  risk reduction, 73
  treatment, 73–74
Diazepam, 224, 235
Dietary Supplement Act of 1994, 203
Digital mammography, 75
Dihydromethysticin, 207
Dihydropyridines, 240
Diltiazem, 239t, 240
Dipeptidylpeptidase 4 (DPP-4) inhibitors, 232
Diphenhydramine, 234t
Direct thrombin inhibitors, 241
Disabilities, women with, 128
Diuretics, 239
Doctor of Nursing Practice (DNP), 20
Dopamine, 81, 205, 212, 295, 310, 326, 330
Doxepin (Sinequan), 318
Drugs, for women wellness and disease prevention
  affecting mental health, 233–235
  to alleviate pain, 236–238
  for asthma, 243
  cardiovascular, 238–241
  for chronic pain syndromes, 238
  for diabetes mellitus, 231–233
  GI disorders/antacid, 241–243
  for insomnia, 235–236, 316t
  to lower blood pressure, 239
  male–female differences response in, 223–225
  related to sex hormones and reproductive health, 228–231
  therapy, 240
  for thyroid dysfunction, 231
  weight-loss, 233
  woman's life span, 225–227
Dual-energy X-ray absorption (DXA), 134
Duloxetine, 234t, 235
Dying. See Death and dying

Dynapenia, 142
Dysgeusia, 167
Dysmenorrhea, 236, 327

E

Early adulthood, puberty through. *See* Well-woman care
Eating disorders (EDs)
    dental erosion with, 175f
    oral health and, 174
    screen for, 48
    ways to prevent, 48
Eating habits, 148–149
Economics, influence on women's health, 270
Ectopic fat, 150t
Education
    influence on women's health, 270
    resources, 23t
Egg protein, 148
Elavil. *See* Amitriptyline
Electro-oculogram, 312
Electroencephalogram (EEG), 312
Electromyogram, 312
Empathy, 286, 301
Employment, health promotion related to, 86–87
Empowerment, 286
Endocrine
    definition, 151t
    drugs, 229t
Energy
    built environment and, 269
    therapy, for preterm infants, 191
Environments, healing, 262–282
    actions fostering individual, community and
        environmental health, 274–279
    built, 262, 263, 263t, 267–270
        energy, 269
        life indoors, 269–270
        transportation, 268–269
        urban development and community
            design, 268
        waste, 269
    health across lifespan in relation to, 271–274
    natural, 262–263, 263t, 265–267
        air, 265
        chemicals and microbes, 267
        climate, 266–267
        food, 266
        land, 266
        water, 265
    role of nurses and health-care professionals,
        279–282
    social, 262, 263, 263t, 270–271
        economic and educational opportunity, 270
        social support and cohesion, 271
        societal attitudes, addictions and media, 271
Epinephrine injection, 244
EpiPen, 242t, 244
Epworth Sleepiness Scale, 315
Escherichia coli fimbriae, 210

Escitalopram, 233
Estazolam, 320t
Estrogen, 84, 102, 240
Eszopiclone (Lunesta), 234t, 235, 319t
Ethinyl estradiol (EE), 229t
Etonogestrel, 229t
Exercises, to enhance body composition, 145–147,
    146–147t
Expressive writing, 300
Extra-osseous fat tissue, 150t
Ezetimibe, 241

F

Family and Medical Leave Act, 88
Family Planning Certificate Nurse Practitioner
    programs, 20
Family planning methods, 41–42
Family Planning Nurse Practitioners, 20
Famotidine, 242–243, 242t
Fat-free mass (FFM), 134
Fatigue, insomnia and, 327–328
Female sex hormones alter processes, 226
Fertility, oral health and, 163
Fexofenadine, 242t, 243
Fiber, 148
Fibrates, 241
Fibroadenomas, 34
Fibromyalgia (FM), 195–196, 327
5,6-dihydrokavain, 207
Five Wishes document, 109
Fletcher, Ron, 249, 250, 251, 253
Fluoxetine, 233, 234t
Fluticasone, 242t, 243
Fluvoxamine, 233
Folic acid supplementation, 43
Food, influence on women's health, 266
Formoterol, 243
Friendship, 53, 296
Fructose, 148
Functional health, of older adults, 104–105
Functional somatic syndromes, 327
Furosemide, 239t, 240
The Future of Nursing, 9

G

Gabapentin, 167, 234t, 238
Garrick, James G., 252
Gastrointestinal disorders, 241–243, 242t
Gender-sensitive resilience, 186
General inpatient care (GIP), Medicare Hospice
    Benefit, 341
Genital herpes, 46
Geriatric health, screening for, 110, 111t
Gestational diabetes mellitus (GDM), 164, 232
Ghrelin, 148
Glipizide, 225, 229t, 232
Glucose intolerance, 151t
Gluteofemoral fat (GF), 137
Glycated hemoglobin (HbA1c), 173
Go Red for Women, 100

Gonorrhea, 45. *See also* Sexually transmitted
    infections (STIs)
Good death, hospice and, 337–339
Government Accounting Office, 15
Graham, Martha, 249
Grief, 348–349
Guggenheim, Peggy, 249
Guidelines for Preconception and Interconception
    Care, 42
Gyrokinesis, 248

H

H₂ blockers, 242
Halcion. *See* Triazolam
Hamilton Anxiety Scale (HAMA), 207
Hamilton Depression Rating Scale (HAM-D)
    scores, 206
Hardship, 289
Hashimoto disease, 177
Head, ears, eyes, nose, and throat (HEENT), 158
Head, ears, eyes, nose, oral cavity, and throat
    (HEENOT), 158
Headache, 327
Healing
    arts, 246–260
    environments, 262–282
    relationships, 285–302
Health
    body composition and, 139–142
    community actions for, 278–279, 278–279t
    personal planetary habits for, 275–277, 275–277t
    promotion of, 8–9
    and relationships, 289–292
        cardiovascular disease, 291
        mental health, 291–292
        morbidity, 290
        mortality, 290
    wellness and, 2
        health care provider's roles in, 4
        holistic/integrated approach to, 2–3
        life-span approach to, 3
        unique aspects of women's, 3–4
Health and Human Services Healthy Marriage
    Initiative, 300
Health care, in 21ˢᵗ century, 7–10
    equal access to high-quality health care, 7–8
    future of nursing, 9–10
    holistic approach to care, 9
    interprofessional health-care workforce, 8
    new roles in health care, 8
    prevention of illness and promotion of
        health, 8–9
Health-care professionals role, in promoting wellness
    advocacy and research, 281
    call to action, 281–282
    education and recommendations, 281
    environmental health, evidence-based
        prescriptions for, 281
    individual and community awareness, raising, 280
    prevention, 279

    social norms, changing, 281
Healthy behaviors, 85–86
Healthy body fat, percentage range of, 135
Healthy lifestyle, 85, 85b
Healthy People 2020, 157
Hearing loss, 103, 104
Heart rate variability (HRV), 288
The Heart Truth, 100
Heide, Wilma Scott, 14
Hematopoietic, 150t
Hepatotoxicity, 208
Hepburn, Katherine, 249
Herbal medicine, women and
    ailments and treatments, 205–217
        depression and anxiety, 205–209
        insomnia, 216–217
        menopause, 214–215
        premenstrual syndrome, 211–213
        urinary tract infections, 210–211
    growth of, 203–205
Herd immunity, 43
Herpes simplex virus (HSV), 46
High cholesterol. *See* Hypercholesterolemia
High density lipoprotein (HDL), 70, 240
Hip circumference (HC), 135, 136b
Hip fracture, 102
Histamine H1 receptor antagonists, 243
Histamine H2 receptor blockers, 242
HMG-CoA reductase inhibitors, 240
Holistic approach, to health and wellness, 2–3, 9
Hormonal contraceptives, 163, 228, 230
Hormone replacement therapy (HRT), 75, 166, 226,
    230–231
Hormone therapy, 82–84, 144, 214, 230, 231, 238
Hospice
    care, 338
    defined, 337
    and good death, 337–339
    interdisciplinary team, 338, 340
    in nursing home, 342
    patients, profile of, 342–343
    quality care, components of, 341
    utilization and payment, 339–341
Hot flashes, 82–83, 324
HPV 16/18 infection, 168. *See also* Sexually
    transmitted infections (STIs)
HPV test, 78, 126
Human, as social animal, 287–289
Human ecology, of sleep, 310–311
Human papilloma virus (HPV), 46–47, 77–79
Hydrochlorothiazide, 239–240, 239t
Hydrocodone, 234t, 237
Hypercholesterolemia, 70
Hyperforin, 205, 206
Hypericum Depression Trial Study Group, 206
Hypericum perforatum. See St. John's wort
Hyperlipidemia, 71b
Hypertension
    guidelines to control, 70b
    in older women, 101

risk factor for heart disease, 69–70
   treatment, 70
Hyperthyroidism, 231
Hypoglycemia, 232
Hyposalivation, 176t
Hypothalamic–pituitary–ovarian axis, 212
Hypothyroidism, 177, 231

I

Ibuprofen, 171, 234t, 236
Idiopathic back pain, 327
IL-6, 139, 151t
IL-15, 139, 151t
Illness, prevention of, 8–9
Imipramine, 205, 234t
Immigrant women, 125–126
Immune system, in older women, 103
Immunizations, 43–44
Imprinting, 256
Individuals with Disabilities Education Act, 300
Infancy
   motivation and ability to environment care, 272
   susceptibility and vulnerability to risk factors, 272
Informal caregiving, 347
Inhaled corticosteroids, 243
Inpatient respite care, Medicare Hospice
   Benefit, 341
Insomnia, 216–217, 313–315
   behavioral therapies for, 317–318
   chronic pain and, 327–328
   delayed sleep onset, 330
   depression and, 325–326
   drugs for, 235–236
   fatigue and, 327–328
   integrative therapies for, 320–321
   medical conditions and, 326–327
   multiple awakenings, 330
   obstructive sleep apnea, 330
   short screening for, 315t
   shortened sleep (sleep loss), 323–324, 330
   sleep-disordered breathing, 323, 324, 325,
      328, 329
   tissue injury and, 326–327
   treatment for, 315–321
   types and features of, 316t
Insomnia Symptom Questionnaire (ISQ), 313
Institute of Medicine (IOM), 4, 7
Insulin, 148, 150t, 151t, 232
Integration, 301
Interdisciplinary team (IDT), 338, 339, 340, 343,
      344, 348
Intermuscular adipose fat tissue, 137
International Classification of Sleep Disorders
      (ICSD-2), 314–315
International Council of Nurses (ICN), 264
International Nurse Coach Association
      (INCA), 22
Interpersonal psychotherapy (IPT), 81
Interprofessional health-care workforce, 7, 8
Interstitial cystitis, 327

Intimate partner violence (IPV), 129–130, 194
Intraoral pain, 170–171
Ionizing radiation, 34
Ipratropium, 242t, 243
Ipsapirone, 207
Irisin, 139, 151t
Irritable bowel syndrome (IBS), 327
Isotretinoin (Accutane), 49

J

Jane Movement, 13
Josiah Macy Foundation, 10

K

Katz, David, 247–248
Kava kava (Piper methysticum), 207–208
   adverse effects and drug interactions, 208
   dosage, 207
   evidence, 207–208
   for insomnia, 321
   potential mechanism of action, 207
Kavain, 207
Keeping Children and Families Safe Act, 300
Kryzanowska, Romana, 249, 250
Kupperman Index score, 215

L

LACE report, 21–22
Land, influence on women's health, 266
Lavender oil, for insomnia, 321
Lean muscle mass, 139
Leptin, 150t
Lesbian, Gay, Bisexual, Transgender, Queer
      (LGBTQ), 51, 114–115, 127
Leukotrienes, 243
Levels of certainty, regarding net benefit, 77t
Levonorgestrel, 229t
Levothyroxine (T₄), 229t, 231
Lewin, Ellen, 15
LI 156 (Sedonium), 217
LI 160 formulation, 206
Licensure, Accreditation, Certification, and
      Education (LACE) Consensus Project, 21
Licensure resources, 23t
Life course perspective (LCP), 30
Life indoors, 269–270
Life-span approach, to health and wellness, 3
Limb movement disorders, 313
Lipoproteins, 70
Lipotoxicity, 141
Living situation, older women and, 109, 113–114
Loneliness, 98, 299
Long-acting reversible contraceptives
      (LARC), 41–42
Loop diuretics, 240
Loratadine, 242t, 243, 244
Lorazepam, 234t, 235
Lorcaserin, 233
Los Angeles Feminist Women's Health Center, 13
Losartan, 239t

Loss of child, coping with, 349–350
Low density lipoprotein (LDL) cholesterol, 70, 240
Lunesta. *See* Eszopiclone
Lung cancer, 102–103
Lyubomirsky, Sonja, 247

M
Macy Foundation, 8
Major depressive disorder, 79
MAO inhibition, 208
Mastalgia, 34
Media, influence on women's health, 271
Medicaid, 116
Medical conditions, insomnia and, 326–327
Medicare, 116, 116t
    advantage plan (managed Medicare), 339
    indemnity (fee for service), 339
    for older women, 110, 110–111t
    part A, 339
Medicare Hospice Benefit, 339, 340
Medication management, older women and, 107–108
Meditation, 188–189, 189b
    for anxiety, 193–194
    for cancer symptom management, 197–198
    for depression, 192–193
    for insomnia, 317
    during menopause, 192
    for mood disorders, 192–194
    for pain, 195–196
    for pediatrics, 190–191
    for posttraumatic stress disorder, 194
    during pregnancy and childbirth, 190
    for stress, 193–194
Medroxyprogesterone, 229t
Meglitinides, 232
Melatonin, 236
Menarche, 31
Menopause, 214–215, 298–299
    Chinese herbal medicine for, 82, 83
    hormone replacement after, 230–231
    oral health and, 166
    therapies for, 192
    transition, 84–85, 324–325
Menopause Rating Scale (MRS), 214
Menstrual changes, 84–85
Menstrual health, 36–37
Mental health, 291–292
    older women, 97–99
    promotion, 89
Mesenchymal stem cells, 150t
Metabolic dysregulation, 140–141
Metabolic syndrome, 140–141, 151t
Metabolically-obese, normal-weight
    (MONW), 141, 151t
Metabolism, 151t
Metformin, 86, 229t, 232
Methimazole, 229t, 231
Methysticin, 207
Metoprolol, 239t, 240
Microbes, influence on women's health, 267

Midlife relationships, 297–298
Midlife women, 68–90
    anxiety, 81–82
    breast cancer, 74–77
    cardiovascular disease, 69–74
    cervical cancer, 77–79
    depression, 79–81
    issues and challenges faced by, 68–69
    menopausal transition and menstrual
        issues, 82–85
    osteoporosis, 74
    promoting health, 85–89
        caregiving, 88
        employment, 86–87
        healthy behaviors, 85–86
        healthy relationships, 89
        healthy self-esteem, 88–89
        mental health promotion, 89
        positive body image, 88–89
        sexuality, 87–88
Mifepristone, 229t, 230
Migraine headache, 238
Mild cognitive impairment (MCI), 98
Military sexual trauma (MST), 125
Military, women in, 124–125
Mindfulness-based stress reduction (MBSR), 189,
    192, 193, 195, 197–198
Mindsight, 301
Monoamine oxidase inhibitors
    (MAOIs), 81–82, 235
Montelukast, 242t, 243
Mood disorders, complementary therapies for,
    192–194
    anxiety, 193–194
    depression, 192–193
    stress, 193–194
Morphine, 225, 234t, 237
Mourning, 348–349
Mouth, anatomy of, 158f
Mucosa, 160
Multiple awakenings, 330
Multiple chemical sensitivity, 327
Multiple chronic conditions (MCCs), 335
Multisymptom illnesses, 327
Muscarinic antagonist, 243
Mutans streptococci (MS), 164
Mutuality, 286
Myocardial infarction, 100
Myocyte, 150t
Myofascial pain syndrome, 327
Myokines, 139, 150t

N
Narcolepsy, 313, 325
Narcotics. *See* Opioid analgesics
National Alliance for Caregiving, 115
National Association of Nurse Practitioners in
    Reproductive Health (NANPRH), 21
National Association of Nurse Practitioners in
    Women's Health (NPWH), 21, 24t

National Association of Professional Geriatric Care
  Managers, 109
National Comprehensive Cancer Network (NCCN), 33
National Council of State Boards of Nursing
  (NCSBN), 21
National Council on Aging, 102
National Fall Prevention Awareness Day, 102
National Health and Nutrition Examination Survey
  (NHANES), 167
National Health Interview Survey (NHIS), 73, 335
National Institute of Health (NIH), 15–16, 99
National Institutes of Health Advisory Committee, 15
National Longitudinal Study of Adolescent
  Health, 52
National Organization for Women, 14
National Organization of Nurse Practitioner Faculties
  (NONPF), 20, 23t
National Osteoporosis Foundation (NOF), 74
National Prevention Council and Strategy, 4
National Scientific Council on the Developing
  Child, 300
National Task Force on Quality Nurse Practitioner
  Education, 21
National Women's Law Center, 270
Natural environment, 262
  components of, 262–263, 263t
  influence on women's health, 265–267
Net benefit, levels of certainty regarding, 76–77t
New conditioning exercise, 183–184
Niacin, 241
Nifedipine, 239t, 240
Night sweats, 82, 324
Nightingale, Florence, 12, 13, 264
Nipple aspirate fluid (NAF), 214
Nocturnal esophageal reflux, 323
Nocturnal periodic leg movements, 323, 325
Nonalcoholic fatty liver disease (NAFLD), 141, 151t
Nonbenzodiazepines, 235
  induce sleep, 234t
  for insomnia, 318, 319t
Non–rapid eye movement (NREM) sleep, 311, 312
Nonrestorative sleep, 327
Nonsteroidal anti-inflammatory drugs
  (NSAIDs), 236
Norepinephrine reuptake inhibitors (SNRIs), 81
Normal blood pressure, 69
Nurses Association of American College of
  Obstetricians and Gynecologists (NAACOG), 20
Nurses role, in promoting wellness
  advocacy and research, 281
  call to action, 281–282
  education and recommendations, 281
  environmental health, evidence-based
    prescriptions for, 281
  individual and community awareness, raising, 280
  prevention, 279
  social norms, changing, 281
Nursing, 14
  future of, in health care, 9–10
  home, hospice in, 342

Nutrition
  to enhance body composition, 148–149
  healthy, guidelines for, 86b
Nytol, for insomnia, 319

O
Obesity
  breast cancer and, 35
  periodontal disease and, 172
  as risk factor for CHD, 72
  risk reduction, 72
  treatment, 72
  ways to preventing, 48
Obstructive sleep apnea (OSA), 330
Office of Research on Women's Health (ORWH), 4,
  15, 16
Older women, 298–299
  functional health, 104–105
  health-care systems for, 115–116
  issues and challenges for, 96
  mental health, 97–99
    anxiety, 97–98
    cognitive aging, 98–99
    depression, 97
  motivation and ability to environment care, 272
  physical health, 99–104
    bone health, 101–102
    cancer, 102–103
    cardiovascular health, 100–101
    immune system, 103
    postmenopausal health, 99–100
    sensory changes, 103–104
  promoting body image, self-esteem and
    relationships, 111–117
    aging and body image, 111–112
    caregiving, 115
    healthy relationships, 112–113
    LGBTQ issues, 114–115
    living situation, 113–114
    sexuality, 112
  promoting healthy behaviors, 105–111
    cognitive and social engagement, 108
    health care and living situation planning, 109
    healthy eating, 106
    medication management, 107–108
    physical activity, 105–106
    screening/vaccinations, 109–110
    substance issues, 106–107
  self-management of chronic conditions, 116–117
  susceptibility and vulnerability to risk
    factors, 272
Olesen, Virginia, 15
Omeprazole, 242–243, 242t
Omnibus Budget Reconciliation Act (OBRA)
  of 1989, 342
On Death and Dying, 337
Opioid analgesics, 237–238
Opipramol, 208
Optimal health, 2
Oral antidiabetic drugs, 229t, 232–233

Oral cancer, 161, 161f
  HPV type 16 infection and, 168
  risk factors for, 168
  signs of, 168
Oral health, 157–177
  in cancer therapy, 169–170
    HIV-infected women, 169
    prevention/treatment, 169–170
  examination, 158–161
    equipment for, 160–161
    oral and dental anatomy, 158–159
    saliva, 159–160
  female hormonal changes affecting, 162–166
    fertility, 163
    menopause, 166
    menses and midlife considerations, 163
    postpartum, 165–166
    pregnancy, 163–165
    puberty, 162–163
  oral–facial pain. See Oral–facial pain, acute and
    chronic
  oral systemic health conditions, 166
    burning mouth syndrome, 166–167
    oral HPV and women, 167–169
Oral Health in Cancer Therapy: A Guide for Health
Care Professionals, 169
Oral HPV infection, 167–169
  prevalence of, 167–168
  prevention/treatment, 168–169
  signs of, 168
  vaccination, 168
Oral–facial pain, acute and chronic, 170
  acute and chronic, 170–177
  bisphosphonates-related osteonecrosis
    of jaw, 171
  eating disorders, 174, 175f
  intraoral pain, 170–171
  osteoarthritis of TMJ, 170
  periodontal disease, 171–174
  Sjögren syndrome, 175–176, 176t
  thyroid disorder, 177
  TMJ disorders, 170
Oropharyngeal cancers (OPCs), 167–168
Oropharyngeal HPV infection, 168
Ospemifene, 229t, 231
Osteoarthritis, 102
  celecoxib for, 237
  of temporomandibular joint, 170
Osteoblast, 150t
Osteocalcin, 150t
Osteoclast, 150t
Osteocyte, 150t
Osteopenia, 101, 141
Osteoporosis, 74, 141, 166
  guidelines to reduce risk of, 74
  in older women, 101–102
  risk reduction, 74
  treatment, 74
Otto, Michael, 247
Our Bodies, Ourselves, 14

Over-the-counter (OTC) drugs, for insomnia,
  319–320
Overweight paradox, 140
Oxycodone, 237
Oxytocin, 288

P
Pain, 247, 248, 342
  chronic neuropathic, drugs for, 238
  COX-2 selective NSAID, 237
  drugs to alleviate, 236–238
  functional health and, 105
  and insomnia, 327–328
  nonsteroidal anti-inflammatory drugs for, 236
  opioid analgesics for moderate, 237–238
Palliative care, 343–344, 349
  defined, 343
  perinatal, 350
Pap test, 78
Paracrine, 151t
Parents
  and adolescent relationship, 52–53
  of adolescents, conversation tips for, 54–55
Parotid salivary glands, 159
Paroxetine, 233, 235
Passionflower (Passiflora app), for insomnia, 321
Patient-Centered Outcomes Research Institute
  (PCORI), 9
Patient Protection and Affordable Care Act
  (PPACA), 9, 25
Patient Self Determination Act (PSDA) of 1990, 345
Pelvic examination, 33
Pelvic press, 256–257
Penduletin, 212
Peptide YY (PYY), 148, 293
Percent body fat (PBF), 134
Perinatal palliative care, 350
Periodic leg movements, 313
  in sleep disorder, 327
Periodic limb movement disorder (PLMD), 330
Periodontal disease, 160, 171–174
  coronary heart disease and, 173
  definition, 171
  diabetes and, 172–173
  obesity and, 172
  prevalence, 171
  risk factors, 172
  treatment and prevention, 173
Periodontitis, 160, 164, 166
Personal planetary habits, for health, 275–277,
  275–277t
Peters, Roberta, 249
Pharmacodynamics, 224
Pharmacogenomics, 225
Pharmacokinetics, 224
Pharmacotherapy, for weight management, 72
Pharynx, 161
Phendimetrazin, 233
Phentermine, 233
Phenytoin, 225

Physical activity, for older women, 105–106
Physical inactivity
   and coronary heart disease, 71–72
   as risk factor, 72
Piercings, 50–51
Pilates, 246–260. *See also* Pilates Method
   alignment, 257–258
   articulation, 255–257
   background/literature on, 246–248
   breathe, 253–258
   center/abdominal connectivity, finding, 255–258
   spinal awareness, 255–257
   tips, 258–260
Pilates, Clara, 249, 253
Pilates, Joseph Hubertus, 249, 250, 253, 254
Pilates Method, 248–253
   fundamentals of, 250
   history of, 249
   inspiration, 252–253
   new beginning, 250–252
Pioglitazone, 229t, 232–233
Piper methysticum. See Kava kava
Pittsburgh Sleep Quality Index (PSQI), 313–314
Planned Parenthood Federation of America, 13, 20
Podwal, Michael, 248
Polycystic ovary syndrome (PCOS), 37, 323
Polysomnography (PSG), 312, 318, 324, 325, 327
Positive body image, health promotion related to, 88
Postmenopausal health, in older women, 99–100
Postmenopausal zest, 274
Postpartum, oral health and, 165–166
Postsurgical pain, complementary therapies for, 196
Posttraumatic growth (PTG), 182
Posttraumatic stress disorder (PTSD), 194
Potassium sparing diuretic, 240
Poverty
   impact on women's health, 270
   women in, 126–127
Preconception care, 30
Pregabalin, 234t, 238
Pregnancy, 292
   delaying/preventing, 41–42
   drugs to prevent, 228–230
   folic acid supplementation, 43
   oral health and, 163–165
   planning, 42
   teratogenic risk during, 227t
Pregnancy Risk Assessment Monitoring System (PRAMS), 39–41
Pregnancy tumor. *See* Pyogenic granuloma
Premenstrual dysphoric disorder (PMDD), 323
Premenstrual syndrome (PMS), 211–213, 323
Prenatal development, 292–293
Proanthocyanidins, 210
Procedural pain, complementary therapies for, 196
Progesterone, 84
Progestin (norethindrone), 228, 229t, 230
Progressive muscle relaxation, for insomnia, 317
Project Northland, 45
Propylthiouracil, 231

Proton pump inhibitors, 242
Psychological stress, 289
   maternal, 293
   and mortality, dose–response relationship between, 290
   short-term, 291
Psychotherapy, for depression, 81
Puberty
   through early adulthood. *See* Well-woman care
   oral health and, 162–163
   sleep in, 321–322
Pyogenic granuloma (PG), 164–165, 165f

Q
Quetelet, Adolphe, 135

R
Raloxifene, 229t, 231
Ramelteon, 234t, 236, 319t
Ranitidine, 242–243, 242t
Rapid eye movement (REM) sleep, 311–312, 321
Reappraisal process, 300
Reciprocity, 286
Regional tissue pain syndrome, 327
Registered nurses (RNs), 21–22
Reiki therapy
   for anxiety, 193–194
   for cancer symptom management, 197–198
   for depression, 192–193
   health-care providers and, 198–199
   history of, 188–189
   during menopause, 192
   for mood disorders, 192–194
   for pain, 195–196
   for pediatrics, 190–191
   for posttraumatic stress disorder, 194
   during pregnancy and childbirth, 190
   self-Reiki, 189b
   for stress, 193–194
Relational health, interventions for promoting, 299–302
Relational paradox, 287
Relationships
   defined, 285–287
   healing, 285–302
   health and, 289–292
      cardiovascular disease, 291
      mental health, 291–292
      morbidity, 290
      mortality, 290
   promoting healthy, 52–57
      bullying prevention, 56–57
      clinicians, 53
      friendships, 53, 55
      parents, 52–53
      romantic relationships, 55–56
   self-silencing within, 288–289
   throughout woman's life span
      adolescence, 295–297
      early childhood, 293–294

Relationships (*continued*)
  menopause/older women, 298–299
  midlife, 297–298
  prenatal, 292–293
  relational health, interventions for promoting,
    299–302
Relaxation therapy, 189, 190
Renin–angiotensin–aldosterone system (RAAS), 291
Repaglinide, 229t, 232
Reproductive life plan (RLP), 37–39
Reproductive years
  motivation and ability to environment care, 273
  susceptibility and vulnerability to risk factors, 273
Resilience, in women, 181–187
  approaches to increasing, 184–186
    accepting change as part of living, 185
    developing realistic goals, 185
    good self-care, 186
    increasing awareness, 184–185
    increasing self-compassion, 185
    keeping things in perspective, 185
    looking for opportunities, 185
    maintaining hopeful outlook, 185
    making connections, 185
    seeing events realistically, 185
    taking actions, 185
  brain change processes and, 183–184
  concept, 181
  definitions, 182–184, 186
  gender-sensitive, 186
  importance of understanding, 181–182
  measuring/assessing, 184
  spirituality and, 183
Resilience Scale™, 184
Respiratory disturbance index (RDI), 329
Restless legs syndrome (RLS), 323, 324, 325,
  327, 330
Restoril. *See* Temazepam
Revised Memory and Behavior Problem Checklist, 194
Rhodiola rosea
  adverse effects and drug interactions, 209
  dosage, 209
  evidence, 209
  potential mechanism of action, 208
Robert Wood Johnson Foundation (RWJF), 9
Roe v Wade decision, 13
Romantic relationships, 55–56
Rosalynn Carter Institute (RCI), 347
Routine home care, Medicare Hospice Benefit,
  340–341
Rozerem, for insomnia, 320t. *See also* Ramelteon

S
Sacred space, 183
Saliva, 159–160
Salivary glands, 159f
Salmeterol, 242t, 243
Sanger, Margaret, 13
Sarcopenia, 142
Saunders, Dame Cicely, 337

SAVA syndemic, 129
School age
  motivation and ability to environment care, 273
  susceptibility and vulnerability to risk factors,
    272–273
SCOFF questionnaire, 48
Second-generation antihistamines, 243
Sedonium. *See* LI 156
Selective estrogen receptor modulators
  (SERMs), 214, 230–231
Self-breast examination (SBE), 33
Self-care
  benefits to health-care providers, 198–199
  cancer symptom management, 197–198
  evidence for use of Reiki and meditation, 190
    Alzheimer disease, 194–195
    menopause, 192
    mood disorders, 192–194
    pain, 195–196
    pediatrics, 190–191
    pregnancy and birth, 190
  history of Reiki and meditation, 188–199
Self-diminishing thoughts, 292
Self-esteem, 350
  health promotion related to, 88–89
  older women and, 112
Self-preservation, 292
Self-Reiki, 189b
Self-silencing within relationships, 288–289
Sensory loss, in older women, 103–104
Serotonin reuptake inhibitors (SSRIs), 81, 233, 235
Serotonin–norepinephrine reuptake inhibitors
  (SNRIs), 81, 234t, 235, 238
Sertraline, 233, 234t, 235
Serum C-reactive protein (CRP), 141, 151t
Severino, Diane, 248
Sexual and reproductive health (SRH), 22, 25
Sexual identity, healthy, 51–52
Sexuality
  health promotion and, 87
  older women and, 112
Sexually transmitted infections (STIs), 45–47
  chlamydia, 45
  genital herpes, 46
  gonorrhoea, 45
  human papilla virus, 46–47, 77–79
Short-acting β2-adrenergic agonists, 243
Shortened sleep (sleep loss) duration,
  323–324, 330
SHR-5, 209
Sinequan. *See* Doxepin
Sitagliptin, 229t, 232
Sjögren syndrome (SS), 175–176, 176t, 327
  salivary gland dysfunction in, 175
  types of, 175
Skeletal muscle, 139
Skin, healthy, 49
Sleep
  in childhood, 321–322
  clinical assessment of, 312–315

cycles of, 311–312
disorders. *See* Sleep disorders
   daytime sleepiness, 315
   insomnia, 313–315
   healthy, promoting, 309–331
   human ecology of, 310–311
   international classification of, 314t
   latency, 312
   movement disorders, 328
   nonrestorative, 327
   NREM, 311, 312
   problem assessment, guidelines for, 314t
   in puberty, 321–322
   -related disorders, 328–330
   REM, 311–312, 321
   during reproductive years, 322–325
   restriction, 317
   short screening for, 315t
   sleep apnea, 313
   sleep parasomnias, 313
   sleep walking, 313
   slow-wave, 321
   stages of, 311–312
   treatment for, 315–321
   and wellness, 309–310
Sleep apnea/hypopnea syndrome
   (SAHS), 329–330
Sleep-disordered breathing (SDB), 323, 324, 325,
   328, 329
Sleep-Eze, for insomnia, 319
Slow-wave sleep (SWS), 321
Smoking, 70–71
   as risk factor for CHD, 70–71
   risk reduction, 71
Social engagement, 298
   older women and, 108
Social environment, 262
   components of, 263, 263t
   influence on women's health, 270–271
Social exclusion, 292
Social isolation, 299
Social rejection, 292
Social support, influence on women's health, 271
Societal attitudes, influence on women's health, 271
Sominex, for insomnia, 319
Sonata. *See* Zaleplon
Spinal awareness, 255–257
Spine, articulation of, 251–252
Spirituality, resilience and, 183
Spironolactone, 239t, 240
St. Christopher's Hospice, 337
St. John's wort (*Hypericum perforatum*), 205–207
   dosage, 207
   evidence, 206
   potential mechanism of action, 205–206
   side effects and drug interactions, 206–207
Stages of Reproductive Aging Workshop
   (STRAW), 84
State Trait Anxiety Inventory (STAI), 207
Statins, 240

Stimulus control, 317
STOP–BANG assessment, 330
Stress, psychological. *See* Psychological stress
Strokes, 100–101
Study of Women Across the Nation (SWAN), 83
Subcutaneous adipose tissue (SAT), 150t
Subcutaneous fat, 137
Sublingual salivary glands, 159
Submandibular salivary glands, 159
Substance abuse, recovering women from, 128–129
Substance use, 106–107
   reducing, 44–45
Sulfonylureas, 232
Sumatriptan, 234t, 238
Superficial subcutaneous adipose tissue
   (SAT), 137
Synthroid, 229t
Systemic lupus erythematosus, 327

T
Tai chi, 248, 317
Task Force on Opportunities for Research on
   Women's Health, 15–16
Tattoos, 50
Teachable moments, 53
Temazepam (Restoril), 234t, 320t
Temporomandibular joint (TMJ), 160
   disorders, 170, 327
   osteoarthritis, 170
Teratogenic, risk during pregnancy, 227t
Terminally ill, defined, 339
Thelarche, 31
Therapeutic touch (TT)
   for cancer symptom management, 197–198
   for pain, 195–196
   for preterm infants, 191
Thiazide diuretics, 70
Thiazides, 239–240
Thiazolidinediones, 232, 233
Thrombi. *See* Blood clots, drugs for
Thrombosis, 228
Thyroid disorder
   oral manifestations of, 177
   treatment, 177
Thyroid dysfunction, drugs for, 231
Tissue injury, insomnia and, 326–327
Title X Family Planning Program, 13
Tongue, 161
Tooth decay, 164
Topical capsaicin, 167
Topiramate, 233, 234t, 238
Toward a New Psychology of Women, 89
Transitional Care Management Services, 116
Transportation, 268–269
Tranylcypromine, 82, 234t
Triazolam, 234t, 320t
Tricyclic antidepressants, 81, 234t, 235, 238
Trier Social Stress Test, 293
Trimethoprim, 210
Trimethoprim–sulfamethoxole, 210

Triptans, 238
Triterpene glycoside, 215
Type 1 diabetes, 72–73, 151t, 232
Type 2 diabetes, 72–74, 151t, 232

U

Unisom, for insomnia, 319
United States
    death and dying in, 335–336
    National Health Interview Survey 2010, 335
United States Pharmacopeial Convention
    (USP), 204
United States Preventive Services Task Force
    (USPSTF), 33, 58–60t, 101
United States Public Health Service (USPHS), 15
Unsteadiness, 236
Upper airway resistance syndrome (UARS), 329
Urban development, influence on women's
    health, 268
Urinary incontinence (UI), 99–100
Urinary tract infections (UTI), 210–211
US National Center for Health Statistics, 225

V

Vaccination
    for older women, 109–110, 110t
    for oral HPV infection, 168
Vaccinium macrocarpon. *See* Cranberry
Valerian (*Valeriana* spp.), for insomnia, 321
Valerian, 216–217
Valeriana officinalis. *See* Valerian
Vanderbilt, Gloria, 249
Vasomotor symptoms (VMSs), 324, 325
Vasopressin, 288
Venlafaxine, 234t, 235
Verapamil, 239t, 240
Veterans, women in, 124–125
Visceral adipose tissue (VAT), 137, 150t
Visceral fat, 137
Vitex agnus-castus. *See* Chasteberry
Voicing my Choices, 347
von Schiller, Friedrich, 250

W

Waist circumference, 135, 136b
Waist-to-height ratios, 135, 136b
Waist-to-hip ratio, 135, 136b
Wald, Florence, 337
Wald, Lillian, 13
Warfarin, 225, 239t, 241
Waste, 269
Water, influence on women's health, 265
Weight cycling, 146
Weight, healthy, 47–48
Weight-loss
    drugs for, 233
    program for, 72

Well-being, 299
Well-woman care, 31
    behaviors, promoting healthy, 43
        immunizations, 43–44
        preventing sexually transmitted infections,
            45–47
        reducing substance use, 44–45
    body image, promoting healthy, 47
        body art and body modification, 49–51
        healthy sexual identity, 51–52
        healthy skin, 49
        healthy weight, 47–48
    breast health, 33–36
    menstrual health, 36–37
    pelvic examination, 33
    pregnancy
        delaying/preventing, 41–42
        folic acid supplementation, 43
        planning, 42
    relationships, promoting healthy, 52
        clinicians, 53
        friendships, 53–55
        parents, 52–53
        preventing bullying, 56–57
        romantic relationships, 55–56
    reproductive life span, 37–39
    risk assessment and counseling, 39–41
Wellness and disease prevention, in women
    antiallergy, 243–244
    drugs
        affecting mental health, 233–235
        to alleviate pain, 236–238
        for asthma, 243
        cardiovascular, 238–241
        for chronic pain syndromes, 238
        for diabetes mellitus, 231–233
        GI disorders/antiacid, 241–243
        for insomnia, 235–236
        male–female differences response in, 223–225
        related to sex hormones and reproductive
            health, 228–231
        for thyroid dysfunction, 231
        weight-loss, 233
        woman's life span, 225–227
    pharmacogenomics, 225
Wellness, sleep and, 309–310
Weltman, Art, 247
White adipose tissue, 137, 150t
Women
    with disabilities, 128
    health
        contemporary challenges to, 22–25
        development of, 12
        history of, 12–14
        organizational resources for, 24t
        practice, 20–22
        redefined, 14–16

scholarship, 16–20
    timeline of significant events in, 17–19
    and wellness of, 3–4
healthy aging for. *See* Older women
immigrant, 125–126
LGBT, 127
in military and veterans, 124–125
in poverty, 126–127
in recovery, 128–130
    intimate partner violence, 129–130
    substance abuse, 128–129
resilience in, 181–187
special populations of, 124–130
USPSTF recommendations for, 58–60
Women's Army Corps (WACs), 124
Women's Health and Healing Program, 15
Women's Health Equity Act, 15
Women's Health Initiative (WHI) study, 83, 214
Women's health nurse practitioner (WHNP),
    20, 22, 25
World Health Organization (WHO), 4, 203, 264,
    265, 267, 343
WS 1490, 207

X
Xerostomia, 167, 174
    inventory, 175
    questionnaire, 175
    salivary and nonsalivary causes of, 176t
    tools to evaluate, 175
    treatment strategies for, 176, 176t

Y
Yangonin, 207
Yellow adipose tissue, 150t
Yoga, 248
    for insomnia, 317
Youth population, risky behavior in, 31, 32f

Z
Zafirlukast, 243
Zaleplon (Sonata), 235, 319t
Zileuton, 242t, 243
Zolmitriptan, 238
Zolpidem (Ambien, and Ambien CR), 234t, 235,
    316, 319t
Zumba dance, 248